DISEASES OF CATTLE

By

Drs. Atkinson, Dickson, Harbaugh, Law, Lowe, Mohler, Murray, Pearson, Ransom and Trumbower

BIOTECH

2016

Biotech Books

New Delhi - 110 002

Revised Edition, 1942
Indian Impression **2016**

ISBN10 81-7622-048-5
ISBN13 978-81-7622-048-4

Published by : **BIOTECH BOOKS**
4762-63/23, Ansari Road, Darya Ganj,
New Delhi - 110 002
Phone: +91-011-23262132
e-mail: biotechbooks@yahoo.co.in

Laser Typesetting : **Classic Computer Services**
Delhi - 110 035

Printed at : **Chawla Offset Printers**
Delhi - 110 052

PRINTED IN INDIA

Contents

Illustrations

PLATES

ILLUSTRATIONS

TEXT FIGURES

Foreword

This book supplies general information to cattle owners concerning diseases or ailments of their animals. Aside from the treatment of minor ailments and the administration of first aid in emergencies, it is not advisable for the stock owner to give drugs or attempt to perform surgical treatment. Such procedures (except by trained practitioners) involve serious risk to the health or even life of animals treated; and the authors of this book disclaim responsibility for results in such cases. However, stockmen can do much to protect the health of their animals along preventive lines, especially by their proper feeding, care, and management.

In administering first aid or engaging in other treatment, the stock owner should seek to prevent unnecessary suffering in his animals. Considerate treatment of livestock is desirable both from a humane standpoint and because greater returns may be expected from animals that receive good care.

In most parts of the United States the services of a competent veterinarian are available, and it is advisable to call such a practitioner when medical or surgical attention is needed. In the case of infectious diseases, the stockman should call a veterinarian at the first indication of symptoms that are of suspicious character in order to avoid unnecessary spread of infection in the herd or to other herds in the neighborhood. A careful study of the discussions concerning symptoms of such diseases will aid the herd owner in recognizing them when they first make their appearance.

JOHN R. MOHLER,
Chief, Bureau of Animal Industry,
United States Department of Agriculture.

Administration of Medicines

By Leonard Pearson, B. S., V. M. D.

[Revised by L. T. Giltner, D. V. M., M. S.]

Medicines may be administered to cattle in many ways. The channel and method of administration depend on whether a general or local effect is desired, the condition of the animal, and the nature of the medicine that is to be given. The easiest method, and therefore the most common, is to give ordinary remedies by the mouth with the feed, with drink, or separately. There are, however, some conditions in which medicines administered in this way will not act promptly enough, or wherein a desired effect of the medicine on a distant part of the body is wholly lacking unless it is applied in some other way.

Following are the various methods of administering medicines to cattle.

By the mouth.—The simplest way to give medicines by the mouth is to mix them with the feed or water. This can be done when the medicine is in the form of a powder or fluid, if but a small quantity is to be given, if it does not have a taste that is disagreeable to the animal and is not so irritating as to injure the lining membranes of the mouth and throat.

The usual method of administering bulky or unpalatable doses is to mix them with a fluid, such as water, milk, molasses, or broth, and give from a bottle. A dose given in this way is known as a drench. In administering a drench the head of the animal should be elevated a little by an assistant. This is best accomplished by standing at the left side of the cow's head and by grasping the nose with the thumb and fingers of the right hand inserted in the nostrils; with the left hand beneath the chin the head is further raised and supported. If the animal is unruly, it may be tied in a stall or placed in a stanchion. The medicine can now be poured into the mouth by inserting the neck of the bottle between the lips on the right side. Care must be taken to avoid getting the bottle between the back teeth. The mouth of the bottle should be inserted as far as the middle of the tongue and the contents poured slowly. If the cow coughs, the head must as once be lowered to permit the fluid to escape from the larynx. If medicine is given during coughing, some of the dose may pass down the windpipe to the lungs and cause a severe or a fatal pneumonia. This is especially to be guarded against when the throat is partly paralyzed or insensitive, as in parturient apoplexy (milk fever). In this disease drenches may flow into the lungs, thus killing the cow.

The quantity of fluid to be given in a drench depends on the effect desired and the nature of the medicine. In impactions of the stomach very large quantites of fluid may be given—as much as several gallons at a time. Usually, however, it is not customary or desirable to give more than 1 to 2 quarts at a dose, and not more than a pint unless it is necessary to lessen the irritating quality of the drug.

Soluble medicines should be completely dissolved before they are given. Insoluble ones should be finely divided by powdering or by shaking and should be well agitated and mixed immediately before they are given. In the latter case a menstruum with considerable body, such as molasses or flaxseed tea or milk, will help to hold solids or oils in suspension until swallowed.

Balls are large pills adapted for the larger animals. Powders or gums are sometimes mixed with an adhesive substance and rolled into balls for convenience of administration. Balls are not used so much and are not so well adapted to the medication of cattle as of horses. The process of solution is slower in the paunch of a cow than in the stomach of a horse. If the cow is so sick as to have stopped ruminating, a ball may get covered up and lost in the mass of material in the paunch and so lie for days, producing no effect whatever.

Capsules are shells or envelopes made of soluble gelatin in which powders or liquids may be enclosed. Capsules and balls are administered by being placed on the tongue well back in the mouth while the tongue is drawn forward and the mouth is held open by a block of wood between the back teeth. The capsule or ball should be dropped, the tongue released, and the block removed as nearly simultaneously as possible, so that the backward carriage of the tongue will throw the capsule or ball into the throat and lead to its being swallowed. In introducing the medicine, care must be taken to avoid having the hand cut or crushed. After a little experience it is possible to do away with the block of wood.

By the stomach.—Medicines are introduced directly into the first stomach by the use of an esophageal tube or through the cannula of a trocar passed into the paunch through the side. This method is used in the treatment of diseases of digestion.

By the rectum.—Medicines are usually administered by the rectum for the purpose of controlling the bowels and for the treatment of local diseases. Sometimes, however, medicines that have a general effect are given in this way when, for any reason, it is not possible or convenient to give them through the mouth. Only drugs that are readily absorbed should be given by the rectum for a general effect and in somewhat larger dose or more frequently than when given by the mouth. Such stimulants as ether, alcohol, or the aromatic spirits of ammonia, diluted with 4 to 6 times their bulk of warm water, may be used in this way.

Rectal injections, or enemas, are used in the treatment of constipation. If it is the purpose of the injection to soften hardened fecal masses, the water should be comfortably warm and may have a little clean soap in it. If it is the purpose of the injection to stimulate sluggish bowels to contraction, the water may be cold.

In giving rectal injections a rectal syringe may be used, or, better, a piece of ½- to ¾-inch rubber hose 5 feet long with a tin funnel attached to one end. The hose is soaped or oiled and introduced slowly and gently into the rectum 2 or 3 feet. The fluid is then slowly poured into the funnel and allowed to gravitate into the rectum. The same apparatus may be used for feeding by the rectum.

By the vagina.—Medicines are inserted into the vagina, and through the vagina into the womb, in a manner similar to that of rectal administration. Most of the medication made use of in this way is for the local treatment of these organs. Following calving, during outbreaks of abortion, and in an infectious disease of the vagina, such injections become necessary.

By the udder.—Injections of filtered air or oxygen into the udder are made in the treatment of parturient apoplexy (milk fever). (See section under Milk Fever.)

Injections into the udder are sometimes made in the treatment of garget, but such procedures should be undertaken only by a veterinarian.

By the nostrils.—An animal may be caused to inhale medicine in the form of gas or vapor to snuff up a fine powder. Sometimes for the purpose of local treatment fluids are injected into the nose.

A medicine inhaled may have either a local or a general effect.

Medicated steam, carrying the volatile products of such agents as creosote, oil of eucalyptus, and compound tincture of benzoin may be liberated beneath the nostrils of a cow so that she must inhale these vapors, but such treatment is not so common for cattle as for horses. In producing general anesthesia, or insensibility to pain, the vapor of chloroform or ether is administered by the nostrils. As a preliminary to this it is necessary to cast and confine the animal. Great care is necessary to avoid complete stoppage of the heart or breathing.

By the trachea.—Medicines are injected into the trachea, or windpipe, in the treatment of some forms of diseases of the lungs, and especially in that form of bronchitis or pneumonia that is caused by lungworms. For this injection a large hypodermic syringe, fitted with a very thick, strong needle, is used. The needle is to be inserted about the middle of the neck and between the cartilaginous rings of the trachea.

By the skin.—Although a number of drugs, notably mercury, are so readily absorbed by the skin of cattle as to render poisoning easy, medicines are not given in this way for their general or constitutional but only for their local effect.

Diseases of the skin and superficial parasites are treated or destroyed by applications in the forms of washes, ointments, dips, and powders. Liniments and lotions are applied to the skin for the relief of some near-lying part, such as a muscle, tendon, or joint. Blisters are applied to the skin for the purpose of obtaining the effect of counterirritation upon a neighboring region or organ. Cold water may be applied to the skin to reduce the temperature and to diminish congestion or inflammation in a superficial area or to reduce the temperature of the whole body. High fever and heat strokes are treated in this way.

By the tissue beneath the skin.—Hypodermic or subcutaneous injections are often made for the purpose of introducing a drug, reagent, or vaccine directly into the connecting tissue beneath the skin. Introduced in this way, the substance is quickly absorbed, none of it is lost, and its whole effect is obtained, often within a few minutes.

Numerous precautions are necessary in making a subcutaneous injection, most of which have to do with cleansing and sterilization. It is also important to select a proper site for the injection, so that blood vessels, joints, and superficial nerves, organs, or cavities may all be avoided. With due regard for the necessary precautions, there is practically no danger in such an injection, but it should be attempted only by those who are able to carry it through in a surgically clean way. Only certain drugs can be given subcutaneously, and dosage must be accurately graduated.

In certain diagnostic and vaccination procedures the intradermic method of injection is used. This consists in inserting the needle into the corium, or true layer of the skin, where the material to be injected is deposited.

By the veins.—Certain medicines act most promptly and surely when introduced directly into the blood by injecting them into a vein, usually the jugular. Some vaccines and antitoxins are administered in this way. Intravenous injection should be practiced only by experienced veterinarians.

Diseases of the Digestive Organs

By A. J. Murray, M. R. C. V. S.

[Revised by C. D. Stein, V. M. D.]

CHARACTER OF FEEDS AND FEEDING

Diseases of the digestive organs are very common among cattle and may often be traced to defects in feeding. The first three stomachs of the larger ruminants hold the feed for a long time, during which period it is subjected to macerating, mixing, and straining processes in preparation for entrance into the fourth, or true, stomach. The straining is accomplished through the medium of the manyplies, whereas the paunch, or rumen, with its adjunct, the waterbag, is concerned in the macerating, kneading, and mixing, as well as in regurgitation for rumination, or the chewing of the cud. The action of the first three stomachs is merely preparatory to digestion. Thus it would seem that as a result of their complex anatomical and functional arrangement of the stomachs, the feed of cattle, when of good quality and wholesome, is in the most favorable condition possible for the digestive process when it reaches the fourth stomach, where true digestion first takes place. The location and arrangement of the stomachs are shown in plates I and II.

If the feed is of improper character or is so given that it cannot be cared for by the animal in a normal way, false fermentations arise, causing indigestion, and possibly, later, organic disease. In feeding cattle there are a number of important considerations apart from the economy of the ration, and some of these are noted below.

Feeds must not be damaged by exposure to the weather, by frost, by molds, or by deleterious fermentations.

Damaged feeds retard or prevent digestion, and sometimes they contain or cause to be generated substances that irritate the digestive tract or are distinctly poisonous to the animal. For example, hay that was rained on severely during curing has not only lost a part of its nutritive value through a washing-out process, but what remains is not so readily available as in good hay. Roots that have been frozen are likely to irritate and injure the digestive tract Grass eaten with frost on it may cause severe indigestion. Although all moldy feeds are not injurious, it is considered prudent to regard such feeds with suspicion and to withhold them from the ration.

Feeds must not contain too large a proportion of woody fiber or of indigestible substances. If the dry matter ingested or the bulk of the feed is very great on account of the small proportion of digestible matter, it is impossible for the great mass to be moistened properly with and attacked by the digestive juices. In consequence, abnormal fermentations arise, causing indigestion and irritation of the digestive organs. On the other hand, a ration too concentrated, and especially too rich in protein, is not suitable, because, after a meal, the animal must have a certain feeling of fullness in order to be comfortable and quiet, and the digestive organs require a relatively large volume of contents to fill them to the point at which secretion is properly stimulated and their activity is most efficient. If too much protein is in the ration there is a waste of expensive feed, and the tendency is for the animal to become thin. It is evident that a cow cannot thrive on concentrated feeds alone, even though they contain in assimilable form all the nutritive materials needed for perfect support. It is because bulk is necessary that the standard of about 25 pounds of dry matter per cow per day has been reached by experimenters. There is no objection to feeding grain or meal separately to a cow, provided enough bulky feed is fed at another time in the day to keep the digestive tract sufficiently distended.

In changing the ration, and especially in making radical changes, as at the beginning and the end of the pasturing season, the change should be made gradually, so that the digestive organs may accommodate themselves to it. After the digestive organs and juices have from long practice become adjusted to the digestion of a certain feed, which is then suddenly withheld and another of quite different character and properties is substituted. the second feed is not well digested; it may even irritate the digestive canal. It is often observed that cattle lose from 25 to 100 pounds when turned on pasture from dry, stable feed. This loss can readily be prevented by making a gradual change in the diet.

Regularity in feeding has much to do with the utilization of the ration, and gross irregularity may cause indigestion and serious disease.

Water for livestock should be as free from contamination and as nearly pure as that used for household purposes. When practicable it is well to warm the water in the winter to about 50° F. and allow cattle to drink often.

DISEASES OF THE MOUTH

WOUNDS AND CONTUSIONS OF THE LIPS, AND SNAKE BITE

The lips may become inflamed from contusions, which are sometimes produced by a blow from the horns of another animal, or by other means. While cattle are grazing, especially when they are in woods, they may be bitten on the lips by insects or serpents.

Symptoms.—As a result of a contusion the lips become thick and swollen, and if treatment is neglected the swelling may become hard and indurated, or an abscess may form. This condition renders it difficult for the animal to get feed into its mouth, on account of the lips having lost their natural flexibility. In such cases the animal will use its tongue more in the taking of feed to make up for the incapacity of the lips. In cases of snake bite the swelling is soft or puffy and its limits are not well defined.

Treatment.—In the case of a bruise, the affected part should be bathed with hot water 2 or 3 times daily. In recent cases no other treatment will be required, but if the swelling is not recent and has become hard or indurated the swollen part should be treated each day by painting it with tincture of iodine. In snake bite a straight incision penetrating into the flesh or muscle should be made across the center of the swelling and in the direction of the long axis of the face to promote free bleeding. After this has been done a small wad of cotton batting should be pressed against the wound until the bleeding has almost stopped. Afterward the following lotion may be applied to the wounds several times a day: Potassium permanganate, half a dram; distilled water, 1 pint. As snake bites are usually attended with considerable depression, which may terminate in stupor, it is advisable to give a stimulant. Small doses of alcoholic stimulants or 1 ounce of aromatic spirits of ammonia mixed with a pint of water should be given, and the dose should be repeated in half an hour if the animal is becoming stupified or unconscious. Repetition of the dose must depend on the symptoms that the animal shows. It must be borne in mind that the object of treatment is to ward off the stupor, which is one of the results of snake bite. Specific treatment for snake bites, except those of the water moccasin, consists in administration of antivenin, which should be given by a veterinarian. The swelling from an insect bite should be bathed with ammonia water as soon as noticed and then treated with frequent applications of hot water.

SALIVATION

Salivation is a symptom of some general or local disorder. It may be a symptom of a general disease, such as rabies, or it may be a purely local trouble, as when copious secretion of the salivary glands is produced by the eating of irritating plants, such as wild mustard. When saliva dribbles from the mouth, that part should be carefully examined by introducing into the mouth an instrument such as a balling iron, or, if one is not at hand, by grasping the tongue and partially withdrawing it from the mouth, and by placing a block of wood between the back teeth, while all parts of the mouth are exposed to a good light, so that the presence of any foreign substance may be detected. The cause is sometimes found to be a short piece of wood becoming fixed on the palate, its two ends resting on the upper molar teeth of each side; or it may be a needle, thorn, or splinter of wood embedded in the tongue. Sometimes a sharp piece of tin or other metal may become partially embedded in the inner surface of the cheek. Hay occasionally possesses some quality, usually dependent on its having heated in the mow or having become moldy, which produces salivation. Second-crop clover and some irritating weeds in the pasture or forage may cause salivation. Cattle rubbed with mercurial ointment may swallow enough mercury in licking themselves to bring about the same result. (See Mercury Poisoning, p. 60.) Such cases, of course, arise from the constitutional action of mercury, and, on account of the common habit that the animals have of licking themselves, indicate the danger of using such preparation externally. Mercury is also readily absorbed through the skin, and as cattle are very susceptible to its action it is thus easy for them to be poisoned by it even without licking it from the surface. Cases of mercurial poisoning sometimes follow disinfection of cattle stables with the usual 1 to 1,000 solution of mercuric chloride.

Treatment.—If salivation depends on the irritation and inflammation set up by the ingestion of acrid plants or of forage possessing some peculiar stimulating property, the feed must be changed, and a lotion composed of an ounce of powdered alum dissolved in a quart of water may be syringed into the mouth twice a day, half a pint of the solution being used each time. If, however, the salivation is due to the presence of a thorn, splinter of wood, or any other foreign substance embedded in the cheek or tongue, the offending object should be removed and the mouth washed occasionally with a weak solution (2 percent) of carbolic acid and tepid water. When salivation is produced by mercurial poisoning, the treatment appropriate to that condition should be applied.

IRREGULARITIES OF THE TEETH

Irregularities of the teeth may be caused by the unequal wearing of some of the teeth or by some of the incisors being broken, which may happen when cattle are pastured on sandy or gravelly soil. The molar teeth may also show irregular wear from similar causes or from a disease or malformation of the jaw. Their edges may become sharp, or a molar tooth may have been accidentally fractured. Perhaps a supernumerary tooth may have developed in an unusual position, thereby interfering with the natural and regular mastication of the feed.

Treatment.—The mouth may be examined by grasping the animal's tongue with one hand and partially withdrawing it from the mouth, so as to expose the incisor and molar teeth to inspection. When it is desired, however, to examine the molar teeth with the fingers, so as to obtain an idea of their condition, an instrument like the balling iron that is used for the horse should be introduced into the mouth, so as to separate the jaws and keep them apart while the examination is being made. Any sharp edges of the molars must be removed by the tooth rasp, such as is used for horses. Any supernumerary tooth that interferes with mastication or any tooth that is fractured or loose should be extracted. In performing such operation it is desirable to throw, or cast, the animal, and to have its head held securely, so as to enable the operator to do what is necessary without difficulty.

CARIES OR DECAY OF THE TEETH

The presence of caries may be suspected if the mouth exhales a bad odor and if the animal during mastication occasionally stops as if it were in pain. The existence of caries in a molar tooth may be ascertained by examining the mouth in the manner already described. If one of the molars is found to be carious, it should be extracted. When the crown of the tooth has been destroyed and only the stump or root is left, extraction is impracticable. In case the animal has special value the root stumps may be removed by a veterinarian by the operation of trephining; otherwise, it is best to sell the animal to the butcher.

ACTINOMYCOSIS OF THE JAWBONES (BIG JAW OR LUMPY JAW)

[See Actinomycosis, p. 383]

INFLAMMATION OF MUCOUS MEMBRANE OF MOUTH (STOMATITIS)

The membrane of the mouth may become inflamed by eating some irritating substance or plant, or little vesicles may form in the mouths of calves when they are affected with indigestion, constituting what is termed "aphtha."

Symptoms.—The saliva dribbles from the mouth, and when the mouth is examined the surface of the tongue and other parts appear red and inflamed. When young animals are affected with the form of disease termed "aphtha," small red elevations are observed on the tongue and other parts of the mouth, having little white points on their centers, which consist of the epithelium of the mucous membrane raised into vesicles. These white patches are succeeded by ulcerated surfaces, which are caused by the shedding of the white patches of epithelium.

Treatment.—When there is merely a reddened and inflamed condition of the mucous membrane of the mouth, it will suffice to syringe it out several times a day with 4 ounces of the following solution: Alum, 1 ounce; water, 2 pints. When the edges of the tongue and other parts of the mouth are studded with ulcers, they should be painted over once a day, until the affected surface is healed, with a solution made by mixing 1 dram of potassium permanganate in 1 quart of water. When indigestion is associated with an ulcerated condition of the mouth, separate treatment is required.

ULCERATIVE STOMATITIS (OR ULCERS IN THE MOUTHS OF YOUNG CALVES)

[See Necrotic Stomatitis, p. 412]

MYCOTIC STOMATITIS (SORE MOUTH)

[See p. 417]

VESICULAR STOMATITIS

[See p. 422]

INDURATION OF THE TONGUE (ACTINOMYCOSIS)

[See Actinomycosis, p. 383]

DISEASES OF THE PHARYNX AND GULLET

PHARYNGITIS (SORE THROAT)

Pharyngitis is an inflammation of the mucous membrane lining the pharynx. It is frequently associated with inflammatory diseases of the respiratory tract, such as laryngitis and bronchitis or pleurisy.

Symptoms.—The muzzle is dry and the saliva dribbles from the corners of the mouth; the animal swallows with difficulty or not at all and holds its neck in a stiff, straight position, moving it as little as possible. The eyelids are half closed, the white of the eye is bloodshot, and the animal occasionally grinds its teeth. After masticating the feed the animal drops it out of its mouth as if to avoid the pain of swallowing, and also evinces pain when pressure is applied externally on the pharynx and tries to prevent the pressure from being applied.

Causes.—Pharyngitis may be produced by a sudden cooling of the surface of the body, as when cattle are exposed to a cold wind or a cold rain, or by swallowing irritating substances.

Treatment.—The throat should be syringed three times a day with an ounce of the following solution: Silver nitrate, 1½ drams; distilled water, 1 pint. Bland and soothing drinks, such as linseed tea or oatmeal and water, should occasionally be offered. Diet should consist of soft feed, such as bran mashes with a little linseed meal mixed in them. Dry hay and fodder should not be given. Fresh, green grass or sound ensilage may be fed in small quantities. The upper part of the throat and the space between the jaws should be well rubbed once a day with the following liniment: Liquor ammonia fortior, 4 ounces; oil of turpentine, 4 ounces; olive oil, 4 ounces; mix. When evidence of blistering appears the application of the liniment should be stopped and the skin anointed with petrolatum. Under the treatment described above, the inflammation of the throat will gradually subside and the animal will be able to swallow as usual in 5 or 6 days. During its treatment the sick animal should be kept in a comfortable stable.

PAROTITIS

Inflammation of the parotid gland may arise from the inflammation extending to it when an animal is affected with pharyngitis or laryngitis, or the inflammation may commence in the salivary ducts and may depend on some influence the nature of which is unknown. Parotitis sometimes arises from a blow or contusion severe enough to set up inflammation in the structure of the gland. Tuberculosis and actinomycosis may infrequently be characterized by the lodgment of their parasitic causes in the parotid glands, in which case parotitis may be a symptom of either of these diseases.

Symptoms.—There is an elongated, painful swelling, beginning at the base of the ear and passing downward along the posterior margin of the lower jaw. The swelling is sometimes limited to one side, and when both are swollen it is generally larger on one side than on the other. The secretion of saliva is increased, the appetite is poor, the neck is stiff, so that it is painful to raise the head, and feed is swallowed with difficulty. In many cases the swelling of the glands, when properly treated, disappears in a comparatively short time. In other cases, however, the glands remain enlarged, even after the animal recovers its appetite. In tuberculosis, lymphatic glands beneath the parotid glands are sometimes enlarged, thus causing the appearance of enlarged parotid glands.

Treatment.—A warm bran poultice, made by mixing bran with a hot, 2-percent compound cresol solution in water, should be applied on the swollen gland and kept in place by means of a bandage. Whenever the poultice has cooled it should be replaced by a new one. This treatment should be continued until the pain is less and the swelling is reduced or until there is evidence of pus formation, which may be ascertained by examining the surface of the gland with the fingers. When, on pressing any part of the surface, it is found to fluctuate or "give," it may be concluded that there is a collection of pus at that place. It is well not to open the abscess until the fluctuation is well marked, as at this stage the pus is near the surface and there is less trouble in healing the wound than if the pus is deep seated. The abscess should be opened with a clean, sharp knife. The poulticing should then be continued for 2 or 3 days, but the form of the poultice should be changed by replacing the bran with absorbent cotton and pouring the compound cresol solution on the cotton. At all times the wound should be kept clean and the cavity injected once or twice daily with a solution of 1 dram of carbolic acid in 8 ounces of water. Under this treatment the pus may cease and the wound heal without complications. Saliva may issue from the orifice and result in the formation of a salivary fistula. This requires operative treatment by a competent veterinarian. When poulticing fails to reduce the swelling or to produce softening, the inflamed area may be rubbed once daily with camphorated oil, compound iodine ointment, or painted twice daily with Lugol's solution of iodine. The diet should be as recommended under Pharyngitis (p. 10).

PHARYNGEAL POLYPI

Tumors frequently form in the pharynx and may give rise to a train of symptoms varying according to their size and location. The tumor may be so situated that by shifting its position a little it may partially obstruct the posterior nares (nostrils), when, of course, it will render nasal breathing noisy and labored. In another situation its partial displacement may impede the entrance of air into the larynx. In almost any part of the pharynx, especially near the entrance of the gullet, tumors interfere with swallowing. As they are frequently attached to the wall of the pharynx by a pedicel or stalk, they may readily be displaced in different directions so as to produce the symptoms before described. Enlarged postpharyngeal lymphatic glands are common in tuberculosis, and by pressing on the wall of the pharynx and restricting the lumen of this organ they cause difficulty in both breathing and swallowing. Such enlarged glands may be differentiated from tumors by passing the hand into the cow's throat after the jaws are separated by a suitable speculum or gag.

Treatment.—The method of treatment in such cases is to separate the animal's jaws with an instrument termed a "gag," and then, after drawing the tongue partially forward, to pass the hand into the pharynx and to twist the tumor gently from its attachment. When the attachment is too strong to be severed in this way an instrument such as a thimble, but possessing a sharp edge at the end, may be used to effect the same purpose, or the base of the tumor may be severed by the use of a crushing instrument known as an écraseur.

CHOKING

Choking usualy occurs from attempting to swallow too large an object, such as a turnip, potato, beet, apple, or pear, though in rare cases it may occur from bran, chaff, or some other finely divided feed lodging in and filling a portion of the gullet. This latter form of the accident is most likely to occur in animals that are greedy feeders.

Symptoms.—The symptoms vary somewhat according to the part of the gullet or throat in which the obstruction occurs. In most cases there is a discharge of saliva from the mouth; the animal coughs frequently, and when it drinks the water is soon ejected. The cow stops eating and stands back from the trough, the expression is troubled, breathing is accelerated, and often there is bloating as a result of the retention of gas in the paunch. These symptoms, however, are not always present, for if the obstacle does not completely close the throat or gullet, gas and water may pass, thus ameliorating the discomfort. If the obstruction is in the neck portion of the gullet, it may be felt as a lump in the left jugular furrow.

Treatment.—If the object is in the throat, it is advisable to put a gag in the animal's mouth, and, while the head is held in a horizontal direction by two assistants, to pass the hand into the pharynx, grasp the foreign body, and withdraw it gradually and steadily. When the substance is lodged in the upper part of the gullet, pressure should be made by an assistant in an upward direction against the object while the operator passes his hand into the pharynx, and if the assistant cannot by pressure dislodge the substance from the gullet, the operator, by passing his middle finger above and partly behind the substance, may gradually slide it into the pharynx and then withdraw it by the mouth.

The presence of an obstructing substance in the cervical (neck) portion of the gullet may be ascertained by passing the hand along the left side of the neck, when a hard and painless swelling will be found to indicate the presence of the foreign body. In such cases, by gentle persevering pressure with the thumb and next two fingers, an attempt should be made to slide the obstructing substance gradually upward to the pharynx. To facilitate this it is well to give the animal a half pint of raw linseed or olive oil before the manipulations described are commenced. When the substance has been brought into or nearly into the pharynx, the mouth gag should be used, the tongue drawn partially forward with the left hand, and the right hand passed backward into the pharynx to withdraw the obstruction.

When bran or chaff causes the trouble it is best to give a little oil to lubricate the walls of the gullet, and then by gentle and persevering pressure, to endeavor to separate and divide the mass and to work it downward toward the stomach. This will be assisted by pouring small quantities of oil and water down the animal's throat. It is not advisable to use the probang (pl. III, figs. 2 and 3) to push down any soft material, such as oats or chaff, as this generally condenses and renders firmer the obstructing substance by pressing its particles or elements together, so that it forms a solid mass that cannot be moved.

In some cases the foreign body, either because it is in the chest portion of the esophagus, and so beyond reach, or because it is too firmly seated, cannot be dislodged from the neck by pressing and manipulating that part externally. In such event use must be made of the probang. This is a flexible instrument which adapts itself to the natural curvature of the gullet, and if used cautiously there is not much risk of injury. Before passing the probang, a gag that has an aperture at each end, from which straps pass to be buckled at the back of the head below the horns, is introduced into the mouth (pl. III, fig. 4). The probang should then be oiled, and, the animal's head and neck being held in a straight line by two assistants, the tongue must be partly drawn out of the mouth, the probang cautiously passed along the roof of the mouth into the pharynx and thence into the gullet, through which it is passed down. If resistance is met, gentle and continuous pressure must be used, under the influence of which the object generally passes into the stomach in a short time. One must be careful not to pass the probang into the larynx and thence into the windpipe, as an animal may readily be killed in this way. This accident is indicated by efforts to cough and by violent disturbed breathing. If such symptoms arise the probang must be withdrawn at once. To avoid a wrong passage, the end of the tube should be pressed very slowly through the throat until its presence in the esophagus is assured. After it is once in the esophagus care is still necessary, because the walls of this tube may easily be torn.

Some writers have advised that when the obstruction is lodged in the cervical (neck) portion of the gullet, it should be struck with a mallet to crush it and thus alter its shape so that it may easily slip down into the stomach. If the obstructing substance is hard, this will be a dangerous operation, but if soft—as in the case of a ripe pear, for example—this procedure may be adopted safely.

In all cases, if pressure applied on the neck fails to move the obstruction and the probang also fails to move it, it may be divided by a subcutaneous operation, or the gullet may be opened and the obstructing substance removed through the wound. In such cases the assistance of a veterinarian or a surgeon must be obtained.

WOUNDS AND INJURIES OF THE GULLET

Sometimes the walls of the gullet may be more or less lacerated or abraded by the rash and too forcible use of the probang, and the animal consequently swallows with pain and difficulty. In such cases dry feed must be withheld for 5 or 6 days so as to allow the injured parts to heal, and the diet must be limited to linseed tea, hay tea, and thin oatmeal gruel and molasses. The same kind of diet must be fed after the operation of cutting into the gullet has been performed.

Sometimes the gullet is ruptured and lacerated to such an extent that treatment of any kind is hopeless. This has been known to occur when the handle of a pitchfork or buggy whip has been pushed down a cow's throat to remove an obstruction. When such treatment has been applied it is best to slaughter the animal without delay, as the flesh may be utilized so long as there is no fever or general disease, and remedial treatment would be hopeless. Whatever substitute may be used for a probang, which sometimes is not at hand, it should be flexible and possess a smooth surface. A piece of new rope with the end closely wrapped and waxed and then oiled, a piece of thin garden hose, or a well-wrapped twisted wire may be used in emergencies.

DISEASES OF THE STOMACHS

ACUTE TYMPANITES (HOVEN, OR BLOATING)

Tympanites is a distention of the rumen or paunch with gases of fermentation and is manifested outwardly by swelling in the region of the left flank.

Causes.—Tympanites may be caused by any kind of feed that produces indigestion. When cattle are first turned onto young clover they eat so greedily of it that tympanites frequently results. Turnips, potatoes, cabbage, or the discarded pulp from sugar-beet factories may also cause it. Middlings and corn meal also frequently give rise to it.

Care is necessary in turning animals into fields of clover or stubble fields in which there is a strong growth of volunteer grain. It is always better to keep them from such pasturage while it is wet with dew, and they should be taken out when they have eaten a moderate quantity. When cattle are fed pulp from sugar beets, germinated malt, or similar feeds, they should be given moderate quantities until they have become accustomed to it, as any of these feeds may give rise to severe bloating.

An excessive quantity or too hasty eating of any of the before-mentioned feeds may bring on this disorder. Sometimes the quality of the feed is at fault. Grass or clover when wet by dew or rain frequently brings on tympanites; frozen roots or pastures covered with hoar frost are also dangerous. When feed has been eaten too hastily or when it is cold and wet, the digestive process is imperfectly performed and the feed in the paunch ferments, during which process large quantities of gas are formed. The same result may follow when a cow is choked, as the obstruction in the gullet prevents the passing up of gas from the stomach, so that the gas continues to accumulate until tympanites results.

Symptoms.—The swelling of the left flank is very characteristic, as in well-marked cases the flank at its upper part rises above the level of the backbone and when struck with the tips of the fingers emits a drumlike sound. The animal has an anxious expression, moves uneasily, and is evidently distressed. If relief is not obtained in time, it breathes with difficulty, reels in walking or in standing, and in a short time falls and dies from suffocation. The distention of the stomach may become so great as to prevent the animal from breathing, and in some instances the case may be complicated by rupture of the stomach.

Treatment.—If the case is not extreme, it may be sufficient to drive the animal at a walk for a quarter or half an hour, or cold water by the bucketful may be thrown against the cow's sides. In some cases the following simple treatment is successful: A rope or a twisted straw band is coated with pine tar, wagon grease, or other unsavory substance and is placed in the cow's mouth as a bit, being secured by tying behind the horns. The efforts of the animal to dislodge this object result in movements of the tongue, jaws, and throat that stimulate the secretion of saliva and swallowing, thus opening the esophagus, which permits the exit of gas and at the same time peristalsis is stimulated reflexly.

In urgent cases the gas must be allowed to escape without delay, and this is best accomplished by the use of the trocar. The trocar is a sharp-pointed instrument incased in a cannula or sheath, which leaves the sharp point of the trocar free (pl. III, figs. 5*a* and 5*b*). In selecting the point for using the trocar, a spot on the left side equally distant from the last rib, the hipbone, and the transverse processes of the lumbar vertebrae must be chosen. Here an incision about three-fourths of an inch long should be made with a knife through the skin, and then the sharp point of the trocar, being directed downward, inward, and slightly forward, is thrust into the paunch (pl. I). The cannula or sheath of the trocar should be left in the paunch as long as any gas continues to issue from it. If the cannula is removed while gas is still forming in the paunch and the left flank becomes considerably swollen, it may be necessary to insert it again. It is well, accordingly, to observe the cannula closely, and if gas is found to be issuing from it, the cannula should not be removed. When gas issues in considerable quantities the sound accompanying its escape renders the exact condition obvious. It is occasionally necessary to keep the cannula in the stomach for several hours. When this is necessary a piece of stout cord should be passed around the neck of the cannula immediately below the projecting rim and then around the animal's body and tied in a secure knot, and a careful attendant must remain with the cow during the entire period that the instrument is in place. The rim surrounding the mouth of the cannula should be in contact with the skin. Whenever the person in charge of the cow is convinced that gas has ceased to issue from the cannula the instrument should be removed.

The trocar is to be used only in extreme or urgent cases, though everyone who has had much experience in treating indigestion in cattle realizes that he has saved the lives of many animals by its prompt application.

When the tympanitic animal is not distressed and the swelling of the flank is not great, or when the most distressing condition has been removed by the use of the trocar, it is best to use internal medicine. Two ounces of aromatic spirits of ammonia should be given every half hour in a quart of cold water, or 1 ounce of creolin in 2 quarts of tepid water may be given at one dose or carefully injected through the cannula directly into the paunch to stop fermentation and the consequent formation of gas. It is generally necessary to give a moderate dose of purgative medicine after bloating has subsided, as animals frequently show symptoms of constipation after attacks of indigestion. For this purpose 1 pound of Glauber's salt may be used.

The animal should be carefully fed easily digested feed for several days after the bloating has subsided, so that all fermenting matter may pass out of the stomach.

CHRONIC TYMPANITES

Cattle, especially those that have been kept in the stable all winter, are likely to suffer from chronic tympanites. In this form, they bloat after feeding but seldom swell so much as to cause any alarm. The chronic form of indigestion may also follow an acute attack like that previously described. This is also a symptom of tuberculosis, when the lymphatic glands lying between the lungs are so enlarged as to press upon and partly occlude the esophagus. It may develop in calves as a result of the formation of hair balls in the stomach.

Treatment.—Treatment should be preceded by a moderate dose of purgative medicine: 1 pound of Epsom salts or Glauber's salt, half an ounce of powdered Barbados aloes, 1 ounce of powdered ginger, 1 pint of molasses. The salts and aloes should be dissolved by stirring for a few minutes in 2 quarts of lukewarm water, then the molasses should be added, and after all the ingredients have been stirred together for about 10 minutes the dose should be administered. After the operation of the purgative it is generally necessary to give some tonic and antacid preparation to promote digestion, which is imperfectly performed in such cases. The following may be used: Powdered gentian, 3 ounces; powdered bicarbonate of potash, 3 ounces; powdered ginger, 3 ounces; powdered capsicum, 1 ounce. Mix and divide into 12 powders, one of which should be given three times a day before feeding, shaken up with 1½ pints of water. It is also advantageous in such cases to give two heaping teaspoonfuls of wood charcoal, mixed with the animal's feed three times a day. The animal should also go out during the day, as want of exercise favors the continuance of this form of indigestion. If the dung is hard, the constipation should be overcome by feeding a little flaxseed twice daily or by giving a handful of Glauber's salt in the feed once or twice daily, as may be necessary. Roots, silage, and other succulent feeds are useful in this connection. If tuberculosis is suspected as the cause of chronic bloating, a skilled veterinarian should make a diagnosis, using the tuberculin test if necessary. Until it is settled that the cow does not have tuberculosis, she should be kept apart from the other members of the herd.

DISTENTION OF RUMEN OR PAUNCH WITH FEED

This form of indigestion is caused by the animal's gorging itself with feed and arises more from the animal's voracious appetite than from any defect in the quality of the feed supplied to it. The condition is, however, more severe if the feed consumed is especially concentrated or difficult of digestion. In cases of this kind there is comparatively no great formation of gas, and the gas that is formed is diffused through the stomach instead of accumulated in a layer in its upper part. On pressing the flank with the closed fist the indent of the hand remains for a short time in the flank, as if the rumen were filled with a soft, doughy mass.

This form of indigestion should be treated by stimulants, such as aromatic spirits of ammonia.

If the formation of gas is not great and the distention with solid material is somewhat limited, the animal may be drenched through a piece of ordinary garden hose, one end inserted in the mouth and the other end fitted with a funnel, use being made of 1½ pounds of Epsom salts or Glauber's salt dissolved in 2 gallons of water, at a single dose. Immediately after this treatment the left side of the animal, extending below the median line of the abdomen, should be powerfully kneaded with the fist, so that the impacted food mass will be broken, allowing the water to separate it into small portions that can be carried downward for the process of digestion. But if the treatment fails and the impacted or overloaded condition of the rumen continues, it may become necessary to resort to surgical operation by a competent veterinarian.

IMAGINARY DISEASES (HOLLOW HORN; LOSS OF CUD; WOLF IN THE TAIL OR HOLLOW TAIL)

It appears quite in place here, in connection with the diseases of the stomach and intestines of cattle, to consider the three old fallacies or superstitions known by the above names, since these names, whenever and wherever used, seem to be invariably applied to some form of digestive derangement or disease having its origin in the stomach and bowels.

Hollow horn.—In the first place, the horns of all cattle are hollow. The horn cores are elongations of the frontal bones of the skull, and the frontal sinuses, which are the larger of the air spaces of the head, are prolonged into the horn cores. When a cow is sick, if the horns are hot it is an evidence of fever; if they are cold it indicates impaired circulation of the blood; but these manifestations of sickness are to be regarded as symptoms of some constitutional disorder and do not in themselves require treatment. The treatment should be applied to the disease that causes the abnormal temperature of the horns. The usual treatment for the supposed hollow horn, which consists of boring the horns with a gimlet and pouring turpentine into the openings thus made, is not only useless and cruel but is likely to set up an acute inflammation and result in an abscess of the sinus.

Loss of cud.—The so-called loss of cud is simply a cessation of rumination, frequently one of the first indications of some form of disease, since ruminants stop chewing the cud when they feel sick. Loss of cud is a symptom of many diseases, and when it is detected it should lead the observer to try to discover other symptoms on which to base a correct opinion as to the nature of the disease from which the animal suffers. No local treatment is required. To restore the cud, laymen sometimes employ such treatment as forcing the animal to swallow a salt herring or old dishrag, which is of no value and may cause further trouble.

Wolf in the tail or hollow tail.—This term also seems to be vaguely applied to various disturbances of the digestive function or to some disease that is in reality in the stomach or bowels.

VOMITING

Vomiting is not to be confounded with rumination, though some writers have advanced the opinion that it is merely a disordered and irregular rumination. It is not of common occurrence in cattle.

Symptoms.—Animals that vomit are frequently in poor condition.

After having eaten tranquilly for some time the animal suddenly becomes uneasy, arches the back, stretches the neck and head, and then suddenly ejects 10 to 12 pounds of the contents of the rumen. After having done this the uneasiness subsides and in a short time the animal resumes eating as if nothing had happened.

Cause.—The cause of this disordered state of the digestive system in cattle is usually obscure, but has in some cases been traced to a partial closure of the opening into the second stomach or to a distention of the esophagus. It has been found to occur when there was cancerous disease of the fourth stomach, and experimentally it has been shown that a suspension of digestion or great derangement of this stomach produces considerable nervous disorder of the rumen and sometimes vomiting or attempts to vomit.

Treatment.—Easily digested feed and plenty of water should be given. Fear and excitement, chasing, or hurrying animals after they have eaten heartily are likely to bring on this result. As a rule medicinal treatment is not successful.

DEPRAVED APPETITE (PICA)

Cattle suffering from this disease have a capricious and variable appetite for their ordinary feed but evince a strong desire to lick and eat substances for which healthy cattle show no desire. Alkaline and saline-tasting substances are especially attractive to cattle having a depraved appetite, and they frequently lick lime, earth, coal, gravel, and even the dung of other cattle. Cows in calf and young cattle are especially likely to develop these symptoms. Animals affected in this way lose condition, the coat is staring, gait slow, and small vesicles containing yellow liquid form under the tongue; the milk given by such cows is thin and watery. Such animals become restless and uneasy, as is indicated by frequent bellowing. The disease may last for months, and the animal ultimately dies emaciated and exhausted. Depraved appetite frequently precedes the condition in which the bones of cattle become brittle and fracture easily, which is known as osteomalacia.

Cause.—From the fact that this disease is largely one of regions, it is generally believed that some dietetic cause, especially mineral deficiency of the soil and water and of the local vegetation, is largely responsible for it. Faulty metabolism likewise may be involved. The condition is more prevalent some years than others and is most common in old pastures, where the soil is more or less depleted. Cattle pastured on low, swampy land become predisposed to it. Occasionally, however, one individual in a herd suffers though all are fed alike. In such cases the disease must arise from the affected animal's imperfect assimilation of the nutritive elements of the feed that is supplied to it.

Treatment.—The affected animals should be supplied with the minerals that are lacking. Usually a good quality of bone meal with a little common salt tends to correct the condition.

HAIR CONCRETIONS

Hair concretions, or hair balls, sometimes result from the habit of some cattle of licking themselves or other animals. As a result, the hairs that are swallowed are carried around by the contractions of the stomach and gradually assume the form of a small pellet or ball. This increases in size as additional quantities of hair are introduced into the stomach and adhere to the surface of the ball. More often hair balls are formed of indigestible, fibrous vegetable matter, such as barley and wheat beards and the bristlelike appendages of certain other grasses.

These balls are found most frequently in the reticulum or second stomach (pl. II, *B*) and sometimes in the rumen. Occasionally the masses become coated with a deposit of salts to form calculi or concretions. In calves, hair balls are generally found in the fourth stomach. There are no certain symptoms by which the presence of hair balls in the stomach can be determined, and therefore no treatment can be recommended for such cases. In making post mortem examinations of cattle, the walls of the reticulum have sometimes been found transfixed with nails or pieces of wire, and yet the animal had shown no symptoms of indigestion but died from maladies not involving the second stomach.

INDIGESTION (DYSPEPSIA, OR GASTROINTESTINAL CATARRH)

Tympanites, already described, is a form of indigestion in which the chief symptom and most threatening condition is the collection of gas in the paunch. This symptom does not always accompany indigestion, so it is well here to consider other forms under a separate head. If indigestion is long continued, the irritant abnormal products developed cause catarrh of the stomach and intestines—gastrointestinal catarrh. On the other hand, irritant substances ingested may cause gastrointestinal catarrh, which, in turn, will cause indigestion; hence, these conditions are usually found together.

Causes.—Irritant feed, damaged feed, overloading of the stomach, or sudden changes of diet may cause this disease. Want of exercise predisposes to it, or feed that is coarse and indigestible may produce it after a time. Feed that possesses astringent properties and tends to check secretion may also act as an exciting cause. Excessive quantities of feed may lead to disorder of digestion and to this disease. It is likely to appear toward the end of protracted seasons of drought; therefore, a deficiency of water must be regarded as one of the conditions that favor its development.

Symptoms.—These are diminished appetite, irregular rumination, coated tongue, slimy mouth, passing of dung with a bad odor and indicating poorly digested feed, dullness, and fullness of the flanks. The disease may in some cases assume a chronic character, and in addition to the foregoing symptoms slight bloating or tympanites of the left flank may be observed, the animal breathes with effort and each respiration may be accompanied with a grunt, the ears and horns are alternately hot and cold, rumination ceases, the usual rumbling sound in the stomach is not audible, the passage of dung is almost entirely suspended, and the animal passes only a little mucus occasionally. Sometimes there is alternating constipation and diarrhea. There is low fever in many cases.

The disease continues a few days or a week in mild cases, whereas severe cases may last several weeks. In the latter form emaciation and loss of strength may be great. There is no appetite, no rumination, no peristalsis. The mouth is hot and sticky, the eyes have receded in their sockets, and milk secretion has ceased. In such cases the outlook for recovery is unfavorable. The animal falls away in flesh and becomes weaker, as is shown by the fact that one frequently finds it lying down.

On examining animals that have died of this disease, it is found that the lining membrane of the fourth stomach and the intestines, particularly the small intestine, is red, swollen, streaked with deeper red or bluish lines, or spotted. The lining of the first three stomachs is more or less softened and may easily be peeled off. The third stomach (psalter) contains dry feed in hard masses closely adherent to its walls.

In some cases the brain appears to become disordered, probably from pain and weakness and from the absorption of toxins, generated in the digestive canal. In such cases there is weakness and an unsteady gait, the animal does not appear to take notice of and will consequently run against obstacles; after a time it falls and gives up to violent and disordered movements. This delirious condition is succeeded by coma or stupor, and death ensues.

Treatment.—Small quantities of roots, sweet silage, or selected grass or hay should be offered several times daily. Little feed should be allowed. Aromatic and demulcent drafts may be given to produce a soothing effect on the mucous lining of the stomachs and to promote digestion. Two ounces of camomile flowers should be boiled for 20 minutes in a quart of water and the infusion on cooling should be given to the affected animal. This may be repeated 3 or 4 times a day. When constipation is present the following purgative may be administered: One pound of Glauber's salt dissolved in a quart of linseed tea and a pint of molasses. After this purgative has acted, if there is a lack of appetite and the animal does not ruminate regularly, the powder mentioned in remarks on the treatment of chronic tympanites may be given according to directions. The diet must be rather laxative and of an easily digestible character after an attack of this form of indigestion. Feed should be given in moderate quantities, as excess by overtaxing the digestive functions may bring on a relapse. Ice-cold water should be avoided.

INDIGESTION FROM DRINKING COLD WATER (COLIC)

This disorder is produced by drinking copiously of cold water, which arrests digestion and produces cramp of the fourth stomach, probably of the other stomachs, and also of the bowels.

Causes.—It is not customary for cattle to drink much water at one time. They usually drink slowly and as if they were merely tasting the water, letting some fall out at the corners of the mouth at every mouthful. It, therefore, seems to be contrary to the habits of cattle to drink copiously; but during hot weather, if an animal is very thirsty and consequently drinks a large quantity of cold water it may be immediately taken with a very severe colic. Cows that are fed largely dry hay drink copiously and also become affected with colic. In such cases they are seized with a chill or fit of trembling before the cramps appear.

Symptoms.—There is some distention of the abdomen but no accumulation of gas. As the distention and pain occur immediately after the animal has drunk the water, there can be no doubt as to the exciting cause.

Treatment.—Walk the animal about for 10 minutes before administering medicine. This allows time for a portion of the contents of the stomach to pass into the bowel and renders it safer to give medicine. Then a tablespoonful of powdered ginger may be administered in a pint of warm water. In many cases the walking exercise and the diarrhea bring about a spontaneous cure of this disorder, without resort to medicinal treatment.

INDIGESTION IN CALVES (GASTROINTESTINAL CATARRH, DIARRHEA, OR SCOUR)

Calves are subject to a form of diarrhea to which the foregoing designations have been applied.

Causes.—Calves that suck their dams are not frequently affected with this disease, though it may be occasioned by their sucking at long intervals and thus overloading the stomach and bringing on indigestion, or from improper feeding of the dam on soft, watery, or damaged feeds. Suckling the calf at irregular times may also cause it. Exposure to damp and cold is a potent predisposing cause. Calves separated from their dams and fed considerable quantities of cold milk at long intervals are likely to contract this form of indigestion. Calves fed on artificial feed, used as a substitute for milk, frequently contract it. Damaged feed, sour or rotten milk. milk from dirty cans, skim milk from a dirty creamery skim-milk vat, or skim milk hauled warm, exposed to the sun, and fed from unclean buckets may cause this disease.

Symptoms.—The calf is depressed, appetite is poor, sometimes there is fever, the extremities are cold. The dung becomes gradually softer and lighter in color until it is cream colored and little thicker than milk. It has a most offensive odor and may contain clumps of curd. Later it contains mucus and gas bubbles. It sticks to the hair of the tail and buttocks, causing the hair to drop off and the skin to become irritated. There may be pain on passing dung and also abdominal or colicky pain. The calf stands about with the back arched and belly contracted. There may be tympanites. Great weakness ensues in severe cases, and without prompt and successful treatment death soon follows.

Treatment.—Remove the cause. Give appropriate feed of best quality in small quantities. Make sure that the cow furnishing the milk is healthy and is properly fed. Clean all milk vessels. Clean and disinfect the stalls. For the diarrhea give two raw eggs or a cup of strong coffee. If the case is severe, give 1 ounce of castor oil with a teaspoonful of creolin and 20 grains of subnitrate of bismuth. Repeat the bismuth and creolin with flaxseed tea every 4 hours.

Calves artificially fed whole or skim milk should receive only such milk as is sweet and has been handled in a sanitary manner. Milk should always be warmed to the temperature of the body before feeding. When calves artificially milk-fed develop diarrhea, the use of the following treatment has given excellent results in many cases: Immediately after milking or the separation of the skim milk from the cream, 1 part of formalin may be added to each 4,000 parts of milk used in feeding. This is equivalent to about 4 drops of formalin to each quart of milk. This medicated milk should be fed to the calf in the usual quantity. When the diarrhea is not controlled in 3 or 4 days by this treatment, the additional use of some of the agents recommended above may assist in a recovery.

INFECTIOUS DIARRHEA; WHITE SCOUR

[See chapter on Diseases of Young Calves, p. 212]

GASTROENTERITIS

Gastroenteritis, or inflammation of the walls of the stomachs and intestines, follows irritations more severe or longer continued than those that produce gastrointestinal catarrh.

Causes.—Severe indigestion may be followed by gastroenteritis, or it may be caused by swallowing irritant poisons, such as arsenic or corrosive sublimate or irritant plants. Exposure to cold or inclement weather may produce the disease, especially in debilitated animals or animals fed improperly.

Symptoms.—These are dullness, drooping of the ears, dryness of the muzzle, dry skin, staring coat, loins morbidly sensitive to pressure, fullness of the left flank, which is caused by the distention of the fourth stomach by gas. The pulse is weak, and the gait is feeble and staggering. Each step taken is accompanied with a grunt, and this symptom is especially marked if the animal walks in a downhill direction. There is loss of appetite, and rumination is suspended. The passages at first are few in number, hard, and are sometimes coated with mucus or with blood. Later a severe diarrhea sets in, when the passages contain mucus and blood and have an offensive odor. There is evidence of colicky pain, and the abdomen is sensitive to pressure. Pain may be continuous. There is fever and acceleration of pulse rate and respirations. Mental depression and even insensibility occur before death. The disease is always severe and often fatal.

Postmortem appearances.—The mucous membrane of the fourth stomach has a well-marked red color and is sometimes ulcerated. The wall is thickened and softened, and similar conditions are found in the walls of the intestines. The red discoloration extends in spots or large areas quite through the wall and shows on the outside.

Treatment.—Small quantities of carefully selected feed should be given and the appetite must not be forced. Protect the animal well from cold and dampness. Internally, give linseed tea, boiled milk, boiled oatmeal gruel, or rice water. These protectives may carry the medicine. Subnitrate of bismuth in doses of 1 to 2 drams may be given. If the bowel movements are not free, one may give from a pint to a quart of castor or raw linseed oil or mineral oil.

TRAUMATIC INFLAMMATION OF THE STOMACH

This disease results from the presence of a foreign body. This condition is rather common in cattle, because these animals have the habit of swallowing their feed without careful chewing. Therefore, nails, screws, hairpins, ends of wire, and other metal objects may be swallowed unconsciously. Such objects gravitate to the second stomach, where they may be caught in the folds of the lining mucous membrane, and in some instances the wall of this organ is perforated. From this accident, chronic indigestion results. The symptoms, more or less characteristic, are pain when getting up or lying down; grunting and pain on sudden motion, especially downhill; coughing;

77431 O—51——3

pain on pressure over the second stomach, which lies immediately above the cartilaginous prolongation of the sternum. If the presence of such a foreign body is recognized, it may be removed by a difficult surgical operation, or, as is usually most economical, the animal may be killed for beef, if there is no fever.

DISEASES OF THE BOWELS

DIARRHEA AND DYSENTERY

[See also Gastrointestinal Catarrh, p. 21]

The word "dysentery," as it is commonly used in relation to the diseases of animals, signifies a severe form of diarrhea.

Causes.—Diarrhea is a symptom of irritation of the intestines, resulting in increased secretion or increased muscular contractions, or both. The irritation is sometimes the result of chilling from exposure, improper feeding, irritant feeds, indigestion, organic diseases of the intestines, or parasites.

Symptoms.—Passages from the bowels are frequent, at first consisting of thin dung, but as the disease continues they become watery and offensive smelling, and may be even streaked with blood. At first the animal shows no constitutional disturbance, but later it becomes weak and may exhibit evidence of abdominal pain by looking around to the side, drawing the feet together, lying down, or moving restlessly. Sometimes this malady is accompanied with fever, great depression, loss of strength, rapid loss of flesh, and it may terminate in death.

Treatment.—When the disease is caused by irritating properties of the feed that has been supplied to the animal, it is advisable to give a mild purgative, such as a pint of castor or linseed oil. When the secretions of the bowels are irritating, an ounce of magnesium carbonate should be shaken up in a quart of linseed tea and given to the animal three times a day until the passages have a natural appearance. When there is debility, want of appetite, no fever, but a continuance of the watery discharges from the bowels, an astringent may be given. For such cases the following is serviceable: Tannic acid, 1 ounce; powdered gentian, 2 ounces; mix and divide into 12 powders, 1 powder to be given 3 times a day until the passages have a natural appearance. Each powder may be mixed with 1½ pints of water. Useful household remedies are raw eggs, strong coffee, parched rye flour, or decoction of oak bark. In all cases the feed must be given sparingly, and it should be carefully selected to insure good quality. Complete rest in a box stall is desirable. When diarrhea is a symptom of a malady characterized by the presence of a blood poison, the treatment appropriate to such disease must be applied.

SIMPLE ENTERITIS

[See Gastroenteritis, p. 24]

CROUPOUS ENTERITIS

Under certain conditions, severe irritation of the digestive canal may cause in cattle, a form of inflammation of the intestines (enteritis) that is characterized by the formation of a false membrane on the surface of the lining membrane of the intestines, particularly the large ones.

Symptoms.—There are fever, depression, loss of appetite, diarrhea, and in the fecal masses shreds of leathery false membrane may be found. These shreds are sometimes mistaken for parasites or for portions of the wall of the intestine.

Treatment.—Give, as a purgative, a pound of Glauber's salt, followed by sodium bicarbonate in doses of 2 ounces four times daily.

ENTERITIS (OBSTRUCTION RESULTING FROM INVAGINATION, OR INTUSSUSCEPTION, TWISTING, AND KNOTTING OF THE BOWELS)

Inflammation may arise from a knot forming on some part of the small intestine if the portion of the bowel becomes twisted on itself, or if one part of the bowel slips into another, which is termed invagination. This form of enteritis occurs occasionally in animals of the bovine species.

Causes.—The small intestine, which in cattle rests on the right side of the rumen, is, from the position which it occupies, predisposed to this accident. Animals showing symptoms of this malady may have trotted, galloped, or made other violent exertions in coming from drinking, or they may have been chased by dogs or by animals of their own species while on pasture. The accident is most likely to occur among cattle on very hilly pastures. The danger of jumping or running is greatest when the rumen is distended with food.

Symptoms.—This form of enteritis or obstruction is manifested by severe, colicky pains; the animal scrapes and strikes the ground with its front and hind feet alternately; keeps lying down and getting up again; keeps its tail constantly raised and turns its nose frequently to its right flank; is frequently bloated, or tympanitic, on that side. It refuses feed and does not ruminate and for some hours suffers severe pains. At first the animal frequently passes thin dung and also urinates frequently but passes only a little urine at a time. On the second day the pains have become less acute; the animal remains lying down and moans occasionally; its pulse is weak and quick; it still refuses feed and does not ruminate. At this stage it does not pass any dung, but sometimes a small quantity of bloody mucus. The animal passes little urine. This condition may continue for a considerable time, as cattle so affected sometimes live for 15 or even 20 days.

Post mortem appearance.—At death the bowels are found to be misplaced or obstructed, as mentioned above, and inflamed, the inflammation always originating at the point where the intestine has been invaginated, twisted, or knotted. Sometimes the part is gangrenous, circulation being prevented by the compression of the blood vessels.

Treatment.—Purgatives, anodynes, and other remedies are of no service in such cases, and bleeding also fails to produce any benefit. Indeed, usually in such cases medicinal treatment is useless. In certain cases the condition may be corrected by surgical interference. Such procedure, of course, should be undertaken only by a competent veterinarian.

CONSTIPATION

Constipation is to be regarded rather as a symptom of disease or of faults in feeding than as a disease in itself. It occurs in almost all general fevers unless the bowels are involved in local disease, in obstructions of all kinds, from feeding on dry, bulky feed, and other causes. In order to remove the constipation, treatment must be applied to remove the causes that give rise to it. Calves sometimes suffer from constipation immediately after birth, when the meconium that accumulates in the bowels before birth is not passed. In such cases, give a rectal injection of warm water and an ounce of castor oil shaken up with an ounce of new milk. The mother's milk is the best food to prevent constipation in the newborn calf, as it contains a large quantity of fatty matter that renders it laxative in its effects.

It is usually better to treat habitual constipation by a change of diet than by medicine. Flaxseed is a good laxative. If the constipation has lasted long, repeated small doses of purgatives are better than a single large dose.

INTESTINAL WORMS

[See chapter on the Parasites of Cattle, p. 449]

RUPTURES (VENTRAL HERNIA)

Ventral hernia, or rupture, is an escape of some one of the abdominal organs through a rupture in the abdominal muscles, the skin remaining intact. The rumen, the small intestine, or part of the large intestine, and the fourth stomach are the parts that usually form a ventral hernia in bovine animals.

Causes.—Hernia is frequently produced by blows of the horns, kicks, and falls. In old cows hernia may sometimes occur without any direct injury.

HERNIA OF THE RUMEN

Hernia of the rumen is generally situated on the left side of the abdomen, on account of the situation of the rumen. In exceptional cases it may take place on the right side, and in such cases some folds of the intestine generally pass into the hernial sac. Hernias have been classified as simple or complicated, recent or old, traumatic (from mechanical injury) or spontaneous.

In recent traumatic hernia there is swelling on the left side of the lower part of the abdomen. The swelling is greatest in hernia situated on the lower part of the abdomen. Unless an examination is made immediately after the injury has been inflicted it is difficult, and sometimes impossible, to ascertain the exact extent of the rupture, owing to the swelling that subsequently takes place. Frequently there is no loss of appetite, fever, or other general symptoms attending the injury. From the twelfth to the fifteenth day the swelling has generally subsided to such an extent that it is possible by an examination to determine the extent of the rupture.

In old cows, what is termed spontaneous hernia may sometimes take place without any direct injury. The occurrence of this form of hernia is due to the increase in the size of the abdomen, which takes place in an advanced stage of pregnancy, causing a thinning and stretching of the muscular fibers, which at last may rupture, or give way. Such hernias frequently occur about the end of the period of gestation and in some instances have contained the right sac of the rumen, the omentum, the small and large intestines, a portion of the liver, and the pregnant uterus.

In old hernias the swelling is soft and elastic, and if they have not contracted adhesions to the sides of the laceration, they can be made to disappear by pressure carefully applied. Sometimes this accident is complicated by a rupture of the rumen, constituting a complicated hernia. If a portion of the contents of the rumen escapes into the abdomen, the case will be aggravated by the occurrence of peritonitis.

HERNIA OF THE BOWEL

When the intestines (pl. III, fig. 6) form the contents of the hernia, it will be situated at the right side of the abdomen. In an intestinal hernia the swelling is usually not painful and is of a doughy consistence or elastic, depending on whether the intestine contains alimentary matter. This swelling can generally be made to disappear by pressure, and when it has been reduced one can easily recognize the direction and extent of the hernial opening. Hernias of the bowel when situated at the upper and right side of the abdomen are usually formed by the small intestine. They are less easily reduced than a hernia in a lower situation, but when reduction has been effected they are less readily reproduced than those occurring lower. In hernias of the small intestine, adhesion of the protruding parts to the walls of the opening, or strangulation, sometimes takes place. If adhesion has taken place the hernia cannot be reduced by pressure, and when strangulation has occurred the animal shows symptoms of pain—is restless, turns its nose to the painful part, and shows those symptoms that are usually collectively designated under the term "colic." If relief is not afforded, the animal will die.

HERNIA OF THE RENNET, OR FOURTH STOMACH

This disease occasionally occurs in calves and is usually caused by a blow from a cow's horn on the right flank of the calf. After such an accident a swelling forms on the right flank near the last rib. This swelling may be neither hot nor painful, even at first, and is soft to the touch. It can be made to disappear by careful pressure, when the sides of the aperture through which it has passed can be felt. The application of pressure so as to cause the disappearance of the hernia is best made immediately after the occurrence of the accident, or when the edema which accompanies the swelling has disappeared.

Treatment.—When a hernia is reducible—that is, can be pushed back into the abdomen—if it is of recent occurrence, it is advisable to maintain the natural position of the parts by bandaging and to allow the walls of the laceration to grow together. The bowels should be kept reasonably empty by avoiding the use of bulky feed, and the animal must be kept quiet.

The following method of bandaging is recommended:

> First prepare a bandage (must be of strong material), about 10 yards long and between 3 and 4 inches broad, and a flexible and solid piece of pasteboard adapted in size to the surface of the hernia. The protruding organ must then be replaced in the abdomen and maintained in that position during the application of the bandage. This being done, a layer of melted pitch and turpentine is quickly spread on the skin covering the seat of the hernia, so as to extend somewhat beyond that space. This adhesive layer is then covered with a layer of fine tow, then a new layer of pitch and turpentine is spread on the tow, and the piece of pasteboard is applied on the layer of pitch, its outer surface being covered with the same preparation. Lastly, the bandage, adhering to the piece of pasteboard, to the skin, and to the different turns that it makes around the body, is carefully applied so as to form an immovable, rigid, and solid bandage that will retain the hernia long enough for the wound in the abdominal walls to heal permanently.

If the hernia is old and small it may be treated by injecting a strong solution of common salt about the edges of the tear. This causes swelling and inflammation, which, respectively, forces the protruded organ back and closes the opening. There is some risk attached to this method of treatment.

In small, old, ventral hernias the method of compressing and sloughing off the skin has been used successfully. If the hernia is large or strangulated, a radical operation will be necessary. This operation is performed by cutting down on the hernia, restoring the organ to the abdominal cavity, and then closing the wound with two sets of stitches; the inner stitches, in the muscular wall, should be made with catgut and the outer stitches, in the skin, may be made with silk or silver wire. The strictest surgical cleanliness must be observed. Bleeding vessels should be tied. Then a compress composed of 10 or 12 folds of cloth must be placed smoothly over the seat of injury and a bandage applied around the body, the two ends being fastened at the back. In the smaller kinds of hernia, nitric acid may sometimes be applied with success. This treatment should not be applied until the swelling and inflammation attending the appearance of the hernia have subsided. Then, the contents of the hernia having been returned, the surface of skin corresponding to it is sponged with a solution of 1 part of nitric acid to 2 of water. This treatment excites considerable inflammation, which causes swelling, thus frequently closing the hernial opening and preventing the contents of the sac from returning. A second application should not be made until the inflammation excited by the first has subsided. In what is termed "spontaneous hernia" it is useless to apply any kind of treatment.

UMBILICAL HERNIA

The umbilicus, or navel, is the aperture through which the blood vessels pass from the mother to the fetus, and naturally the sides of this aperture ought to adhere or unite after birth. In very young animals, and sometimes in newborn calves, this aperture in the abdominal muscles remains open and a part of the bowel or a portion of the mesentery may slip through the opening, constituting what is called umbilical hernia. The wall of the sac is formed by the skin, which is covered on the inner surface by a layer of cellular tissue, and within this there is sometimes, but not always, a layer of peritoneum. The contents of the hernia may be formed by a part of the bowel, by a portion of the peritoneum, or may contain portions of both peritoneum and bowel. When the sac contains only the peritoneum it has a doughy feel, but when it is formed by a portion of the bowel it is more elastic on pressure.

Causes.—In the newborn animal the opening of the navel is generally large and may sometimes give way to the pressure of the bowel on account of the weak and relaxed condition of the abdominal muscles. This defective and abnormal condition of the umbilicus is frequently hereditary. It may be occasioned by roughly pulling away the umbilical cord, through kicks or blows on the belly, or through any severe straining by which the sides of the navel are stretched apart. In newborn calves it is best to tie the umbilical cord tightly about 2 inches from the navel, and then to leave it alone, when in most cases it will drop off in a few days, leaving the navel closed.

Treatment.—Many, especially the smaller, umbilical hernias heal spontaneously, that is, nature effects a cure. As the animal gets older the abdominal muscles become stronger and possess more power of resistance to pressure, and the bowels are larger and do not pass so readily through a small opening. Therefore, from a combination of causes there is a gradual growing together or adhesion of the sides of the navel. In cases of umbilical hernia in which there are no indications that a spontaneous cure will take place, the calf should be laid on its back; immediately on this being done the hernia will often disappear into the abdomen. If it does not, its reduction may be brought about by gentle handling, endeavoring, if need be, to empty the organs forming the hernia before returning them into the abdomen. After the hernia has been returned, the hair should be clipped from the skin covering it and a compress composed of 10 or 12 folds of linen or cotton should be applied. First, the skin should be smeared with pitch and then a bandage about 3 inches wide should be passed around the body to retain the compress in position. The lower part of the compress as well as those portions of the bandage that pass over it, should be smeared with pitch to keep the compress solid and prevent it from shifting. In some cases the contents of the sac cannot be returned into the abdomen, generally because some part of the contents of the sac has grown to or become adherent to the edges of the umbilical opening. In such a case the skin must be carefully laid open in the long direction, the adhesions of the protruding organs carefully separated from the umbilicus, and after the protruding parts have been returned into the abdomen, the sides of the umbilicus must be freshened if necessary by paring, and then the edges of the opening brought together by catgut stitches. The wound in the skin must then also be brought together by stitches. It must be carefully dressed every day and a bandage passed around the body to cover and protect the part operated on.

In small hernias nitric acid has been used successfully in the same manner as has been described in the treatment of ventral hernia. Sulfuric acid has also been used for a similar purpose, diluted to 1 part of acid to 3 or 5 of water. In thin-skinned animals the weaker preparations are preferable, and caution must be exercised in using such preparations so as not to destroy the tissues on which they are applied.

Another method of treatment is as follows: After the contents of the sac have been returned into the abdomen, tie a piece of strong, waxed cord around the pendulous portion that formed the outer covering of the hernia. The string is likely to slacken after 2 or 3 days, when a new piece of cord should be applied above the first one. The constriction of the skin sets up inflammation, which generally extends to the umbilicus and causes the edges to adhere, and by the time the portion of skin below the ligature has lost its vitality and dropped off, the umbilicus is closed and there is no danger of the abdominal organs protruding through it. This is what takes place when this method has a favorable result, though if the umbilicus does not become adherent and the skin sloughs, the bowels will protrude through the opening.

GUTTIE (PERITONEAL HERNIA)

In peritoneal hernia of cattle a loop or knuckle of intestine enters from the abdomen into a rent in that part of the peritoneum situated at the margin of the hipbone, or it passes under the remains of the spermatic cord, the end of which may be grown fast to the inner inguinal ring. The onward pressure of the bowel, as well as the occasional turning of the latter around the spermatic cord, is the cause of the cord's exercising considerable pressure on the bowel, which occasions irritation, obstructs the passage of excrement, and excites inflammation, terminating in gangrene and death.

The rent in the peritoneum is situated at the upper and front part of the pelvis, nearer to the sacrum than the pubes.

Causes.—Among the causes of peritoneal hernia considerable importance is attached to a method of castration practiced in certain districts, that is, the tearing or rupturing of the spermatic cord by main force instead of dividing it at a proper distance above the testicle in a surgical manner. After this violent and rough method of operating, the cord retracts into the abdomen and its stump becomes adherent to some part of the peritoneum, or it may wind around the bowel and then the stump becomes adherent, resulting in strangulation of the bowel. The rough dragging on the cord may also cause a tear in the peritoneum, the result of which need not be described. The exertion of drawing heavy loads or fighting may also give rise to peritoneal hernia.

Symptoms.—The animal suddenly becomes very restless, stamps its feet, moves backward and forward, hurriedly lies down, rises, moves its tail uneasily, and kicks at its belly with the foot of the affected side. The pain evinced may diminish but soon returns. In the early stage there are frequent passages of dung, but after the lapse of 18 to 24 hours this ceases, the bowel apparently being emptied to the point of strangulation, and the passages now consist only of a little mucus mixed with blood. When injections are given at this time the water passes out of the bowel without even being colored. The animal lies down on the side where the hernia exists and stretches out its hind feet in a backward direction. These two symptoms serve to distinguish this affection from enteritis and invagination of the bowel. As time passes the animal becomes quieter, but this cessation of pain may indicate that gangrene of the bowel has set in, and may, therefore, under certain circumstances, be considered a precursor of death. Gangrene may take place in from 4 to 6 days, when perforation of the bowel may occur and death result in a short time.

Treatment.—In the first place the animal should be examined by passing the oiled hand and arm into the rectum; the hand should be passed along the margin of the pelvis, beginning at the sacrum and continuing downward toward the inguinal ring, when a soft, painful swelling will be felt, which may vary from the size of an apple to that of the two fists. This swelling will be felt to be tightly compressed by the spermatic cord. There is rarely any similar swelling on the left side, though in such cases it is best to make a thorough examination. The bowel has sometimes been released from its position by driving the animal down a hill or by causing it to jump from a height of 2 feet to the ground. Trotting the animal also has been resorted to with the hope that the jolting movement might bring about a release of the bowel. If the simple expedients mentioned fail, the hand being passed into the rectum should be pressed gently on the swelling in an upward and forward direction in an endeavor to push the imprisoned portion of the bowel back into the abdomen. While this is being done the animal's hind feet should stand on higher ground than the front to favor the slipping out of the bowel by its own weight, and at the same time an assistant should squeeze the animal's loins to bend the bowel downward and so relax the band formed by the spermatic cord. If the imprisoned portion of bowel is freed, which may be ascertained by the disappearance of the swelling, the usual sounds produced by the bowels moving in the abdomen will be heard, and in a few hours the feces and urine will be passed as usual. If the means mentioned fail to release the imprisoned portion, an incision about 4 inches long must be made in the right flank in a downward direction, the hand introduced into the abdomen, the situation and condition of swelling exactly ascertained, and then a probe-pointed knife inserted between the imprisoned bowel and band compressing it, and turned outward against the band, the latter being then cautiously divided and the imprisoned bowel allowed to escape. If necessary, the bowel should be drawn gently from its position into the abdomen. The wound in the flank must be brought together in the same way as in the wound made in operating for impaction of the rumen.

WOUNDS OF THE ABDOMEN

A wound of the abdomen may merely penetrate the skin; but as such cases are not attended with much danger nor their treatment with much difficulty, only those wounds are considered here that penetrate the entire thickness of the abdominal walls and expose to a greater or less extent the organs contained in that cavity.

Causes.—Such accidents may be occasioned by falling on fragments of broken glass or other sharp objects. A blow from the horn of another animal may penetrate the abdomen. Exposure and protrusion of some of the abdominal organs may also be occasioned by the incautious use of caustics in the treatment of umbilical or ventral hernia. The parts that generally escape through an abdominal wound are the small intestine and floating colon.

Symptoms.—When the abdominal wound is small, the bowel exposed has the appearance of a small round tumor, but in a few moments a loop of intestine may emerge from the opening. The animal then shows symptoms of severe pain by pawing with its feet, which has the effect of accelerating the passage of new loops of intestine through the wound, so that the mass which they form may even touch the ground. The pain becomes so great that the animal now not only paws but lies down and rolls, thus tearing and crushing its bowels. In such cases it is best to slaughter the animal at once; but in a valuable animal in which tearing and crushing of the bowels have not taken place, the bowels should be washed with freshly boiled water reduced to the temperature of the body and returned, and the wounds in the muscle and skin brought together in a manner somewhat similar to that described for ventral hernia.

DISEASES OF THE LIVER AND SPLEEN

JAUNDICE (THE YELLOWS, OR CONGESTION OF THE LIVER)

When jaundice exists, there is a yellow appearance of the white of the eyes and of the mucous membrane of the mouth. A similar aspect of the skin may also be observed in animals that are either partly or altogether covered with white hair. Jaundice is then merely a symptom of disease and ought to direct attention to ascertaining, if possible, the cause or causes giving rise to it. A swollen condition of the mucous membrane of that part of the bowel called the duodenum may produce jaundice, as that mechanically closes the orifice of the biliary duct. In constipation there is an inactive or torpid condition of the bowel, and the bile that passes into the intestine may be absorbed and cause the yellow staining of jaundice. Jaundice is one of the symptoms of cattle-tick fever. It may also arise from the presence of parasites or gallstones in the ducts, forming a mechanical obstruction to the flow of bile. The conditions under which jaundice most commonly calls for treatment are when cattle have been highly fed and kept in a state of inactivity. At such time there is an excess of nutritive elements carried into the blood, this associated with increased fullness of the portal vein and hepatic artery. When continued high feeding has produced this congested state of the liver, the functions of that organ become disordered, so that a considerable portion of the bile, instead of being excreted and passing into the intestine, is absorbed by the hepatic veins. The structure of the liver is shown in plate IV.

Symptoms.—This disease, although rare, occurs most frequently among stall-fed cattle. Pressure along the margin of the short ribs on the right side produces pain; the appetite is poor and the animal shows little inclination to drink; the mucous membranes of the eye and mouth are yellow; the urine has a yellow or brown appearance; the animal lies down much and moves with reluctance, moans occasionally, and has a tottering gait. The ears and horns are alternately hot and cold; in cows the secretion of milk is much diminished, and that which is secreted has a bitter taste; sometimes the animal has a dry, painful cough and a dull, stupefied appearance.

Treatment.—In such cases it is advisable to produce free action of the bowels to remove the usually congested condition of the liver and portal vein. For this purpose the administration of the following dose is recommended: Sodium sulfate, 16 ounces; molasses, 1 pint; warm water, 1 quart. The sodium sulfate is dissolved by stirring it in tepid water. Following this the animal should have a heaping tablespoonful of artificial Karlsbad salt in the feed three times daily. This laxative treatment may be assisted by giving occasional injections of warm water and soap. The diet should be laxative and moderate in quantity and may consist of coarse bran mash, pulped roots, grass in season, and hay in moderate quantity.

HEPATITIS (INFLAMMATION OF THE LIVER)

Hepatitis is an inflammation of the liver and usually occurs as a complication of some infectious disease. It may also occur as a complication of gastrointestinal catarrh or in hot weather from overheating or putrid or fermented feeds.

Symptoms.—The symptoms are sometimes obscure and their real significance is frequently overlooked. The most prominent symptoms are yellowness of the white of the eye and of the membrane lining of the mouth. The appetite is poor, the body is emaciated, the feces are light colored, whereas the urine is likely to be unusually dark. There is thirst, and pain is caused by pressing over the liver. The gait is weak and the animal lies down more than usual and while doing so frequently rests its head on the side of its chest.

Treatment.—Give a purge of Glauber's salt, and after it has operated give artificial Karlsbad salt in each feed, as described under Jaundice. Give green feed and plenty of water. Oil of turpentine rubbed in well once a day over the region of the liver may be helpful. The skin on which it should be applied extends from the false ribs on the right side to 6 inches in front of the last one, and from the backbone to 12 inches on the right side of it.

FLUKE DISEASE

[See Parasites of Cattle, p. 481]

SPLENITIS (INFLAMMATION OF THE SPLEEN)

This disease occurs almost solely as a result of some infectious disease, and the symptoms caused by it merge with the symptoms of the accompanying causative disease. The spleen is seriously involved and becomes enlarged and soft in cattle-tick fever, anthrax, and blood poisoning.

DISEASES OF THE PERITONEUM

PERITONITIS

Peritonitis consists in an inflammation of the peritoneum, which is the thin, delicate membrane that lines the abdomen and covers the abdominal organs.

Causes.—Wounds are the usual cause in cattle. The wound may be of the abdominal wall or of the intestines, stomach, or uterus; or inflammation may extend from one of the organs of the abdominal cavity to the peritoneum. Therefore, this disease may complicate enteritis or inflamed womb. A sharp metal body may perforate the second stomach and allow the gastric contents to escape, irritating the peritoneum. This disease may follow castration or operation for hernia.

Symptoms.—These are as follows: A continuous or occasional shivering; the animal lies down but appears uneasy; it frequently turns its head toward its belly and lows plaintively; pressure on the flanks produces pain; it has no appetite; muzzle is dry and no rumination; while standing, its legs are placed well under its body; pulse weak and hard. The evacuations from the bowels are dry and hard. If this disease is complicated by the presence of inflammation of the bowels, the pain is more severe and the animal is more restless. The skin is cold and dry in the early stage of this disease, but in a more advanced stage this condition may be succeeded by heat of the skin and quick breathing. The fits of trembling, uneasiness, weak and hard pulse, and tension of the left flank are symptoms the presence of which would enable one to reach the conclusion that peritonitis exists.

Post mortem appearance.—The membrane lining the abdomen and covering the surface of the bowels is reddened to a greater or less extent, and there is usually considerable serous, or watery, fluid in the abdomen.

Treatment.—When peritonitis resulting from an injury is involved, as when the horn of another animal has been thrust through the abdominal walls, this lesion must be treated in accordance with directions before given, but the general treatment must be similar to that which follows. Peritonitis resulting from castration or from parturient fever must also be treated in connection with the special conditions that give rise to it, as the general treatment of this disease must be modified to some extent by the exciting cause.

The aim must be to discover and remove the cause, which must be treated according to its nature. To bring on evacuations of the bowels it is better to give rectal injections than to administer purges. The strength may be sustained by coffee or camphor.

The body should be warmly covered, and it is advisable, when practicable, to have a blanket that has been wrung out of hot water placed over the abdomen, then covered by several dry blankets, which are maintained in position by straps or ropes passing around the body. The wet blanket must be changed as it cools, the object of treatment being to warm the surface of the body and to bring as much blood to the skin as possible. The diet should consist of laxative feed and drinks, such as linseed tea. If peritonitis assumes chronic form the diet should be nutritious, such as selected clover hay, linseed cake, and grass. Potassium iodide given three times a day in gram doses dissolved in a pint of water may be helpful in the resorption of the inflammatory exudate.

DROPSY OF THE ABDOMEN (ASCITES)

In this disease there is a serous, or watery, effusion in the cavity of the abdomen.

Causes.—When old animals are fed on innutritious feed or when they are reduced by disease, they become anemic; in other words, their blood becomes impoverished and dropsy may follow. An innutritious and insufficient diet produces the same effect in young animals. It is one of the results of peritonitis and may also arise from acute or chronic inflammation of the liver, such as is of common occurrence when flukes are present in the liver in large numbers. Heart disease and chronic lung disease may be followed by ascites. It is sometimes, in calves, a symptom of infestation with worms.

Symptoms.—These are as follows: A gradual increase in the size of the abdomen at its lower part whereas the flanks become hollow, pallor of the mucous membrane of the mouth and eyes, weak and sluggish gait, want of appetite, and irregularity in ruminating. On percussion or tapping the surface of the abdomen with the fingers, a dull sound is produced. If the hand and arm are oiled and passed into the rectum as far as possible, on moving the hand from one side to the other the fluctuation caused by the presence of fluid in the abdomen may be felt.

Treatment.—If possible the cause must be discovered and removed. The diet should be nutritious, and in those cases involving merely anemia (the bloodless state) arising from insufficient diet, the use of tonics and diuretics, at the same time keeping the skin warm, may bring about a gradual absorption of the fluid contained in the abdomen. One of the following powders may be mixed with the animal's feed three times a day; or, if there is any uncertainty as to its being taken in that way, it should be mixed with sirup, so as to form a paste, and smeared well back on the animal's tongue with a flat wooden spoon: Carbonate of iron, 3 ounces; powdered gentian, 3 ounces; powdered potassium nitrate, 3 ounces; mix and divide into 12 powders. The administration of purgatives that promote a watery discharge from the mucous surface of the bowels also tends, by diminishing the serum of the blood, to bring about absorption and a gradual removal of the fluid in the abdomen. Large doses should not be given, but moderate ones should be administered morning and night to produce a laxative effect on the bowels for several days. To attain this end the following may be used: Sodium sulfate, 8 ounces; powdered ginger, half an ounce; to be mixed in 2 quarts of tepid water and given at one dose.

DISEASES OF THE DIGESTIVE ORGANS

DESCRIPTION OF PLATES

PLATE I. Position of the first stomach (rumen or paunch) on the left side. The area enclosed by heavy dotted lines represents the rumen; the elongated, shaded organ is the spleen resting upon it. The skin and muscles have been removed from the ribs to show the position of the lungs and their relation to the paunch.

PLATE II. Stomach of ruminants.

Figure 1. Stomach of the full-grown sheep, ⅕ natural size (after Thanhoffer, from R. Meade Smith's Physiology of Domestic Animals): *A*, Rumen, or first stomach; *B*, reticulum, or second stomach; *C*, omasum, or third stomach; *D*, abomasum, or fourth stomach; *E*, esophagus, or gullet, opening into the first and second stomachs; *F*, opening of fourth stomach into small intestine; *G*, opening of second stomach into third; *H*, opening of third stomach into fourth.

The lines indicate the course of the food in the stomachs. The incompletely masticated food passes down the esophagus, or gullet, into the first and second stomachs, in which a churning motion is kept up, carrying the food from side to side and from stomach to stomach. From the first stomach regurgitation takes place; that is, the food is returned through the gullet to the mouth to be more thoroughly chewed, and this constitutes what is known as chewing the cud. From the second stomach the food passes into the third, and from the third into the fourth, or true stomach, and from there into the intestines.

Figure 2. Stomach of bovine (after Colin, from R. Meade Smith's Physiology of Domestic Animals): *A*, Rumen; *B*, reticulum; *C*, omasum, *D*, abomasum; *E*, esophagus; *F*, opening of fourth stomach into small intestine.

Fürstenberg calculated that in an ox of 1,400 pounds weight the capacity of the stomach is as follows:

	Percent
Rumen, 149.25 quarts, liquid measure	62.4
Reticulum, 23.77 quarts	10
Omasum, 36.98 quarts	15
Abomasum, 29.05 quarts	12.6

According to Colon—

	Quarts
The capacity of a beef's stomach is	266.81
Small intestine	69.74
Cecum	9.51
Colon and rectum	25.58

PLATE III. Instruments used in treating diseases of digestive organs.

Figure 1. Clinical thermometer, ⅘ natural size. This is used to determine the temperature of the animal body. The thermometer is passed into the rectum after having been moistened with a little saliva from the mouth, or after having had a little oil or lard rubbed upon it to facilitate its passage. There it is allowed to remain 2 or 3 minutes, then withdrawn, and the temperature read as in any ordinary thermometer. The clinical thermometer is made self-registering; that is, the mercury in the stem remains at the height to which it was forced by the heat of the body until it is shaken back into the bulb by taking hold of the upper portion of the instrument and giving it a short, quick swing. The normal temperature of cattle varies from 100° to 103° F. In young animals it is somewhat higher than in old. The thermometer is a very useful instrument and frequently is the means by which disease is detected before the appearance of any external sign.

Figure 2. Simple probang, used to dislodge foreign bodies, such as apples, potatoes, and eggs, which have become fastened or stuck in the esophagus or gullet.

Figure 3. Grasping or forceps probang. This instrument, also intended to remove obstructions from the gullet, has a spring forceps at one end in the place of the cuplike arrangement at the end of the simple probang. The forceps are closed while the probang is being introduced; their blades are regulated by a screw in the handle of the instrument. This probang is used to grasp and withdraw an article that may have lodged in the gullet and cannot be forced into the stomach by use of the simple probang.

Figure 4. Wooden gag, used when the probang is to be passed. The gag is a piece of wood that fits in the animal's mouth; a cord passes over the head to hold it in place. The central opening in the wood is intended for the passage of the probang.

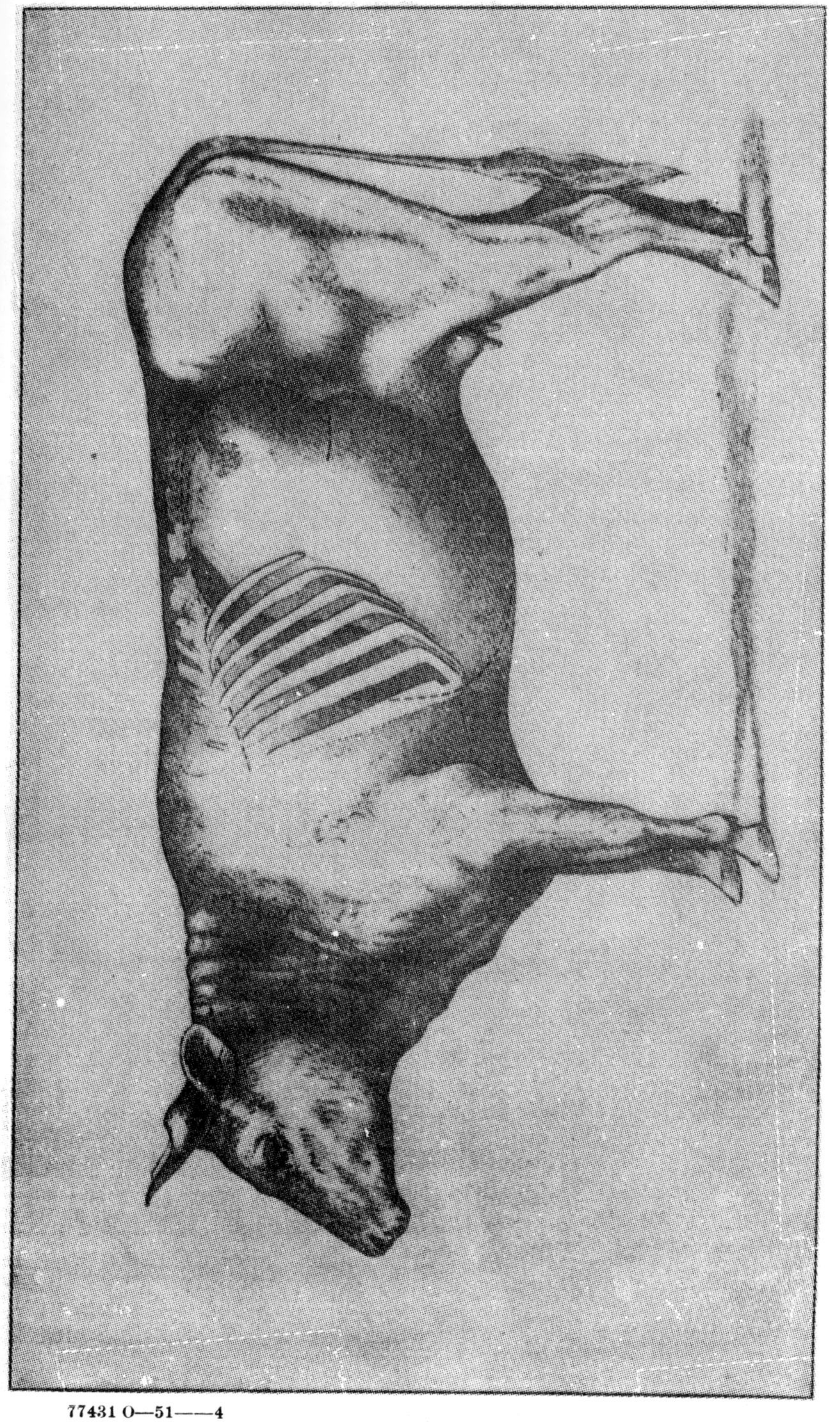

THE RUME

77431 O—51——4

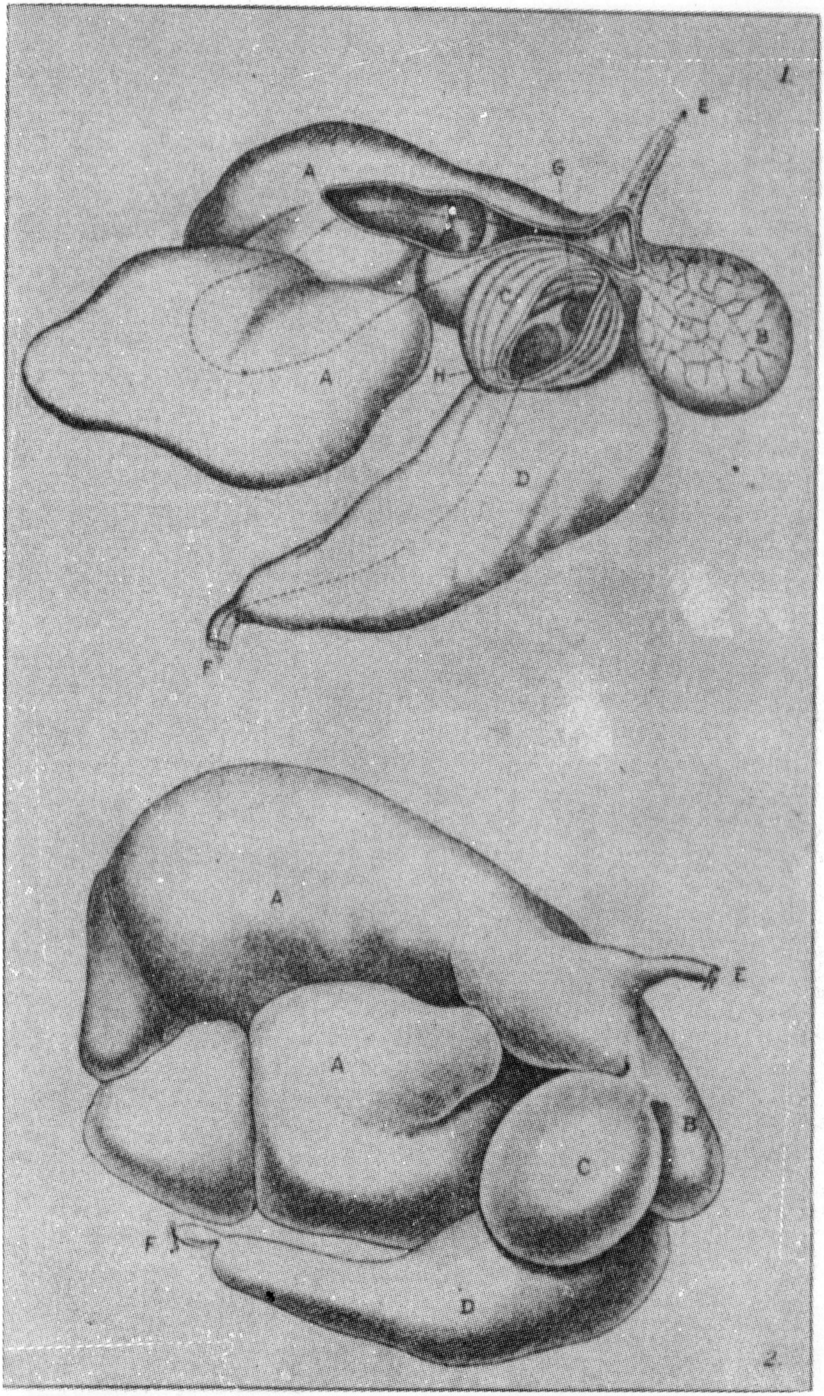

STOMACH OF RUMINANTS.

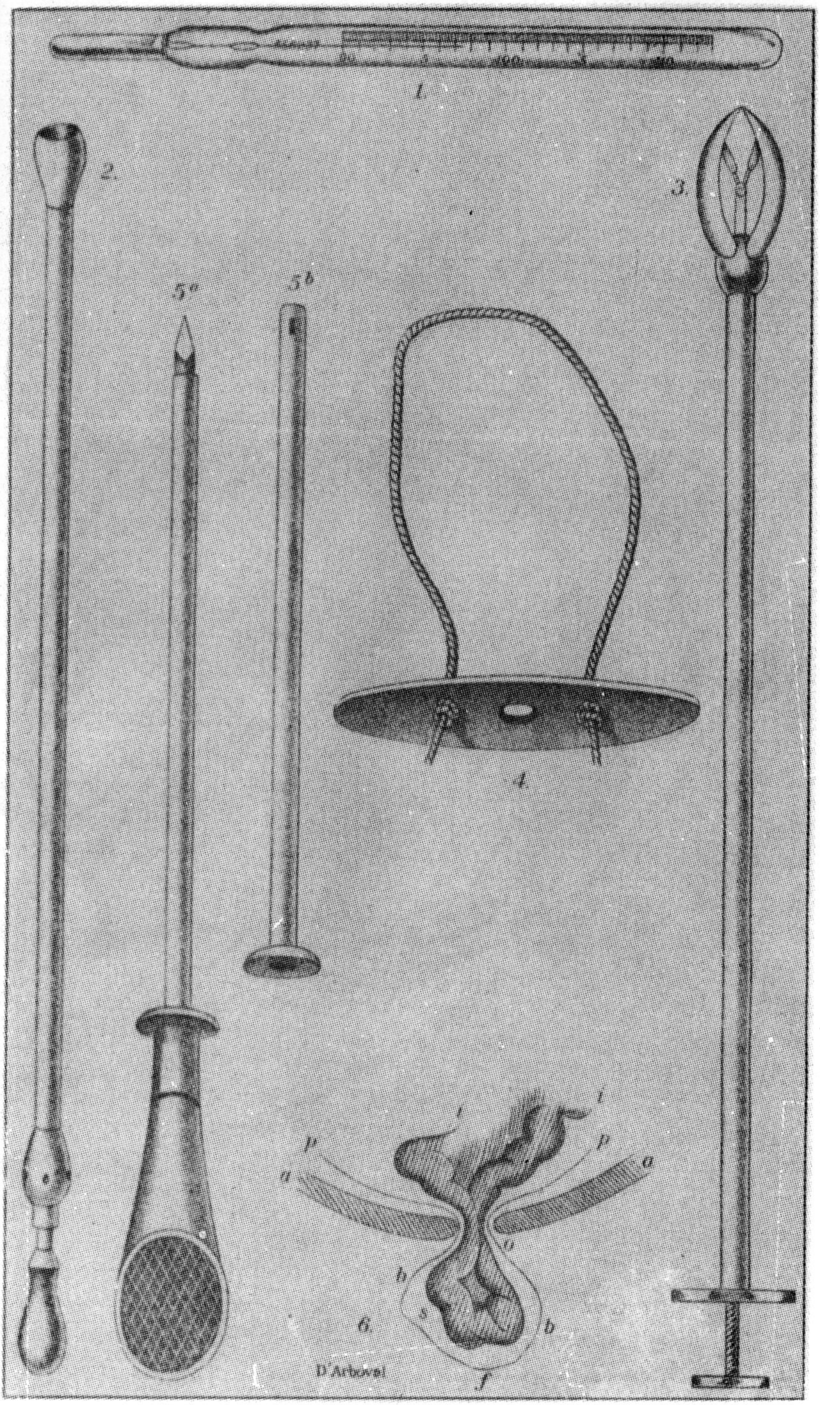

INSTRUMENTS USED IN TREATING DISEASES OF DIGESTIVE ORGANS.

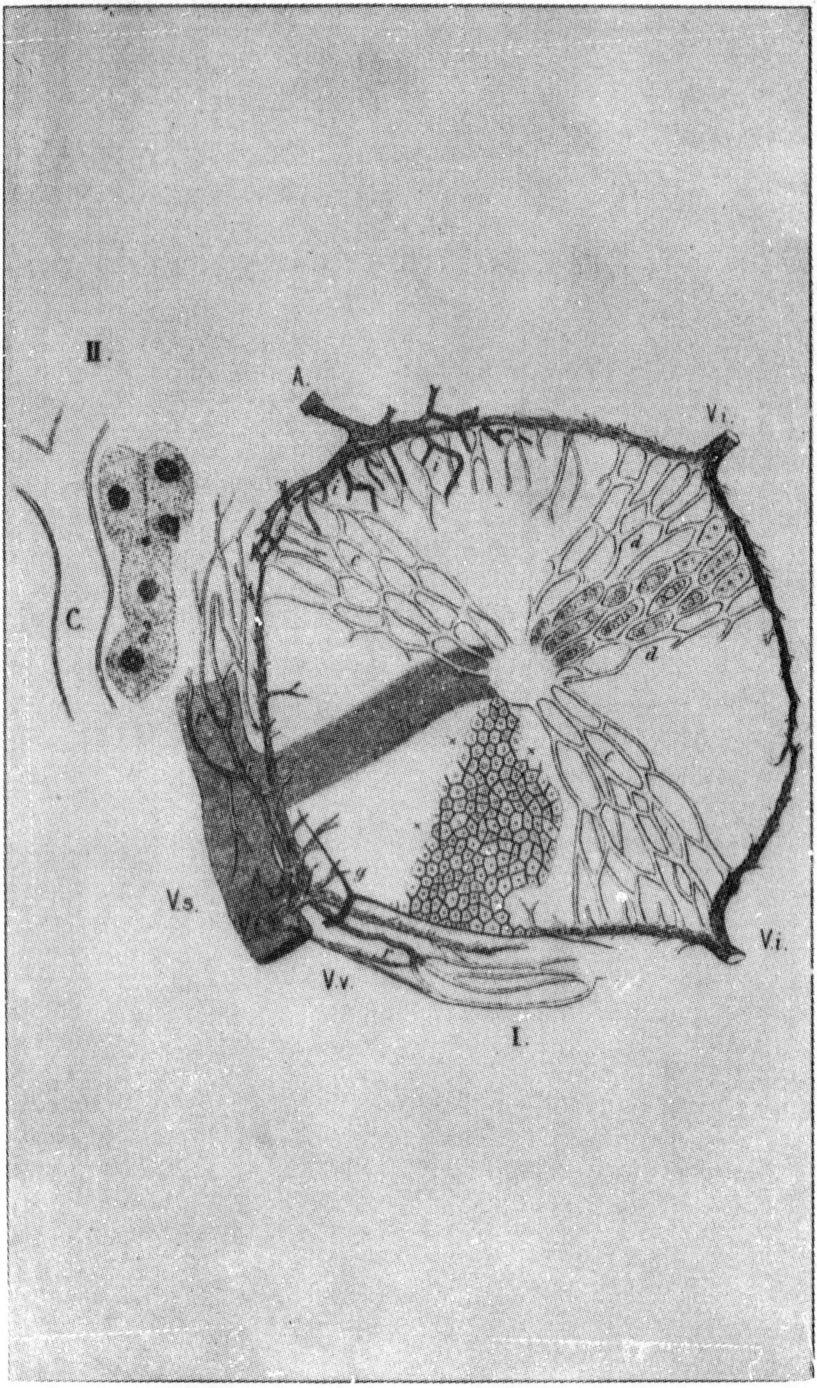

MICROSCOPIC ANATOMY OF THE LIVER.

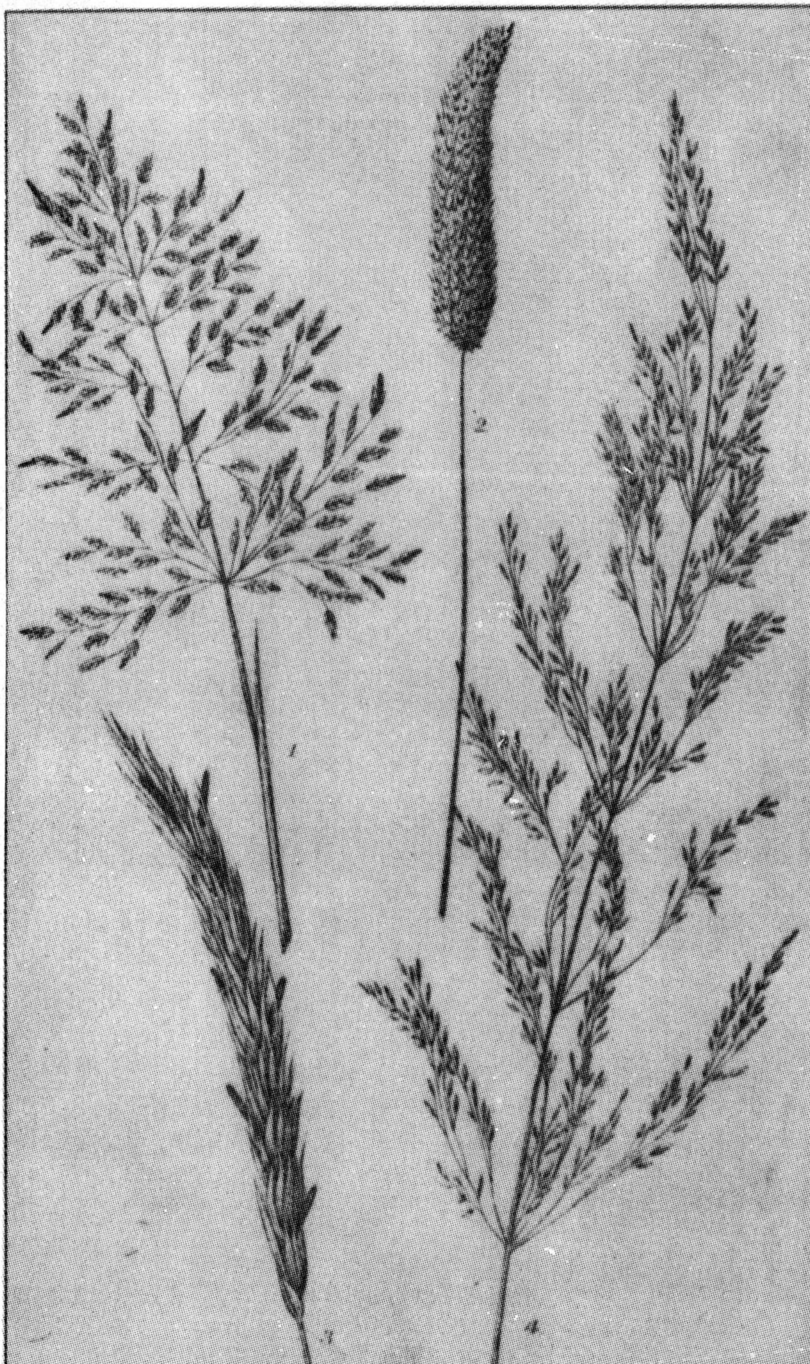

ERGOT IN HAY.

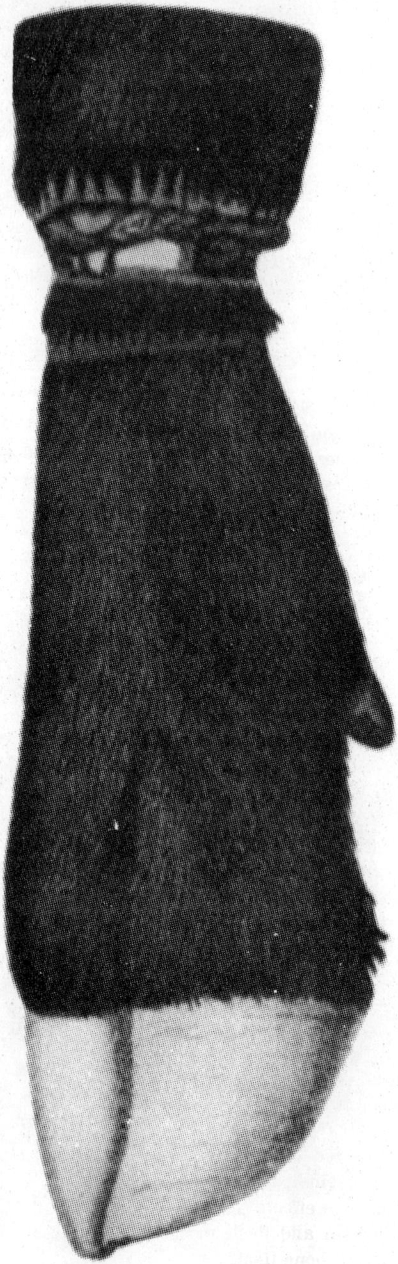

MARX, FROM NATURE.

ERGOTISM.

Figures 5*a* and 5*b*. Trocar and cannula; 5*a* shows the trocar covered by the cannula; 5*b*, the cannula from which the trocar has been withdrawn. This instrument is used when the rumen or first stomach becomes distended with gas. The trocar covered by the cannula is forced into the rumen, the trocar withdrawn, and the cannula allowed to remain until the gas has escaped.

Figure 6. Section at right angles through the abdominal wall, showing a hernia or rupture. (Taken from D'Arboval. Dictionnaire de Médecine, de Chirurgie de Hygiene): *a a*, The abdominal muscles cut across: *o*, opening in the abdominal wall permitting the intestines *i i* to pass through and outward between the abdominal wall and the skin; *p p*, peritoneum, or membrane lining the abdominal cavity, carried through the opening *o* by the loop of intestine and forming the sac *s*, the outer walls of which are marked *b f b*.

PLATE IV. Microscopic anatomy of the liver. The liver is composed of innumerable, small lobules, from one-twentieth to one-tenth inch in diameter. The lobules are held together by a small quantity of fibrous tissue, in which the bile ducts and larger blood vessels are lodged.

Figure I illustrates the structure of a lobule: *V. v.*, interlobular veins or the veins between the lobules. These are branches of the portal vein, which carries blood from the stomach and intestines to the liver; *c c*, capillaries, or very fine blood vessels, extending as a very fine network between the groups of liver cells from the interlobular vein to the center of the lobule and emptying there into the intralobular vein to the center of the lobule; *v c*, intralobular vein, or the vein within the lobule. This vessel passes out of the lobule and there becomes the sublobular vein; *V. s.*, sublobular vein. This joins other similar veins and helps to form the hepatic vein, through which the blood leaves the liver; *d d*, the position of the liver cells between the meshes of the capillaries; *A A*, branches of the hepatic artery to the interlobular connective tissue and the walls of the large veins and large bile ducts. These branches are seen at *r r* and form the vena vascularis; *V. v.*, vena vascularis; *i i*, branches of the hepatic artery entering the substance of the lobule and connecting with capillaries from the interlobular vein. The use of the hepatic artery is to nourish the liver, whereas the other vessels carry blood to be modified by the liver cells in certain important directions; *g*, branches of the bile ducts, carrying bile from the various lobules into the gall bladder and into the intestines; *x x*, intralobular bile capillaries between the liver cells. These form a network of very minute tubes surrounding each ultimate cell, which receives the bile as it is formed by the liver cells and carried outward as described.

Figure II. Isolated liver cells: *C*, blood capillary; *a*, fine bile capillary channel.

PLATE V. Ergot in hay: 1, Bluegrass; 2, timothy; 3, wild rye; 4, redtop. Ergot is a fungus that may affect any member of the grass family. The spore of the fungus, by some means brought in contact with the undeveloped seed of the grass, grows, obliterates the seed, and practically takes its place. When hay affected with ergot is fed to animals it is productive of a characteristic and serious affection or poisoning known as ergotism.

PLATE VI. Ergotism, or the effects of ergot. The lower part of the leg of a cow, showing the loss of skin and flesh in a narrow ring around the pastern bone and the exposure of the bone itself.

Poisons and Poisoning

By V. T. Atkinson, V. S.

Revised by Ward T. Huffman, D. V. M.

To define clearly the word "poison" is somewhat difficult. A definition is likely to include either too much or too little. The common conception of a poison is any substance that, in small quantity, will destroy life, except such as act by purely mechanical means, as, for example, powdered glass. The following definition is given by Dorland in The American Illustrated Medical Dictionary: "Any substance applied to the body, ingested, inhaled, or developed within the body, which causes or may cause damage or disturbance of function."

Some substances, such as drugs or common salt, which produce beneficial results when introduced into the body in small quantities, may act as poisons when taken in larger quantities. Other substances, such as distilled water, milk, or glycerin, which are harmless when taken into the body in the usual way, are poisonous if injected into the circulation. Living organisms, such as disease-producing bacteria, are not considered as poisons in this section.

Poisoning of cattle may result from many causes although the following in about the order mentioned are the principal ones:

Poisonous plants on the ranges and in the pastures or feed.—Probably more animals are poisoned from this source than from all others combined. Plant poisoning may result from a shortage of more palatable feed, allowing hungry animals to graze in areas where poisonous plants exist, or carelessness in leaving poisonous plant material, such as roots of water hemlock or branches that have been trimmed from cherry, yew, or oleander, in accessible places.

Poisonous substances in places accessible to animals.—These include poisons used for the following purposes: Spraying trees and noxious weeds; killing insects or vermin, disinfecting pens and barns, dipping cattle and sheep, and painting. They also include carelessly discarded poisons used for other purposes and the deposits from smelter fumes.

Damaged feeds.—Many cases of poisoning are due to the use of feeds that have become moldy or spoiled. Poisoning of this class includes botulism, forage poisoning, and poisoning by sweetclover hay.

Errors in medication.—Some animals are poisoned or injured by the use, as remedies, of the wrong substances, by giving too large doses, by lack of skill in administering them, or by external application without proper dilution.

Stings or bites of poisonous insects or animals.—The fatal poisoning of cattle from these sources is probably rare, although occasionally an animal may die as the result of a snake bite.

Malicious poisoning.—Many cases of malicious poisoning of livestock are reported, but a thorough investigation nearly always reveals that carelessness in handling or disposing of poisonous substances is the cause, or that poisonous plants are responsible for the trouble.

Action of poisons.—The principal or most apparent action of several poisons is local, the tissues with which they first come in direct contact being affected. These substances, such as strong acids, alkalies, and several plant poisons, either cause a more or less serious destruction of cells and tissues by a corrosive action or irritation, or set up local inflammation that may eventually lead to tissue destruction. The other poisons produce their principal effects only after entering the circulation and being carried to the particular organ or organs on which they act, and often not then unless they have reached a certain minimum degree of concentration in the blood stream. They exert their effect on such organs of metabolism and excretion as the liver and kidneys, may act directly on the organs of circulation, as the heart and blood vessels or, as is true of many poisons, may exert their effect by acting on the various portions of the nervous system. Most poisons act on more than one group of organs, and many have both a direct, local, irritating effect and a secondary effect after being absorbed into the blood.

Several factors modify or influence the action of all poisons. The most important of these factors are the following: The quantity of poison present, consumed, or administered; the strength or concentration of the solution or mixture; the part of the body with which it comes in contact or its method of gaining access; the relative rates at which it is absorbed and eliminated; and to some extent the physical condition of the animal.

Some poisons, such as hydrocyanic acid and the poisonous alkaloids of larkspur, which produce fatal results if administered in small quantities within a short time, may be given in much larger quantities without harm, provided their administration is spread over a longer period. In the latter case, the excretion of the poison or its modification in the body is sufficiently rapid that it does not reach a dangerous or effective degree of concentration in the blood. On the other hand, some poisons or their effects accumulate in the animal's body so that even minute quantities administered or consumed at more or less frequent intervals and for prolonged periods produce harmful results eventually. This is true of lead. of the poisonous substances contained in the locoweeds, and of some of the groundsels. Although some substances act almost immediately after they have been consumed or have gained entrance to the body, a few set up series of changes in the body that do not become apparent until some days or even weeks after they have been administered or consumed.

Certain poisons, such as snake venom, which are very active if injected directly into the blood or beneath the skin, or if they come in contact with serous membranes, are relatively harmless if taken into the stomach, where they are modified by the action of the digestive fluids. Other substances may be very poisonous if injected into the blood but when taken into the alimentary tract are absorbed slowly and eliminated through the kidneys in a relatively short time and may not become sufficiently concentrated in the blood to produce harmful results.

Symptoms and lesions.—Naturally there is a relatively close correlation between the injurious effects or lesions produced on the organs and tissues by poisons and the symptoms manifested by the effected animal. Although no sharp line can be drawn between the symptoms and lesions produced by poisons and those accompanying disease, the more prominent or apparent effects are limited and to a considerable extent can be classified into groups. By basing conclusions on these characteristics and a knowledge of the effects of the different known poisons, it is often possible to determine, with a fair degree of certainty, the type of poison and sometimes the specific one that has caused a given case. Thus, if within a few minutes after the animals have been feeding on some plants and plant material, symptoms develop, including an increasingly rapid and later a labored respiration, muscular weakness, cyanosis, and spasms, they may usually be ascribed to cyanide or a cyanogenetic or hydrocyanic acid-producing plant, such as cherry leaves or one of the sorghums.

Nausea, salivation, and vomiting are likely to follow the ingestion of a substance having an irritating effect on the inner wall of the alimentary tract with secondary effects on other organs, particularly the central nervous system. Such substances and poisons as mustard oil, death camas, and the laurels are in this group. Severe depression, evidence of pain, labored irregular breathing, and a fast pulse are likely to accompany poisoning by substances that have a severely irritating or corrosive action on the stomach and intestines, or that produce severe injury to such internal organs as the liver and kidneys. Effects of this type are produced by strong acids, alkalies, phenols, common salt, and several plant poisons such as cocklebur, some of the milkweeds, and oak brush. The illness may be accompanied with severe constipation or equally pronounced scouring, or the scouring may follow the constipation. Trembling, weakness, and staggering, followed by collapse occur after the ingestion of such poisons as white snakeroot, rayless goldenrod, larkspur, and some of the lupines and, although liver lesions sometimes occur as in the case of white snakeroot, the effects are doubtless largely the result of the action of the poisons on the central nervous system. Severe spasms, usually accompanied with a very rapid pulse rate and frequently culminating in death, are characteristic of poisoning by such plants as the whorled milkweed and water hemlock.

For a correct diagnosis one must associate the symptoms and lesions with a knowledge of what the affected animals have consumed or may have had access to not only immediately before but for a considerable period preceding the time they became ill.

Treatment.—The proper and safe treatment of poisoned animals involves a knowledge of and correct interpretation of symptoms and of the conditions accompanying the poisoning, as well as a knowledge of the specific effects of the drugs used and considerable skill in administering them. In many cases of poisoning, either the cause is at the time obscure or the illness has progressed so far before being noticed that the administration of drugs is of little value. Also, when treatment is attempted by untrained individuals, they may either use the wrong drug or improper administration and, therefore, do more harm than good. Thus, if given as a drench, especially if the animal is very ill, the remedy instead of going into the stomach sometimes gets into the trachea and lungs and sets up a mechanical pneumonia that eventually causes death. In some cases of poisoning, especially when many animals are exposed, some or most may be saved by an entire change of feed, thus preventing their eating more of the poisonous substance. In some instances, especially if the poison has been consumed with the water or feed, liberal doses of a purgative such as castor oil, linseed oil, or Epsom salts may be of benefit in expelling the unabsorbed poison. With poisoning from plants forming hydrocyanic acid, beneficial results may be obtained by intravenous injections of solutions of sodium nitrite or sodium thiosulfate, or a combination of the two substances, provided not more than 3 grams per 500 pounds of animal weight of the former substance is used. Although potassium permanganate and tannic acid are frequently recommended for animals poisoned by plants, their use for poisoned cattle has not proved satisfactory. Such specific remedies or remedial measures as have been found beneficial will be mentioned in connection with the various poisons.

STOCK-POISONING PLANTS

There are many plants, native and introduced, in the United States that are poisonous and at times are eaten by cattle and other animals in sufficient quantities to produce injurious or fatal results. Losses from this source have been greatest in the western stock-raising States where conditions conducive to the eating of the less palatable plants sometimes develop. Although less common in the Middle and Eastern States, the losses caused by plant poisoning are probably greater than is commonly realized. The plants most likely to poison cattle in the United States are listed and their effects described briefly in the following pages. So far as possible, they are arranged in groups and according to the botanical relationships. Exceptions are made of those plants whose poisonous qualities are due to cyanide or hydrocyanic acid (also known as prussic acid). As a few plants owe their toxicity to the rare metal selenium, this subject is included with the poisonous plants.

No satisfactory methods of treatment are known for most plant poisons. The principal reliance should be placed on so managing the animals that they will not eat the harmful species.

BRACKEN (PTERIDIUM AQUILINUM)

Many cases of the poisoning of cattle by bracken, or bracken fern, have occurred in England and in continental Europe, and a considerable number have occurred in various places in the United States. There is some difference of opinion as to the way the fern acts but none as to the final result. The symptoms in cattle, which usually come on suddenly but after the animals have had access to fern for some days, are a very high temperature, bloody discharges from the mouth, nose, and rectum, collapse, and death. On post mortem examination, numerous hemorrhages are found throughout the body. No treatment is known that is effective after symptoms have developed.

Prevention of bracken poisoning is comparatively simple since the plant is not palatable and is seldom eaten by cattle when other forage is available.

YEW (TAXUS SP.)

The European yew (*Taxus baccata*) is one of the well-known poisonous plants of Europe. It has been introduced into the United States, where it appears to have caused a few cases of poisoning. The leaves and berries of *T. canadensis*, a form growing in North America, are looked upon with suspicion but are rarely eaten by grazing animals. The symptoms of yew poisoning, which are trembling, respiratory paralysis, staggering and collapse, come on very quickly and death may occur within 5 minutes. After death the liver, spleen, and lungs are engorged with blood.

CYANOGENETIC PLANTS

As several plants owe their poisonous character to the formation of cyanide or hydrocyanic acid, they are considered together. Of these, the principal plants that poison cattle are arrowgrass (*Triglochin maritima*), sorghum (*Sorghum vulgare*), Johnson grass (*S. halepense*), Sudan grass (*S. vulgare* var. *sudanense*), chokecherries (*Prunus melanocarpa*, or *P. demissa*, and *P. virginiana*), and flax (linseed) (*Linum usitatissimum*).

Hydrocyanic acid does not ordinarily exist as such in the plants but is formed by the interaction of two substances both of which under certain conditions are contained in the plants mentioned. This interaction may take place in the plant before it is consumed, as it is said to do in wilting and frosting, or in the stomachs of the animals after the plants have been eaten. As the presence of abundant moisture and a somewhat elevated temperature, such as are encountered in the animal's stomach, are both conducive to the rapid interaction of the two substances and the resultant formation of hydrocyanic acid, and as the action is further accelerated by the crushing of the plant in eating, the latter condition of poisoning is the more common. When absorbed into the blood in sufficient quantities, the cyanide soon causes an increase in the pulse rate and in both the rate and the depth of respiration. Respiration becomes faster and deeper and then labored, the animal staggers and soon falls, usually going over on its side. Soon respiratory paralysis, cyanosis, and spasms develop and the animal may die within a few minutes after it has eaten the plant that is responsible for the poisoning. If absorbed quickly, as little as 0.0002 percent of the animal's weight of hydrocyanic acid may be fatal for cattle. Cyanide acts principally on the central nervous system and visible lesions are not always apparent.

Although death may occur within a few minutes, the illness may progress much more slowly. In such cases it is possible to save many cattle by intravenous injections of 2 to 3 grams of sodium nitrite in solution, or 10 to 20 grains of sodium thiosulfate, or better yet, the two substances together. In cases of emergency, the common photographic "hypo," or hyposulfite of soda, which is a commercial form of sodium thiosulfate, may be used.

Arrowgrass grows normally in wet or swampy ground and is apparently only slightly toxic under such conditions. However, when this excess of water is not present, as is often the case under drought conditions, growth is retarded and this plant may become highly toxic. The green leaves are the most poisonous part of the plant and they remain toxic during the entire growing season. When cut and dried, arrowgrass may retain its poisonous properties for some weeks or months, although there is usually a gradual loss in toxicity.

The leaves of wild cherry are poisonous during the spring and summer but lose most of their toxicity at maturity or after light freezes. The plant is most poisonous during late spring and early summer and becomes less dangerous as the season advances. Poisoning may result from grazing on the green growing leaves or on branches cut from trees. To produce a toxic effect, a definite quantity of leaves must be eaten in a short time in order that the hydrocyanic acid content of the blood will reach a certain level. If eaten in smaller quantities over a longer period of time, no effect is produced. Cherry is seldom eaten in toxic quantities when other feed is available although it is potentially dangerous along trails or on overgrazed ranges.

CORNSTALK DISEASE

Considerable losses of cattle have occurred when they were turned on cornfields in the fall. Death is very sudden and there is no opportunity to apply remedies. It has been thought that these fatalities, like those from sorghum, were caused by hydrocyanic acid, but there is good reason to think that this is not true, and at the present time there is no accepted explanation of this disease, although there seems to be no doubt that it is connected in some way with the condition of the corn. Whether a given field is poisonous or not can be determined only by experiment, and the wise farmer will keep his cattle under close observation when they are first turned into a cornfield. Results of recent experiments indicate that the stalks lose their poisonous qualities after being cut or after prolonged standing in the field.

DEATH CAMAS (ZIGADENUS SP.)

Several species of death camas are poisonous and occasionally affect cattle. These are meadow death camas (*Zigadenus venenosus*) of the northwestern Pacific Coast States, grassy death camas (*Z. gramineus*) of Montana and Wyoming, foothill death camas (*Z. paniculatus*) of Utah and Nevada, and Nuttall death camas (*Z. nuttallii*) of Oklahoma and adjoining parts of Texas and Kansas. All parts of the plants are poisonous and if eaten in sufficient quantity will cause salivation, nausea, vomiting, prostration, and sometimes death.

STAGGER GRASS (AMIANTHIUM MUSCAETOXICUM)

Stagger grass, a plant known also as fly poison or crow poison, that grows in patches on sandy, damp soils and in open woods, causes considerable loss of cattle in the Southeastern States. The plant is related to death camas and produces similar symptoms.

OAKS (QUERCUS SP.)

Although the leaves, young shoots, and acorns of some species of oaks are valuable feeds, they sometimes cause the death of cattle.

In England, Germany, and to a less extent the United States, many cattle are reported to have died as a result of eating considerable quantities of acorns. However, this is probably due to overeating a highly concentrated feed rather than to any toxic substance contained in the acorns. Heavy losses have occurred in the United States among cattle feeding almost exclusively on the leaves and young, growing shoots of oaks. The most serious losses from this source have occurred in some of the Western and Southwestern States where, during the early spring months, the scrub oak (*Quercus gambelii*) and the "shinnery" oak (*Q. havardi*) form a large proportion of the available forage. Most of the cases develop after the cattle have been feeding on the oak leaves and shoots for 10 days or more. The symptoms of oak-brush poisoning are emaciation, edema, and severe constipation followed by equally severe diarrhea in which the feces contain mucus and blood. Microscopically, the kidneys contain numerous casts and many distended tubules. No remedy is known except a change in feed, which must be made before the animals become so ill that they will not eat.

BUCKWHEAT (FAGOPYRUM ESCULENTUM)

White cattle, or those with white areas, when fed on green flowering buckwheat, sometimes become so affected that their skin is peculiarly sensitive to sunlight. The grain, chaff, straw, and bran may cause the same symptoms although not so pronounced. The skin, especially about the head and ears, is inflamed and edematous or swollen. When the animals are severely affected, small vesicles may develop on the edematous areas of the skin. These may break and allow a clear exudate to cover and form crusts on the skin. The swollen, inflamed areas are irritating to the animals and cause them to shake and rub their heads. The affected animals also may be uneasy and show evidence of excitement. This or very similar effects, which are known as photosensitization, are sometimes caused by a few other plants, among which are alsike clover (*Trifolium hybridum*) and St. Johnswort (*Hypericum perforatum*). A disease of sheep, commonly called bighead or in some areas swellhead, has some of the same characteristics. The only known treatment is an entire change of feed and protection from sunlight.

LARKSPUR (DELPHINIUM SP.)

Throughout the Western States, especially in the mountainous areas, the larkspurs cause heavy losses to cattle owners. A few cases of poisoning occur in the Eastern States. The losses are largely confined to cattle, usually in the spring and early summer months. Although there appears to be some difference in the poisonous qualities of the different species of larkspur, it is safest to consider them all as dangerous for grazing cattle. They are most poisonous when the plants are young, that is, before flowers develop. Most cases of poisoning are due to the eating of the leaves and stemps. As the plants grow older they become progressively less toxic and are relatively harmless for cattle after they have formed seed. The seeds, which are very poisonous, are rarely eaten in sufficient quantity to cause trouble.

Symptoms.—When the animal is closely observed, the first symptoms noticed are a slight uneasiness and, when standing, a tendency to shift the weight of the body from one foot to another. Definite weakness soon develops and the poisoned animal may fall suddenly. Often the forelegs appear weaker than the hind ones. In mild cases the animal, after falling, may get to its feet in a few minutes and appear to be normal, or it may fall several times in succession. In more severely poisoned animals illness and weakness may persist for several hours. The animal may become nauseated and vomit. Dyspnea may develop, and if vomiting occurs while the animal is prostrate the vomited material may be drawn into the trachea and lungs and cause death. Death is caused by respiratory failure and the general collapse of the animal.

Treatment.—As exercise causes the illness to be more severe, poisoned animals should never be disturbed more than is absolutely necessary to prevent them from getting into dangerous positions and the vomited material from being drawn into the lungs. Hypodermic injections of physostigmine salicylate (1 grain), pilocarpine hydrochloride (2 grains), and strychnine sulfate (half grain), will save a large proportion of such cases.

SWEETSHRUB (CALYCANTHUS SP.)

Two species, the smooth sweetshrub (*Calycanthus fertilis*) of the southern Allegheny Mountains and California sweetshrub (*C. occidentalis*), of northern California, are said to poison cattle. The plants are rarely eaten and consequently not many animals are affected. The seeds are very poisonous and when eaten cause weakness followed by spasms.

SQUIRRELCORN (DICENTRA CANADENSIS) AND DUTCHMAN'S-BREECHES (D. CUCULLARIA)

Both the squirrelcorn and dutchman's-breeches at times poison cattle. The losses occur in the early spring when there is a shortage of other green plants. The symptoms are similar to those produced by the poisonous larkspur.

LOCO (ASTRAGALUS SP. AND OXYTROPIS LAMBERTII)

Probably no other group of plants in the United States has caused such heavy losses of cattle, horses, and sheep as plants known as loco. There are several species of these plants, all belonging to the genera *Astragalus* and *Oxytropis*. Several other species of *Astragalus* are poisonous but do not cause loco symptoms. The best known locoweeds are white loco (*Oxytropis lambertii*), a widely distributed plant in the Great Plains States; purple loco (*Astragalus mollissimus*), also of the Great Plains States but less widely distributed; blue loco (*A. diphysus*) of Arizona, Utah, and New Mexico; and a western Texas species, Big Bend loco (*A. earlei*). The two locoweeds in California, the gray loco (*A. menziesii*) and spotted loco (*A. lentiginosus*), also are said to poison cattle. These plants are poisonous at all stages of growth.

The loco plants contain cumulative poisons and illness develops after the animals have been feeding on them, either in a green or dry state, for many days, weeks, or, in some cases, months. Many cattle acquire a liking for locoweed and will eat these plants in preference to other types of forage.

Symptoms.—The effects, which are primarily on the central nervous system, vary considerably in different animals. Cattle poisoned by loco often show pronounced nervousness, trembling, nervous shaking of the head, an apparent lack of muscular control, and impaired vision. The coat becomes rough, the eyes staring, and the animals grow weak. They also become severely constipated, cease to eat, and gradually lose flesh until they eventually die of starvation. Pregnant cows that become locoed frequently abort.

Treatment.—Before the disease reaches the final stage, cattle usually will improve greatly and many of them will eventually recover if they are kept away from loco and given an abundance of some nutritious laxative feed, such as green alfalfa or cottonseed cake. Epsom salts is useless in relieving the constipation, and a general stimulant, such as daily hypodermic injections of one-eighth to one-fifth of a grain of strychnine sulfate, will hasten recovery. Cattle that have once developed the loco-eating habit should never be allowed access to the weed.

Several species of *Astragalus* that are poisonous to cattle do not produce typical symptoms of loco poisoning. These plants are the straight-stem poison vetch (*A. sabulosus*) in northern New Mexico and Arizona, the two-grooved loco (*A. bisulcatus*) of Wyoming, and the timber-poison vetch (*A. hylophilus*) of Wyoming and Utah. The symptoms by these plants are those of acute poisoning.

77431 O—51——5

SWEETCLOVER (MELILOTUS SP.)

Sweetclover hay that has been allowed to spoil, even though this spoilage is not pronounced, sometimes becomes poisonous for cattle.

Just why some lots of spoiled hay are poisonous and others are not, is not known. The poison apparently is cumulative, as illness rarely occurs until the cattle have been feeding on the spoiled hay for 10 days or longer. The poison causes changes in the blood resulting in its failure to clot normally. If they are dehorned or castrated, or if in other ways blood vessels are cut or ruptured, affected animals bleed to death. In severely affected cattle the blood leaks through the walls of the blood vessels and accumulates in various places in the tissues. Treatment consists in entirely changing the feed and giving intravenous injections of defibrinated blood from normal cattle. In the hands of a competent veterinarian, the latter procedure is often highly successful.

LUPINES (LUPINUS SPP.)

Although lupines have for years been considered as poisonous only for sheep, it is now known that at least two species are poisonous for cattle. These are *Lupinus caudatus*, a species growing in parts of Utah, Nevada, and California, and *L. laxiflorus* var. *silvicola*, of northern California. Both have been associated with the losses of cattle on the ranges and have been shown by experimental feeding to be poisonous for these animals. Although most cases of poisoning are thought to have occurred when fruit was present, the plants are poisonous at all stages of growth. The symptoms produced in cattle by these two species are very similar to, and difficult to distinguish from, those produced by species of larkspur. Cattle rarely eat lupines in harmful quantities when they can readily obtain other and more palatable feed.

HORSE CHESTNUT; BUCKEYE (AESCULUS SPP.)

The bark, leaves, and fruit of all species of *Aesculus*, the group of plants to which the horse chestnut and buckeye belong, are poisonous at least during certain seasons of the year. The plants are said to cause incoordination of movements, staggering, muscular twitching, paralysis, and death. They are also said to cause abortion.

WATERHEMLOCK (CICUTA SP.)

Waterhemlock, which grows in damp or wet places throughout most of the United States, is the most poisonous plant in North America and is often eaten by cattle. As the roots and root stocks, and perhaps the very young shoots, contain much larger quantities of the poisonous substances than the tops, most cases of poisoning are due to the eating of these portions of the plant. In feeding on closely grazed areas, along ditches, and in wet places, or where the roots and root stocks of waterhemlock have been uncovered, cattle sometimes get portions of them and are fatally poisoned. The most marked symptoms of waterhemlock poisoning are the violent spasms that sometimes appear within 2 hours after the plant has been eaten. They are intermittent and in fatal cases increase in violence.

HEATHS (ERICACEAE)

Several species of the heath family, some of which are called laurels, are poisonous. Although sheep are more commonly affected, cattle also are said to be poisoned. The principal plants of this group by which animals are poisoned in the United States are mountain-laurel (*Kalmia latifolia*), sheep laurel (*K. angustifolia*), and drooping leucothoe (*Leucothoe catesbaei*) in the Eastern States; and western azalea (*Rhododendron occidentale*), blacklaurel (*Leucothoe davisiae*), and coast rhododendron (*Rhododendron californicum*) in the Pacific Coast States. The symptoms caused by all these plants are the same and consist of nausea, salivation, more or less profuse vomiting, weakness, and in some cases prostration and death. Often breathing becomes labored. In some cases linseed oil and whole milk have been given to poisoned animals with beneficial results.

MILKWEED (ASCLEPIAS SP.)

Several species of milkweeds native to the United States are poisonous to cattle. The most poisonous of these is *Asclepias labriformis*, but, owing to its limited distribution (a portion of southeastern Utah), the loss caused by it is not so great as by some of the others. Two of the narrow-leaved or whorled milkweeds at times poison cattle. These are the horsetail milkweed (*Asclepias galioides*) found in Colorado, Utah, New Mexico, and Arizona, and the Mexican milkweed (*A. mexicana*) found in the Pacific Coast States. The horsetail milkweed is more toxic and poisons more animals than the Mexican milkweed. Both sometimes grow in hay fields and as the dry leaves are more palatable, although somewhat less toxic than when green, serious losses may occur from using hay containing these plants. The most noticeable symptoms caused by milkweeds are staggering, followed by violent spasms. Animals in which spasms develop usually die. No effective treatment is known.

YERBA DE PASMA (BACCHARIS PTERONIOIDES)

This plant, a low shrub found in western Texas and the southern parts of New Mexico and Arizona, is poisonous to cattle. Although not ordinarily palatable, it sometimes poisons cattle on overgrazed ranges, especially in the late fall and early winter after the other plants have largely been grazed off. Poisoned animals are much depressed.

WHITE SNAKEROOT (EUPATORIUM RUGOSUM) AND RAYLESS GOLDENROD (APLOPAPPUS HETEROPHYLLUS)

Although very different in appearance and found in widely separated parts of the United States, white snakeroot, and rayless goldenrod contain the same poisonous substances and, therefore, have the same effect on cattle. White snakeroot grows principally in Illinois, Indiana, Ohio, Kentucky, Tennessee, and North Carolina. Rayless goldenrod is found in parts of western Texas, New Mexico, and Arizona. In the eastern area the illness in cattle due to their having eaten white snakeroot is known as trembles or slows. In the western region the similar illness, but caused by the rayless goldenrod, is spoken of as alkali disease and sometimes as milk sickness and trembles. The symptoms are constipation, weakness, muscular trembling, and in severely poisoned animals, coma and death. Cows during lactation excrete the poisonous substance of these plants with their milk, and the milk and milk products from such cows are rendered poisonous for human consumption, especially if not diluted by being mixed with the milk from other cows. Human beings poisoned from this source are said to have milk sickness. Cattle, especially milk cows, should not be pastured where either of these plants is growing.

GROUNDSEL (SENECIO SP.)

Several species of groundsels or ragworts are poisonous and some of them have been known to affect cattle. The ones that are more evidently associated with cattle poisoning in the United States are *Senecio longilobus* and *S. riddellii*, both of which grow in areas in the western half of the United States. The poison is cumulative and the effects do not appear until the animals have been feeding on the plants for some time. The symptoms of poisoning are loss of appetite or a depraved appetite, emaciation, uneasiness, jaundice, and sometimes discolored areas on the skin and on the visible mucous membranes. The affected areas are irritating to the animals. The poison affects the liver and produces cirrhosis.

TARWEED (AMSINCKIA INTERMEDIA)

Amsinckia intermedia, known locally as tarweed, grows abundantly in the dry-land wheat areas and along roadsides in eastern Washington and northern Idaho and is found to some extent in other sections of the Northwest. Poisoning occurs when the seeds of this plant become mixed with wheat screenings or chaff and these products are fed to livestock. When screenings constitute a portion of the rations in feed lots, cattle become affected after a feeding period of 30 to 60 days. This plant affects the animal in much the same way as groundsel, causing liver destruction and fibrosis.

COPPERWEED (OXYTENIA ACEROSA)

This plant grows in alkaline areas in many sections of the Colorado River drainage and, under adverse feed conditions, has caused considerable loss of cattle. The leaves are toxic so that a hungry animal can eat a lethal quantity in a very short time. The symptoms, which usually consist of depression, weakness, incoordination, and coma, may appear within a few hours and death often occurs in less than a day after the plant is eaten. The primary action of the toxic substance appears to be on the liver.

When ample feed is available there is little danger of cattle eating copperweed in sufficient quantities to be dangerous.

COCKLEBUR (XANTHIUM SP.)

Cockleburs are widely distributed in the United States and sometimes poison cattle. All poisoning is caused by the young plants when they first come up or are in the cotyledon stage. The symptoms of cocklebur poisoning are depression, extreme weakness, labored respiration, and gasping. These are associated with a severe irritation of the wall of the fourth stomach and a very much congested and degenerated liver.

PLANTS GROWN ON SOIL CONTAINING SELENIUM

In the cretaceous soils of a number of restricted areas, selenium occurs in sufficient quantities to be taken up by certain plants in toxic quantities, and poisoning occurs when cattle feed on vegetation that has been grown on soils containing this element. In certain localities this type of poisoning is commonly known as alkali disease. Forage plants or other nontoxic vegetation may become seleniferous, and a few plants that are poisonous in other locations may have their toxicity increased and their effects complicated by the presence of selenium in the soil. When this element occurs in cultivated land, the crops grown on these areas are likely to be injurious to livestock. Symptoms consist of irregular and deformed hoofs, lameness, loss of hair especially of the tail, unthriftiness, and emaciation that may result in death. Prevention consists in removing the cause and supplying feed free from selenium.

FUNGI

Although much has been written about the poisoning of animals by fungi and fungus-infected feeds, there is little definite information about the poisonous properties of most of them. It is known that ergot (*Claviceps purpurea*) at one time caused serious outbreaks of poisoning. Within recent years the poisoning of cattle in the United States from this source has been comparatively rare. Ergot may grow on a considerable number of grasses and grains but most commonly occurs on rye. The fungus growth is on the seeds where it appears as black, elongated bodies attached to and larger than the natural seed.

Prolonged feeding on ergot causes a degeneration and obstruction of the smaller arteries, which shut off the circulation of distal portions of the body, as the ears, tail, and feet. Such areas then undergo degenerative changes and dry gangrene may set in, or the part may mummify. Ergot may also cause a serious irritation of the digestive system and also act on the nervous system, causing lethargy and paralysis.

Various feeds, such as straw, hay, grain, and silage, when improperly cured, or that have undergone spoilage as a result of exposure to moisture or other causes, may be unsafe for animal consumption. Although this is apparently due to the growth of molds or other fungi or saprophytic bacteria in them, the exact effect of the growth of the various organisms in animal feeds or other food products is unknown.

POISONING BY CHEMICALS

ARSENIC

The preparations of arsenic likely to be accessible to cattle are arsenious oxide, also called white arsenic and arsenious acid; paris green, an arsenite of copper used as an insecticide; arsenical weed killers; lead arsenate and calcium arsenate much used in spraying; arsenical dips; and rat poisons containing arsenic. A concentrated form of Fowler's solution used in veterinary medicine has occasionally caused arsenic poisoning. Lead arsenate may cause arsenical poisoning, but more commonly the serious effects are due to the lead that it contains. The use of arsenical pastes to remove tumors, warts, proud flesh, or scar tissue has resulted in acute arsenic poisoning.

The toxicity of an arsenical preparation depends to a large extent on its form and readiness of absorption. In cases in which the arsenic is in solution, absorption takes place readily and smaller doses are effective. Comparatively insoluble forms of arsenic are slower in their action but are still very toxic. The toxic doses of arsenious oxide for cattle are 15 to 30 grams (225 to 450 grains) by mouth or, when introduced through wounds, 2 to 4 grams (30 to 60 grains).

Symptoms.—Two types of arsenic poisoning are the acute and chronic. In acute cases the symptoms are those of severe colic.

There is salivation, thirst, vomiting, great uneasiness, feeble and irregular pulse and respiration. The animal stamps, lies down, and gets up. The odor of garlic may be detected on the breath. There is diarrhea with a garlic odor and the feces are sometimes bloody. The animal becomes exhausted, collapses, and death follows in a few hours or the animal sometimes survives for several days. Coldness of the ears and horns may be noticed, and sometimes there are subnormal temperature, trembling, stupor, and convulsions.

Chronic poisoning caused by small doses taken over a long period is characterized by a dullness, lack of appetite, wasting, eventual paralysis, a chronic cough, continual diarrhea, and death. There may be a chronic eczematous condition of the skin and abortion or sterility.

Treatment.—The antidote for arsenic is freshly prepared ferric hydroxide suspended in water. This may be made by adding any alkali to any ferric salt and is most advantageously prepared by mixing a solution of ferric chloride or of ferric sulfate with an excess of milk of magnesia, or powdered magnesia suspended in water. The thick magma produced should be introduced into the stomach and repeated doses given. Meanwhile the strength of the animal should be supported by stimulants and mucilaginous drinks or oils to soothe the injured mucous membranes of the digestive tract.

LEAD

Lead poisoning in cattle results from the licking of freshly painted surfaces or of old paint that has begun to flake off; from discarded paint cans and paint brushes; from fodder that has been stored in bins or silos that have been painted on the inside; from water that has been conducted through lead pipes or stored in lead-lined tanks; from lead arsenate sprays; and infrequently from eating lead bullets (shot) scattered by hunters, from litharge, or from sugar of lead. Cattle are much more susceptible to lead poisoning than are other classes of livestock, and although the toxic and lethal doses have not been well established, it is estimated that from 1.5 to 3 ounces of sugar of lead will cause death.

Symptoms.—Acute and chronic cases of lead poisoning are observed. In the acute cases the symptoms are colic, salivation, severe abdominal pain, constipation, blindness, fetid breath, ropy urine, tremors, coma, and death, sometimes in convulsions. The period of illness is variable. Symptoms come on slowly and the animal may be sick a week or more before dying.

In chronic cases produced by small quantities of lead that accumulate in the system, there are weakness, digestive derangement, constipation alternating with diarrhea, a tucked up abdomen, staring and dull eyes, and gradual wasting and prostration. Paralysis sets in followed by convulsions, coma, and death. A blue line may appear on the margins of the gums, but this is not always present.

Treatment.—In acute cases sulfates such as Epsom salts or Glauber's salt, which form insoluble lead sulfate, should be given with linseed or castor oils to purge, and mucilaginous drinks or feeds to soothe the mucous lining of the stomach and intestines. Potassium iodide is recommended in chronic cases.

COPPER

Salts of copper in large doses are very irritant to the stomach and intestines, and several instances of fatal poisoning of cattle by copper salts have been reported. The commonest copper compound is the sulfate, also known as blue vitriol, or bluestone. This substance is used in a variety of ways and also enters into the composition of bordeaux mixture. Plant material that has been sprayed with copper compounds should never be left where cattle can obtain access to it. The symptoms of copper poisoning include those of intestinal irritation such as short breathing, choking, colic, loss of appetite, purging, blue-tinged feces, rapid pulse, elevated temperature, weakness, muscular spasms, coma, convulsions, and paralysis with death from exhaustion. Copper poisoning should be treated with powdered iron followed by magnesia and mucilaginous drinks.

ZINC

Soluble zinc salts are irritant poisons and act much the same as copper salts. Zinc dissolved from the linings of galvanized iron buckets by acid liquids has been suspected of causing poisoning. The symptoms and treatments are similar to those for copper poisoning.

PHOSPHORUS

Yellow phosphorus was at one time used extensively for rat poisons and in the manufacture of matches. The latter use has now almost entirely ceased, and phosphorus as a rat poison has been superseded by more effective yet less dangerous substances. The symptoms of phosphorus poisoning are loss of appetite, colic, diarrhea, weakness, difficult breathing, rapid pulse, fever, irritation of the mouth and throat, paralysis of the throat, delirium, stupor, convulsions, and death often after several days. The feces and urine may be luminous in the dark. A jaundiced condition may be noticed especially in cases of long standing. Treatment is directed toward oxidizing the phosphorus to harmless phosphates and to overcoming the systemic effects of the poison. Old oil of turpentine is the favored antidote. Potassium permanganate may be given also. Stimulants should be administered as needed. As fatty substances such as oils, milk, melted lard, or bacon grease dissolve the phosphorus and promote its absorption, they should never be given to an animal suffering from phosphorus poisoning.

POTASSIUM BICHROMATE

This substance, known also as bichromate of potash, is sometimes used in making battery fluid and for tanning hides. It is a violent poison producing a corrosive gastroenteritis and nephritis. The symptoms are weakness, loss of appetite, stiffness, rapid and irregular pulse, lowered temperature, slow respiration, intense thirst, and abdominal pain, followed by coma, convulsions, and death in a few hours. The urine may contain albumin and blood. Treatment is symptomatic. Drenching with large quantities of magnesia or lime water should be of assistance by converting the chromate into an insoluble form.

SALTPETER

Both potassium nitrate (saltpeter) and sodium nitrate (Chile saltpeter) are poisonous to cattle. These substances are used for preserving meats and as fertilizers. They may be administered in a drench by error in place of Glauber's salt, or they may be left within reach of cattle and thus be eaten. Sodium nitrate is often stored for use as fertilizer and, being rather palatable, has frequently caused losses when cattle have had access to it. The toxic dose varies considerably but if given in solution on an empty stomach, as little as 3 ounces of saltpeter (potassium nitrate) may be fatal to a cow. More of the Chile saltpeter (sodium nitrate) is required to cause serious trouble. Symptoms are severe gastroenteritis, colic, tympanites, diarrhea, excessive urination, weakness, trembling, convulsions, collapse. Treatment is the same as for poisoning by common salt.

SODIUM CHLORATE

Sodium chlorate has been introduced as a very effective weed killer. Although it is not highly dangerous in small doses, its salty taste is attractive to cattle and may induce them to eat the substance or vegetation that has been sprayed with it, even plants that ordinarily are not palatable, especially if the cattle are hungry for salt. In the blood stream it produces a methemoglobinemia and interferes with the oxygenation of the blood so that, in severe cases, the animal suffocates. Symptoms are rapid breathing, increased temperature, prostration, and death. The veins of the eyeball may be chocolate brown in color. After death the blood and muscle tissues are chocolate color and do not become red on exposure to the air. Treatment is of little avail.

SODIUM CHLORIDE (COMMON SALT)

Three to five pounds of common salt will produce well-marked signs of poisoning in cattle. This quantity of salt will not be taken by cattle except under unusual conditions. If the feed is poor in salt or if none has been given for a long time, there is an intense hunger for it that may lead an animal to eat a sufficient quantity to be poisoned. Herring and mackerel brine and pork pickle are also poisonous to cattle and are especially dangerous for hogs. Sometimes saltpeter is present in such brines. Symptoms of salt poisoning are great thirst, abdominal pain, diarrhea, poor appetite, redness and dryness of the mouth, increased urination, paralysis of the hind legs, weak pulse, general paralysis, coma, and death in 6 to 8 hours. In treating a poisoned animal, allow as much warm water as the animal will drink. Give protectives, such as linseed tea. Linseed or olive oil may be given. To keep up the heart action give stimulants.

MERCURY

Cattle are very susceptible to mercury poisoning, and antiseptics containing this metal, such as mercuric chloride or corrosive sublimate, should be used on cattle with caution. Calomel should be used sparingly with cattle. Mercury compounds cause intense inflammation of all tissues with which they come in contact. The first effect is corrosion of the stomach lining and inflammation of the intestines. The animal is nauseated, is in great pain, and there is watery and bloody diarrhea. Collapse follows with weak pulse, irregular respiration, lowered temperature, and death by shock. If the case is more prolonged, salivation may be observed and the animal finally dies from exhaustion. White of egg beaten in water and given sparingly is the accepted antidote. If poisoning has occurred by absorption through the skin or from a mercurial ointment applied to a wound, the area should be thoroughly cleansed of the ointment or lotion. Supportive treatment should be given to meet the symptoms as they arise.

FLUORINE

Fluorine poisoning may result from several causes, but probably the most common are insecticides and rock phosphates. Acute poisoning may result from the accidental ingestion of fluorine in the form of insecticides on account of the more concentrated form in which it occurs. Chronic poison may occur following the use of rock phosphates as a source of phosphorus in the rations of dairy cows. Experimental work has shown that some rock phosphate contains sufficient fluorine to affect the teeth and bones and interfere with normal growth, nutrition, and reproduction.

MINERAL ACIDS

The mineral acids, including nitric, sulfuric, and hydrochloric, when used in a concentrated form destroy the animal tissues with which they come in contact and in this respect differ from most of the poisons previously described. When they are taken into the stomach the mucous membrane of the mouth, pharynx, esophagus, and stomach is likely to be destroyed. If such acids are taken in large quantities, death is likely to result so speedily that nothing can be done to relieve the patient. Even if the action of the acid can be arrested, it cannot be done until considerable and, perhaps, irreparable damage has been done. In a less concentrated form acids exert an irritant effect. In this form they may not do much harm unless taken in considerable quantity. Any of the alkalies may be used as an antidote. Most convenient of these are chalk, baking soda, marble dust, magnesia, lime, soap, or plaster from a wall. Mucilaginous drinks should be given in large quantities.

VEGETABLE ACIDS

Oxalic acid in particular is corrosive in its action when taken in concentrated solution, and irritant when more dilute. It also exerts a specific effect on the heart, frequently causing death from syncope. Taken in the form either of the crystals or solution, it is likely to cause death in a short time. Failure of heart action and the attendant weak pulse, body weakness, staggering, and convulsions are the more noticeable symptoms. Strong acetic acid is irritant to the gastrointestinal tract and may cause sudden paralysis of the heart. The action of the acid should be counteracted by the use of alkalies, as advised for mineral acids, by limewater or lime or plaster given promptly, by protectives to the digestive tract, and by stimulants.

CARBOLIC ACID

Phenol (carbolic acid), creosote, coal-tar dips, and cresol disinfectants in poisonous doses produce similar effects. When they are taken internally or used externally in concentrated form over a large surface of the body, poisoning may result.

Symptoms.—These poisons cause whitening, shrinking, and numbness of the structures with which they come in contact, and, besides their irritant effect, exert a strong influence on the nervous system. Being readily absorbed, they produce effects whether swallowed, injected into the rectum, inhaled, or applied to wounds, or even to a large tract of unbroken skin. Used extensively as a dressing, these disinfectants may produce nausea, dizziness, and smoky or blackish-colored urine. The last symptom is nearly always noticeable where the poisonous effect is produced. In more concentrated form or in larger quantities, convulsions, followed by fatal coma, are likely to take place. Even in smaller quantities, dullness, trembling, and disinclination for feed often continue for several days. Any of these products in concentrated solution coagulates albumin and acts as an astringent.

Treatment.—As an antidote internally, a solution of sodium sulfate or magnesium sulfate (Glauber's salt or Epsom salts) may be given. The white of egg is also useful. Stimulants may be given if needed. When the poisoning occurs through too extensive applications to wounds or the skin, as in treatment of mange, cold water should be applied freely to wash off any of the acid that may still remain unabsorbed. As a surgical dressing a 3-percent solution is strong enough for ordinary purposes. Water will not hold more than 5 percent in permanent solution. No preparation stronger than the saturated solution should be used medicinally under any circumstances.

ALKALIES

The carbonates of potash and soda and the alkalies themselves in concentrated form cause symptoms of intestinal irritation similar to those produced by mineral acids. Animals are most frequently exposed to ammonia, caustic soda, caustic potash (lye), washing soda, and lime. The extent of their caustic, irritant effects depends on their degree of concentration. When they reach the stomach the symptoms are nearly as well marked as in the case of the acids. The irritation is even more noticeable, and purgation is likely to be a more prominent symptom. If death does not follow, irritation of the gastrointestinal tract and malnutrition will continue for a long time. Treatment consists in neutralizing the alkali by an acid, such as dilute sulfuric acid (1 percent) or strong vinegar. The effect of such an antidote must be carefully watched during administration. When bloating occurs it may be relieved by opening the flank, permitting the gas to escape. (See Acute Tympanites, or Bloating, p. 15). Flaxseed or slippery elm decoction and oils must be given to soothe the inflamed mucous surface.

LOIN DISEASE

A condition known as loin disease causes the loss of a considerable number of cattle, particularly those more than 18 months of age, in certain range areas of the country. Although this disease is not due to any toxic substance contained in the plants, inferior grass and other forage growing on low, poorly drained, more or less flat lands appear to be conducive to the trouble. Such forage is likely to contain less mineral matter than is necessary for health, and animals may develop bone diseases on such feed. Although mature animals possess the power to draw on the mineral matter that has been deposited in the skeleton, the need for a balance in the body induces a craving for mineral salts, particularly those containing phosphorus. To satisfy this craving range animals instinctively resort to the licking and chewing of bones. Many ranges, in addition to being overgrazed, are allowed to accumulate carcasses of dead animals. Wild animals consume some of these carcasses, and the remaining parts become infested with blowflies and myriads of germs thrive in the tissues. Some such bacteria form poisonous substances or toxins as a result of their growth.

Bone chewing by cattle is prevalent in many grazing areas of the West, and when the bones are clean and free from putrefaction no particular harm results except occasionally from choke, but when fragments of decomposing flesh are still attached to the bones a severe toxemia may result. This latter condition appears to be responsible for loin disease.

Symptoms.—In the early stages of loin disease, animals lag behind the herd during drives or when trailing to water. They graze poorly, lie down much of the time, and have some difficulty in getting on their feet. Later, often within a few hours, the animals cannot rise, they lie on the brisket, appear to be bright, and usually accept feed and water put before them. Soon, however, the feces become coated with mucus and are sometimes bloody, the sick animal slumps to its side, and a gradually developing paralysis is plainly evident. Before reaching this stage, some animals only slightly poisoned will slowly improve and eventually recover if carefully nursed. After marked paralysis and failure of the appetite develop, however, recovery occurs in only a few cases.

Prevention.—Since loin disease is caused basically by deficiencies in the soil and vegetation, efforts should be made to improve these by such treatment as is advised by soil experts. Pending the remedy of this situation, 1 or 2 parts of steamed bonemeal may be added to each 2 parts of salt fed to the cattle. A lesser proportion of bonemeal may be advisable if the animals are inclined not to eat the mixture, and grain supplements such as wheat bran or cottonseed cake may be fed. Dead animals should always be disposed of promptly by deep burial or burning on the spot. This practice will eliminate the bones and other tissues that are a potential source not only of loin disease but of dangerous infectious diseases as well.

VEGETABLE POISONS USED AS MEDICINE

Many drugs and preparations used in medicines are derived from plants, and most of these are poisonous when given in excessive quantities. Many of the more familiar preparations are used as remedies for cattle and, when their use is advisable and they are properly administered, are often highly beneficial. However, if an overdose is given or the wrong medicine is used, additional injury or death may result. Each drug or preparaton has a more or less specific action and the indications for their uses are determined by the symptoms or conditions to be treated. In many cases it is safer to postpone treatment until a qualified veterinarian can be called. Of the many vegetable poisons used as medicine, only two, strychnine and aconite are discussed here.

STRYCHNINE (NUX VOMICA)

Strychnine, the active poison of nux vomica, is a very concentrated poison and produces its effect quickly, usually only a few minutes being necessary if given in sufficient dose and in such a way that it will be absorbed at once. When strychnine is used as a medicine, minimum doses, as a rule, should be given as cattle are susceptible to its effects and may be killed by the maximum doses prescribed for some other species in the common manuals of veterinary medicine.

In addition to its use in medicine, strychnine is used extensively as a poison for rodents and predatory animals. In preparing rodent poison the strychnine is frequently added to grain, and if carelessly disposed of or left within reach of cattle, lethal quantities may easily be eaten. Many cases of poisoning from this cause have been reported.

Symptoms.—The first noticeable symptom is evidence of unrest or mental excitement. At the same time the muscles over the shoulder and croup may be seen to quiver or twitch, and later a more or less well-marked convulsion occurs. The head is jerked back, the back arched, the legs extended, and the eyes drawn backward. The spasm continues only a few minutes, when it relaxes and another occurs in a short time. The return is hastened by excitement and continues to reappear and disappear until death results. As the poisonous effect advances, the intervals between the spasms become shorter and less marked and the spasms more severe until the animal dies in violent struggles.

Treatment.—The best method is to put the patient under the influence of chloroform, ether, chloral, or one of the barbitals and keep it there continuously until the effect of the poison has passed off.

ACONITE

Aconite is one of the most deadly poisons known. It produces paralysis of motion and sensation, depresses the heart's action, and causes death by paralysis of respiration. In large doses it causes profuse salivation, champing of the jaws, and attempts at swallowing. If the dose is not sufficient to cause death, the result is impaired appetite with more or less nausea for some time after. In poisonous doses it causes the animal to tremble violently, to lose power to support itself, and brings on slight convulsions, with perspiration. The pulse is depressed, irregular, and afterwards intermittent. The chemical antidote is tannic acid, which forms an insoluble compound with the aconitine. The depressing effect on the heart should be counteracted by the use of appropriate heart stimulants.

COAL-OIL POISONING

Coal oil is sometimes administered as a treatment for intestinal parasites. If given in large doses it produces poisonous effects, which are likely to be manifested sometime after the administration. It acts as an irritant to the digestive tract, causing driveling of ropy saliva from the mouth, diarrhea, straining, and loss of appetite, with increased temperature and cold extremities. Visible mucous membranes are congested, pupils of the eyes are contracted, and there is a watery discharge from the eyes and nostrils. Remotely it exerts a depressing influence on the functions of the brain and slight coma, and occasionally convulsions, from which the animal is easily aroused. The kidneys are also affected and the urine is dark colored and has the characteristic odor of coal oil. Death may result from gastroenteritis or convulsions. The patient's strength should be supported by frequent administration of mild stimulants, of which aromatic spirits of ammonia is perhaps the best. Soft feed and mucilaginous drinks should be given.

Crude coal oil is sometimes applied to the skin to kill parasites. If too much is used, especially in hot weather, great weakness and depression may be caused and in some cases death may result.

Diseases of the Heart, Blood Vessels, and Lymphatics

By W. H. Harbaugh, V. S.

[Revised by L. T. Giltner, D. V. M., M. S.]

THE CIRCULATORY SYSTEM

In cattle, as in human beings, the heart, blood vessels, and lymphatics constitute the circulatory apparatus.

The heart is in the thoracic cavity (chest). It is conical in form, with the base or large part uppermost, and the apex, or point, rests just above the sternum (breastbone). It is situated between the right and left lungs, the apex inclining to the left, and owing to this fact the heart beats are best felt on the left side of the chest, behind the elbow. The heart may be considered as a hollow muscle containing four compartments, two on each side. The upper compartments are called auricles and the lower ones ventricles. The right auricle and ventricle are completely separated from the left auricle and ventricle by a thick septum or wall, so that there is no communication between the right and left sides of the organ.

At the bottom of each auricle is the auriculoventricular opening, each provided with a valve to close it when the heart contracts to force the blood into the arteries. In the interval between the contractions these valves hang down into the ventricles.

The muscular tissue of the heart belongs to that class known as involuntary, because its action is not controlled by the will.

The cavities of the heart are lined by a serous membrane, called the endocardium, which may be considered as a continuation of the veins and the arteries, forming their internal lining. The walls of the ventricles are thicker than those of the auricles, and the walls of the left ventricle are much thicker than those of the right.

The heart is enveloped by a fibrous sac (or bag), called the pericardium, which assumes much of the general shape of the outer surface of the heart.

The action of the heart is similar to that of a pump and its function is to keep the blood in circulation. The auricles may be considered as the reservoirs or receivers of the blood and the ventricles as the pump chambers. During the interval between contractions, the heart being in momentary repose, the blood pours into the auricles from the veins; the auriculoventricular orifices being wide open, the ventricles also receive blood. The auricles contract and the ventricles are filled; contraction of the ventricles follows; the auriculoventricular valves are forced up by the pressure of the blood and close the auriculoventricular opening and prevent the return of blood into the auricles; the contraction of the ventricles forces the blood from the right ventricle into the lungs through the pulmonary artery and its branches, and from the left ventricle into the aorta, thence through the arteries to all parts of the body. After the contraction of the ventricles the heart is again in momentary repose and is being filled with blood, while the valves in the aorta and pulmonary artery close to prevent the return of blood into the ventricles (pl. VII).

The weight of the heart of a mature bovine animal is said to be 3½ to 5 pounds, but owing to the many breeds and sizes of cattle it varies in different animals.

The vessels that convey the blood from the heart to all parts of the body are called arteries; those that return the blood to the heart are called veins. The arteries divide and subdivide (like the branches of a tree), become smaller and smaller, and ultimately ramify into every part of the body. Between the ultimate ramifications of the arteries and the beginning of the veins there is an intermediate system of very minute vessels called capillaries, which connect the arterial with the venous system of the circulation. The walls of the arteries possess a certain amount of rigidity, sufficient to keep the tubes open when they are empty.

The blood leaves the left ventricle through a single vessel, the common aorta, consisting of the anterior and posterior aortas, which give off the large arteries.

The veins take the blood from the capillaries in all parts of the body. They begin in very small tubes, which unite to become larger in size and fewer in number as they approach the heart.

In its course an artery is usually accompanied with a vein and in many situations with a nerve. The more important arteries are placed deep within the body. When they are superficial, however, they are generally found where least exposed to injury, as, for example, on the inner side of the legs. Arteries are less numerous than veins, and their total capacity is much less than that of the veins. A great number of veins are in the tissue immediately beneath the skin and do not generally accompany arteries.

77431 O—51——6

The blood, throughout its course in the heart, arteries, capillaries, and veins, is enclosed within these vessels. Except where the large lymphatics empty into the venous blood, there is no opening into the course of the blood.

All the arteries except the pulmonary and its branches carry bright-red blood, and all the veins, except the pulmonary veins, carry dark-red blood. The impure dark-red blood is collected from the capillary vessels and carried to the right auricle by the veins. It passes down into the right ventricle, and thence into the pulmonary artery and through its branches to the capillaries of the lungs, where carbonic acid gas and other impurities are given up to the air in the air cells of the lungs (through the thin walls between the capillaries and the air cells), and where it absorbs from the air oxygen necessary to sustain life. The oxygen changes it to the bright-red, pure blood. It passes from the capillaries to the branches of the pulmonary veins, which convey it to the left auricle of the heart. It then passes through the auriculoventricular opening into the left ventricle, the contraction of which forces it through the common aorta into the posterior and anterior aortas, and through all the arteries of the body into the capillaries, where it parts with its oxygen and nutritive elements and where it absorbs carbonic acid gas and becomes dark colored. (See theoretical diagram of the circulation, pl. VII.)

The branches of certain arteries in different parts unite again after subdividing. This reuniting is called anastomosing and assures a quota of blood to a part if one of the anastomosing arteries should be tied in case of hemorrhage or should be destroyed by accident or operation.

THE BLOOD

The various kinds of food, after being digested in the alimentary canal, are absorbed and carried into the blood by the lymphatics, and by the blood to the places where nutrition is required. The blood takes from all parts of the body all that is no longer required, and carries it to the different organs through which it is eliminated from the body. It contains within itself all the elements that nourish the body.

The blood may be considered as a fluid holding in solution certain inorganic elements and having certain bodies suspended in it. To facilitate description, the blood may be considered as made up of the corpuscles and the liquor sanguinis. The corpuscles are of two kinds, the red and the white, the red being the more numerous. The color of the blood is caused by the coloring matter in the red corpuscles, which are the oxygen carriers. Both kinds are very minute bodies, which require the aid of the microscope to recognize them. The liquor sanguinis is composed of water containing in solution salts, albumin, and the elements of fibrin.

The lymphatics, or absorbents, are the vessels that carry the lymph and chyle in the blood. They begin as capillaries in all parts of the body, and gradually unite to form larger trunks. Placed along the course of the lymphatic vessels are glands, in some situations collected into groups; for example, in the groin. These glands are often involved in inflammation arising from the absorption of deleterious matter.

Absorption is the function of the lymphatics. The liquor sanguinis passes from the blood capillaries to supply nutrition to the tissues. All the liquor sanguinis that is not required is absorbed by the lymphatic vessels and conveyed back to the blood by the lymphatic ducts. The lymphatics that proceed from the intestines convey the chyle into the blood during digestion. As a rule, the lymphatic vessels follow the course of the veins. All the absorbent vessels convey their contents to the thoracic duct and right great lymphatic vein, which empty into the anterior vena cava, where the lymph and chyle mix with the venous blood and thus maintain the supply of nutritive elements in the blood.

THE PULSE

As previously explained the heart pumps the blood throughout the arterial system. The arteries are always full and each contraction of the ventricle pumps more blood into them. This process distends their elastic walls and sends along them a wave that gradually becomes less perceptible as it nears the very small arteries. This wave constitutes the pulse and is lost before the capillaries are reached. The sensation or impression given to the finger when placed on the artery shows the force exerted by the heart and some important facts concerning the condition of the circulation. In adult cattle the average number of pulsations in a minute is 40 to 60 and in dairy cows is as high as 70. The pulse is faster than normal after exercise, excitement, on hot days, as a result of pain, or of fullness of the stomach In old animals it is slower than in the young and in males slightly slower than in females. In fevers and inflammations and in local diseases of the heart the pulse rate is increased. If the rate is greater than 100 or 110 to the minute the outlook for recovery is not good.

Other variations of the pulse are known as infrequent pulse, which means that the number of pulsations in a given time is less than normal. The irregular or the intermittent pulse indicates one in which the pulsations do not follow in regular order. The strong pulse and the feeble pulse refer to the strength or weakness of the pulsation. The pulse is said to be hard when the vessel feels hard and incompressible; the soft pulse is the opposite. By dicrotic pulse is meant that kind of pulsation which makes each beat seem double, and therefore it is generally called the double pulse.

The venous or "jugular pulse" is the pulsation frequently observed in the jugular vein of cattle and is particularly noticeable while they are ruminating—"chewing the cud." It is not always associated with disease but may be a symptom of some disease of the heart; in such cases the jugular pulse is continuous.

The place selected for feeling the pulse in cattle is where the submaxillary artery winds around the lower jawbones, just at the lower edge of the flat muscle on the side of the cheek; or, if the cow is lying down, the metacarpal artery on the back part of the fore fetlock is very convenient for the purpose.

EXAMINATION OF THE HEART

Corresponding to the beats of the heart two sounds are emitted that are of a definite type in healthy animals. The first is produced by the contraction of the heart and the flow of blood out of it; the second, by the rebound of blood in the aorta and the closure of the valves that prevent it from flowing backward into the heart, whence it came. The first sound is the longer and louder of the two, though of low pitch. The second sound is sharper and shorter and is not always easy to hear. There is a brief interval between them.

To distinguish these sounds, the ear is placed against the left side of the chest, a little above the point where the elbow rests when the animal is standing in a natural position and about opposite the sixth rib. Both heart sounds are reduced in intensity when the animal is weak or when the heart is forced away from the chest wall by collections of fluid or by tuberculous or other growths. Nonrhythmical heart sound is often caused by pericarditis or by disease of the valves. It may also be attributable to overfilling of the heart on the right side, as occurs in severe congestion of the lungs and in some febrile diseases.

In pericarditis, sounds like scraping, rubbing, or splashing may be heard, entirely apart from the two normal sounds described.

The impulse of the heart, as felt by placing the hand against the chest, is of some consequence in reaching a conclusion in respect to disease of the heart; but it must be remembered that the impulse may be very much increased by diseases other than those of the heart, as, for example, inflammation of various organs and severe pains. The impulse may be increased also (when disease does not exist) by work, exercise, fright, or any cause of excitement, or, in general, by anything that causes acceleration of the pulse.

The impulse of the heart may be felt and the sounds may be heard fairly well in lean cattle, but in fat ones it is difficult and often impossible to detect either impulse or sound with any degree of satisfaction.

PALPITATION

When the impulse of the heart is excessive—that is, when it beats more or less tumultuously—the familiar expression "palpitation of the heart" is applied; by many it is called thumps. The hand or ear placed against the chest easily detects the unnatural beating. In some cases it is so violent that the motion may be seen at a distance. Palpitation is but a symptom and in many instances not connected with disease of the structure of the heart or its membranes. A badly frightened animal may have palpitation. When it comes on suddenly and soon passes away, it deepnds on some cause other than diseases of the heart. When it is gradually manifested, however, and becomes constant, although more pronounced at one time than another, heart disease may be suspected, especially if other symptoms of heart disease are present.

INJURY TO THE HEART BY FOREIGN BODIES

Cattle chew and swallow many objects not intended as articles of food, a fact that is well known by butchers. Among the great variety of objects that have thus found their way into the stomachs of cattle are the following: Finger rings, knitting needles, old shoes, table knives, wood, pieces of leather, pieces of wire, buttons, hairpins, brushes, nails, and coins. The more sharply pointed objects sometimes penetrate the wall of the stomach, and in some cases cause gastric irritation enough to produce indigestion, gradually work their way through the diaphragm toward the heart, pierce the pericardium (bag enclosing the heart), wound the heart, and thus are fatal to the animal. Cases are recorded in which the foreign body had actually worked its way into one of the cavities of the heart. Instances are known, however, in which the object took a different course and finally worked its way toward the surface and was extracted from the wall of the chest. Although the foreign body may pierce the wall of different parts of the alimentary canal, as it frequently does that of the rumen (paunch), it is thought that in most cases it passes through the wall of the reticulum (smaller honeycombed compartment, or second stomach) and is drawn toward the heart by the suctionlike action of the chest. Post mortem examinations have demonstrated the course it pursued, as adhesions and other results of the inflammation caused by it were plainly to be seen. All manner of symptoms may precede those showing involvement of the heart, depending on the location of the foreign body and the extent of inflammation caused by it. Severe indigestion may occur; stiffness and difficulty in moving about owing to the prods of the sharp body following muscular contraction; pain on pressure over the front, lower, or right side of the abdomen; coughing and difficult, quick breathing. In most cases the foreign body does not penetrate to the heart, nor even to the pericardium.

Symptoms.—The symptoms are as follows: The animal is disinclined to move actively, the step is restricted and cautious, sudden motion causes grunting, the attitude is constrained, the feet are drawn somewhat together, the back is arched, the face has an anxious expression. If the disease is of several days' duration, there is likely to be soft swelling (edema) beneath the neck, in the dewlap, and under the chest, between the forelegs. Breathing is short and difficult; it may clearly be painful. The pulse is rapid, 80 to 120 a minute. The muscles quiver as though the animal were cold. Rumination and appetite are depressed or checked. The dung is hard, and to void it appears to cause pain. These symptoms usually develop gradually and vary considerably in different animals, depending on the size and location of the foreign body and the irritation it causes.

In recent years operative treatment has been undertaken by veterinarians and the results obtained have been very encouraging. The abdominal cavity is opened under aseptic conditions and a manual search for the offending foreign body is made. In favorable cases the foreign substance may be removed and the wound closed by appropriate sutures. If veterinary service is not available, it is usually most economical to slaughter the affected animal. Knowing that cattle are prone to swallow such objects, care should be taken in keeping their surroundings as free of them as possible.

PERICARDITIS

Inflammation of the pericardium (heart bag) is often associated with pneumonia and pleurisy, rheumatism, and other constitutional diseases, or with an injury. It also occurs independently owing to causes similar to those of other chest affections, as exposure to cold or dampness and changes of the weather.

Symptoms.—The disease may begin with a chill, followed by fever of more or less severity; the animal stands still and appears dull, with head hanging low, and anxiety expressed in its countenance. The pulse may be full, perhaps hard; there is also a venous pulse. The hand against the chest will feel the beating of the heart, which is often irregular, sometimes violent, and in other instances weak, depending in part on the quantity of fluid that has transuded into the pericardial sac. The legs are cold, the breathing is quickened and usually abdominal; if the left side of the chest is pressed on or struck, the animal evinces pain. There may be spasms of the muscles in the region of the breast, neck, or hind legs. After a variable time swelling may also appear in the legs and under the chest and brisket.

In those animals in which the heart sounds may be heard somewhat distinctly, the ear applied against the chest will detect a to-and-fro friction sound, corresponding to the beats of the heart. This sound is produced by the rubbing of the internal surface of the heart bag against the external surface of the heart. During the first stages of the inflammation these surfaces are dry, and the rubbing of one against the other during the contraction and relaxation of the heart produces this sound. The dry stage is followed by the exudation of fluid into the heart sac, and the friction is not heard until the fluid is absorbed sufficiently to allow the surfaces to come in contact again. But during the time that the friction sound is lost, a sound that has been called a churning noise may take its place.

The friction sound of pericarditis cannot be mistaken for the friction sound of pleurisy if the examination is a careful one, because in the heart affection the sound is made in connection with the heart beats, whereas in the pleuritic affection the sound is synchronous with each respiration or breath of air taken in and expelled from the lungs.

Treatment.—When pericarditis is complicated with other diseases, the latter must be treated as directed in the description of them. Keep the animal in a quiet, comfortable place, where it will be free from excitement. Apply warm blankets to the body, and rub the legs until the circulation in them is reestablished, and then bandage them snugly. The feed should be nutritive and in moderate quantity.

In extreme cases tapping the pericardium with a trocar and cannula to draw off the fluid is resorted to, but the operation requires exact anatomical knowledge.

After death from pericarditis there is always more or less fluid in the pericardium; the surfaces are rough and covered with a yellow-colored exudate. In many cases there are adhesions to a greater or less extent between the heart and pericardium.

MYOCARDITIS

Inflammation of the muscular structure of the heart occurs in limited, circumscribed areas, as shown by post mortem examination, and it is probably always somewhat involved in connection with pericarditis and endocarditis. It may readily be inferred that if the whole organ were inflamed death would ensue immediately. Usually myocarditis results from the preexistence of blood poisoning or of some infectious febrile disease.

Symptoms.—The chief symptoms are those of heart weakness. The heart beat is fast, weak, and often irregular. Respiration is difficult and rapid. There is great general weakness and depression. Death comes suddenly.

Treatment.—Treatment consists in supporting the animal by the use of stimulants, such as ammonia, coffee, digitalis, or camphor. Complete quiet must be provided, and the general care should be as in pericarditis.

ENDOCARDITIS

When the membrane that lines the cavities of the heart—the endocardium—suffers inflammation, the disease is called endocarditis. The real cause is some other disease, during which substances that irritate the lining of the heart are produced and admitted into the circulation. These substances are usually living organisms, but in some cases they are chemical irritants. Endocarditis occurs as a complication of, or sequel to, pneumonia, blood poisoning, inflammation of the womb, rheumatism, or severe wounds or abscesses. The symptoms are much the same as those of pericarditis, and it is difficult to discriminate between the two affections. There is a jugular pulse, the legs may become dropsical, and there is a tendency to faint if the head is elevated suddenly. The bellowslike sound is more distinct than it is in pericarditis. It is the most fatal of heart diseases, because of the likelihood of formation of clots, which may adhere to the valves; change in the structure of the valves; and often a complication with an abnormal condition of the blood. Clots may be formed in the heart and, being carried to other parts, prove fatal by interrupting the circulation in some vital organ.

Treatment similar to that recommended for myocarditis may be followed in this disease.

VALVES OF THE HEART

The valves are subject to abnormal growths and structural changes in chronic endocarditis or as a result of acute endocarditis. Sometimes valves are torn by sudden, extreme muscular effort or a congenital abnormality. Cases are also reported in which they have been found ruptured.

Symptoms.—The general symptoms are those of heart weakness, accompanied with edema and congestion of the lungs.

Treatment.—Relief is sometimes afforded, but usually only temporarily, by the use of stimulants, especially digitalis.

RUPTURE OF THE HEART

Sudden effort, blows, or disease may lead to rupture of the heart. The first cause does not operate so often in cattle as in horses. Tuberculosis or ulceration from other causes, such as a foreign body, is the most common source of this accident. Rupture is shown by sudden fainting, followed very shortly by death.

HYPERTROPHY AND DILATATION OF THE HEART

This is an enlargement of the heart and may consist in the thickening of the walls alone, or at the same time the cavities may be either enlarged or diminished. Dilatation of the cavities has been noticed as existing independently of thickened walls. In hypertrophy the sounds of the heart are loud and pronounced, may be heard on both sides of the chest distinctly, and palpitation occurs to a greater or less extent. Fortunately, both conditions are very rare in cattle.

ATROPHY

Atrophy is the technical term for wasting of the muscular tissue. Atrophy of the heart is very rare among cattle and is usually a result of other diseases.

FATTY DEGENERATION OF THE HEART

This condition of the heart is met with in some very fat cattle, but the accumulation of fat around the heart is not referred to by this designation. In fatty degeneration the elements of the muscular tissue are replaced by fatty or oily granules. The muscle becomes weak, the heart contractions are insufficient, and heart weakness is shown by general weakness, shortness of breath, and weak rapid pulse.

CYANOSIS

Owing to the most prominent symptoms, cyanosis is also called blue disease and is seen occasionally in newborn calves. It is recognized by the blue color of the mucous membrane (easily seen by looking within the mouth and nostrils), the coldness of the surface of the body, and rapid, labored breathing. It is caused by nonclosure of the foramen ovale, connecting the right with the left side of the heart, and the consequent mixing of the venous with the arterial blood. Calves so affected live but a short time.

MISPLACEMENT OF THE HEART

Cases are recorded in which the heart has been found out of its natural position, sometimes even outside the chest. This is a congenital condition for which there is no remedy. A heifer calf with the heart entirely outside the thoracic cavity and beneath the skin in the lower part of the neck was kept for 2 years at the veterinary hospital of the University of Pennsylvania, during which time it grew to be a well-developed cow.

WOUNDS OF ARTERIES AND VEINS

When a blood vessel is opened a glance will tell whether it is an artery or a vein by simply remembering that bright-red blood comes from arteries and dark-red blood from veins. When a vein or a very small artery is severed the blood flows from the vessel in a continous and even stream, but when one of the larger arteries is severed the blood comes in intermitting jets or spurts corresponding to the beats of the heart. The dark-red blood that flows or oozes from a wound soon becomes bright red, because it gives up its carbonic acid gas to the air and absorbs oxygen from the air, which is the same change that it undergoes in the capillaries of the lungs.

The general treatment of wounds is discussed in another section; here it is necessary only to refer briefly to some of the most practical methods used to arrest hemorrhages, as instances occur in which an animal may lose much strength from the loss of blood or even bleed to death unless action is prompt.

BLEEDING (HEMORRHAGE)

The severity of a hemorrhage depends on the size of the vessel from which the blood escapes, though it is more serious when arteries are severed. If the wound in an artery is in the direction of its length, the blood escapes more freely than if the vessel is completely severed because in the latter instance the severed ends retract, curl in, and may aid very much in arresting the flow. When the blood merely oozes from the wound, and even when it flows in a small stream, the forming of the clot arrests the hemorrhage in a comparatively short time.

Slight hemorrhages may be checked by the continuous application of cold water, ice, or snow, to the wound, as cold causes contraction of the small vessels. Water from a hose may be thrown on a wound or dashed on it from the hand or a cup, or folds of cotton cloths may be held on it and kept wet. Ice or snow may be held against the wound or be put into a bag and conveniently secured in position.

Hot water of an average temperature of 115° to 120° F. injected into the vagina or womb is often efficient in arresting hemorrhages from those organs. Tow, raw cotton, lint, or sponges may be forced into a wound and held or bound there with bandages. This is an excellent method of checking the flow of blood until the arrival of a veterinarian. If the flow persists, these articles may be saturated with tincture of iron, but it is not advisable to use it unless necessary, as it is a caustic and retards healing by causing a slough. In cases of necessity, the articles may be saturated with vinegar, tannic acid, or alum dissolved in water. Whatever article is used should be left in the wound sufficiently long to make sure that its removal will not be followed by a renewal of the hemorrhage. Sometimes it must remain there 1 or 2 days.

An iron heated white and then pressed on the bleeding vessel for 3 or 4 seconds is occasionally used. It should not be applied longer, or the charred issue will come away with the iron and thus defeat the purpose of its application.

Compression may be applied in different ways, but only the most convenient will be mentioned. To many wounds bandages can easily be applied. The bandages may be made of linen, muslin, or similar material, sufficiently wide and long, according to the nature of the wound and the region to be bandaged. Bed sheets torn in strips the full length make excellent bandages for this purpose. Cotton batting, tow, or a piece of sponge may be placed on the wound and firmly bound there with the bandages.

Many cases require ligating, which is almost entirely confined to arteries. A ligature is a piece of thread or string tied around the vessel. Veins are not ligated unless very large (and even then only when other means are not available) on account of the danger of causing phlebitis, or inflammation of a vein. The ligature is tied around the end of the artery, but in some instances this is difficult and it is necessary to include some of the adjacent tissue, although care should be taken not to include a nerve. To apply a ligature it is necessary to have artery forceps (tweezers or small pincers may suffice) by which to draw out the artery in order to tie the string around it. To grasp the vessel it may be necessary to sponge the blood from the wound so that the end will be exposed. In case the end of the bleeding artery has retracted, a sharp-pointed hook, called a tenaculum, is used to draw it out far enough to tie. The ligature should be drawn tightly, so that the middle and internal coats will be cut through.

Another method of checking hemorrhage is called torsion. It consists in catching the end of the bleeding vessel, drawing it out a little and then twisting it around a few times with the forceps, which lacerates the internal coats so that a check is affected. This is very effective in small vessels and is preferable to ligatures, because it leaves no foreign body in the wound. A needle or pin may be stuck through the edges of the wound and a string passed around between the free ends and the skin (pl. XXVII, fig. 10), or it may be passed around in the form of a figure 8, as is often done in checking bleeding from the jugular vein.

ANEURISM

A circumscribed dilatation of an artery, constituting a tumor that pulsates synchronously with the beats of the heart, is called aneurism.

It is caused by disease and rupture of one or two of the arterial coats. The true aneurism communicates with the interior of the artery and contains coagulated blood. It is so deeply seated in cattle that treatment is out of question. Such abnormalities are ascribable to severe exertion, to old age, to fatty or calcareous degeneration, or to parasites in the blood vessels. Death is sudden when caused by the rupture of an aneurism of a large artery, owing to internal hemorrhage. Sometimes spontaneous recovery occurs. As a rule no symptoms are caused in cattle by the presence of deep-seated aneurisms, and their presence is not known until after death.

A false aneurism results from blood escaping from a wounded artery into the adjacent tissue, where it clots, and the wound, remaining open in the artery, causes pulsation in the tumor.

THROMBOSIS (OBSTRUCTION) OF THE ARTERIES

Arteries become obstructed as a result of wounds and other injuries to them, as those caused by the formation of an abscess or the extension of inflammation from surrounding structures to the coats of an artery. Arteries are also obstructed by the breaking off of particles of a plug or clot, partly obstructing the aorta or other large artery. These small pieces (emboli) are floated to an artery that is too small to permit them to pass and are there securely held, producing obstruction. These obstructions are shown by loss of power in the muscles supplied by the obstructed artery and by excitation of the heart and by respiration after exercise. The loss of power may not come into evidence until after exercise.

Symptoms.—While standing still or when walking slowly the animal may appear to be normal, but after more active exercise a group of muscles, a leg or both hind legs may be handled with difficulty, lameness results, and later there is practically a local paralysis. These symptoms disappear with rest. In some cases the collateral circulation develops in time, so that the parts receive sufficient blood and the symptoms disappear.

INFLAMMATION OF VEINS (PHLEBITIS)

When blood is taken from an animal without proper care or with an unclean instrument, inflammation of the vein may result, or it may be caused by the animals rubbing the wound against some object. When inflammation follows the operation, the coats of the vein become so much enlarged that the vessel may feel hard and knotted beneath the skin, and pressure produces pain. A thin, watery discharge, tinged with blood, issues from the wound. The blood becomes coagulated in the vessel. In inflammation of the jugular the co-

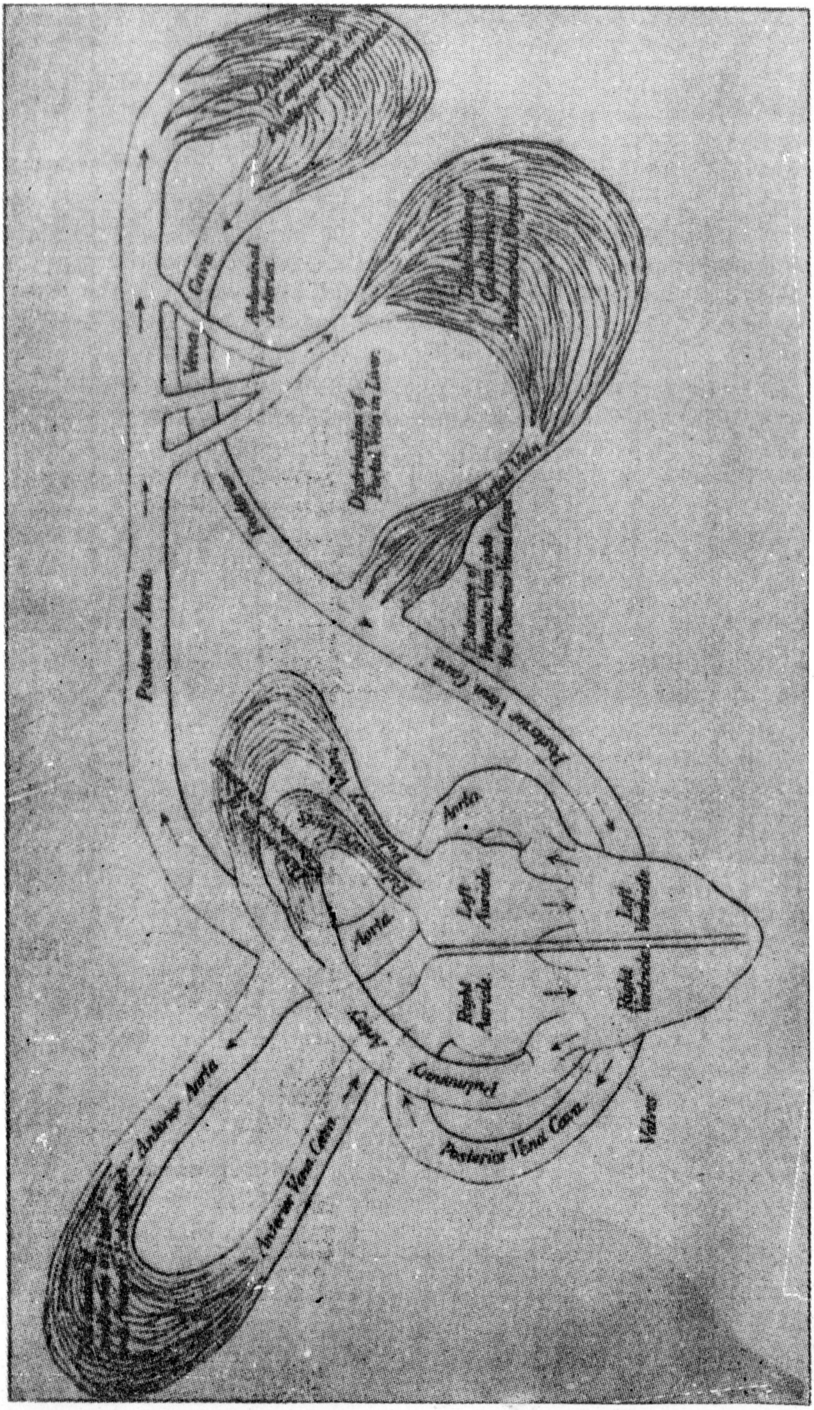

DIAGRAM OF THE CIRCULATION OF THE BLOOD.

agulation extends from the wound upward to the first large branch. Abscesses may form along the course of the vein. The inflammation is followed by obliteration of that part in which coagulation exists. This is of small import, as cattle have an accessory jugular vein that gradually enlarges and accommodates itself to the increased quantity of blood it must carry.

Treatment.—The treatment for inflammation of the vein is to clip the hair from along the course of the affected vessel and apply a blister, such as the cerate of cantharides. Abscesses should be opened as soon as they form, because there is a possibility of the pus getting into the circulation.

In any surgical operation the instruments should be clean, sterile, and free from rust. If the skin is not sufficiently opened, or when in closing the wound the skin is drawn out too much, blood may accumulate in the tissue, in which case it should be removed by pressing absorbent cotton or a sponge on the part. Care should also be used in opening the vein, so that the instrument may not pass entirely through both sides of the vein and open the artery beneath it.

DISEASES OF THE HEART, BLOOD VESSELS, AND LYMPHATICS

DESCRIPTION OF PLATE

PLATE VII:

Diagram illustrating the circulation of the blood. The arrows indicate the direction in which the blood flows. The valves of the heart, situated between the right auricle and ventricle, and left auricle and ventricle, and between the ventricles and large arteries, are represented by curved lines. These valves are intended to prevent the flow of blood in a direction contrary to that indicated by the arrows.

Noncontagious Diseases of the Organs of Respiration

By William Herbert Lowe, D. V. S.

[Revised by Maurice S. Shahan, D. V. M.]

In the determination of disease in the human body, the physician in making his diagnosis is aided by both subjective and objective symptoms, but the veterinary physician in most cases is obliged to rely almost solely on objective symptoms, and perhaps in no class of diseases is this more true than in the exploration of those under consideration. This condition has a strong tendency to develop observation and discernment in the veterinarian. Usually the successful veterinary practitioner is a very accurate diagnostician. In order to make a differential diagnosis, however, it is not only necessary to know the structure and functions of the organs in health, but also to adopt a rigid system of details of examination.

History.—The history of a case is of great assistance to the veterinarian in establishing a diagnosis. Often the information obtained from the owner or caretaker is unsatisfactory or not to be depended on, because of the layman's inability to weigh the evidence from every point of view.

A knowledge of the origin and development of a disease is important, both in making a diagnosis and in formulating the treatment. Exposure to cold and dampness is frequently the cause of affections of the organs of respiration. Such exposure is a common occurrence during fall and winter shipments.

The experienced practitioner is always sure to ascertain whether the particular animal he is called on to attend is the only one in the stable or on the premises that is similarly affected. If several animals are similarly affected, the disease may have a common cause, which may or may not be of an infectious nature.

Another thing that the experienced practitioner ascertains is what previous treatment, if any, the animal has had. Medicine given in excessive doses sometimes produces symptoms resembling those of disease due to infectious or other causes.

The hygienic and sanitary conditions must always be considered in connection with the cause as well as the treatment of disease.

Much of the disease that occurs in large dairies and elsewhere could be prevented if owners and those in charge of animals had proper regard for the fundamental laws of animal hygiene and modern sanitation. Disregard for these laws is the cause of most of the diseases under consideration in this chapter.

Attitude and general condition.—The feeling of pain in animals suffering from serious affections of the organs of respiration is expressed to the close observer in no uncertain language—by their flinching when the painful part is touched; by the care with which they move or lie down; by walking or standing to "favor" the part; by the general attitude and expression of the eyes; by the distress and suffering apparent in the face; and by other evidences.

The general physical condition and attitude of the sick animal tell the careful observer much that aids him in making a diagnosis and prognosis. Cows suffering from affections of the organs of respiration usually assume a position or attitude that is characteristic, well known to experienced stockmen as well as to veterinarians. When an animal has a fever or is suffering from an inflammation, the skin is one of the first parts to undergo a change that is apparent to the average observer, for it soon loses its elasticity and tone, and the hair becomes dry and staring.

From the general condition or state of nutrition one is able to judge the effect that the disease has already had on the animal and to estimate the strength remaining for its restoration to health; from the degree of emaciation one can approximate the length of time that the animal has been ill. The age and breed of the animal, as well as its constitution and temperament, must be taken into account in making a diagnosis and in attempting to overcome the disease.

The mucous membranes.—Examination of the mucous membranes should be made. This can be readily done by everting the eyelids or by an inspection of the lining membrane of the nostrils, mouth, rectum, or vagina.

Paleness of the mucous membranes indicates weak circulation or poor blood and may result from disease, hemorrhage, or inappropriate feed.

In healthy animals increased redness of the mucous membranes occurs from pain, excitement, or severe exertion and in such instances is always transitory. In certain pathological conditions, such as fevers and inflammation, increased redness of the membrane will also be observed. This lasts for the duration of the fever or inflammation.

A bluish or blue mucous membrane indicates that the blood is imperfectly oxidized and contains an excess of carbon dioxide. This condition is seen in serious diseases of the respiratory tract, such as pneumonia, and in heart weakness.

77431 O—51——7

Icterus or yellowness of the membranes indicates poor functioning of the liver or intestines or a serious blood condition.

The secretions.—The secretions may be diminished, increased, or perverted. In the early stage of an inflammation of a secretory organ its secretion is usually diminished. In the early stage of pleurisy the serous membrane is dry, and as the disease advances the membrane becomes unnaturally moist. The products of secretion are sometimes greatly changed in character from the secretion in health, as they become excessively irritant and yield evidence of chemical and other alterations in the character of the secretion.

Coughing.—Coughing depends on a reflex nervous action and may be primary when the irritation exists in the lungs or air passages, or secondary when caused by irritation of the stomach, intestines, or other parts having nervous communications with the respiratory apparatus. A cough is said to be dry, moist, harsh, hollow, difficult, paroxysmal, suppressed, or sympathetic, according to its character. It is a very important symptom, often being diagnostic in diseases of the respiratory organs.

Respiration.—In making an examination of an animal the depth, frequency, quickness, facility, and the nature of the respiratory movements are observed. They may be quick or slow, frequent or infrequent, deep or imperfect, labored, unequal, or irregular, each of which indication has its significance to the experienced veterinarian.

Exercise, sleep, rumination, pregnancy, and other conditions modify the respiratory movements even in health. Respiration consists of two acts—inspiration, or inhaling, and expiration, or exhaling. The function of respiration is to take in oxygen from the atmosphere, which is essential for the maintenance of life, and to exhale the deleterious gas known as carbon dioxide.

The frequency of the respiratory movements is determined by observing the motions of the nostrils, chest wall, or flanks. The normal rate of respiration for a healthy animal of the bovine species may vary from 10 to 30 times a minute. The extent of the respiratory system makes it likely to become affected by contiguity to many parts and its nervous connections are very important.

Rapid, irregular, or difficult breathing is known as dyspnea, and in all such cases the animal has difficulty in obtaining as much oxygen as it requires. Among the conditions that give rise to dyspnea are a restricted area of active lung tissue, due to the filling of portions of the lungs with inflammatory exudate, as in pneumonia; painful movements of the chest, as in fractured rib or pleurisy; fluid in the chest cavity (hydrothorax); adhesions between the lungs and chest walls; compression of the lungs or loss of elasticity; excess of carbon dioxide in the blood; weakness of the respiratory passages, tumors of the nose

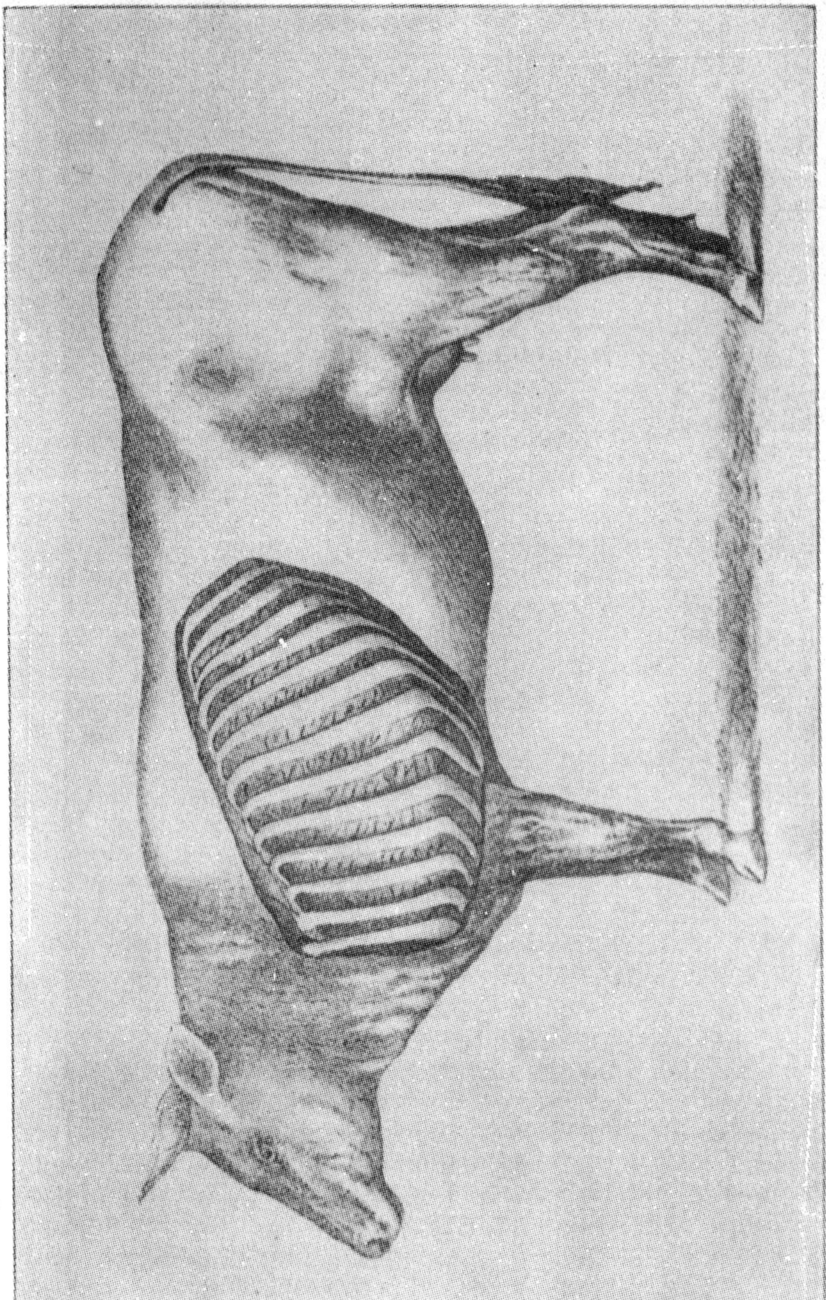

and paralysis of the throat; swellings of the throat; foreign bodies and constriction of the air passages leading to the lungs, and fevers.

As already stated, only careful and constant examination of animals in health will enable one to recognize abnormal conditions. One must become familiar with the frequency and character of the pulse and of the respirations and know the temperature of the animal in health, before changes in abnormal conditions can be appreciated.

Temperature.—The temperature should be taken in all cases of sickness. Experienced practitioners can approximate the patient's temperature with remarkable accuracy, but it is advisable to use the self-registering clinical thermometer, which is a valuable instrument in diagnosing diseases (pl. III, fig. 1). It is advisable to get a tested instrument, as some thermometers are inaccurate. The thermometer should be inserted into the rectum and kept against the walls of the passage for about 3 minutes. The normal temperature of the bovine is 101° to 102° F., which is higher than that of the horse. Furthermore, the cow breathes faster, its heart beats faster, and its internal temperature is higher. Ordinary physiological influences, such as exercise and digestion, give rise to slight variations of internal temperature, but if the temperature rises 2° or 3° above normal a diseased condition is indicated.

Pulse.—A discussion of this subject is given on page 69 in connection with "Diseases of the Heart, Blood Vessels, and Lymphatics."

Auscultation.—Auscultation and percussion are the chief methods used to determine the various pathological changes that occur in the respiratory organs. Auscultation is the act of listening and may be either mediate or immediate. Mediate auscultation is accomplished by aid of an instrument known as the stethoscope, one extremity of which is applied to the ear and the other to the chest of the animal. In immediate auscultation the ear is applied directly to the part. Immediate auscultation will answer in most cases. Auscultation is resorted to in cardiac and certain abdominal diseases, but it is mainly used for determining the condition of the lungs and air passages. Animals cannot describe the feelings experienced in the various phases of respiration, as can the patients of the human practitioner. The organs themselves are less accessible than in man, owing to the greater bulk of tissue surrounding them and the pectoral position of the fore extremities, all of which render it more difficult in determining pathological conditions (pl. VIII).

The air going in and out of the lungs makes a certain soft, rustling sound, known as the vesicular murmur, which can be heard distinctly in a healthy animal, especially on inspiration. There are, however, normal lungs in which the usual murmur is scarcely detectable or not demonstrable. Exercise and excitement accelerate the rate of respiration and intensify this sound. The vesicular murmur is heard only when the lung contains air and its function is active. The vesicular murmur is weakened as inflammatory infiltration takes place and when the lungs are compressed by fluids in the thoracic cavity and disappears when the lung becomes solidified in pneumonia or the chest cavity is filled with fluid. The bronchial murmur is a harsh, blowing sound, heard under normal conditions by applying the ear over the lower part of the trachea, and may be heard to a limited extent in the anterior portions of the lungs after severe exercise. The bronchial murmur when heard over other portions of the lungs generally signifies that the lung tissue has become more or less solidified or that fluid has collected in the chest cavity.

Other sounds, known as mucous râles, are heard in the lungs in pneumonia after the solidified parts begin to break down in the later stages of the disease, in bronchitis when there is an excess of secretion, and in other conditions. Mucous râles are of a gurgling or bubbling nature. They are caused by air rushing through tubes containing secretions or pus. They are said to be large or small as they are distinct or indistinct, depending on the quantity of fluid that is present and the size of the tubes in which the sound is produced. According to their character, mucous râles may be either dry or moist. The friction sound is produced by the rubbing together of roughened surfaces and is characteristic of pleurisy.

Percussion.—Percussion is that mode of examination by which sounds are elicited by striking or tapping over the part. It may be direct or indirect. If a finger of the left hand is placed firmly on the chest and smartly tapped or struck with the ends of the fingers of the right hand, the sound will be noticed to be more resonant and clear than when the same procedure is practiced on a solid part of the body. This is because the lungs are not solid but, in health, always are well expanded with air. In certain pulmonary diseases, however, as in pneumonia, the lungs fill up and become solid, when percussion produces a dull sound, like that on any other solid part of the animal. When fluid has collected in the lower part of the chest cavity the sound will also be dull on percussion. When there is an excess of air in the chest cavity, as in emphysema or in pneumothorax, the percussion sound becomes abnormally loud and clear. By practice on healthy animals the character and boundaries of the sounds can be so well determined that any variation from them will be readily detected, and will sometimes disclose the presence of a diseased condition when nothing else will.

Percussion is sometimes practiced with the aid of a special percussion hammer and an object known as a pleximeter to strike upon. A percussion hammer is made of rubber or has a rubber tip, so that when the pleximeter, which is placed against the side of the animal, is struck the impact will not be accompanied with a noise.

CATARRH (COLD IN THE HEAD)

Nasal catarrh is an inflammation of the mucous membranes of the nostrils and upper air passages. Simple catarrh is not a serious disease in itself but if neglected is likely to be complicated with laryngitis, bronchitis, pneumonia, pleurisy, or other serious and sometimes fatal diseases of the respiratory organs. Catarrh is a common disease among cattle, particularly calves. It is often caused by sudden exposure to wet and cold after the animals have been accustomed to shelter. It may arise from inhalation of irritating gases, dust, or stable odors. It may assume an enzoötic form. Catarrh of the head, sometimes called summer snuffles, occurs particularly in certain dairy cows during the summer months when on pasture. It appears to be similar to hay fever in man and is probably attributable to abnormal sensitiveness to the pollen of certain plants. The more severe forms of catarrh are very debilitating and require prompt and judicious treatment. Malignant catarrhal fever is to be considered in such cases.

Symptoms.—Redness of the mucous membranes of the nose and redness and watering of the eyes are symptoms of nasal catarrh. The mucous membrane first becomes dry; afterward a watery discharge appears, and later, in severe cases, the discharge becomes mucopurulent. In mild cases there is little or no fever, but in severe attacks the temperature may be high. The animal becomes dull, languid, and is not inclined to move about, and the appetite may be impaired; there is also variable temperature of the horns and ears. If in a cow giving milk the secretion diminishes, the mucus from the eyes and nose becomes thicker and yellower. Afterward, as the symptoms increase in severity, the discharge becomes mucopurulent.

Treatment.—The animal should be housed in a well-ventilated place, with good hygienic surroundings. In cold and damp weather it should be kept warm with blanketing, and, in severe cases, hot, medicated inhalations may be given. A fourth of a pound of Epsom salts in 1 to 2 gallons of water containing 2 to 6 tablespoonfuls of common salt to the gallon may be given as a drench but more conveniently by way of the stomach tube. Diffusible stimulants are beneficial in some cases. Too much importance cannot be attached to good nursing.

Catarrh of the nasal passages should not be regarded lightly as it may be an indication of infectious disease of dangerous nature. It is commonly seen in advanced cases of tuberculosis. Generally speaking, warm clean quarters do not encourage the condition. Dairy cows susceptible to summer snuffles are best confined to the corral or stable during the season when they are affected.

EPISTAXIS (BLEEDING FROM THE NOSE)

Bleeding from the nostrils is rather rare in cattle. It may arise from any one of a variety of causes but usually results from disease or injury to the mucous membranes or to violent exertions in coughing, sneezing, or running. It is seldom serious. It generally occurs in drops from one nostril only, accompanied with sneezing, and without frothing. Bleeding from the lungs comes from both nostrils, is bright red, frothy, and accompanied with a cough.

Treatment.—In many cases the bleeding will cease spontaneously if the animal is kept quiet and the head and nostrils bathed with cold water. The cause of the bleeding should be determined and the treatment governed accordingly. In severe and exceptional cases, when the hemorrhage is persistent and long continued, the animal's head should be tied to a high rack or beam and cold water or ice applied. The veterinarian may pack the nasal chamber with gauze or other material and may resort to the injection of various styptic solutions or coagulating substances.

LARYNGITIS (SORE THROAT)

An inflammation of the mucous membrane lining the larynx is known as laryngitis. It may be either a primary or a secondary disease, complicated or uncomplicated. In the absence of specific infectious disease it is attributable to some form of exposure, a sudden change from warm to cold surroundings, or exposure to cold storms. It may also result from inhaling irritating gases or from external violence. The infectious disease known as calf diphtheria commonly causes severe lesions in the larynx of young animals.

In an acute attack of laryngitis there is an elevation of temperature, pain on pressure over the region of the larynx, violent paroxysms of coughing, and difficult and noisy respiration. The nostrils are dilated, the nose extended, the tongue protruded, and the animal has a frightened expression. The symptoms of acute laryngitis are sometimes suggestive of obstruction of the esophagus, or choke. There is marked difficulty in swallowing. A harsh, dry cough may persist for weeks, particularly in cattle that are continuously stabled during the winter. Such animals may not recover till milder weather appears and pasture is available.

Treatment.—A warm, dry stall free from drafts is most desirable. If an injury is responsible for the attack, cold water or ice packs may be all that is necessary to bring about prompt recovery. In other cases, treatment consists of hot applications over the throat.

Stimulating liniments, mustard mixed with cold water and well rubbed in with a stiff brush, or other forms of counterirritation may be applied in severe cases. Hot inhalations may be resorted to and often afford much relief to the suffering animal. In this disease medicines should be given, so far as possible, in the form of electuaries (soft solid) or by the stomach tube on account of the difficulty of swallowing. Large drafts of medicines have a tendency to produce violent spells of coughing and in this way retard recovery. The bowels should be kept open and the diet should be such that the patient can easily swallow. Warm, wet mashes, boiled oatmeal gruel, linseed tea, and the like are suitable substances. If the animal is threatened with suffocation during the course of the disease, tracheotomy should be performed without delay. The operation is described under the head of Surgical Operations (p. 245).

When the disease assumes a chronic form, strong counter irritation is advisable. In some cases it will be necessary to repeat the treatment.

PLEURITIS (PLEURISY)

Pleurisy is an inflammation of the serous membrane known as the pleura, which lines the chest cavity and envelops the lungs. It is somewhat rare as an independent disease, but it often complicates pneumonia; its causes, in general, are the same as those of pneumonia. (See Pneumonia, p. 89.) It may arise from exposure to cold or wet or from external violence, and is usually present in some degree in cases in which the ribs have been fractured with or without a wound perforating the chest cavity.

Symptoms.—In the first stage there is great pain, aggravated by movement, and the animal is usually stiff as though foundered, the pulse is quick and hard, the breathing abdominal, the chest being fixed so far as possible, the inspiration short and jerky, the expiration longer. The pain is caused by the friction of the dry, inflamed pleural surfaces of the lung and chest on each other. At this stage the ear detects a dry friction murmur, resembling somewhat the sound made by rubbing two pieces of sole leather together. Pressure between the ribs causes pain and the animal usually flinches and grunts. The muzzle is hot and dry, the mouth slimy, and the secretions scanty. After a day or two the severity of the symptoms is usually much lessened; the temperature, which during the first days may have been as high as 106° F., falls to 103° or 104°; the pain decreases; the stiffness disappears, and the patient eats a little. The pulse softens but remains quicker than normal. At this stage the patient gradually loses strength, the friction sound disappears as the exudation moistens the pleural surfaces, percussion shows a horizontal line of dullness that day by day rises higher in the chest the respiration grows more frequent and labored, the countenance is anxious and haggard, the eyes sink somewhat in their sockets, and in unfavorable cases death occurs during the first or second week from either asphyxia or heart failure.

In pleurisy, as in pneumonia, the elbows are usually turned outward. Care must be taken to differentiate pleurisy from traumatic pericarditis. In the latter condition the area of dullness of the heart is much increased, and usually a splashing sound is heard at each beat of the heart. Another diagnostic symptom of traumatic pericarditis is painful but not difficult respiration, and the respiratory rate is much increased on movement. In both conditions considerable swelling of the dewlap may be noticed in the later stages. Since pleurisy in cattle is usually secondary to some other disease, the outlook varies with the type of infection present but it is usually a grave condition.

Chronic pleurisy, on the other hand, although frequent in old cattle, rarely causes marked symptoms or threatens the life of the animal, except in the case of tuberculosis, and here of course other severe lesions are usually present.

Treatment.—In acute cases, the same general care as for bronchitis or pneumonia is recommended. The bowels should be kept relaxed and the kidneys secreting freely. There is no specific remedy for pleuritis, but cough-controlling and stimulant drugs are advantageous. If collapse of the lung is threatened, a surgical operation, termed paracentesis thoracis, is sometimes performed; this consists in puncturing the chest cavity and drawing off a part of the fluid. The instruments used are a small trocar and cannula, which are usually introduced between the eighth and ninth ribs. The skin is prepared as for any surgical operation and, after incision, it is drawn to one side so that the external wound does not communicate directly with the puncture of the chest and thus permit the entrance of air. Only a portion of the fluid is usually removed. The animal gets immediate relief, but it is generally only temporary as the fluid has a tendency to accumulate again.

BRONCHITIS

Bronchitis is an inflammation of the mucous membrane of the bronchial tubes. When a primary disease, it is generally the result of what is commonly known as catching cold and usually occurs when the animals are housed in cold, damp, poorly ventilated stables that are not exposed to sunlight. It may be secondary to, or complicated with, many of the diseases of the respiratory system. It may also be caused by breathing irritating gases, or by the introduction of foreign bodies into the bronchial tubes, which sometimes results from injudicious and careless drenching when the larynx is temporarily relaxed. It may be acute or chronic and is divided, according to the seat of the inflammation, into bronchitis proper when the large tubes are affected, or capillary bronchitis when the trouble is in the smaller ones.

Symptoms.—Usually there are loss of appetite and elevation of temperature, generally 104° or 105° F. The inspiration is incomplete, short, and painful and the expiration is prolonged. The pulse is increased in frequency and is hard. A characteristic, painful cough is present, but it is paroxysmal and incomplete. Auscultation and percussion greatly aid in a diagnosis. A normal sound is given on percussion. On auscultation, in the early stages, rhonchal râles are detected if the larger tubes are affected, and sibilant râles if the smaller ones are affected. Later mucous râles are noted, and sometimes all sounds in certain parts are absent owing to the plugging up of the tubes. This plugging, if extensive enough, sometimes causes death, or death may result from extension of the disease to the lungs or pleura.

Treatment.—The animal should be placed in a light, well-ventilated box stall and the bowels kept open by enemas or other suitable means. Violent purgatives should not be used. If warm quarters have been made available, a mustard plaster, composed of equal parts of mustard and flour, mixed with sufficient lukewarm, but not hot, water to form a paste, may be gently rubbed through the coat down to the skin over the chest walls. This is then covered with paper, which will usually stick to the moistened hair. The dried, encrusted paste may be removed later by a thorough grooming. The body should be kept warm by blanketing. Medicinal treatment necessarily varies according to the character and stage of the disease.

The feed should be light and nutritious. Bronchitis is likely to become chronic if not treated properly in the earliest stage. In this case remedial treatment is of little value.

PNEUMONIA

Pneumonia is an inflammation of the lung substance. When diseased, the lungs probably have more varieties of inflammation than any other organ. The classification of pneumonia presents considerable difficulty, but for practical usage the disease is usually called either lobar pneumonia or bronchopneumonia (pl. XXX). These forms, however, can be differentiated only by the expert; therefore, for the purpose of the present discussion the subject is treated under the general head of pneumonia.

This condition in cattle is most common in the disease known as hemorrhagic septicemia and more particularly in those forms of hemorrhagic septicemia known as stockyards pneumonia or shipping fever, and in calves affected with so-called enzootic calf pneumonia.

Most other forms of pneumonia of cattle, which occur usually in only a few animals on one farm, are attributable to various micro-organisms that are present in such conditions as mastitis, metritis, infections due to the perforation of the stomach wall by foreign bodies, or other acute and chronic infections. Another frequent cause is the inhalation of feeds, water, or medicines that well-meaning but untrained persons give to animals in drenches. Pneumonia commonly follows attempts to force feed or to medicate animals that are prostrate or that have paralysis of the throat and cannot swallow.

Acute bronchopneumonia of undetermined cause has been known to affect considerable numbers of cattle, particularly calves in a given area. Invariably chilling, exposure to severe weather, overexertion, and other debilitating influences have been observed to precede such outbreaks and there is little doubt that such situations influence the occurrence of pneumonia. Cattle in feed lots sometimes develop what is called pulmonary edema, the accumulation of watery inflammatory exudates in the lungs. This has been attributed to various micro-organisms but is believed by some to be connected with feeds to which the animal, for various reasons, cannot adapt itself. Pneumonia is sometimes due to infestations with parasites in the lungs, especially in calves. It also results from certain types of mold infections and sometimes develops in tuberculosis as a complicating condition.

Symptoms.—In the first stage, that of congestion, the disease is usually ushered in by a chill, although this may not always be observed by the attendant. This is followed by an elevation of temperature, usually 105° to 106° F., or it may be even higher. The respirations are quick and shallow, the nostrils are dilated, the pulse is full and hard. Coughing may or may not appear in this stage. The nose is hot and dry, the tongue sometimes protrudes and is slimy, the coat is staring and the skin dry and harsh. The urine is usually diminished in quantity and highly colored, and the bowels constipated. The animal stands with the forelegs wide apart to facilitate respiration. On auscultation crepitation will be observed over the portion of the lung affected. The sounds elicited on percussion are practically normal in this stage.

In the second stage the temperature generally drops 1° or 2°, and respiration is performed with much difficulty. Coughing is usually frequent and painful. The animal still stands with the forelegs wide apart and the elbows turned outward. If it lies down, it rests on the sternum. All secretions, particularly the milk, are more or less suspended. The animal has a haggard appearance, and the pulse becomes weak and wiry at this period. The extremities are hot and cold alternately; the crepitation that was present in the first stage is now absent, and no sound on auscultation is heard, unless it is a slight wheezing or whistling noise. On percussion dullness over the diseased lung is manifested, indicating consolidation. The affected portion of the lung has now assumed a characteristic liverlike appearance.

In the third stage, if the disease is to terminate favorably, the cough becomes loose, the animal improves, the appetite returns, and the above symptoms rapidly subside; if, on the other hand, resolution is not progressing, the lung substance degenerates, and becomes clogged up. The gravity of the illness may be shown by hemorrhages from the lungs (hemoptysis). In fatal cases the breath has a peculiar, fetid, cadaverous odor and is taken in short gasps; the horns, ears, and extremities become cold and clammy, and the pulse is imperceptible. On auscultation, when suppuration is taking place and the lung structure is breaking down, a bubbling or gurgling crepitation, caused by the passage of air through pus, is heard.

Treatment.—Good hygienic surroundings, with shelter in inclement weather, and good nursing are essential in connection with the medicinal treatment. The probability of recovery depends largely on the extent of the lung tissue involved, as well as on the intensity of the inflammatory process and the nature of the underlying primary disease. Although in the past, febrifuges (drugs that tend to lower fever) were usually administered, it is now generally believed that such medication may impair the resistance of the animal and it is used only when the fever is exceptionally high and continued. Indeed, efforts are sometimes made by various means to increase the temperature in the tissues of the diseased areas in pneumonia and other diseases to hasten recovery. So, although aconite, sweet spirits of niter, and other so-called febrifuges frequently have a place in the treatment of pneumonia, they are no longer so generally employed as formerly. Good care and nursing are of first importance in this disease. The animal should be kept warm and have plenty of fresh air and sunshine when possible. A mustard plaster or other counterirritant is sometimes of benefit in the early stage of the disease. Diffusible stimulants, such as strong, black coffee (1 to 2 pints), whiskey or brandy (2 to 4 ounces), or aromatic spirits of ammonia (1 ounce), are advisable in certain phases of pneumonia. It is preferable to promote elimination by mild means, as by giving small doses of table salt in water and in bran mashes, rather than by giving drastic purgatives. The salt increases thirst and the drinking of water. Green. succulent feed or silage in small quantities may be offered whenever available. If the veterinarian attributes the condition to hemorrhagic septicemia, immune serum is usually administered. In some cases a blood transfusion may be given.

PULMONARY EMPHYSEMA (HEAVES)

Pulmonary emphysema is an accumulation of air in the lung tissue, outside the bronchi and air vesicles. It is caused by the rupture of the air sacs, which may be induced by attacks of asthma, continued severe coughing from any cause, or extreme exertion. Many aged milk cows are found at slaughter to have small areas of emphysema that caused no particularly noticeable symptoms before the animals were killed. Larger areas of emphysema, however, cause an interference with breathing, in which there is a shortened inspiration and a prolonged, interrupted expiration. The severity of the symptoms depends on the extent of the lesions. In such cases there is no fever, and the acceleration in breathing may be little noticed under ordinary conditions. The symptoms become more marked in hot weather or after exercise, and under these circumstances may be accompanied by a feeble but shrill, dry cough. Advanced cases may become thin despite a ravenous appetite, and the milk flow may decrease materially. Finally, the animal becomes emaciated and "hidebound," with a staring coat. In rare instances after a particularly severe attack of difficulty in breathing, the air may even escape from the thoracic cavity and permeate the tissues beneath the skin (subcutaneous emphysema).

Treatment.—The disease is incurable, and only a palliative form of treatment can be carried out. The destruction of the animal is often advisable, from a humane as well as from a financial point of view.

PULMONARY CONGESTION

Cattle that are overdriven are liable to pulmonary congestion in an acute form and sometimes to pulmonary apoplexy. In such cases they should be allowed to rest immediately, and if the weather is hot, they should be put in a shady place. Stimulants are given internally or hypodermically.

HEMOPTYSIS (BLEEDING FROM THE LUNGS)

Extensive bleeding from the lungs usually is shown by the presence of bright red, frothy blood in both nostrils and the mouth, but in some instances the blood is clotted. There is usually a cough by which the blood, mixed with considerable mucus, is discharged. The blood comes from one or more ruptured blood vessels. If the vessel is a minute capillary, a slight flow of blood results, but if a larger vessel is ruptured the flow is usually profuse. One of the more common causes of hemoptysis in cattle is multiple pulmonary abscess formation. In acute pneumonia of cattle, extensive pulmonary hemorrhage forecasts death. Continued, free hemorrhage results in pale mucous membranes, progressive weakness, and finally convulsions and death but, except in pneumonia, there is a tendency for the bleeding to cease of its own accord. If it continues the animal should be kept perfectly quiet. Cold applications over the sides may partially arrest the hemorrhage until a veterinarian can reach the case and institute treatment of the underlying cause of the bleeding. The success of treatment depends on the nature and extent of the lesion from which the flow of blood comes.

ABSCESS OF THE LUNG

Abscess of the lung is a common fatal complication of acute pneumonia. It sometimes occurs in pulmonary tuberculosis, in infestations of the lung with parasites and in general pyemic infections. Particularly in pyemic infections such as metritis, mastitis, navel ill, and traumatic perforations of the stomach, abscesses may form in other organs besides the lungs. Some cattle develop lung abscess without showing symptoms. One of the first indications of severe abscess formation in the lungs is hemoptysis, caused by a ruptured blood vessel.

The temperature is usually elevated to above 104° F. and the pulse and respiration are fast. There is usually a cough and mucous râles may be detected over the lungs. The animal may refuse feed and water and the chest wall is often very sensitive. With the passing of the acute stage, the animal loses flesh rapidly, eats sparingly, and moves about with a stiff gait and arched back. There is a general septic condition. Such animals go from bad to worse and as a rule, their prompt destruction is to the interest of the owner.

HYDROTHORAX

Hydrothorax, or dropsy of the chest, is not a disease in itself but is simply a condition in which an effusion takes place in the chest cavity and is the result or effect of some disease, usually pleurisy. It can be easily diagnosed by physical signs. A loss of the respiratory murmur will be noticed on auscultation, and on percussion dullness or flatness on a line as high as the effusion has taken place. When a large amount of effusion is present, tapping with the trocar and cannula is generally resorted to. The operation is described under the head of Pleurisy, p. 87.

PNEUMOTHORAX

An accumulation of gas in the pleural sac is known as pneumothorax. The presence of air may result from an injury of the lung, a wound communicating from the exterior or, in rare instances, from severe pulmonary emphysema. Treatment calls for the removal of any foreign body that may have penetrated, prevention of further entrance of air into the cavity by the closure of the external opening, and the use of antiseptics and adhesive dressings. The air already in the cavity will in most cases be absorbed. In pneumothorax caused by rupture of emphysematous lungs, healing of the lesion is unlikely and the animal should be destroyed in a humane manner.

Diseases of the Nervous System

By W. H. Harbaugh, V. S.

[Revised by John R. Mohler, A. M., V. M. D., D. Sc.]

THE NERVOUS SYSTEM

The nervous system is the distinguishing feature of animal life. Without it there can be no intelligence, no instinct, no sensibility, no perception; in fact, existence would be nothing more than vegetable life.

The senses—touch, taste, sight, hearing, smell—all depend on the nervous system. Motion depends on it. A muscle cannot contract without receiving the stimulus from the nervous system. For example, if a nerve passing from a nerve center to a muscle is severed, the particular muscle that is supplied by the cut nerve is paralyzed.

The nervous system is often studied in two divisions—the cerebrospinal division and the sympathetic division.

The cerebrospinal division consists of the brain and spinal cord, nerves, and ganglia. The nerves of this division convey the impulses of motion and sensation and supply all parts that are under the control of the will. For example, the voluntary muscular tissue includes all the muscles that act as the will directs. Another example: If anything comes in contact with any part of the skin, the impression is immediately perceived. All the special senses belong to this division.

The sympathetic division consists of nerves and ganglia. The muscular tissue, which acts independently of the will—as, for example, the stomach, intestines, womb, heart, blood vessels, and ducts is called involuntary muscular tissue and receives nervous stimulus from the sympathetic division.

The brain, spinal cord, and the ganglia are the central organs of the nervous system. The nerves conduct the nervous influence. The nerves terminate differently according to their function. The terminations are called end organs. The terminal end organs in the skin and other parts endowed with sensation receive the impressions, which are conveyed to the brain. They are so sensitive that the most gentle zephyr is perceived. They are so abundant that the point of the finest needle cannot pierce the skin without coming in contact

77431 O—51——8

with them, and the sensation of pain is instantly conveyed to the brain. The terminal end organs of the nerves that supply the muscles are different, as they give the impulse that is conveyed by the motor nerves to the elements constituting the muscles, and this impulse is the excitation that causes the muscle to contract. The terminal end organs of the special senses of taste, smell, etc., receive their special impressions, and their respective nerves carry the impressions to the brain.

There are two divisions of nerves, the afferent and efferent.

The afferent nerves convey the impression to the nerve centers. All the sensory nerves belong to this division.

The efferent nerves convey the nervous impulse outward from the nerve centers, and they are further classified according to the function of their respective centers. For example, motor fibers carry the impulse from the nerve center to a muscle to cause contraction. Vasomotor fibers carry the impulse to the muscular tissue in the blood vessels, which regulates their caliber. The secretory fibers convey the impulse to the cells of the glands and excite the activity of the gland, and its particular product is secreted or evolved, as for instance, milk in the mammary gland. Inhibitory fibers control or inhibit the action of the organ to which they are distributed, as, for instance, the heart.

Nerve centers may be considered as a collection or group of nerve cells. Both the cerebrospinal and the sympathetic divisions have nerve centers. The centers derive their special names from their functions. The brain is the great center of the nervous system, as it is the center of intelligence and perception. The centers of all the special senses, as well as the centers of various functions, are located in different parts of the brain. Nerve centers also exist in the spinal cord and in connection with the sympathetic system.

A nerve is a cord consisting of a certain number of fibers of nerve tissue, enclosed in a sheath of connective tissue. Nerves divide and subdivide, sending off branches, which ramify in all parts of the body, and, as they near their terminations, they contain but one or two fibers.

The brain and spinal cord are contained within a bony canal, which forms a protective covering for them.

The spinal cord, or spinal marrow, contained in the spinal canal, or hollow of the backbone, is continuous with the brain anteriorly, and terminates in a point in the sacrum (that part of the spinal column which immediately precedes the tail). The spinal cord gives off branches at each of the spaces between the segments of the backbone (vertebral column). These branches form nerve trunks that carry both sensory and motor impressions and impulses. The spinal cord is a grand nerve trunk to carry messages to or from the brain and to and from the reflex centers contained within itself.

The brain is contained within the cavity of the skull and is continuous with the spinal cord; there is nothing to mark the place where one leaves off and the other begins. The brain is the seat of reason and intelligence. Voluntary effort originates from the brain. Coordination, or harmony of movement, is controlled by the rear portion of the brain, known as the cerebellum.

The meninges are the membranes, three in number, that envelop the brain and spinal cord and separate them from the bones forming the walls of the cranial cavity and spinal canal. Between the outer and middle membranes is a delicate film of fluid originating in the blood and serving as a cushion for the brain and spinal cord. This so-called cerebrospinal fluid has certain other protective properties and during inflammation of the central nervous system may be so increased in quantity as to cause great pressure on the nervous tissue.

The sympathetic, also called the ganglionic, division of the nervous system consists of two chains of ganglia, reaching from the head to the tail, situated beneath the spinal column, one on either side. The presence of the ganglia or enlargements on the cords gives them their chainlike appearance.

The sympathetic nerves are closely connected with the cerebrospinal nerves but are not under the control of the will.

Symptoms of nervous diseases.—Inflammation and other disease conditions of the nervous tissue cause symptoms that may be grouped as follows: (1) Disturbances of consciousness, as shown either by depression, somnolence, delirium, or excitement; (2) indications of excessive irritation of the motor centers or motor nerves, such as twitching and spasms; (3) disturbance of the senses, such as blindness, itching, or impaired hearing; (4) partial or complete paralysis; (5) ataxia, or incoordination of movements.

ENCEPHALITIS (INFLAMMATION OF THE BRAIN, STAGGERS)

Inflammation of the brain is technically termed "encephalitis" and of its membranes "cerebral meningitis," but as both conditions usually occur together (cerebromeningitis), and since it is practically impossible to distinguish one from the other by the symptoms observed in the diseased animal, they are considered together here as varieties of the same disease. Staggers, coma, and frenzy are terms that are sometimes applied to this disease in its different forms or stages.

Causes.—Severe blows on the head with a hard object, the head coming violently in contact with the ground or other hard substance in a fall, or severe horn injuries, causing increased pressure on the cranial cavity, may be followed by encephalitis. Irritation caused by tumors in the brain may produce inflammation. Highly nitrogenous feeds are sometimes blamed for causing this disease. Acute indigestion and inflammations of the intestines sometimes cause symptoms of cerebromeningitis. Parasites, mineral and narcotic poisons, hot weather, and severe exertion or excessive excitement may cause this condition. Inflammation of the brain may occur as a complication of some infectious disease, such as tuberculosis, anthrax, blackleg, or hemorrhagic septicemia. Virus infections, such as rabies, specific bovine encephalitis, and pseudorabies, cause inflammation of the brain. Infections in which pus formation occurs—infections of the sinuses following dehorning, navel ill in calves, septic metritis, infections of the body cavities due to the perforation of the stomach wall by foreign bodies—may travel to the central nervous system and there set up inflammation. In many localities certain plants have the reputation of causing staggers. Conditions in which the blood salts are decreased in quantity (milk fever, grass tetany) frequently result in symptoms of severe cerebral disturbance.

Symptoms.—The symptoms vary much, but a careful observer will detect any trouble connected with the nervous system without much uncertainty. The first signs may be those of frenzy, but generally at the beginning the animal is dull and sleepy, with little or no inclination to move about; the head may be pressed against the wall or fence and the legs kept moving, as if the animal were endeavoring to walk through the obstruction; the body, especially the hind part, may be leaned against the side of the stall or stable, as if for support. There may be either constipation or diarrhea; the urine, when passed, is often limited in quantity and darker in color than natural. There may be trembling and even spasms of muscles in different parts. In the dull stage the animal may breathe less frequently than is natural, and each breath may be accompanied with a snorelike sound. The pulse may be full and less frequent than normal. If suddenly aroused from the drowsy state, the animal appears startled and stares wildly. When moving about it may stagger, and the hindquarters sway from side to side.

If delirium ensues, the cow is commonly said to be mad. She may bellow, stamp her feet, run about wildly, grate her teeth, and froth at the mouth. If she is confined in the stable, she rears and plunges; the convulsions are so violent in many instances that it is dangerous for one to attempt to render aid. She may fall; the muscles twitch and jerk; often the head is raised and then dashed against the ground until blood issues from the nose and mouth; the eyes may be bloodshot and sightless; the legs stiff and outstretched, or they may kick about aimlessly; the head may be drawn back and the tail drawn up; the urine may be squirted out in spurts; and often the "washer" nictitating membrane is forced over the eye. When the convulsions cease they may be followed by a period of quiet unconsciousness (coma) more or less prolonged, when the animal may gradually regain consciousness, get up on its feet, and perhaps quietly partake of feed, if there be any within reach, whereas at other times it arises with much difficulty and staggers blindly about the stall or field.

All the foregoing symptoms are not always seen in the same case. In cases usually designated as "sleepy staggers," the general symptoms of drowsiness are present, whereas in other cases the symptoms of frenzy cause the affection to be called "mad staggers." In other cases there are symptoms of paralysis, swaying of the hind quarters, and inability to rise, and sometimes these symptoms of paralysis are the most striking manifestations and continue until death. Acute cases are usually accompanied with fever.

When the disease follows injuries to the head symptoms may not be manifested until 2 or 3 days or longer after the accident. Since the disease may be rabies or another disease dangerous to man and because of other obvious advantages, it is particularly desirable that a veterinarian be in attendance whenever possible.

Treatment.—Although the prospects of the final outcome depend considerably on the basic cause, recoveries are rare in spite of careful attention. To be of any service whatever, treatment must be prompt. In the very early stage, when the pulse is full, a few cases will admit of bleeding. Four quarts of blood may be taken from the jugular vein of an average-size cow. However, all animals having symptoms of an affection of the brain or its membranes are not to be bled indiscriminately; the loss of blood in some cases may be absolutely detrimental to the animal's chance of recovery. Drenching, however, is not to be undertaken if the animal has any difficulty in swallowing. The use of the stomach tube is preferable in such cases, or medication may be administered hypodermically. No medication should be attempted without veterinary direction.

About 2 quarts of warm water containing 2 teaspoonfuls of common salt, or warm soapsuds, may be injected with a syringe into the rectum every 3 or 4 hours. It is best to keep the animal in a quiet, sheltered place, where it will be free from noise or other cause of excitement. All the cold water the animal will drink should be allowed, but feed should be withheld, except bran slops occasionally in small quantities, or grass, if in season, which may be cut and carried fresh to the patient.

The skull should be examined, and if sign of injury is found, appropriate surgical treatment is to be provided.

During the convulsions all possible efforts should be made to prevent the animal's injuring itself. The head should be held down on the ground and straw kept under it. Cold water may be continuously poured on the head, or bags filled with ice broken in small pieces may be applied to the head. Different authorities recommend different remedies to allay the convulsions, but for two reasons it will be found extremely difficult to administer medicines during the convulsions: (1) While the animal is unconscious the power to swallow is lost, and therefore the medicine is more likely to go down the windpipe to the lungs than to the paunch; (2) the convulsions are often so violent that it would be utterly useless to attempt to drench the animal. Furthermore, during this stage the functions of digestion and absorption are suspended, and as a consequence the medicine, provided it finds its way to the paunch, is likely to remain there unabsorbed and therefore useless. Sedative drugs are sometimes administered hypodermically or into the vein, in such cases. If the spasms or convulsions are due to lack of sufficient calcium, salts of that element are usually put into the animal's body by way of a vein.

The rubbing of a stimulating liniment, such as soap liniment, over the loins, along the spine, and back of the head on each side of the neck may be beneficial, especially if paralysis is present. In such cases, nerve stimulants, such as strychnine, may be prescribed by the attending veterinarian. Purgatives may or may not be indicated.

In those cases in which recovery takes place, it is often only partial, as there is generally a sequel that remains, such as partial paralysis. In some such cases, the animal may be fattened for slaughter under inspection, the latter to insure its suitability for food.

Post mortem examinations may reveal congestion of the brain and its membranes, but microscopic examination is frequently necessary to show pathological changes. In animals having much paralysis of the hind legs before death, the cord may be congested in the lumbar region (loins). When the disease has been caused by injury to the head, the congestion and extravasated blood may be found inside the cavity in the location corresponding to the place where the injury was inflicted externally. In some cases pus is also discovered. In practically all animals that have died from this affection the lungs are found to be very much congested. This may lead the superficial observer to suppose that the disease was a lung affection, but it is only a natural consequence when death ensues from brain disease.

APOPLEXY

That form of congestion of the brain known as parturient apoplexy, or parturient paresis, which is frequently associated with the period of calving, is described in another part of this work. (See Milk Fever, p. 200.)

Cerebral apoplexy, not connected with parturition, is a rare disease among cattle. However, it may occur as the result of so-called hardening or degeneration and consequent rupture of a blood vessel in the brain.

The attack is sudden; the animal in most cases falls as if it had received a blow on the head. It may stagger and reel for some time before going down. After falling, the animal has convulsive movements of the legs or becomes insensible. There may be remissions in the severity of the symptoms, but the pressure resulting from the continued escape of blood soon causes death. Rest, friction to the legs and surface, frequent turning of the animal, and cold applications to the head may be provided pending arrival of the veterinarian.

CONGESTION OF THE BRAIN

Although congestion of the brain, of a greater or less extent, occurs in practically all diseases of that organ, there is a form of congestive apoplexy affecting cattle that are in a plethoric condition. The congestion, or overfilling with blood, causes pressure on the brain substance and disorganizes its function. It occurs mostly in hot weather. In this disease the symptoms are somewhat similar to those of encephalitis, but the onset is more sudden, the duration is shorter, and there is less fever. There may be frenzy or coma, or alternations one with the other. There are diminished intelligence, staring eyes, bracing with the legs, pressing against the stall partition or manger, and red mucous membranes. This condition usually terminates in recovery.

This is one of the few diseases in which the withdrawal of blood from the body may be advantageous. Purgatives or other medication should not be given indiscriminately.

Cold applications to the head and the general treatment recommended for encephalitis are generally applicable.

CONCUSSION OF THE BRAIN

Severe blows on the head, striking the head against some hard object while running, or falling on the head may fracture bones of the cranium and produce compression of the brain.

Symptoms and treatment.—The symptoms and the treatment advised differ little from those for congestion of the brain and for encephalitis. In some cases it may be necessary to operate to remove a piece of bone that is pressing on the brain or to remove a clot of blood under the area that received the blow.

EPILEPSY (FALLING SICKNESS, FITS)

The term "epilepsy" applies to a chronic nervous disorder in which repeated attacks of convulsions, or so-called fits, followed by unconsciousness, occur. The seizures occur at intervals throughout life. The disease appears to be associated with heredity but the actual cause is unknown. Cattle are more often affected than some other species, horses for example. The disease closely resembles inflammations of the brain and its membranes. Convulsions due to poisoning, intoxications, infections, teething, or worm infestations are not to be confused with true epilepsy.

The animal as a rule shows signs of a coming attack before the actual seizure occurs. A general nervousness, twitching of the ears or facial muscles, and tossing of the head are some of the early symptoms in cows that are subject to the disease. The actual attack usually lasts only a few minutes, after which the animal dazedly regains its feet and is soon again apparently normal. However, the attacks may appear without warning after a variable interval and human beings, as well as other animals, may be endangered by the violence of the movements of the affected animal. Breeding such animals is inadvisable and they are usually best disposed of by slaughter, under inspection.

SUNSTROKE (PROSTRATION FROM HEAT)

Owing to the fact that cattle are seldom put to work at which they have to undergo severe exertion, as are horses, they are not frequently prostrated by the extreme heat of the summer months. When in pasture they select the coolest places in the shade of trees or in water when the heat becomes oppressive and thereby avoid, as much as possible, the effects of it.

However, cattle that are driven some distance in very hot weather are sometimes prostrated. For this to occur it is not necessary for the animal to be exposed to the rays of the sun, as those confined in hot, close places may suffer. This often happens in shipping, when the animals are crowded together in cars or trucks and sometimes at shows.

Symptoms.—The premonitory signs are those of exhaustion—dullness, panting, frothing at the mouth, tongue hanging out, irregular gait, uneasiness, palpitation—when, if the circumstances that tend to the prostration are not mitigated, the animal staggers or sways from side to side, falls, struggles for awhile, and then gradually becomes quiet, or the struggles may continue, with repeated but ineffectual efforts to regain a standing position. In serious cases the attack may be very sudden and unconsciousness may occur without continued or distressing premonitory symptoms. In animals that have died following heat stroke, the blood clots poorly or not at all, the veins are distended, and the lungs and brain are usually very much congested.

Treatment.—At first, if the case is not very serious, removal to a quiet, sheltered place, with a few days on a reduced diet and plenty of salt is all that need be done. When the animal has fallen, apply cold water or ice to the head; rub the body and legs with cloths or wisps of straw and continue the rubbing for a considerable time. If the ability of swallowing is not lost, which may be ascertained by pouring a little cold water into the mouth, 1 to 2 drams of liquor of ammonia, diluted with a quart of cold water, may be given as an emergency treatment. Be very careful in drenching the animal when lying down. This may be repeated in a half hour and an hour after the first one has been given if a veterinarian is not available. Instead of the ammonia, a drench composed of 2 ounces of spirits of nitrous ether in a pint of water may be given, if more convenient, but the ammonia drench is generally preferable. If unconsciousness continues, so that a drench cannot be administered, the same quantity of ammonia and water may be injected with a syringe into the rectum. The popular aqua ammonia, commonly called hartshorn, will do as well as the stronger liquor of ammonia, but as it is weaker than the latter the dose for a cow is about ½ ounce, which should be diluted with a quart of water before it is given to the animal, either as a drench or an enema.

As soon as the animal is able to rise it should be assisted and slowly and quietly moved to the nearest shelter. All the cold water it will drink should be allowed, but only in small quantities at one time. The diet should be limited for several days to bran slops and a little grass. The flesh of an animal that is suffering from heat stroke should not be prepared for use as food. On account of the fever with which the animal suffers, the flesh contains toxins that may render it poisonous to the consumer.

INJURIES TO THE SPINAL CORD

The spinal cord is liable to concussion from blows and falls, and paralysis, to a greater or less extent, may be the result. Fracture with displacement, or disease with distortion, of the bones (vertebrae) that form the spinal column, by compressing the spinal cord, produces paralysis varying in its degree and effect according to the part of the cord that is compressed and the extent of the pressure. If the abnormality is above the middle of the neck, death soon follows, as communication between the brain and diaphragm (the essential muscle of inspiration) is stopped. When the injury is farther down in the neck, posterior to the origin of the phrenic nerve, breathing continues, but there is paralysis in all parts posterior to the fracture, including the legs. When the fracture is in the region of the loins the hind legs are paralyzed, but the forelegs are not. If the fracture is in the sacrum (the division of the spinal column between the loins and the tail), the tail alone is paralyzed.

As a matter of course, when the back is broken there is usually no practicable remedy; the animal may best be killed at once.

PARALYSIS

Paralysis, or loss of motion in a part, may be due to a lesion of the brain, of the spinal cord, or of a nerve. It may also be caused by reflex irritation. Paralysis may occur in connection with parturient apoplexy, lead poisoning, ergotism, and other causes. Abscesses due to navel ill infection in calves or tuberculosis in older cattle have been found to be the cause of spinal paralysis in some cases.

When the paralysis affects both sides of the body, posterior to a point, it is further designated by the name "paraplegia." When one side of the body (a lateral half) is paralyzed, the term "hemiplegia" is applied to the affection. When paralysis is caused by a lesion of a nerve, the paralysis is confined to the particular part supplied by the affected nerve.

An injury to one side of the brain may produce paralysis of the same side of the head, but usually the opposite side of the body (hemiplegia) is affected. Local paralysis, paralysis of a leg or other part of the body, may occur as a result of injuries, infections, or other inflammations that involve, directly or indirectly, the nerves supplying the part. In encephalitis and various forms of poisoning or intoxication, the nerves controlling the throat may be particularly affected and inability to swallow is the result.

CONGESTION OF THE SPINAL CORD

Paraplegia, or paralysis of the rear part of the body, is a dominant symptom in congestion or inflammation of the spinal cord. The cause is variable and is often difficult to determine. In some cases it is thought that a toxic influence (poison) may be responsible for its development.

Symptoms.—The symptoms usually appear suddenly and consist in inability to stand. Sometimes this is preceded by a period of excitement. The animal usually lies quietly, but sometimes it groans and tosses its head about in a way that indicates pain. Cows heavy with calf are sometimes affected with a form of paraplegia, which usually attacks them from about a month to a few days before calving. Apparently they are in good health in every respect except the inability to stand on account of the paralysis of the hindquarters. This form is generally attributed to feeds containing insufficient protein and ash. It is most likely to occur in cows that are weak and thin. With good care and feed combined with stimulants, recovery usually occurs.

Treatment.—The animal should be given a soft, dry bed under shelter and in a quiet, airy place. Turn the cow two to four times daily and rub the legs well each time.

In spite of all efforts that are made to compel the cows to stand, there are instances when they will persist in lying down, when it cannot really be said that they are paralyzed. They have sensation in all parts; they can move all their feet and change their position; in fact, every function seems to be normally performed, but they obstinately refuse to rise or even make an effort to do so. Such cows have been killed, as it was impossible to get them on their feet. However, there are instances when a cow, after refusing to rise when all other means had been tried, quickly jumped to her feet and showed fright on the appearance of a dog or other terrifying object.

RABIES (HYDROPHOBIA)

(See Infectious Diseases, p. 358)

PSEUDORABIES (MAD ITCH)

(See Infectious Diseases, p. 362)

LIGHTNING STROKE (ASPHYXIA ELECTRICA)

When an animal is struck by lightning or comes into contact with electrical currents of very high voltage, the shock is instantaneously expended on the nervous system, and as a rule death occurs immediately. However, when the shock is not fatal, animation is suspended to a greater or less extent, as shown by prostration, unconsciousness, and paralysis.

Symptoms.—When the shock is not fatal, the symptoms vary greatly according to the severity of the shock. The animal usually falls, as from an apoplectic attack, and the symptoms are such as are generally manifested in connection with concussion of the brain. The muscular system may be completely relaxed, the legs limber, the muscles flabby and soft to the touch; or there may be convulsions, spasms, and twiching of the muscles. Breathing is generally labored, irregular, or interrupted, and slower than normal. In most instances the electricity leaves its mark by singeing the hair or by inflicting wounds, burns, or blisters.

Treatment.—As long as the beating of the heart is perceptible, the endeavor to revive the animal should be continued. Dash cold water over the head and body, rub the body and legs, whip the body smartly with wet towels or switches. Mustard, mixed with water, may be well rubbed over the legs and back of the head on each side of the neck. It is also advisable to inject, into the rectum, 1½ ounces of ammonia water (hartshorn) diluted with a quart of warm water. An uncorked bottle of the undiluted ammonia water may be cautiously held to the nostrils, so that some of it is inhaled, but care should be taken that too much is not suddenly inhaled. If the animal is unconscious, hypodermic injections of stimulants are usually advised.

When the animal revives sufficiently to be able to swallow, 1½ ounces of the ammonia water or 4 to 6 ounces of brandy or whisky diluted with a quart of cold water may be given as a drench, and the dose may be repeated every 3 or 4 hours if necessary. Care must be used in drenching.

If any paralysis remains, certain stimulants may be prescribed by the veterinarian. The wounds, burns, or blisters should be treated antiseptically.

TUMORS IN THE BRAIN, ETC.

Tumors of different kinds have been found within the cranial cavity, and in many cases no well-marked symptoms were manifested during the life of the animal to lead one to suspect their existence. Cases are recorded in which bony tumors were found in the brains of cattle that died suddenly, but during life no signs of disease were manifested. Post mortem examinations disclosed tubercles in the membranes of the brain. (See Tuberculosis, p. 363.) Abscesses, usually the result of inflammation of the brain, were found on post mortem. For the description of hydrocephalus, or dropsy of the brain, of calves the reader is referred to the section on parturition. (See Water in the Head, p. 155.)

Chorea, constant twitching and irregular spasmodic movements of the muscles, has been noticed in connection with or as a sequel to other affections, as, for example, parturient apoplexy.

Various diseases, the description of which are found in other sections of this work, affect the nervous system to a greater or less extent—for example, ergotism, lead poisoning, uremia, parturient apoplexy, colic and other affections associated with cramps, or spasms. Disease of the ovaries or of the spinal cord, by reflex irritation, may cause nymphomania. (See Excess of Sexual Desire, p. 125.)

METABOLIC DISEASES

Metabolism consists of the chemical and physical processes that take place in the utilization of feeds and the nourishment of the living animal. The metabolism of the normal animal is definitely modified by diet and other factors, including infection. If, from any cause, the vital processes are so much disturbed that the normal constituents of the blood stream are greatly changed in their relationship one to another, or are so altered that toxic products accumulate, so-called metabolic disease develops.

Cattle are no less susceptible to such conditions than other animals, but a cow that is heavy with calf or that has recently calved seems to be particularly prone to develop such so-called intoxications, which regularly cause symptoms of disease of the nervous system.

Calcium, phosphorus, magnesium, and other minerals are required for health. For example, the calcium content of a normal cow's blood serum varies from 9 to 12 milligrams, and of inorganic phosphorus from 2 to 9 milligrams per 100 cubic centimeters. An increase in the quantity of one results in a relative decrease of the other until the latter is promptly restored to its normal level. These elements must not only be present in the feed in adequate quantities but must also be in a certain ratio to each other. If the intake of either calcium or phosphorus is too low or too high, the absorption of the other element is interfered with. Excess or deficiency of certain other food elements also affects the assimilation of the required minerals. The normal utilization of the minerals also demands the presence of vitamin D and sunshine or a substitute.

Growing and pregnant animals, as well as those being milked, require liberal quantities of calcium and phosphorus in their diet. If these are not supplied, rickets may develop in young animals. Older animals, usually the best-producing dairy cows, which may not have the proper balance between the minerals, draw upon the minerals in the bones for a time. If the deficiencies continue, a point is finally reached at which the bones can no longer supply these. Under modern conditions of domestication, dairy cows are generally bred and fed for the production of large quantities of milk, and hypocalcemia—a state in which the blood calcium is below normal—frequently develops. The predominant symptom of hypocalcemia is disturbance of the nervous system. Milk fever is generally believed to be such a disease. (See p. 200.) A condition known as grass tetany results when high-producing cows that have been fed for some time on concentrated rations consisting chiefly of grain or that are approaching calving time or have recently calved, are turned out on luxuriant grass pastures. There appears to be a relationship between the high-protein content of the feed and the low-calcium and magnesium content of the depleted system. Nervousness, resulting in the animal's cringing when touched, may be observed early in the disease. Other cases develop suddenly, and a marked irritability and excitement may be shown by twitching of the muscles of the shoulder or the head, a tendency to charge, blinking of the eyes, and other nervous symptoms. The appetite is usually lost; clamping or grinding of the teeth, an unsteady gait, and a generally wild appearance are evident. The symptoms are variable in degree and nature and may pass off, but usually the animal finally goes down. It may thrash about considerably but later loses consciousness and has, in many instances, the appearance of a case of milk fever. The condition is treated by the injection into the vein, of sterile solutions of calcium or mixtures of calcium and magnesium.

Another metabolic disease, affecting milk cows chiefly, is known as acetonemia. In this disease an acid condition of the body (acidosis) results from the accumulation of the byproducts of incomplete metabolism of fats. These products, known as ketones, one of which is acetone, are believed to form through the failure of proper burning or assimilation of carbohydrates (starches, sugars) or as a result of a shortage of these constituents in the ration. Because of this, there is a marked decrease in the sugar content of the blood. Acetonemia in its typical form occurs in well-nourished, mature cows within 7 to 10 days after parturition. A few cases among nonpregnant animals have been reported, and the disease has been observed in animals before calving. There is a more or less gradual loss of appetite and a rapid loss of condition. After a few days the milk flow may be reduced one-half or more. Later or in some cases developing suddenly, severe nervous symptoms such as excitement, spasms, convulsions, or paralysis occur. In the course of the disease such symptoms as reluctance to move, the eating of litter or trash, dry and mucus-coated feces, arched back, half-closed or wild staring eyes, and difficult swallowing may be observed. In severe attacks the characteristic, chloroformlike sweetish odor of acetone in the urine, milk, and the breath is detectable. The odor may be noticeable only in the urine. Chemical tests may be necessary to determine whether acetone is present in sufficient quantity to account for the illness.

Few animals die as a result of acetonemia, particularly if they are promptly and properly treated. Sterile sugar solutions are injected into the blood stream. Sometimes the administration of insulin beneath the skin is resorted to. Chronic cases or those for which a veterinarian's attendance cannot be obtained may be benefited by receiving 1 to 2 pints of molasses or corn syrup three times daily. Common baking soda, to counteract hyperacidity of the stomach, may be placed on the feed, in the drinking water, or given as a drench. Four to six ounces of soda may be given daily. When feeding is resumed, excess fats and proteins in the feed should be avoided. A plentiful supply of water should be available.

Cattle that have been driven great distances or that have been shipped by train or truck sometimes develop a condition known as railroad sickness (not to be confused with shipping fever or hemorrhagic septicemia). This is an affection that somewhat resembles an attack of milk fever. It occurs chiefly during the summer in cows in advanced or recently terminated pregnancy. Often the animals affected are from pasture, but they are usually in good condition. Anxiety, restlessness, staggering, spasms, and grinding of the teeth are rapidly followed by stupor and collapse, in which state the case particularly resembles one of milk fever. The exact cause is not known. Usually, as with other similar conditions, if medicines are to be administered, it is best to give them by means of the stomach tube or hypodermically. Placing the cow in a cool, well-ventilated place and gently spraying the body with cool water may be advantageous. Solutions containing glucose may be injected intravenously. Strong coffee is sometimes used if the animal swallows without difficulty, or stimulants may be administered hypodermically. Removing the cows from pasture a few days before shipment and feeding clean, bright, legume hay may assist in preventing some of the trouble. Careful, quiet loading and regular feeding of hay in transit likewise appear to be beneficial. Animals placed in a field rather than in a small pen, after shipment, appear less likely to develop the disease than otherwise.

Diseases of the Urinary Organs

By James Law, F. R. C. V. S.
[Revised by Maurice S. Shahan, D. V. M.]

Of the materials that have served their purpose in building up the animal body or in sustaining the body temperature, and that are now to be thrown out as waste, the greater part is expelled from the system through the lungs and the kidneys, but the materials passing out from these two channels differ in the main from each other. Thus from the lungs, in the form of carbon dioxide—the same gas that comes from burning of coal or oil—there escapes most of the waste material resulting from the destruction in the system of fats, sugars, starch, and such other foods as are wanting in the element nitrogen, and do not form fibrous tissues, but go mainly to support animal heat or maintain functional activity. From the kidneys, on the other hand, are thrown out the waste products resulting from the destruction of the foods and tissues containing nitrogen—of, for instance, albumin, fibrin, gluten, casein, gelatin, and woody tissue. Although much of the waste material containing nitrogen leaves the body by the bowels, this is virtually only such of the albuminoid foods as has failed to be fully digested and absorbed; this has never formed a true constituent part of the body itself or of the blood but is so much waste food, like that which has come to the table and again carried away unused. If the albuminoid food element has entered the blood, whether or not it has been built up into a constituent part of the structure of the body, its waste products, which contain nitrogen, are in the main expelled through the kidneys, so that the latter become the principal channels for the expulsion of all nitrogen-containing waste.

It would be in error, however, to infer that all nitrogenous food, when once digested and absorbed into the blood, must necessarily leave the system in the urine. On the contrary, in the young and growing animal, all increase of the fibrous structures of the body is gained through the building up of those flesh-forming constituents into their substance. In the pregnant animal the growth of the offspring and its envelopes has a similar origin, and in the dairy cow the casein or curd of the milk is a means of elimination of these nitrogen-containing agents. Thus, in the breeding cow, and, above all, in the milking cow, the womb or udder carries on a work in one sense equivalent to that otherwise performed by the kidneys. Not only are these organs alike channels for the secretion or excretion of albuminous products, but they are also related to each other structurally and by nervous sympathy, so that disorder in the one is likely to induce some measure of disturbance in the other.

As in the case of other mammals, this nitrogenous waste matter is present mainly in the urine of cattle in the form of urea, but also, to some extent, as hippuric acid, a derivative of vegetable food which, in the herbivora, replaces the uric acid found in the urine of man and carnivora. Uric acid, however, is found in the urine of suckling calves that have practically an animal diet, and it may also appear in the adult in case of absolute, prolonged starvation, and in diseases attended with complete loss of appetite and rapid wasting of the body. In such cases the animal lives on its own substance, and the product is that of the wasting flesh. The other products containing nitrogen are present in only small quantities and need not be specially referred to.

The urine of cattle contains much less carbonates than that of horses and effervesces less on the addition of an acid. As the carbonates form a large proportion of the solid deposits (gravel, stone) from the horse's urine, there is less likelihood for these deposits to form in the urine of a cow, yet even in this animal the carbonates become abundant or scanty, according to the nature of the feed, and therefore gravel, formed by carbonate of lime, is not infrequent in cattle. When cattle are fed beets, clover hay, or bean straw, carbonates are present in large quantities, these aliments being rich in organic acids and alkaline carbonates; whereas when they are fed oat straw, barley straw, and, above all, wheat straw, carbonates are present in small quantities. When calves are fed milk alone no carbonates are found in the urine.

Phosphates, usually in combination with lime, are, as a rule, present only in traces in the urine of cattle. However, when a diet of wheat bran or other feed rich in phosphates is fed, these minerals may be present in large quantities and, as a result, they render the liquid cloudy or are deposited in solid crystals.

The urine of a cow fed on hay and potatoes contained:

	Parts
Urea	18.5
Potassic hippurate	16.5
Alkaline lactates	17.2
Potassium bicarbonate	16.1
Magnesium carbonate	4.7
Lime carbonate	0.6
Potassium sulphate	3.6
Common salt	1.5
Silica	Trace
Phosphates	0.0
Water and undetermined substances	921.3
Total	1,000.0

The specific gravity of the urine of healthy cattle varies from 1.030 to 1.045; the specific gravity of water is 1.000. Milk-cow's urine commonly falls in lower ranges. This urine is transparent, with a yellowish tinge, and has a characteristic musky smell. The chemical reaction is alkaline, turning red litmus paper blue. The quantity passed in 24 hours varies from 1½ to more than 5 gallons and increases not only with the water consumed but also with the albuminoids taken in with the feed and the urea produced. If a solution of urea is injected into the veins the secretion of urine is greatly augmented. Similarly, excess of minerals, such as potassium carbonate, in the feed, or of sugar, increases the action of the kidneys.

Only about 20 percent of the water swallowed escapes in the urine. The remaining 80 percent passes mostly from the lungs and to a slight extent through the bowels. The skin of the bovine does not perspire so readily nor so freely as that of the horse; hence the kidneys and lungs are called on for extra work. The influence of an excess of water in the feed is most remarkable in cattle fed on distillery byproducts. Such animals urinate profusely and frequently yet often thrive and fatten rapidly.

Among the other conditions that increase the flow of urine is overfilling of (internal pressure in) the blood vessels of the kidneys; hence the contraction of the blood vessels of the skin by cold drives the blood inward, tends to dilate the blood vessels of the kidneys, and to increase the secretion of urine. Nervous conditions, such as excitement and fear, or congestion, or structural injuries to the back part of the base of the brain, have a similar result. Cows in estrum urinate frequently. Bacteria and their products are commonly expelled by the kidneys and become sources of local infection, irritation, and disease.

The mutual influence of the kidneys and other important organs tends to explain the way in which disease in one part supervenes on preexisting disorder in another. The introduction of albuminoids in excess into the blood results in the formation of an excess of urea and a more profuse secretion of urine, of a higher specific gravity, and with a greater tendency to deposit its solid constituents, as gravel, in the kidneys or bladder. A torpid action of the liver, leaving the albuminoids in transition forms less soluble than the urea into which they should have been changed, favors the deposit of such albuminoid products in the kidneys, the formation of a deep-brown or reddish urine, and congestion of the kidneys. Any abnormal activity of the liver in the production of more sugar than can be burned in the circulation or impaired metabolism of the pancreas overstimulates the kidneys and produces increased flow of a heavy urine with increased sugar content. This increased production of sugar may be primarily due to disease of the brain, which, in its turn, determines the disorder of the liver. Disease of the right side of the heart or of the lungs, by obstructing the onward flow of blood from the veins, increases the blood pressure in the kidneys and produces disorder and excessive secretion. Inactivity of the kidneys results in increase in the blood of waste products, which become irritating to different parts and produce skin eruptions, itching, dropsies, and nervous disorders. Sprains of the loins may produce bleeding from the kidneys and disease of the spinal cord and sometimes terminate in albuminous or milky-looking urine.

The kidney of the bovine (pl. IX, fig. 1) is a compound organ made up of 15 to 25 separate lobules like so many separate kidneys, but all pouring their secretion into one common pouch (pelvis) situated in an indentation in the center of the lower surface. Although the cow is the only domesticated quadruped that maintains this divided condition of the kidney after birth, this condition is common to all such animals while at an early stage of development in the womb. The cluster of lobules making up a single kidney forms an ovoid mass flattened from above downward, and extending from the last rib backward beneath the loins and to one side of the solid chain of the backbone. The right is more firmly attached to the loins and extends farther backward than the left. Deeply covered in a mass of fat, each kidney has a strong outer, white, fibrous covering, and inside this two successive layers of kidney substance, of which the outer is that in which the urine is mainly separated from the blood and poured into the fine, microscopic urinary ducts (pl. X, fig. 1). These latter, together with blood vessels, lymph vessels, and nerves, make up the second, or internal, layer. The outer layer is composed mainly of minute globular clusters of microscopic, intercommunicating blood vessels (Malpighian bodies), each of which is furnished with a fibrous capsule that is only the dilated commencement of a urine tube. These practically microscopic tubes follow at first a winding course through the outer layer (Ferrein's tubes), then form a long loop (doubling on itself) in the inner layer (Henle's loop), and finally pass back through the inner layer (Bellini's tubes) to open through a conical process into the common pouch (pelvis) on the lower surface of the organ (pl. X, figs. 1, 2, 3).

The tube (ureter) that conveys the urine from the kidney to the bladder is like a white, round cord, about the size of a goose quill, prolonged from the pouch on the lower surface of the kidney backward beneath the loins, then inward, supported by a fold of thin membrane, to open into the bladder just in front of its neck. The canal passes first through the middle (muscular) coat of the bladder, and then advances perceptibly between that and the internal (mucous) coat, through which it finally opens. By this arrangement in overfilling the bladder, this opening is closed like a valve by the pressure of the urine, and the return of liquid to the kidney is prevented. The bladder (pl. IX, fig. 2) is a dilatable, egg-shaped pouch, closed behind by a strong ring of muscular fibers encircling its neck, and enveloped by looped, muscular fibers extending on all sides around its body and closed anterior end. Stimulated by the presence of urine, these last contract and expel contents through the neck into the urethra, which is the tube leading backward along the floor of the pelvic bones and downward through the penis. In the bull this canal of the urethra is remarkable for its small caliber and for the S-shaped bend that it describes in the space between the thighs and just above the scrotum. This bend is attributable to the fact that the retractor muscles are attached to the penis at this point, and in withdrawing that organ within its sheath they double it upon itself. The small size of the canal and this S-shaped bend are serious obstacles to the passing of a catheter to draw the urine. Yet by extending the penis out of its sheath the bend is effaced, and a small, gum-elastic catheter, not more than one-fourth of an inch in diameter, may with care be passed into the bladder. In the cow the urethra is very short, opening in the median line on the floor of the vulva about 4 inches in front of its external orifice. Even in the cow, however, the passing of a catheter is a matter of no little difficulty, as the opening of the urethra is very narrow and encircled by the projecting membranous and rigid margins, and on each side of the opening is a blind pouch (canal of Gärtner) into which the catheter will almost invariably find its way. In both male and female, therefore, the passing of a catheter is an operation which demands special skill.

General symptoms of urinary disorders.—These are not so prominent in cattle as in horses, yet they are of a similar kind. There is a stiff or straddling gait with the hind legs and some difficulty in turning or in lying down and rising, the act causing a groan. The frequent passage of urine in driblets, its continuous escape in drops, the sudden arrest of the flow when in full stream, the rhythmic contraction of the muscles under the anus without any flow resulting, the swelling of the sheath, the collection of hard, gritty masses on the hair surrounding the orifice of the sheath, the occurrence of dropsies in the limbs under the chest or belly, or in either of these cavities, and finally the appearance of nervous stupor, may indicate serious disorder of the urinary organs. The condition of the urine passed may likewise lead to suspicion. It may be white, from crystallized carbonate of lime; brown, red, or even black, from the presence of blood or blood-coloring matter; yellow, from biliary coloring matter; frothy, from contained albumin; cloudy, from phosphates; glairy, from pus; it may also show gritty masses from gravel. In many cases of urinary disorder in cattle, however, the symptoms are by no means prominent, and unless special examination is made of the loins, the bladder, and the urine the true nature of the malady may be overlooked.

BLOODY URINE (RED WATER, HEMATURIA, HEMOGLOBINURIA)

Bloody urine is technically classed as a hematuria when the urine contains clots or, when observed under the microscope, blood cells. In hemoglobinuria, sometimes called smoky water, the urine contains the blood coloring matter known as hemoglobin. Both hematuria and hemoglobinuria are, strictly speaking, only symptoms of disease. The color of the urine in either condition may vary from a faint pink to a coffeelike, brownish black. The presence of blood cells in the urine is the direct result of structural disease of the kidneys or urinary passages (inflammation, stone, or gravel, tumors, hydatids, kidney worms, sprains of the loins, etc.), whereas urine that is stained is usually the result of some general disease in which the red blood cells are destroyed in the circulating blood and the coloring matter dissolved in and diffused through the whole mass of the blood and of the urine secreted from it. Since the blood constituents excreted in the urine contain albumin, actually both a hemoglobinuria and an albuminuria are present.

Many factors are to be considered in the determination of the cause of bloody urine. The fact that the condition is common in tick fever, anthrax, and other acute infectious diseases should prompt the stockman to consult a veterinarian immediately. Hemoglobinuria is a characteristic of the infectious disease known as bacillary hemoglobinuria, caused by an anaerobic micro-organism, which occurs in certain sections of the western part of the United States. The mortality is high in untreated cases, and a vaccine for prevention and a serum for prophylaxis and treatment have been used in such areas.

In certain areas of the United States, particularly on poorly drained, wooded, or recently cleared lands, bloody urine is a common affection of cattle. The cause has not been determined in all cases, but stagnant water containing large quantities of decaying vegetable matter and certain species of bracken and the specific micro-organism mentioned previously have been implicated as causes. Scattered cases of hemoglobinuria occur in high-producing dairy cows a short time after calving. In these cases, less than normal quantities of phosphorus have been found in the blood. Cattle in fattening pens sometimes develop hemoglobinuria, apparently owing to a toxic state brought about by gastrointestinal disturbances or, possibly, the concentrated ration on which they are often fed. In these instances, the individual animal's constitution may play a part. Turnips and some other roots, when frozen and fed in large quantities, appear to have been the cause of bloody urine in several reported instances.

Many mineral poisons and some medicinal agents when taken to excess are responsible for hematuria or hemoglobinuria. Such metallic salts as those of mercury, arsenic, and lead have been so involved under certain conditions. Overdoses of such drugs as turpentine, cantharides, squill, and iodine occasionally produce hematuria or hemoglobinuria. Several varieties of acrid plants have been suspected also, but positive proof is generally lacking.

Finally, cattle sometimes are the victims of a condition similar to azoturia in horses, and in such cases the urine contains large quantities of pigment. This condition has been observed in young cattle turned out to pasture in the spring and in draft oxen that have been worked after a period of idleness with undiminished rations.

The specific symptom of bloody urine is a very patent one. It may or may not be associated with fever, abdominal tenderness as shown by pressure applied manually, pale or yellow mucous membranes, and general weakness. So-called parturient hemoglobinuria of dairy cows results in an immediate reduction in milk flow, and in severe, protracted cases, necrosis or gangrene of the extremities may appear. When direct damage to the kidneys, bladder, vagina, sheath, or penis is the immediate cause of the disease, the urine may be passed often in a small quantity at a time and with considerable straining. When the active cause is some irritant substance, abominal tenderness, colic, and other signs of bowel inflammation are common features. Small calculi, known as gravel, as well as intact blood cells, will settle to the bottom in a receptacle of collected urine.

Treatment.—Treatment varies according to the cause. If the disease is caused by a known chemical agent, antidotes of proper character should be administered, together with such symptomatic treatment as the case demands. The irritant should be eliminated as rapidly as possible, but drastic saline purgatives (Epsom or Glauber's salt) and severe diuretics are sometimes harmful, particularly in very weak, anemic animals. Frequently the bowels are highly inflamed and a diarrhea is present, in which case 2 to 4 pints of olive oil or, if necessary, 1 to 2 pints of raw linseed oil or castor oil may be given. In addition to this treatment, the animal should receive succulent, nourishing feed, and possibly enemas of warm water containing a moderately heaped teaspoonful of table salt to a quart of water. It is not advisable to attempt further treatment except under veterinary direction.

If the disease is caused by sprained loins, fractured vertebrae, inflamed kidneys, and gravel, the treatment should be that given for these conditions, so far as possible.

The infectious diseases involving bloody or smoky urine are to be dealt with according to their nature.

NEPHRITIS

By nephritis is meant an inflammation of the kidneys. It may be either acute or chronic. Acute nephritis is a common complication of several of the acute infectious diseases of cattle; otherwise the condition is rarely diagnosed except by chemical and microscopic examination. Feeds such as distillery byproducts or garbage or those particularly high in protein content may place a heavy burden on the kidneys through which much of the waste materials must pass. Injuries incurred by cows ridden by other animals that are in heat may cause a transitory inflammation of the loin region involving the kidneys. As a result of these conditions or some chronic septic or toxic states, nephritis may develop.

The extent of the damage to the kidneys and its character largely determine the nature of the symptoms. Cattle may be affected in mild or arrested form and show no indications of illness. On the other hand, high fever, loss of appetite, and suspended rumination, symptoms observed in other diseases, may be noted. Arching of the back, frequent passage of small quantities of cloudy or highly colored urine, abnormal tenderness over the loins, and symptoms of colic may be indicative of acute nephritis, as well as other diseases. Microscopically, the urine usually contains varying quantities of albumin, perhaps casts of the small tubules of the kidney, and frequently large numbers of cells that have been sloughed from the lining of the urinary channels, as well as white and red blood cells. Undue exposure to cold or abrupt chills may increase the severity of this and other kidney conditions and make the symptoms more pronounced. In severe, chronic cases, loss of flesh and swellings along the belly or of the legs may appear.

Treatment.—The first consideration is the removal of the cause. Deleterious feeds or chemicals should be eliminated and the animal placed on a nutritious but not too concentrated diet. Laxative feeds and succulent roughage should form a large part of the ration. Pasturing is advisable in mild weather but at other times stabling is better. The animal should have access to plenty of fresh, clean water. Hot fomentations over the loins or the hollow of the flank may be beneficial in acute, painful attacks. Urinary antiseptics, tonics, or stimulants may be prescribed by the veterinarian.

ALBUMINURIA

Albumin in the urine is a frequent occurrence in many diseases. It is a common symptom of practically all forms of inflammation of the kidneys and in a variety of disease conditions of distant organs, as well as in most of the acute infectious diseases. Therefore, albuminuria does not indicate the existence of any one specific disease, and it must be looked upon as a symptom of the several diseases in which it may occur. Albumin may be detected in urine if the fluid is boiled in a test tube and a few drops of dilute acetic acid is added and the mixture again boiled, when the presence of albumin will cause the clouding of the contents of the tube, the degree of cloudiness being an indication of the quantity of albumin present.

Except for the transitory albuminuria that may occur in healthy animals after feeding, the condition is to be considered as an indication of disease. Determination should be made of the disease involved and treatment given for this disease.

SUGAR IN THE URINE (DIABETES MELLITUS)

The sugar content of normal cow's blood is 0.04 to 0.06 gram per 100 cubic centimeters. Fasting in cattle causes a marked decrease in the blood sugar, which does not return to normal for several days. Increases in blood sugar may follow the excessive consumption of feeds containing much glucose (sugar). Ordinarily, the liver and muscles store the excess sugars, but if this process is long continued these parts of the body may be overtaxed and the surplus sugar is then excreted in the urine. The utilization of sugar is controlled chiefly by the pancreas, the so-called abdominal sweetbread, which produces a secretion governing the use of that food by the body, but it may also be regulated by a center in the brain. The secretion of the adrenal gland, which is poured into the blood stream, together with the internal secretions of other glands, is also believed to have a part in sugar metabolism. Certain diseases of the kidney, as well as of the several organs mentioned, may upset the functional balance between the organs, thus causing a glycosuria (the presence of glucose in the urine), which if continued becomes diabetes mellitus. True diabetes mellitus is not an uncommon disease in man and has been found in other animals. The disease has rarely been diagnosed in cattle. Animals having the disease should receive a ration in which carbohydrates and sugars are at least greatly reduced. In particularly valuable animals, treatment with insulin, an expensive extract made from the pancreas, may be tried.

PUS IN THE KIDNEY

The formation of pus in the kidney, caused by the presence of pus-forming organisms in that organ, is a much more serious condition than simple, uncomplicated nephritis. The kidney may have small or large abscesses that are caused by the circulation in the blood of such organisms as streptococci and staphylococci. These bacteria often enter the circulation through the umbilical cord at or shortly after birth. In some such cases calves not uncommonly develop an inflammation of the navel, the joints, and the liver, as well as kidney abscesses, and a rapid loss of flesh and death result. Older animals, particularly dairy cows, sometimes develop abscesses in the kidneys and other organs due to infection of the blood with pyogenic bacteria from purulent inflammation of the stomach or heart sac caused by puncture by foreign bodies such as nails, wire, and needles, infections of the uterus, or other acute or chronic suppurative conditions.

There is also a specific disease, known as pyelonephritis, which also causes pus in the kidney. This disease is caused by a germ (*Corynebacterium renale*) that gains entrance to the kidneys through the urinary passages, or possibly by way of the blood stream, and produces a highly fatal, chronic, purulent inflammation of not only the pelvic portion of the kidneys but also the ureters and bladder. This condition occurs chiefly in cows but has been found in bulls and in some unbred heifers and even calves.

Symptoms.—Pus in the kidney and, more specifically, pyelonephritis do not always cause clear-cut symptoms, as there is often only a gradual loss of flesh over a period of weeks during which time the milk flow gradually decreases. Some cases have the symptoms of purulent inflammation of the uterus or of the bladder. Either or both of these conditions may exist simultaneously with pus in the kidney. A mixture of blood and pus is often excreted with the urine, and in the case of pyelonephritis the specific causative organism can usually be demonstrated in stained smears under the microscope or may be recovered in cultures of the fluid. Many animals affected with pyelonephritis appear to be suffering from an acute attack of colic. The cow is very restless, may strain and groan considerably, go off feed, show pain over the kidneys, and commonly discharges a reddish urine. The animal may shift its weight from leg to leg, kick at the belly, and is often "tucked up" in the abdomen. Some cases appear to improve temporarily, only to suffer another acute attack. There are apparently very few recoveries, although there is evidence that some animals may be carriers of the organism without showing symptoms. Evidence that the organism causing pyelonephritis may be widespread in nature has been presented by some investigators. Diagnosis of either abscessed kidney or pyelonephritis may be made in most instances by the veterinarian through the recognition of the above-mentioned symptoms, by laboratory tests, and by means of manual examination through the rectal wall.

Treatment.—In pyelonephritis or abscessed kidneys, treatment is often unsatisfactory, and unless the animal is a valuable one it may be advisable to fatten it as well as possible and market it for slaughter.

It is not wise to slaughter such an animal for food purposes if a competent inspection service is not available as the diseased condition may extend to other parts of the body and render the carcass unfit for food. Attempts to cure valuable animals may be made through the use of general supportive treatment, good care, and possibly the injection into the blood stream of certain antiseptic chemicals. Some cases of abscess involving only one kidney, if the condition can be relieved temporarily by proper treatment, may be subjected to a surgical operation, such as drainage or removal of the entire kidney.

RETENTION OF THE URINE

Inability to pass urine may come from one or more of several conditions: (1) Obstruction of the urethra by calculi (stones), inflammation, or tumors (occurs chiefly in males); (2) paralysis or rupture of the body of the bladder; and (3) spasm of the neck of the bladder. Partial suppression of the flow of urine or scanty urine may occur in acute febrile conditions with catarrh of the bladder in acute poisoning by certain metals or turpentine, and in other severe toxic conditions.

In cattle the commonest cause of retention of the urine is obstruction, by calculi of the urinary channel, usually in the urethra of steers on fattening rations. Generally speaking, the formation of calculi (plate XI) appears to attend the heavy feeding of rich feeds or the use of feeds or water that contain particularly high concentrations of certain salts. Other factors, including heritable constitution, none of which are thoroughly understood, are believed by some to play a part. Briefly, when the urine contains an excess of certain salts, some of these are deposited upon any foreign body that may be present in the urinary passages. Such a foreign element is usually the product of inflammation and may be in the form of a clump of sloughed-off cells from the tubules, or casts, blood clots, pus, fibrin, or shreds of necrotic tissue. In some sections of the United States minute calculi, so-called gravel, are not uncommon, being found in the form of a sandlike sediment in the pelvis of the kidney, in the bladder, along the urethra, or within the sheath. Accumulations in the bladder or kidney of cattle rarely become of sufficient size to impair the animal's health seriously. However, in some animals, such as those on soils particularly rich in lime or fed large quantities of potatoes, sugar beet wastes, mangel beets, or feeds particularly rich in phosphorus, such as bran, the formed deposits of more or less insoluble salts accumulate considerably and the particles may attain a size sufficient to block the narrower parts of the urinary passages.

The early symptoms in those animals in which the deposits are confined to the kidneys or are relatively small are usually overlooked since alarming symptoms rarely develop. Minute granules, such as powdered chalk or fine sand, are easily flushed out with the urine. Larger particles may lodge in the urethra, sometimes at its opening into the bladder or where it turns downward over the pelvis, but usually in the S-shaped curve of the penis. In the event of such obstruction, some urine may dribble from the sheath after considerable straining. Later, the obstacle becomes imbedded and the inflammatory swelling of the tissues fixes it firmly and prevents the passage of any urine. The animal becomes fretful, stamps its feet, refuses feed, lies down and gets up anxiously, raises and switches the tail, and shows other so-called colicky symptoms. The animal shows extreme sensitiveness along the course of the penis, and the urethra and bladder, if not ruptured by the accumulation of urine, are found to be greatly swollen, tense, and painful on rectal examination. In cases of rupture of the bladder, which permits the urine to escape into the abdominal cavity, there is usually a temporary but deceptive appearance of improvement. In such an event, the urine, which is rarely free of bacteria, may later cause an active suppurative inflammation of the lining membrane or the outflow of large quantities of fluid into the cavity. The last condition, commonly called water belly, is a frequent occurrence in calves suffering from stoppage of the urethra. Such animals, or those in which the urine accumulates in the very easily stretched urinary bladder, sometimes live for days. Without relief, however, the animal becomes a victim of uremic poisoning known as uremia. Death is certain following continued absorption of urine by the circulating blood. The symptoms of uremia consist of intermittent spasms and extreme drowsiness, lastly unconsciousness, and profuse sweating with the odor of urine strongly present in the exhaled air and sweat from the animal.

Treatment.—The treatment for retention of the urine depends on the cause. If it is due to a calculus obstructing the urinary passages, the occlusion may sometimes be felt and, in some instances, massage and manipulation will dislodge it. All such manipulations, as well as palpations through the walls of the rectum, however, should be undertaken with the greatest care and properly by a competent veterinarian. If the obstacle cannot be dislodged and ejected by gentle manipulation, catheterization or crushing by means of forceps (pl. XI, fig. 4) or an operation called urethrotomy (cutting into the urethra) is resorted to. In animals about ready to go to the market, an incision is made over the urethra below the anus and a permanent opening is created for escape of the urine. Sometimes, as in valuable bulls, the incision may be made over the penis at the site of the obstruction. The stone is removed and the incision is closed by sutures. The success of either operation depends to a considerable extent on the animal's condition at the time. Early in the course of the trouble results are generally good. Catheterization or puncture of the bladder by means of a trocar is frequently necessary to prevent rupture if the urine has been accumulating for some time or if there is a paralysis due to injury of the spine or other causes, and may be advisable in spasm of the neck of the organ. In paralysis or spasms, either stimulants or sedatives may be required to restore the proper functions of the bladder. If the bladder is everted, or thrown into the vagina or outside the body as a result of prolonged labor at calving or through continued straining from other causes, anesthetics are usually required to effect its replacement.

TUMORS AND CYSTS OF THE KIDNEY

Cattle are sometimes affected with tumors and cysts of the kidney. Most of such growths originate in the embryo in the uterus. They do not often cause serious illness and are most commonly encountered after the animal is slaughtered. These tumors, as well as those developing after birth, may be suspected, however, because of indications of kidney disease and are sometimes diagnosed by palpation through the walls of the rectum. Malignant or cancerous tumors may cause enlargements of other organs, including the regional lymph nodes. Cysts (renal dropsy) occasionally develop in adult cattle as a result of inflammatory and circulatory changes and may eventually cause an atrophy or shrinking of the organ, thus placing a greater burden on the remaining normal tissue. Before intensive tuberculosis-eradication work was instituted, nodular swellings of the kidney due to tuberculosis were not uncommon but are now unusual. The nature of such swellings may be disclosed by means of the tuberculin test or by laboratory examinations.

If tumors or cysts of the kidney are recognized, the organ may in some cases be removed by a surgical operation.

DISEASES OF THE URINARY ORGANS

DESCRIPTION OF PLATES

PLATE IX. Kidney and male generative and urinary organs.

Figure 1. Kidney of a bovine. (From Handbuch des Vergleichenden Anatomie des Haus Säugethiere, vol. 7, 1890.) *A*, Renal artery carrying blood into the kidney; *V*, renal vein carrying blood from the kidney back to the heart, *H*, ureter, the tube carrying the urine from kidney to bladder. It is formed by the union of a number of branches that begin as cups (calices), each enclosing the tip of a conical mass of tissue from which the urine exudes.

Figure 2. Genital and urinary organs of the bull. (From Leisering, Mueller, and Ellenberger, Handbuch des Verg. Anat. des Haus Säugethiere.) 1, Scrotum, or the pouch containing the testicles; 2, tunica vaginalis,

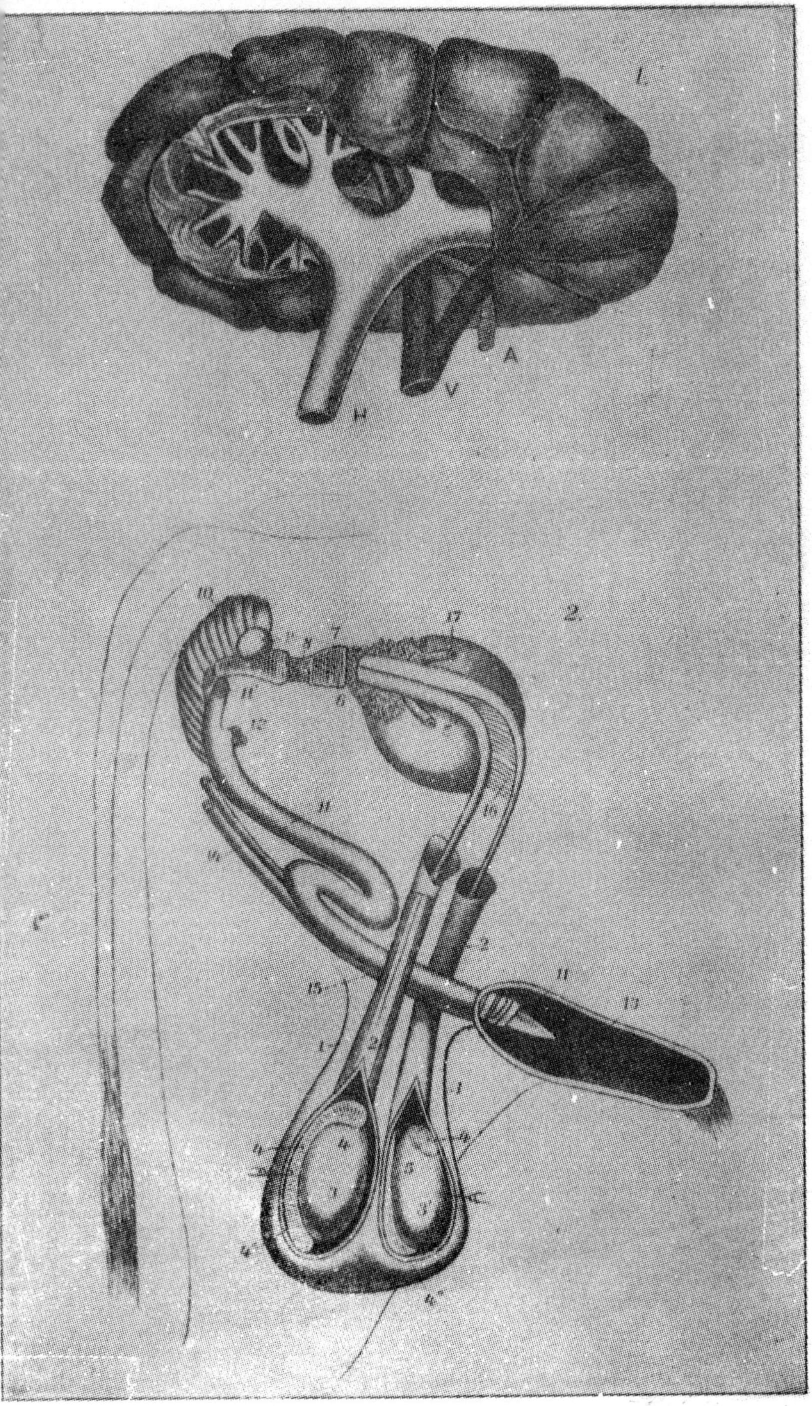

KIDNEY AND MALE GENERATIVE AND URINARY ORGANS.

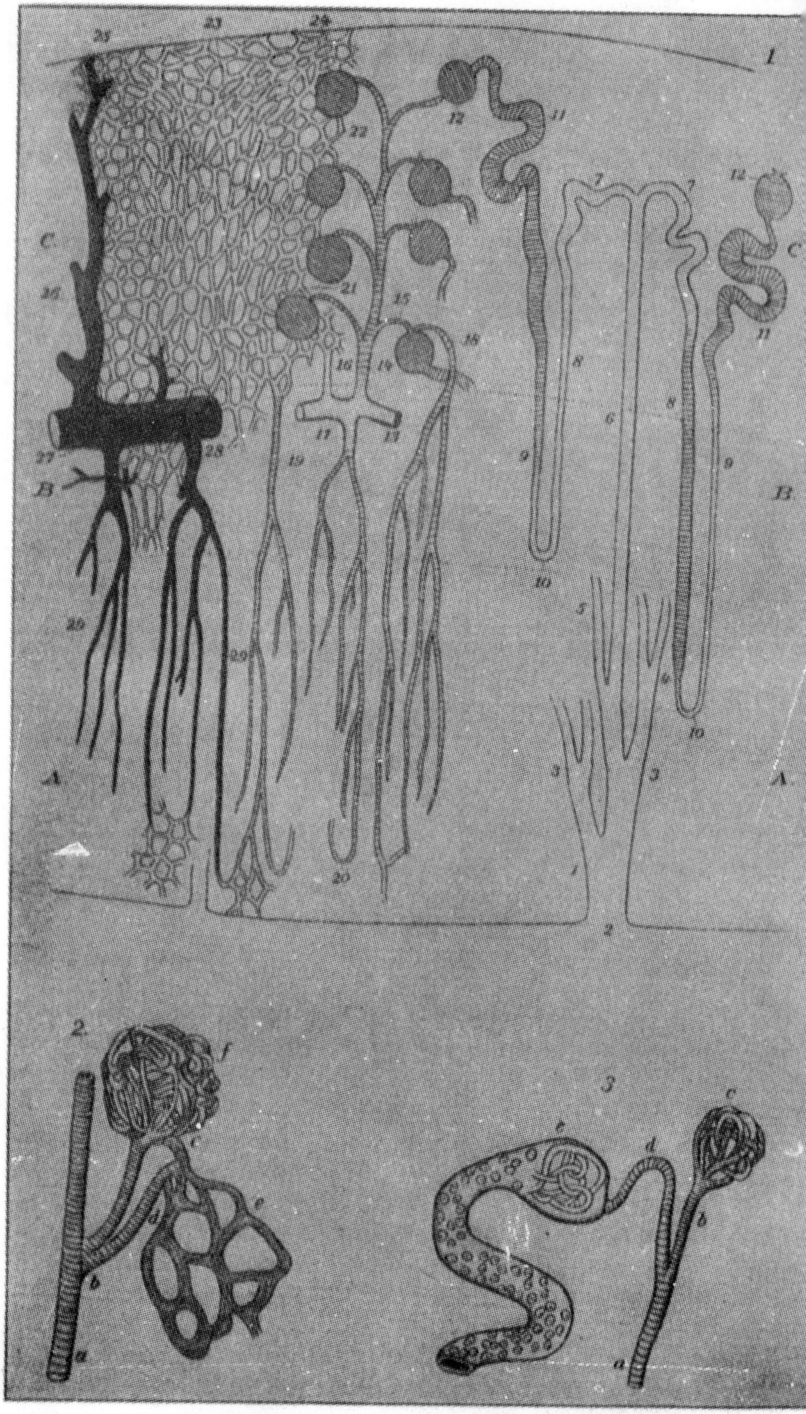

MICROSCOPIC ANATOMY OF THE KIDNEY.

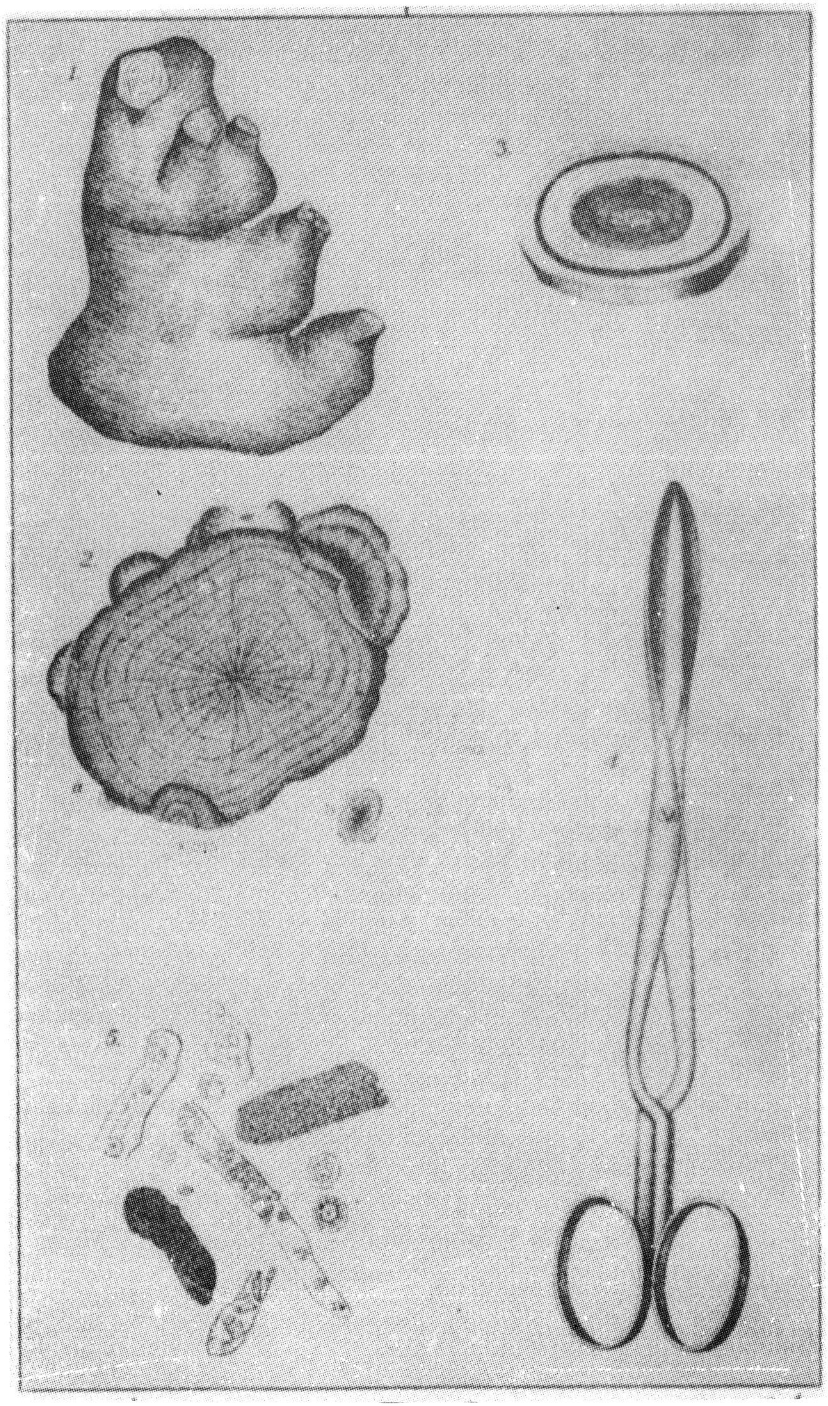

CALCULI OF KIDNEY AND BLADDER.

the serous membrane enveloping the testicles; 3, the right testicle, outer view; 3′, left testicle, inner view; 4, epididymis, or the beginning of the excretory canal of the testicle; 4′, globus major, or the head of the epididymis; 4″, globus minor, or the tail of the epididymis; 5, vas deferens, the duct through which the seminal fluid reaches the ejaculatory ducts; 5′, pelvic dilation of the vas deferens; 6, vesicula seminalis. The vesiculae seminalis are two oval pouches, which, in addition to their own secretions, receive the semen conveyed by the seminal ducts and hold it in reserve until copulation; 7, membranous or intrapelvic portion of the urethral canal covered by Wilson's muscle; 8, part of the prostate gland, covered by Wilson's muscle; 9, Cowper's gland. This gland, like the prostate gland, secretes a fluid that is thrown into the urethral canal in abundance immediately before ejaculation; by this means the expulsion of the semen is facilitated; 10, accelerator urinae muscle; 11, penis; 11′, cut portion of same; 12, cut suspensory ligaments of penis; 13, sheath, or prepuce laid open; 14, retractor muscles of sheat; 15, cremaster muscle cut at superior extremity; 16, duplicature of peritoneum; 17, ureters carrying urine from the kidneys to the bladder.

PLATE X. Microscopic anatomy of the kidney.

Figure 1 illustrates the minute apparatus for the secretion, collection, and discharge of the urine into the pelvis of the kidney (see pl. IX). The course is as follows: The urine is secreted from the blood vessels in the little round bodies called glomeruli (12), and by the minute cells in the curved tubes (11, 9, 10, 8), and passes through the convoluted and straight tubes (7, 6) into the larger tube (1), and then out into the pelvis, thence through the ureters into the bladder. The fluid and salts dissolved in the urine are taken from the blood, and the minute blood vessels are therefore very abundant in the kidneys, as is shown by the branches and network on the left of the figure. The blood passes into the kidney in the artery (13), which then divides into branches that pass into the glomeruli (12) and also forms a network around the secreting tubules (11, 9). The urine and salts pass from these vessels through the cells lining the tubules into the latter, and are discharged as described above. The blood is again collected in veins drawn black in the figure.

Figure 2 illustrates the manner in which the blood is distributed in the glomerulus (*f*), and also to the secreting tubules (*e*).

Figure 3 shows the relation between the blood vessel in the glomerulus (*e*), the tubule that conducts the urine therein secreted from the blood vessel; (*c*) represents a glomerulus from which the urinary tubule has been removed.

PLATE XI. Calculi of kidney and bladder.

Figure 1. Calculus, or stone, from the kidney. These are in the pelvis or portion of the ureter receiving the urine. The prolongations are casts of the branches of the pelvis. See the plates of the kidney for further description.

Figure 2. Calculus made up of oxalate of lime magnified 215 times.

Figure 3. Phosphatic calculus containing a nucleus of uric acid, sawed through to show concentric layers.

Figure 4. Straight forceps used in removing stones from the bladder.

Figure 5. Casts of the minute tubules of the kidney found in the urine in various kinds of kidney disease. Highly magnified.

77431 O—51——10

Diseases of the Genital Organs

By JAMES LAW, F. R. C. V. S.

[Revised by W. E. COTTON, D. V. M., and W. T. MILLER, D. V. M. M. S., Ph. D.]

Owing to the seriousness of various diseases and conditions discussed in this section, the stock owner is reminded of the importance of having a veterinarian make a careful diagnosis and perform or direct necessary treatment or procedures. This applies especially to symptoms that may indicate the presence of infectious abortion and to cases of difficult calving. The information given here is intended principally for aiding those who are not within reach of a veterinarian or who must give immediate attention to animals in distress.

Diseases of the genital organs are confined practically to animals that are kept for reproduction and the dairy. In three respects the castrated male is subject to such diseases: (1) To inflammation and tumefaction of the cut end of the cord that supported the testicle and of the loose connective tissue of the scrotum; (2) to inflammation of the sheath and penis from the accumulation of gravel in the former, from which the penis is not usually protruded in passing water; and (3) to bruising, abrasion, and inflammation of the sheath and penis. Apart from these, the castrated male ox is practically exempt from inflammations and injuries of the genital organs. The same applies to the castrated heifer. Inflammation may occur in the broad ligament of the womb whence the ovary has been removed or infective inflammation in the abdominal cavity (peritonitis) in case the operation has been performed through the flank, as it usually is in the young heifer. Apart from these, the castrated heifer is practically immune from any trouble of the generative apparatus. Even the virgin heifer is little subject to such troubles, though she is not exempt from inflammations, and above all, from morbid growths in the ovaries, which are well developed and functionally very active after the first year, or in precocious animals after the first few months of life. The breeding cow, on the other hand, is subjected to all the disturbances attendant on the gradual enlargement of the womb, the diversion of a large mass of blood to its walls, the constant drain of nutrient materials of all kinds for the nourishment of the fetus, the risks attendant and consequent on abortion and parturition, the dangers of infection from the bull, the risks of sympathetic disturbance in case of serious diseases of other organs, but preeminently of the urinary organs and the udder, and finally the sudden extreme derangements of the circulation and of the nervous functions that result from the sudden withdrawal of a great mass of blood from the walls of the contracting womb into the body at large immediately after calving.

In this class of diseases, therefore, two points should be kept in mind: (1) They are almost exclusively restricted to breeding animals, and (2) in keeping with the absolute difference of the organs in the male and female, there are two essentially distinct lists of diseases affecting the two sexes.

EXCESS OF SEXUAL DESIRE (SATYRIASIS IN MALE, OR NYMPHOMANIA IN FEMALE)

This may occur in the male from too frequent sexual intercourse or from injury and congestion of the base of the brain (vasodilator center in the medulla) or of the posterior end of the spinal cord, or it may be kept up by congestion or inflammation of the testicles or of the mucous membrane covering the penis. It may be manifested by a constant or frequent erection, by attempts at sexual connection, and sometimes by the discharge of semen without connection. In bad cases, feverishness and restlessness lead to loss of flesh, emaciation, and physical weakness.

It is, however, in the female especially that this morbid desire is most noticeable and injurious. A frequent cause is the excitation or congestion of some part of the genital organs. Disease of the ovaries is preeminently the cause, and this may be due to the formation of cysts (sacs containing liquid) or of solid tumors or degenerations or the formation of a tubercle. Indeed, in case of tuberculosis attacking the abdominal organs of cows, the ovaries or the serous membranes that support and cover them (the broad ligaments of the womb) are peculiarly subject to attack, and the animal has constant sexual excitement, incessantly riding or being ridden by other cattle, having no leisure to eat or chew the cud, but moving restlessly about and gradually wasting away. In some localities these cows are known as "bullers", because they are nearly always disposed to take the bull, but they do not conceive, or, if they do, they are subject to early abortions. They are, therefore, useless alike for the dairy and for the feeder, unless the removal of the ovaries subdues the sexual excitement.

Among the other sources of irritation charged with causing nymphomania are tumors and cancers of the womb, rigid closure of the neck of the womb so that conception cannot occur, inflammation, and a purulent discharge from the womb or vagina.

Treatment.—The treatment in each case will vary with the cause and is most satisfactory when that cause is a removable one. The animal may be exercised in an open field or the diseased ovaries may be removed (see Castration, p. 254), catarrhs of the womb and passages overcome by antiseptic, astringent injections (see Leucorrhea, p. 198), and tumors of the womb may often be detached and extracted, the mouth of that organ having been first dilated by sponge tents or otherwise. The rubber dilator (impregnator), sometimes helpful in the mare, is rarely available for the cow, owing to the different condition of the mouth of the womb.

DIMINUTION OR LOSS OF SEXUAL DESIRE (ANAPHRODISIA)

This occurs in either sex from low condition and ill health. Long-standing, chronic diseases of important internal organs, leading to emaciation and weakness, or prolonged semistarvation in winter may be sufficient cause. It is, however, much more common as the result of degeneration or extensive and destructive disease of the secreting organs (testicles, ovaries) that elaborate the male and female sexual hormones, respectively. Such diseases are, therefore, a common cause of sterility in both sexes. The old bull, fat and lazy, becomes sluggish and unreliable in serving and finally becomes useless for breeding purposes. This is not attributable to his weight and clumsiness alone but largely to fatty degeneration of the testicles and their excretory ducts, which prevents the formation and maturation of the semen. If he has been kept in extra high condition for exhibition in the show ring, this disqualification comes upon him sooner and becomes more irremediable.

Similarly the overfed, inactive cow, and above all the show cow, fails to come in heat at the usual times, shows little disposition to take the bull, and fails to conceive when served. Her trouble is the same, namely, fatty degeneration of the ovaries and of their excretory ducts (Fallopian tubes), which prevents the formation or maturation of the ovum or, when it has formed, hinders its passage into the womb. Another common defect in such old, fat cows is a rigid closure of the mouth of the womb, which prevents conception, even if the ovum reaches the interior of that organ.

Preventive.—The true preventive of such condition is to be found in a sound hygiene. The breeding animal should be of adult age, neither overfed nor underfed, but well fed and moderately exercised; in other words, the most vigorous health should be sought, not only that a strong race may be propagated, but that the whole herd, or nearly so, may breed with certainty. One authority gives 79 percent as the general average of cows that are found to breed in one year. Here more than a fifth of the progeny is sacrificed, also a fifth of the product of the dairy. With careful management the proportion of breeders should approach 100 percent. The various local and general obstacles to conception should be carefully investigated and removed. Vigorous health, which comes from a sufficiently liberal diet and abundant exercise, should be sought. In a bull or cow that is becoming unduly fat and showing indications of sexual indifference, the treatment must be active. Turning out on a short pasture where the animal must cover some distance to obtain sufficient feed will often suffice. A bull that cannot be turned out to pasture may sometimes be utilized in the yoke or tread power, or he may be kept a part of the time in a field or paddock chained by a ring in his nose to a strong wire extending from one side of the lot to the other and attached securely to two trees or posts. The wire should be higher than the back of the bull, which will move frequently from end to end. If he is indisposed to take sufficient exercise in this way he may be safely driven.

In case of rigid closure of the mouth of the womb the only resort is dilation. This is far more difficult and uncertain in the cow than in the mare. The neck of the womb is longer, is often tortuous in its course, and its walls so approximated to each other and so rigid that it may be almost impossible to follow it, and there is always danger of tearing its walls or of causing inflammation and a new, rigid, fibrous formation that on healing leaves matters worse than before. The opening must be carefully made with the finger, and when that has entered the womb further dilation may be effected by inserting a sponge tent or by careful stretching with a mechanical dilator (Pl. XX, fig. 6).

STERILITY FROM OTHER CAUSES

The questions as to whether a bull is a sure stock getter and whether a cow is a breeder are so important that it would be wrong to pass over other prominent causes of sterility. Breeding at too early an age is a common source of increasing weakness of constitution, which has existed in certain breeds. When for generation after generation heifers have been bred at less than a year old, the demand for the nourishment of the fetus is too great a drain on the immature animal, which accordingly remains small and stunted. As it fails to develop in size, so every organ fails to be nourished properly. Similarly with the immature bull bred to too many cows; he fails to develop his full size, vigor, or stamina and transfers his acquired weakness to his progeny. An increasing number of barren females and an increasing proclivity to abortions are the results of both courses. When this early breeding has occurred accidentally it is well to dry up the dam just after calving and to avoid having her served again until she is full grown.

The various diseases of the ovaries, their tubes, the womb, the testicles, and their excretory ducts, as referred to under Excess of Sexual Desire, are causes of barrenness. In this connection, the discharges following calving are fatal to the vitality of semen introduced before these have ceased to flow. Hence, service too soon after calving, or to a cow whose womb or genital passages have been injured, resulting in the keeping up of a mucopurulent flow until the animal comes in heat, is likely to fail of conception. Any such discharge should be first arrested by repeated injections as for leucorrhea, after which the cow may be bred.

Feeding a diet rich in carbohydrates, which greatly favors the deposition of fat, seems to have an even more direct effect in preventing conception. Among other causes of barrenness are all those that favor abortion, ergoted grasses, smutty wheat or corn, laxative or diuretic drinking water, any improper or musty feed that causes indigestion, colic, and diseases of the urinary organs, notably gravel, and all irritants of the bowels or kidneys.

Hermaphrodites are barren, of course, as their sexual organs are not distinctly either male or female. The heifer born as a twin with a bull is usually a hermaphrodite and barren, but the animals of either sex in which development of the organs is arrested before they are fully matured remain as in the male or female prior to puberty and are barren. Bulls with both testicles retained within the abdomen may go through the form of serving a cow, but the service fails; the spermatozoa are not fully elaborated. A heifer with a properly formed but very small womb and an extremely narrow vagina and vulva, the walls of which were very muscular, could never be made to conceive. A post mortem examination would probably have disclosed an imperfectly formed ovary incapable of bringing ova to maturity.

A bull and a cow that have been too closely inbred in the same line for generations may be sexually incompatible and unable to generate together, though both are abundantly prolific when coupled with animals of other strains.

Finally, a bull may be unable to get calves, not from any lack of sexual development, but from disease of other organs (back, loins, hind legs), which renders him unable to mount with the energy requisite to the perfect service.

CONGESTION AND INFLAMMATION OF THE TESTICLES (ORCHITIS)

This usually results from blows or other direct injuries but may be the result of excessive service, the formation of some new growth (tumor), in the gland tissue, or local infection resulting from some chronic disease such as tuberculosis or brucellosis (Bang's disease). The bull moves stiffly, with straddling gait, and the right or left half of the scrotum in which the affected testicle lies is swollen, red, and tender, and the gland is drawn up within the sac and dropped again at frequent intervals. It may be treated by rest, by 1½ pounds of Epsom salts given in 4 quarts of water, by a restricted diet of some succulent feed, by continued fomentations with warm water by means of sponges or rags sustained by a sling passed around the loins and back between the hind legs. The pain may be allayed by smearing with a solution of extract of belladonna. Should a soft point appear, indicating the formation of pus, it may be opened with a sharp lancet and the wound treated daily with a solution of a teaspoonful of carbolic acid in a half pint of water. Usually, however, when the inflammation has proceeded to this extent, the gland will be ruined for breeding purposes and must be cut out. (See Castration, p. 254.)

INFLAMMATION OF THE SHEATH

Although this may occur in bulls from infection during copulation and from bruises, blows, and other mechanical injuries, the condition is more common in the castrated male in connection with the comparative inactivity of the parts. The sheath has a very small external opening, the mucous membrane of which is studded with sebaceous glands secreting a thick material with a strong, heavy odor. Behind this orifice is a distinct pouch, in which this secretion is likely to accumulate when the penis is habitually drawn back. Moreover, the sheath has two muscles (protractors) that lengthen it, passing into it from the region of the navel, and two (retractors) that shorten it, passing into it from the lower surface of the pelvic bones above (pl. IX, fig. 2). The protractors keep the sheath stretched, so that it habitually covers the penis, whereas the retractors shorten it in the act of service, so that the penis can project to its full extent. In stud bulls the frequent protrusion of the erect and enlarged penis and the retraction and dilation of the opening of the sheath serve to empty the pouch and prevent any accumulation of sebaceous matter or urine. In the castrated male, on the other hand, the undeveloped and inactive penis is usually drawn back so as to leave the anterior preputial pouch empty. The sebaceous matter thus has space to accumulate and is never expelled by the active retraction of the sheath and protrusion of the erect penis in service. Again, the castrated animal rarely protrudes the tip of the penis in urination, the urine is discharged into the preputial pouch and lodges and decomposes there, so that there is a great liability to the precipitation of its mineral salts in the form of gravel. The decomposing ammoniacal urine, the gritty crystals precipitated from it, and the fetid, rancid, sebaceous matter set up inflammation in the delicate mucous membrane lining the passage. The membrane is thickened, reddened, rendered friable, and ultimately ulcerated, and the now narrowed sheath is blocked by the mass of material. The penis can no longer be protruded, the urine escapes in a small stream through the narrowing sheath, and finally the outlet is completely blocked and the urine distends the back part of the sheath. This will fluctuate on being handled, and soon the inflammation extends on each side of it and causes a thick, doughy, tender swelling under the belly and between the thighs. The next step in the morbid course is overdistention of the bladder, with the occurrence of colicky pains, looking at the flanks, uneasy movements of the hind legs, raising or twisting of the tail, pulsatory contractions of the urethra under the anus, and finally a false appearance of relief, which is caused by rupture of the bladder. Before rupture takes place the distended bladder may press on the rectum and obstruct bowel movements. Two mistakes are therefore probable (1) that the bowels alone are to be relieved, and (2) that the trouble is obstruction of the urethra by a stone. Hence the need of examining the sheath and pushing the finger into its opening to see that there is no obstruction there, in all cases of retention of urine, overdistended bladder, or blocked rectum. The disease may be acute or chronic—the first by reason of acute, adhesive inflammation blocking the outlet, the second by gradual thickening and ulceration of the sheath and blocking by the sebaceous and calculous deposits.

Treatment.—The treatment of this affection depends on the stage. If it is recent, and without instant danger of rupture of the bladder, the narrow opening of the sheath should be freely cut open in the median line below, and the sac emptied out with a finger or spoon, after which it should be thoroughly washed with tepid water. To make the cleansing more thorough a catheter or a small, rubber tube may be inserted well back into the sheath, and water may be forced through it from a syringe or a funnel inserted into the other end of the tube and considerably elevated. A fountain syringe answers admirably. The sheath may be washed out daily with tepid water, with a suds made with Castile soap or with a weak solution of zinc sulphate (one-half dram to a quart of water).

In case the disease has progressed to absolute obstruction, with the bladder ready to rupture at any moment, no time should be lost in opening into the urethra with a sharp knife over the bony arch under the anus, where the pulsations are seen in urinating. This incision is best made in the median line from above downward, but in the absence of a skillful operator a transverse incision with a sharp knife over the bone in the median line until the urine flows with a gush is better than to let the patient die. Considerable blood will be lost and the wound will heal slowly, but the animal will be saved. Then the slitting and cleansing of the sheath can be done at leisure, as described already. If the bladder is ruptured, the case is hopeless.

INFLAMMATION OF THE SHEATH AND PENIS FROM BRUISING

This also is an affection of work oxen, caused by the pressure and friction of the sling if the animals are held in stocks for shoeing. This crushing of both sheath and penis for half an hour or more leads to the development, several hours later, of a hard, hot, and painful swelling, extending from the scrotum as far as the opening of the sheath. Fever sets in, with dry muzzle, red eyes, hard, full, rapid pulse, accelerated breathing, and elevated temperature. The animal stands obstinately with his hind legs drawn apart and urine falling drop by drop from the sheath. Appetite and rumination are suspended. In 24 hours there may be indications of advancing gangrene (mortification), the swelling becomes cold, soft, and doughy and may even crack slightly from the presence of gas. A reddish brown, fetid liquid oozes from the swelling, especially around the edges, and if the animal survives it is only with a great loss of substance of the sheath and penis.

Prevention.—The prevention of such an injury is easy. It is necessary only to see that the slings do not press on the posterior part of the abdomen. They must be kept in front of the sheath.

Treatment.—Treatment, to be effective, must be prompt and judicious. Put around the patient a strap with soft pads in contact with the affected parts, constantly soaked in cold water for at least 24 hours. A pound or two of Epsom salts in 4 quarts of hot water should also be given. The second day the parts may be washed with 1 quart of witchhazel (extract) and 2 drams of sugar of lead, or the cold-water irrigations may be continued if the active inflammation persists. In case the swelling continues to be hard and resistant, it may be pricked at the most prominent points to the depth of one-third of an inch with a lancet first dipped in dilute carbolic acid, and the whole surface should be washed frequently with some antiseptic solution.

When softening occurs in the center of a hard mass and fluctuation can be felt between two fingers pressed on different parts of the softening, it should be freely opened to let out the pus, and the cavity should be syringed often with antiseptic solution.

In bad cases extensive sloughs of dead skin, of the whole wall of the sheath, and even of the penis, may take place, which will require careful antiseptic treatment. The soaking of the urine into the inflamed and softened tissue and the setting up of putrefactive action not only cause great destruction of the tissues from putrid inflammation, but even threaten life itself from a general blood poisoning (septicemia). Every case should have skilled treatment to meet its various phases, but in the severe ones this is most urgently demanded.

INFLAMMATION OF THE URETHRA

Like other males, the bull sometimes suffers from inflammation of the canal that conveys the urine through the penis, and a whitish mucopurulent discharge forms in consequence. It may have originated in gravel, the excitement of too frequent service, infection from a cow with leucorrhea, or from extension of inflammation from the sheath. Besides the oozing of the whitish liquid from the end of the penis and sheath, there are tenderness and pain when handled, and although there is no actual arrest of the urine, its flow is subject to frequent voluntary checks, as the liquid irritates the tender surface.

Treatment.—If the disease is recognized before the discharge sets in, a dose of 1½ pounds of Epsom salts and local, warm fomentations would be appropriate. After the onset of the whitish discharge a daily injection of a solution of 20 grains of potassium permanganate in a pint of water into the penis will be beneficial.

WARTS AND PAPILLARY GROWTHS ON THE PENIS

These growths are not frequent in the bull or the castrated male. They may interfere with the protrusion of the organ from its sheath or with service and always give rise to a bad-smelling discharge.

Treatment.—They may be twisted off with a pair of small tweezers or cut off with a pair of scissors, and the seat burned with a pencil of lunar caustic. To get hold of the penis in the bull, bring him up to a cow. In the castrated animal it will be necessary to push it out by manipulation through the sheath. In difficult cases the narrow opening of the sheath may be slit open.

WOUNDS OF THE PENIS

The most common wounds are those sustained by blows of horns, sticks, or other means. The blood vessels and sacs are ruptured to a greater or less extent, and considerable swellings filled with coagulated blood and inflammatory products occur. These lead to distortion of the organ and sometimes to the impossibility of protruding it.

Treatment.—A lotion of a dram of alum in a quart of water may be applied (injected into the sheath, if necessary), and a large sponge constantly irrigated by a stream of cold water may be kept applied, by means of a surcingle to the outer side of the sheath. Incisions are rarely applicable to the organ, but in an extensive clot that is unlikely to be absorbed the lancet may be resorted to. If the injury leads to paralysis of the penis and hanging out of its sheath, it should be supported in a sling and astringents used freely until inflammation subsides. Then the restoration of power may be sought by a blister between the thighs, or by the careful use of nerve stimulants, such as strychnine, 1 grain twice daily.

ULCERS ON THE PENIS

Sores on the penis of the bull may result from gravel or sebaceous masses in the sheath or from having served a cow having leucorrhea.

Treatment.—These ulcers may be treated by frequent injections into the sheath, of a lotion made with 1 dram of sugar of lead, 60 drops of carbolic acid, and 1 quart of water.

POLYPUS OF THE VAGINA OR UTERUS

A polypus is a tumor growing from the mucous membrane and often connected to it by a narrow neck. A definite cause cannot always be assigned. If growing in the vagina, a polypus may project as a reddish, rounded tumor from the vulva, especially during the act of passing water. It can be distinguished from descent of the womb by the absence of the orifice of that cavity, which can be felt by the oiled hand beyond the tumor in the depth of the vagina. From a vaginal hernia caused by the protrusion of some abdominal organ enveloped by the relaxed wall of the vagina it may be distinguished by its persistence, its firm substance, and the impossibility of returning it into the abdomen by pressure. A hernia containing a portion of bowel gurgles when handled and can be completely effaced by pressure, the gut passing into the abdomen.

A polypus in the womb is less easily recognized. At the time of calving it may be felt through the open mouth of the womb and recognized by the educated touch (it must be carefully distinguished from the mushroom-formed cotyledons (pl. XIII, fig. 2), to which in ruminants the fetal membranes are attached). At other times, unless the womb is opened in the effort to expell it, the polypus can be detected only by examining the womb with the oiled hand introduced through the rectum.

Polypi may cause a mucopurulent discharge, or they may only be suspected when they prove to be an obstacle to parturition. The best way to remove them is to put the chain of an écraseur around the neck, or pedicle, of the tumor and tear it through; or the narrow neck may be torn through by the emasculator, or in an emergency it may be twisted by rotating the tumor on its axis. The removal of the tumor will allow calving to proceed. After this the sore may be treated by a daily injection of ½ dram of zinc sulfate, 1 dram of carbolic acid, and 1 quart of warm water.

SIGNS OF PREGNANCY

If a cow remains for 3 or 4 weeks after service without showing signs of heat (bulling), she is probably pregnant. There are very exceptional cases in which the well-fed cow will accept the bull weeks or months after actual conception and others equally exceptional in which the thrifty nonpregnant female will refuse the male persistently, but these in no way invalidate the general rule.

The bull, no matter how vigorous or how ardent his sexual instinct, usually pays no attention to a cow that is not in heat; hence indications of pregnancy can be had from both the male and female. When she has conceived, the cow usually becomes more quiet and docile and lays on flesh and fat more rapidly, especially during the first 4 months of gestation. The stimulus to digestion and nutrition created by the demands of the growing fetus contributes to this result. Some feeders avail themselves of this disposition to prepare heifers and cows speedily for the butcher.

The enlargement of the abdomen and its dropping so that it bulges below and to each side, whereas it falls in at the flank, between the outer angle of the hipbone and the last rib, are significant features which, though they may be caused by abdominal tumor or dropsy, are usually marks of pregnancy. From the same increasing weight of the abdomen the spine in the region of the loins sinks so that the bones of the croup seem to rise, especially back toward the root of the tail. In the early stages of pregnancy the udder develops slowly, and toward its completion quite rapidly. For a long time there is merely a sense of greater fullness when handled; the wrinkles in the skin become shallower and are effaced, and the teats are materially enlarged. Beginning a few weeks after conception, this tends to a steady development, though slight alterations in the sense of successive growth and shrinkage are not uncommon. In milking cows this does not hold true, as the milk usually tends to a steady diminution and the udder shrinks slowly until near the completion of the period, when it undergoes its sudden, remarkable development and yields at first a serous liquid and then the yellow colostrum, which coagulates when heated. As pregnancy advances the mucous membrane lining the vulva becomes swollen and of a darker, bluish-red hue. The mucous secretion also increases, and becomes very abundant just before calving. When the feeding has not been altered or restricted, a steady diminution of lime is excreted in the urine as the lime is demanded for the growing body of the fetus.

After the fifth month the movements of the calf may often be observed in the right flank, nearly in front of the stifle, when the cow is drinking cold water. The sensation of cold on the side of the first stomach, which lies to the left and directly below the womb (pl. I), stimulates the calf to active movements, which are detected on the sudden jerking outward of the abdominal wall as if from blows delivered from within. In a loose, pendent abdomen in the latter months of gestation the skin may often be seen pushed out at a sharp angle, irrespective of the period of drinking.

Another mode of examination through the flank is by touch. The palm of the hand is pressed strongly inward, about 8 inches in front of the stifle and a little below, several times in succession, and is then brought to rest with the pressure maintained. Presently there are felt distinct and characteristic movements of the fetus, which has been disturbed and roused to action. Another mode is to press the closed fist strongly inward in the same situation and hold it so, forming a deep indentation in the abdominal wall. Presently the knuckles are felt to be struck by a solid body, which is the fetus that has been displaced to the left by the push of the hand and now floats back in its liquid covering (amniotic fluid; see pl. XII) downward and to the right.

Of all the modes of examination by touch, that done through the rectum gives the earliest satisfactory indications. The hand and arm, well oiled, are introduced, and, the excrement having been removed if necessary, the palm of the hand is turned downward and the floor of the pelvis carefully examined. There will be felt in the median line the pear-shaped outline of the bladder, more or less full, rounded, or tense, according to the quantity of urine it contains. Between this and the hand will be felt a soft, somewhat rounded tubular body, which divides in front into two smaller tubes or branches, extending to the right and left into the abdomen. This is the womb, which in its virgin, or unimpregnated, condition is of nearly uniform size from before backward, the main part or body being from 1½ to 2 inches across, and the two anterior branches or horns being individually little over an inch wide. Immediately after conception the body and one of the horns begin to enlarge, the other horn remaining disproportionately small, and the enlargement will be most marked at one point, where a solid, rounded mass indicates the presence of the growing embryo. In case of twins, both horns are enlarged. At a more advanced stage, when the embryo begins to assume the form of the future animal, the rounded form gives place to a more or less irregular nodular mass, while later still the head, legs, and body of the fetus may be distinctly made out. The chief source of fallacy is found in the very pendent abdomen of certain cows, into which in advanced gestation the fetus has dropped so low that it cannot be felt by the hand in the rectum. The absence of the distinct outline of the vacant womb, however, and the clear indications obtained on external examination through the right flank will serve to prevent any mistake. The fetus may still be felt through the rectum if the abdomen is raised by a sheet passed from side to side beneath it.

Still another sign is the beating of the fetal heart, which may be heard in the latter half of pregnancy when the ear is pressed on the flank in front of the right stifle or from that downward to the udder. The beats, which are best heard in the absence of rumbling, are about 120 a minute and easily distinguished from any bowel sounds by their perfect regularity.

DURATION OF PREGNANCY

The average duration of pregnancy in the cow is 285 days. A calf born at the two hundred and fortieth day may live, and a calf born on the three hundred and thirty-fifth day and another in the three hundred and thirty-sixth day have been reported. In most cases of prolonged pregnancies the offspring are males. Although the prevailing tendency is to carry the males overtime, the small and comparatively much less developed females sometimes fail to stimulate the womb to contraction until very far beyond the regular date.

HYGIENE OF THE PREGNANT COW

Among domestic animals considerations of hygiene must be made subservient to profit, and therefore the first consideration is not to obtain the most robust health, but such a measure of vigor and stamina as is compatible with the most profitable utilization of the animal. The breeding cow must carry a calf every year, and this notwithstanding that she is at the same time suckling another large, growing calf. The dairy cow must breed every year and at the same time must furnish a generous flow of milk from 9 to 11 months yearly. If her health is lowered thereby or her life shortened, the question of profit must still hold sway, and, when unprofitable, she must yield her place to another.

There are certain points, however, in which the interests of hygiene may be considered. The pregnant cow should have exercise, and as regards both exercise and feed, nothing is better than a run on a smooth pasture. She should be withheld from all violent excitement, such as being driven by dogs, riding or being ridden by cows in heat, being driven in a herd rapidly through narrow gateways, being forced to jump ditches or fences, subjected to blows with the horns of other cattle, being driven on icy or otherwise slippery ground, being kicked by attendants, or thrown down for operations. The diet should be good, not of a kind to fatten, but with a generous quantity of nitrogenous constituents that will favor both the yield of milk and the nourishment of the fetus. Feeds such as wheat bran or middlings, which are rich in lime and phosphates, can be used to advantage, as there is a constant drain of mineral salts for the building of the body of the calf. Hard, innutritious, and indigestible feeds, musty grain or hay, partly ripened rye grass, millet, Hungarian grass, vetches, peas, or maize are objectionable, as they are likely to cause indigestion or even paralysis; and corn or hay affected by smut or ergot, spoiled by dampness, or overripened and rendered fibrous and innutritious, is equally objectionable. In the main the feed should be laxative, as constipation and straining are likely to cause abortion. Roots and green feed that have been frosted are objectionable, as being likely to cause indigestion, though in their fresh condition they are very wholesome and desirable. Ice-cold water should be avoided, as it may check the flow of milk and derange digestion. A good temperature for the drink of the dairy cow is 55° F.

In the case of the plethoric and heavy-milking cow of mature age and in the prime of life, the hitherto liberal diet must be changed at the last week for the scantiest possible fare, and the bowels must be kept open by laxatives, if need be, if the owner would avoid milk fever. Her stall should not incline downward from shoulder to croup, lest the pressure of the abdominal organs should produce protusion or abortion. Strong purgatives and diuretics are to be especially avoided.

PROTRUSION OF THE VAGINA (PROLAPSUS VAGINAE)

During pregnancy protrusion of the vagina is common from chronic relaxation of the vaginal walls and from lying in stalls that are lower behind than in front. The protrusion is of a rounded form and smooth, and if it embraces both sides of the canal it is double, with a passage between. It may sometimes be remedied by raising the hind part of the stall higher than the front part. If this fails a truss may be applied as for eversion of the womb and worn until the period of calving approaches (pls. XXII, XXIII).

HERNIA (BREACH) OF THE UTERUS

In advanced pregnancy hernia occurs usually from a gradual relaxation and distention of the lower wall of the abdomen in the region of the udder, so that the latter is displaced downward, and in the sac above and in front of it may be felt the form and movements of the fetus. In other cases the womb escapes through a great laceration of the abdominal muscles to one side of the udder, and the hernial mass extends down to one side of the organ. However unsightly, this often allows the animal to complete its pregnancy naturally, and a broad, supporting bandage placed around the abdomen is about all that can be recommended. After calving it is best to fatten the cow for slaughter.

CRAMPS OF THE HIND LEGS

The compression of the nerves by the womb and fetus passing through the pelvis sometimes causes cramp and inability to move the leg, but it disappears under friction and motion and is never seen after calving.

DROPSY OF THE HIND LEGS AND BETWEEN THE THIGHS

In the latter months of pregnancy the hind legs may swell beneath the hocks, or a soft swelling that pits on pressure with the finger appears from the vulva down between the thighs to the udder and in front. It is mainly ascribable to the pressure of the enlarged womb on the blood vessels is not dangerous, and disappears after calving.

DROPSY OF THE MEMBRANES OF THE FETUS (DROPSY OF THE WOMB)

The unimpregnated womb may be filled with a dropsical fluid, but the pregnant womb is more likely to become overdistended by an excess of fluid in the inner water bag in which the fetus floats (pl. XII). From an unhealthy state of this membrane or for other reasons this liquid may go on accumulating until the cow seems almost as broad as she is long. If the trouble has not originated in the ill health of the cow, the result is still to draw on her system, overtax her strength, and derange her digestion, so that the result may prove fatal to both mother and offspring. On the other hand, extreme cases have been known to come to the natural term without help and produce a living calf, after which the dam did well. The natural resort is to draw off a portion of the fluid through a hollow needle passed through the neck of the womb or through its tense wall adjacent. This may be repeated several times, as demanded, to relieve the cow from the injurious distention.

PARALYSIS OF THE HIND PARTS

In ill-fed, weak, unthrifty cows paralysis of the hind legs and tail may appear in the last weeks of pregnancy. The anus and rectum may participate in the paralysis so far as to prevent defecation, and the rectum is more or less completely impacted. Exposure to wet and cold are often accessory causes. The affected animals should be provided with a warm, dry bed, an abundant warm diet, and should be rubbed with straw wisps or with a liniment of equal parts of oil of turpentine and sweet oil on the loins, croup, and legs. The case becomes increasingly hopeful after calving, though some days may still elapse before the animal can support herself upon her legs.

EXTRAUTERINE GESTATION (FETUS DEVELOPING OUTSIDE THE WOMB)

These curious cases are rare and are usually divided into three types: (1) That in which the fetus is formed in or on the ovary (ovarian gestation); (2) that in which it is lodged in the Fallopian tube, or canal between the ovary and womb (tubal gestation); and (3) that in which it is lodged in the abdominal cavity and attached to one or more of its contents from which it draws its nourishment (abdominal gestation). Undoubted cases of the first and last varieties are recorded as occurring in the cow. The explanation of such cases is that the actively moving sperm cells (spermatozoa) entering the womb have made their way through the Fallopian tubes to the ovary. If they met and impregnated an ovum in the tube, and if the consequent growth of that ovum prevented its descent and caused its imprisonment within the tube, it developed there, and became attached to and drew nourishment from the mucous walls. Its development then may be arrested by compression by the undilatable tube, or, bursting through the walls of the tube, it escapes into the abdomen and perishes. If, on the contrary, the spermatozoa only meet and impregnate the ovum on or in the ovary, the development may take place in the substance of the ovary, from which the fetus draws its nourishment, or the impregnated ovum, escaping between the ovary and the open end of the tube, falls into the abdominal cavity and becomes adherent to and draws nourishment from some of the abdominal organs (womb, bowel, liver, stomach, or other organ).

Symptoms.—The symptoms are those of pregnancy, which may be suddenly complicated by inflammation (peritonitis), owing to rupture of the sac containing the fetus; or at full term signs of calving appear, but no progress is made; an examination with the oiled hand in the vagina or rectum finds the womb empty and its mouth closed. Further examination will disclose the fetal sac attached in some part of the abdominal cavity and containing the more or less perfectly developed body of a calf. In the most hopeful cases the fetus perishes at an early stage of gestation, becomes enclosed in a fibrous sac, and is slowly absorbed, its soft parts becoming liquefied and removed and the bones remaining encysted. In some cases the bones have finally sloughed into the rectum or through an artificial opening in the side of the belly.

Treatment.—Little can be done in such cases except to quiet pain and excitement by anodynes (chloral or similar drug) and leave the rest to nature. A fistula discharging bones may be dilated and the bones extracted, the sac being then washed out with a solution of 10 grains of bichloride of mercury in a quart of water. In certain cases

77431 O—51——11

with a live calf, a veterinarian may be justified in cutting into the abdomen and extracting the calf with its membranes.

PROLONGED RETENTION OF THE FETUS

Even when the fetus has developed within the womb it may fail to be delivered at the proper time; labor pains have quickly subsided and the cow resumed her usual health. In such cases the calf dies. Its soft parts are gradually liquefied and absorbed, whereas its bones become enclosed in the remains of the fetal membranes. These may be expelled at any time through the natural channels, or they may remain indefinitely in the womb, not interfering with the general health but preventing conception.

If the condition is recognized at the time of the subsidence of the labor pains, the mouth of the womb may be dilated by the fingers, by the insertion of sponge tents, or by a mechanical dilator (pl. XX, fig. 6), the fetal membranes may be ruptured, and the calf extracted. After the removal of the calf and its membranes the danger of putrid poisoning may be obviated by injecting an antiseptic solution.

ABORTION (SLINKING OF THE CALF)

Technically, abortion is the term used for the expulsion of the offspring before it can live out of the womb. Its expulsion before the normal time, but after it is capable of an independent existence, is premature parturition. In the cow this may be after 7½ months of pregnancy. Cattle owners commonly use the term "abortion" for the expulsion of a dead or weak calf that is not carried to the full term.

Abortion in cows is either infectious or noninfectious. It does not follow that infection is the only cause in every case of infectious abortion. The germs (microbes) of infection vary greatly in virulence at different times, and the animal system also varies in susceptibility to their attack. The causative germ may, therefore, be present in a herd without any manifest injury, its disease-producing power having for the time abated considerably, or the whole herd being in a condition of comparative insusceptibility. At other times the same germ may have become so virulent that few pregnant cows escape its effects, or the herd may have been subjected to other causes of abortion which, though of themselves powerless to cause serious trouble, may yet so predispose the animals that even the weaker germ will operate with destructive effect. In dealing with this disease, therefore, it is the part of wisdom not to be satisfied merely with the discovery and removal of one specific cause, but rather to try to find every existent cause and to obtain a remedy by correcting all the harmful conditions.

NONINFECTIOUS ABORTION

Poor condition and weakness are sometimes predisposing causes of noninfectious abortion. This in its turn may result from poor or insufficient feed, from excessive drain on the system while rearing the previous calf, from the use of feed deficient in certain essential elements, and from chronic wasting diseases. In some cases the nourishment is so deficient that the fetus dies in the womb and is expelled in consequence. Excessive loss of blood, attended as it usually is with shock, becomes a direct cause of abortion.

Acute inflammations of important organs are sometimes causes of abortion, and in most contagious fevers it is a common result. Affections of the chest that prevent due aeration of the blood induce contractions of the womb.

Ergoted grasses have long been considered responsible for abortion in cows. The ergot is familiar as the dark purple or black, hard, spurlike growths that protrude from the seeds of the grasses at the period of their ripening (pl. V). It is especially common in damp localities and cloudy seasons on meadows shaded by trees and protected against the free sweep of the winds. The same is to a large extent true of smut.

The riding of one another by cows is attended by such severe muscular exertion, jars, jolts, mental excitement, and gravitation of the womb and abdominal organs backward that it may occasionally cause abortion in a predisposed animal.

Keeping cows in stalls that slope too much behind (more than 2 inches) acts in the same way, the compression from lying and the gravitation backward pressing more than a predisposed cow can safely bear.

Deep gutters behind the stalls, into which one or both hind legs slip unexpectedly, strain the loins and jar the body and womb injuriously. Slippery stalls in which the flooring boards are laid longitudinally in place of transversely, and on which there is no device to give a firm foothold, are almost equally dangerous. Driving on icy ground, or through a narrow doorway where the abdomen is likely to be jammed, are other probable causes. Aborting cows often fail to expel the afterbirth, and if this remains hanging in a putrid condition it may be a menace to pregnant cows in the near vicinity. The same is true of retained afterbirth in other cows after calving normally. The excitement, jarring, and jolting of a railroad journey may occasionally cause abortion, especially as the cow nears the period of calving.

Irritant poisons may cause abortions by the disorder and inflammation of the digestive organs, and if such agents act also on the kidneys or womb, the effect may be enhanced. Powerful purgatives or diuretics should never be administered to pregnant cows.

Among other causes of abortion are the death or the various illnesses of the fetus, the slipping of a young fetus through a loop in the navel string so as to tie a knot that will tighten later and interrupt the flow of blood with fatal effect, and the twisting of the navel string by the turning of the fetus until little or no blood can flow through the contorted cord. There is in addition a series of diseases of the mucous membrane of the womb and of the fetal membranes (inflammation, effusion of blood, detachment of the membranes from the womb, fatty or other degenerations), that interfere with the supply of blood to the fetus or change its quality so that death is the natural result, followed by abortion.

Treatment.—Even if the first symptoms of abortion have appeared, it does not necessarily follow that it will go on to completion. So long as the fetus has not perished, if the waters have not been discharged, nor the water bags presented, attempts should be made to check its progress. Every appreciable and removable cause should be done away with, the cow should be placed in a quiet stall alone, and agents given to check the excitement of the labor pains. Use potassium bromide or, better, extract of *Viburnum prunifolium* (black haw), 40 grains, at intervals of 2 or 3 hours until five or six doses have been given.

BRUCELLOSIS (BANG'S DISEASE, INFECTIOUS ABORTION)

Brucellosis, also known as Bang's disease, infectious abortion, contagious abortion, abortion disease, and slinking of the calf, is an affection especially prevalent in cattle but occurs to a lesser degree in other domestic animals. It is characterized by an inflammatory condition of the female reproductive organs, which results in the expulsion of the immature young.

History.—This disease has been known in England and continental Europe for many years, and descriptions of it are given in the writings of various investigators. In the early part of the nineteenth century the infectiousness of the disease was recognized, but it was not until 1876 that the disease was produced in healthy, pregnant cows by the introduction of exudate and material from aborting animals. In 1896 Bang, assisted by Stribolt, published their findings regarding infectious abortion of cattle, in which they incriminated a short bacillus as the causative agent. With pure cultures of this bacillus they were able to produce the disease artificially and to recover the same organism from the experimental cases. Since that time many investigators, both in this country and in Europe, have confirmed these findings. For a number of years the germ of

Bang's discovery was known as the bacillus of Bang, or Bang's bacillus.

It was later found to bear a close resemblance to a germ previously discovered by Bruce in the milk of goats on the Isle of Malta. Both germs are now considered as belonging to the same genus, the one of Bang's discovery being known as *Brucella abortus*, and Bruce's as *Br. melitensis*. A third similar germ, known as *Br. suis*, was recovered by Traum in 1914 from swine.

Cause.—Br. abortus is now generally recognized as the causative agent of the disease in cattle.

Natural mode of infection.—This phase of the disease is of greatest importance for a clear understanding of the methods of prevention. Many investigators have demonstrated that the infection is transmitted through the digestive tract by means of contaminated feed and water. The germs are taken up by the body from the intestines with the liquid nourishment, reach the blood, and are carried to the genital organs and udder, where they find conditions best suited to their development.

Brucellosis may occasionally be transmitted from animal to animal by direct contact. Experimentally the disease can be transmitted to susceptible cattle by depositing a small quantity of *Br. abortus* infection on the mucous membrane surrounding the eyeball and also by applying it to the skin whether slightly abraded or intact.

The belief long entertained that the female acquires the disease at the time of copulation as a result of transference of the infection from affected to healthy females on the genital organs of the bull has failed to receive the support of experimental evidence. The view that the disease is spread to any great degree in this way has been largely discredited. Pregnant cows of all ages are more or less susceptible, but young ones in first or second pregnancy seem to contract the disease most readily.

Symptoms.—Brucellosis is a very insidious malady. It develops slowly through several months of the gestation period and results finally in the expulsion of the immature young, this act being simply an indication of the presence of the disease and not the disease itself. Because of this slow development and the fact that the health of the animal is not noticeably influenced, the presence of the disease may not be suspected until it has gained a firm foothold in the herd. The symptoms of approaching abortion are often similar to those preceding normal calving. In addition, there may be observed, a few days previous to abortion, a sticky, sometimes purulent, rusty, and odorless discharge. Abortion occurs most frequently from the third to the seventh month. Calves sometimes are carried almost to full term and are born alive but are sickly and soon die. After abortion there is a dirty, yellowish-gray mucopurulent discharge that persists for 2 or more weeks. If abortion occurs early, the fetus is likely to be surrounded by its membranes, but if late in the period of pregnancy, the membranes are usually retained. Aborting animals are often rendered sterile temporarily, if not permanently.

Lesions.—The most characteristic change is in the uterus in which a dark-brown fluid, purulent or even gluey in consistence and containing grayish-white flakes, separates the maternal membranes from those of the fetus, and prevents that intimate contact between the two which is so necessary for the interchange of fluids and gases by which the fetus is nourished and by which it obtains its oxygen. These being cut off, the fetus dies. The germs producing the disease are found in greatest numbers at this point. In addition there may be inflammatory changes, first in the walls of the uterus and then in the tissues of the fetus. These inflammatory changes seem most intense in the cotyledons and result in the destruction of the minute structure of those bodies, and they appear swollen, pale, and soft. The membrane of the uterus between the cotyledons also may show inflamed and necrotic patches.

Complications.—Serious results sometimes follow abortion, particularly when there is retained afterbirth. The retained membranes decompose, the poisonous products of decomposition and the organisms of decomposition themselves are absorbed, blood poisoning results, and the animal dies. Sometimes, when the animal is able to resist the effects of this decomposition, the uterus becomes the seat of such severe changes that sterility results. The walls of that organ become thickened and hard, the lining membranes become eroded, and conception cannot take place. At other times the ovaries, where the reproductive cells originate, become affected and lose their function. Abortion does not invariably follow infection. The calf may be carried to full term and in these cases retained afterbirth is a common occurrence, even to the extent that frequent retention of afterbirth in a herd may be taken as an indication of the presence of the disease. Suppurative processes often persist for a long time, prevent conception, or sterility may result without apparent cause. A sterile cow is valueless for any purpose except beef. Such an animal may be a source of infection for the others and should not be allowed to remain in the herd.

Diagnosis.—Although the only certain way of determining whether an animal has the disease is to isolate the causative micro-organism from its body, a more practical way of diagnosing the disease in large numbers of animals consists in subjecting their blood to the agglutination test. It is possible, through the use of this test, to determine with reasonable accuracy whether or not animals are affected with the disease. The test sometimes fails to detect cases of recent infection, and it likewise fails to differentiate sharply between infected animals and those that have spontaneously recovered from the disease. The test has nevertheless been widely used as a means of detecting diseased animals in infected herds and of enabling owners to eradicate the disease by the removal of reacting animals.

Treatment.—There is no drug, chemical, or medicinal compound that has been proved to be effective in the prevention or cure of brucellosis. Much effort has been spent by various laboratories and experiment stations to find some substance that could penetrate the tissues invaded by the *Brucella* organisms in a concentration sufficient to destroy the organisms without harmful effect on the tissues themselves. A number of different chemicals and compounds that have proved to be effective in various other diseases were tried in brucellosis, but none proved successful. In 1939 sulfanilamide, a chemical substance that has been very effective in the treatment of streptococcic infections and that has been reported as beneficial in the treatment of brucellosis in man, was tried in cattle with *Brucella* infection of the udder. However, with a concentration in the blood of only slightly less than toxic quantities, the drug had no apparent action in destroying the *Brucella* organisms or reducing their virulence.

Medicinal substances for the treatment of this disease have gained their popularity almost entirely because they were used and their value was judged at a time when the disease had passed its active stage, that is, when the wave of abortions has ceased. If a medicine is used after a cow has aborted credit is likely to be given to the medicine when the animal fails to abort on her next pregnancy, whereas this cessation of abortion was a natural sequence in the disease.

Several widely advertised "cures" or "remedies," for which numerous testimonials were submitted, have been tested under controlled conditions and have been found worthless in the prevention or cure of brucellosis of cattle.

Following abortion or full-term pregnancy in the infected animal, a more or less heavy, persistent discharge from the uterus occurs. Nature may be assisted in relieving this condition by douching the uterus with mild, nonirritating antiseptics or preferably with a solution of common table salt in water in the proportion of 1 ounce of salt to a gallon of water. When douchings are made, boiled water cooled to body temperature with the salt added should be used and all utensils should also be boiled both before and after being used. Care should be taken that the washings from the uterus and the vagina are not expelled in a place to which cattle have access.

After abortion or full-term pregnancy in an infected animal, it may be some time before the inflammation in the walls of the uterus subsides and it is therefore advisable to allow several months' rest before the animal is bred again.

Control.—It is doubtful whether any one method of dealing with infected herds is well adapted to the needs of every herd owner or will be satisfactory with all degrees of infection. Several advantageous methods, therefore, are described.

Test-and-slaughter method.—This method calls for the repeated testing of herds and the prompt elimination for slaughter of the reacting animals. In herds in which the disease is active, the plan may require the sacrifice of many more animals than the results of the original test indicate. This method is likely to be most successful and practical in herds having a low percentage of reactors, those in which the breeding or milk-producing value of the animals is not greatly in excess of their value for beef, and in herds in which the disease is only mildly active.

Test-and-segregation method.—This method, likewise, requires the repeated testing of herds but for the prompt segregation of the reactors rather than the disposal of them for slaughter. It thus permits valuable blood lines to be preserved. It is sometimes practiced at no great additional expense to the owners, and enables them to eliminate reacting animals more gradually and in such a manner as not to affect profits seriously. This method is specially appropriate in larger herds that have access to two or more buildings. Although the herd is separated in accordance with the results of the original test, it is necessary that the nonreacting group of animals be tested at intervals of 30 to 60 days in order that subsequent reactors may be detected and promptly removed before they become sources of infection.

Sanitary management.—Herd owners who are unable to dispose of reactors promptly or even to segregate them can naturally expect to derive some benefit from a system of sanitary management that gives consideration to reducing rather than entirely eliminating the *Brucella abortus* exposure to which the animals of a herd are subjected. This method calls for the temporary isolation of the diseased animals during those times when they are most menacing as spreaders of the causative germs. Make frequent observations of all animals for signs of aborting, such as swelling of the external genitals or udder enlargement, and when such an animal is discovered, place her immediately in a separate stall well away from other stock. If an abortion occurs unexpectedly, isolate the animal in the same manner as soon as the discovery is made. Bury or completely destroy the fetus and afterbirth if the latter has been expelled. Clean and apply disinfectant solutions to areas that may have been grossly contaminated by the abortion products. Place all pregnant animals in individual stalls a week or 10 days before calving and confine them to their calving quarters for a month after calving and as long afterward as uterine discharges can be detected. Avoid carrying germ-laden material from maternity stalls to other parts of premises on hands or clothing. The footwear of the attendant should be well scrubbed with a disinfectant solution after he has been in an infected stall. Refrain from breeding cows for at least 2 months after calving or aborting. Keep aborting animals isolated for 6 weeks to 2 months. Cows with uterine discharges should always be kept away from the rest of the herd, whether they have aborted or not, until they have recovered. Dispose of the bedding used by infected or suspected animals in such a manner as to render it inaccessible to stock free from the disease.

The best results from sanitary management have been obtained in those herds to which no cows nor heifers other than those raised in the herd were added. There are reasons for believing that the introduction even of animals that have never come in contact with the germs may be a detriment. Such animals may acquire the disease more readily than those raised in the herd as the latter have developed increased resistance to the disease through repeated exposure to the casual organisms.

Vaccination.—As a result of many years' experience with vaccine in the prevention of brucellosis, it has been found that the vaccination of calves between 4 and 8 months of age with a *Brucella* germ of reduced virulence is very effective in preventing infection and abortion when these animals as adults receive exposure in infected herds. The vaccination of adult cattle negative to the agglutination test is as effective as in calves. Unfortunately, however, a substance known as agglutinin, which is found in the blood after an animal has been vaccinated, tends to persist in adults, whereas in calves it usually disappears within 6 to 12 months after vaccination. Agglutinin is also found in the blood of naturally infected animals. It is evident, therefore, that the vaccination of adult animals would interfere with all methods of control based on a positive reaction to the agglutination test.

Vaccine should be administered only by veterinarians. Many States have regulations governing the use of vaccine and for that reason it should not be used until permission has been obtained from State livestock sanitary officials or the State veterinarian.

More detailed information concerning brucellosis will be found in Farmers' Bulletin 1871, which may be obtained from the United States Department of Agriculture, Washington, D. C.

INFECTIOUS VAGINITIS (INFECTIOUS GRANULAR VAGINITIS)

The affection to which the foregoing names have been given is a chronic, mild, and apparently contagious disease of cattle, characterized by an inflammatory condition of the mucous membrane of the vagina and the development of nodules on its surface.

This disease is very widespread, but from an economic point of view it does not appear to have great significance. It has been asserted that it is difficult to find a single herd in this country which is free of this disease and that granular vaginitis has a vital relation to abortion. This view, however, has not been substantiated, it being generally accepted that the disease is only rarely responsible for abortion, and further, that it exerts no apparent ill effects on the health of the animal and that it has no effect on the milk yield.

Symptoms.—Natural infection may take place either by direct contact of animals or at the time of service. Most of the cows in the affected herd contract the disease, but the bulls are rarely or very mildly affected. The inflamed condition of the membranes of the vagina results in a catarrhal exudate, and this discharge, which soils the external genitals and the tail, and the uneasiness and sometimes the straining of the animal, are the first and most prominent symptoms observed. On examination, small, hard, grayish nodules can be seen and felt on the inflamed membranes. This acute stage may last for 3 to 4 weeks, then it gradually subsides and assumes the chronic form, only to flare up again as the animal comes in heat.

These nodules are sometimes found on the membranes of the uterus, and some investigators have argued from this fact that it was responsible for abortion and sterility. Others, however, deny this and point out that the *Brucella abortus* can be demonstrated in nearly every case. The importance of the disease is therefore in dispute and the decision must be left to future investigation.

Treatment.—The exaggerated importance that has been attached to this disease resulted in the exploitation of the most varied kinds of remedies for its treatment. It is true that with a protracted and laborious treatment it is possible to effect cures in 1 to 3 months, but with our present knowledge of this disorder it is advisable to limit the treatment to animals that have an acute inflammatory condition of the vagina and vulva with a discharge as a result of the granular affection. The treatment should be local and confined to the application of washes in the form of irrigations. For this purpose a solution of table salt and baking soda, 1 tablespoonful each, in a gallon of warm boiled water is as satisfactory as stronger douches. Daily irrigations should be made until the condition shows improvement.

PARTURITION (CALVING)

SYMPTOMS OF CALVING

In the cow the premonitions of calving are the enlargement of the udder, which becomes firm and resistant to the touch, with more or less swelling in front, and yields a serous, milky fluid; the enlargement and swelling of the vulva, which discharges an abundant, stringy mucus; the drooping of the belly, and the falling in of the muscles at each side of the root of the tail, so as to leave deep hollows. When this last symptom is seen, calving may be counted on in 24 hours or in 2 to 3 days. When the act is imminent the cow becomes uneasy, moves restlessly, stops eating, separates from the herd, lies down and rises again as if in pain, shifts upon her hind feet, moves the tail, and may bellow or moan. When labor pains come on the back is arched, the croup drooped, the belly is drawn up, and straining is more or less violent and continuous. Meanwhile blood may have appeared on the vulva and tail, and soon the clear water bags protrude between the lips of the vulva. They increase rapidly, hanging down toward the hocks, and the fore or hind feet can be detected within them. With the rupture of the bags and escape of the waters the womb contracts on the solid, angular body of the fetus and is at once stimulated to more violent contractions, so that the work proceeds with redoubled energy to the complete expulsion. This is why it is wrong to rupture the water bags if the presentation is normal, as they furnish a soft, uniform pressure for the preliminary dilation of the mouth of the womb and passages, in anticipation of the severe strain put on them as the solid body of the calf passes.

The cow often calves standing, in which case the navel string is broken as the calf falls to the ground. If, however, she is recumbent, this cord is torn through as she rises. The afterpains come on 3 or 4 hours later and expel the membranes.

NATURAL PRESENTATION

When there is but one calf the natural presentation is that of the forefeet with the front of the hoofs and knees turned upward toward the tail of the dam and the nose lying between the knees (pl. XV). If there are twins the natural position of the second is that of the hind feet, the heels and hocks turned upward toward the cow's tail (pl. XVIII, fig. 1). In both of these natural positions the curvature of the body of the calf—the back arched upward—is the same with the curvature of the passages, which descend anteriorly into the womb, ascend over the brim of the pelvis, and descend again toward the external opening (vulva). Any presentation differing from the above is abnormal.

OBSTACLES TO PARTURITION

With a well-formed cow and calf and a natural presentation, as just described, calving is usually prompt and easy. Obstacles, however, may come from failure of the mouth of the womb to dilate; from twisting the neck of the womb; from tumors in the vagina; from dropsy in the womb or abdomen; from overdistention of the rectum or bladder; from undue narrowing of the passages; from excess of fat in the walls of the pelvis; from the disturbance of a nervous cow by noises; from stone or urine in the bladder; from wrong presentation of the calf, its back being turned downward or to one side in place of upward toward the spine of the dam; from the bending backward of one or more legs or of the head into the body of the womb; from presentation of the back, shoulder, or croup, all four legs being turned back; from presentation of all four feet at once; from obstruction caused by an extra head or extra legs or double body on the part of the offspring (pl. XIX); from dropsy or other disease of the calf; from excessive or imperfect development of the calf; from the impaction of twins into the passages at the same time; or at times it may be from the mere excessive volume of the fetus.

GENERAL MAXIMS FOR THE ASSISTANT CONCERNING DIFFICULT PARTURITION

Do not interfere too soon. After labor pains set in, give a reasonable time for the water bags to protrude and burst spontaneously, and interfere only when delay suggests some mechanical obstruction. If there is no mechanical obstruction, let the calf be expelled slowly by the unaided efforts of the cow. Bruises and lacerations of the passages and flooding from the uncontracted womb may come from the too speedy extraction of the calf. When assistance is necessary, the operator should dress in a thick flannel shirt from which the sleeves have been cut off clear to the shoulders. This leaves the whole arm free. Before inserting the hand, it and the arm should be smeared with oil, lard, or petrolatum, care being taken that the oil or lard is fresh, neither salted nor rancid, and that it has been purified by boiling or rendered antiseptic by the addition of a teaspoonful of carbolic acid to the pound. This is a valuable precaution against infecting the cow by introducing infection into the passages and against poisoning of the arm by decomposing discharges in case the calving is unduly protracted. When labor pains have lasted some time without any signs of the water bags, the dropping in at the sides of the rump, and the other preparations for calving being accomplished, the hand should be introduced to examine. When the water bags have burst and neither feet nor head appear for some time, examination should be made. When one forefoot only and the head appear, or both forefeet without the head, or the head without the forefeet, examine. If one hind foot appears without the other, make examination. The presenting leg or head should be secured by a rope with a running noose, so that it may not pass back into the womb and get lost during the subsequent manipulations, but may be retained in the vagina or brought up again easily. In searching for a missing member it is usually better to turn the head of the cow downhill, so that the gravitation of the fetus and abdominal organs forward into the belly of the cow may give more room in which to bring up the missing leg or head. If the cow is lying down, turn her on the side opposite to that on which the leg is missing, so that there may be more room for bringing the latter up. Even if a missing leg is reached, it is vain to attempt to bring it up during a labor pain. Wait until the pain has ceased and attempt to straighten out the leg before the next pain comes on. If the pains are violent and continuous, they may be checked by pinching the back or by putting a tight surcingle around the body in front of the udder. These failing, 1 ounce or 1½ ounces of chloral hydrate in a quart of water may be given to check the pains. If the passages have dried up or lost their natural, lubricating liquid, smear the interior of the passages and womb and the surface of the calf, as far as it can be reached, with pure fresh lard; or pure sweet oil may be run into the womb through a rubber tube (fountain syringe). In dragging on the fetus apply strong traction only while the mother is straining and drag downward toward the hocks as well as backward. The natural curvature of both fetus and passages is thus followed and the extraction rendered easier.

LABOR PAINS BEFORE RELAXATION OF THE PASSAGES

Any of the various causes of abortion may bring on labor pains before time. Straining comes on days or weeks before time, and there is not the usual enlargement, swelling, and mucous discharge from the vulva. There is little or no falling in by the sides of the root of the tail; the abdomen has not dropped to the usual extent, and the udder is less developed and yields little or no milk. In spite of the pains no water bags appear, and the oiled hand cautiously introduced into the vagina finds the neck of the womb firmly closed, rigid, and undilatable. If it is known that the cow has not reached her proper time of calving, the examination through the vagina should be omitted and the animal should be placed in a dark, quiet place by herself, and be given fluid extract of *Viburnum prunifolium* (blackhaw), 1 ounce, if necessary, and repeated in 3 hours. The pains will usually subside.

In some instances the external parts are relaxed and duly prepared, but the neck of the womb remains rigidly closed. In such case the solid extract of belladonna should be smeared around the constricted opening and the animal left quiet until it relaxes.

DISEASED INDURATION OF THE MOUTH OF THE WOMB

From previous lacerations or other injuries the neck of the womb may have become the seat of fibrous hardening and constriction, so as to prevent its dilatation, when all other parts are fully prepared for calving. The enlarged, flabby vulva, the sinking at each side of the rump, the full udder, and drooping abdomen indicate the proper time for calving, but the labor pains effect no progress in the dilatation of the mouth of the womb, and the oiled hand introduced detects the rigid, hard, and, in some cases, nodular feeling of the margins of the closed orifice that no application of belladonna or other antispasmodic suffices to relax. Sponge tents may be inserted or the mechanical dilator (pl. XX, fig. 6) may be used if there is opening enough to admit it, and if not, a narrow-bladed, probe-pointed knife (pl. XXIV, fig. 2) may be passed through the orifice and turned upward, downward, and to each side, cutting to a depth not exceeding a quarter of an inch in each case. This done, a finger may be inserted, then two, three, and four, and finally all four fingers and thumb brought together in the form of a cone and made to push in with rotary motion until the whole hand can be introduced. After this the labor pains will induce further dilation, and finally the presenting members of the calf will complete the process.

TWISTING OF THE NECK OF THE WOMB

This is rather common in the cow, the length of the body of the womb and the looseness of the broad ligaments that attach it to the walls of the pelvis favoring the twisting. It is as if one were to take a long sack rather loosely filled at the neck and turn its closed end over, so that its twisting should occur in the neck. The twist may be one-quarter round, so that the upper surface would come to one side, or it may be half round, so that what was the upper surface becomes the lower. The relation of the womb of the cow to the upper and right side of the paunch favors the twisting. The paunch occupies the whole left side of the abdomen and extends across its floor to the right side. Its upper surface thus forms an inclined plane, sloping from the left downward and to the right, and on this sloping surface lies the pregnant womb.

It is easy to see how, in the constant movements of the paunch upon its contents and the frequent changes of position of the growing fetus within the womb, to say nothing of the contractions of the adjacent bowels and the more or less active movements of the cow, the womb should roll downward to the right. Yet in many cases the twist is toward the left, showing that it is not the result of a simple rolling downward over the paunch, but rather of other disturbances. The condition may be suspected when labor pains have continued for some time without any sign of the water bags, and it is confirmed when the oiled hand, introduced through the vagina, finds the mouth of the womb soft and yielding but furnished with internal folds running forward in a spiral manner. If the folds on the upper wall of the orifice run toward the right, the womb is twisted to the right; if, on the contrary, they turn toward the left, it indicates that the womb is turned in that direction. The direction of the twist must be known before treatment can be undertaken. Then, if the twist is toward the right, the cow is laid on her right side with her head downhill, the hand of the operator is introduced through the spirally constricted neck of the womb, and a leg or other portion of the body of the calf is seized and pressed firmly against the wall of the womb. Meanwhile, two or three assistants roll the cow from her right side over on her back to her left side. The object is to hold the womb and calf still while the body of the cow rolls over. If successful, the twist is undone, its grasp on the wrist is slackened, and the water bags and calf press into the now open passage. If the first attempt does not succeed, it should be repeated until success has been attained. If the spiral folds on the upper wall of the opening turn toward the left, the cow is laid on her left side and rolled over on her back and on to her right side, the hand being, as before, within the womb and holding the fetus, so that all may not rotate with the cow. In introducing the hand it will usually be necessary to perforate the membranes, so that a leg of the calf may be seized direct and firmly held. Among occasional causes of failure with these cases have been first, the previous death and decomposition of the fetus, leading to such overdistention of the womb that it could not be made to rotate within the abdomen, and, second, the occurrence of inflammation and an exudate on the twisted neck of the womb, which hindered it from untwisting.

In obstinate cases, in which the hand can be made to pass through the neck of the womb easily, additional help may be had from the use of the instrument shown in plate XX, figure 5. Two cords, with running nooses, are successively introduced and made fast on two legs of the calf; the cords are then passed through the two rings on the end of the instrument, which is passed into the womb and the cords drawn tight and fixed round the handle. Then, by the use of the handle as a lever, it is turned in the direction opposite to the twist. The hand meanwhile should be introduced into the womb and the snared legs seized and pressed against its walls so as to obtain the rotation of the uterus along with the body of the fetus. The relaxation of the constriction and the effacement of the spiral folds will show when success has been gained, and the different members at one end of the body should then be brought up so as to obtain a natural presentation.

NARROW PELVIS FROM FRACTURE OR DISEASE

In a small cow the pelvis may be too narrow to pass a calf sired by a bull of a large breed, but this is exceptional, as the fetus usually accommodates itself to the size of the dam and makes its extra growth after birth. When the pelvic bones have been fractured repair takes place with the formation of a large permanent callus, which, projecting internally, may be a serious obstacle to calving. Worse still, if the edge of the broken bone projects internally as a sharp spike or ridge, the vaginal walls are cut on it during the passage of the calf, with serious or fatal result. In other cases, in which the cow has suffered from fragility of bone, the thickening of the bone causes narrowing of the long passage of the pelvis, and the crumbling fractures poorly repaired with an excess of brittle new material may form an insuperable obstacle to parturition. Cows affected in any of these ways should never again be bred, but if they become pregnant and reach full time a careful examination will be necessary to determine whether natural parturition can take place or whether the calf must be extracted in pieces. (See Embryotomy, p. 178.)

OBSTRUCTION BY MASSES OF FAT

This is not unknown in old cows of the beef breeds, the enormous masses of fat on and within the pelvis being associated with weakness or fatty degeneration of the muscles. If the presentation is natural, little more is needed than judicious traction on the fetus to compress and overcome the soft, resisting masses.

OBSTRUCTION BY A FULL BLADDER OR RECTUM OR BY STONE

In all cases of delayed or tardy parturition the evacuation of the rectum and the bladder is important, and it is no less so in all difficult parturitions. Stone in the bladder is rare in the cow, but when present it should be removed to obviate crushing and perhaps perforation of the organ during calving.

CALVING RETARDED BY NERVOUSNESS

There is a case on record of a cow at a public fairground having labor pains beginning early in the day and keeping up in a weak and insufficient manner for many hours. When the stall was closed and the cow secluded from the constant stream of visitors and the incessant noise, the pains became strong and effective and the calf was soon born.

COAGULATED BLOOD UNDER THE VAGINAL WALLS

This is common after calving but sometimes occurs before, as the result of accidental injury. The mass may be recognized by its dark hue and the doughy sensation to the touch. It may be cut into and the mass turned out with the fingers, after which it should be washed frequently with an antiseptic lotion (1 dram of carbolic acid in 1 quart of water).

CONSTRICTION OF A MEMBER BY THE NAVEL STRING

In early fetal life the winding of the navel string around a leg may cause the latter to be slowly cut off by absorption under the constricting cord. So at calving the cord wound round a presenting member may retard progress somewhat, and though the calf may still be born tardily by the unaided efforts of the mother, it is likely to be stillborn, because the circulation in the cord is interrupted by compression before the offspring can reach the open air and commence to breathe. If, therefore, it is possible to anticipate and prevent this displacement and compression of the navel string it should be done, but if this is no longer possible, then the extraction of the calf should be effected as rapidly as possible, and if breathing is not at once attempted it should be started by artificial means.

WATER IN THE HEAD OF THE CALF (HYDROCEPHALUS)

This is an enormous distention of the cavity holding the brain, by reason of the accumulation of liquid in the internal cavities (ventricles) of the brain substance. The head back of the eyes rises into a great rounded ball (pl. XIX, figs. 4 and 5), which proves to be an insuperable obstacle to parturition. The forefeet and nose being the parts presented, no progress can be made, and even if the feet are pulled on, the nose cannot by any means be made to appear. The oiled hand introduced into the passages will feel the nose presenting between the forelegs, and on passing the hand back over the face the hard, rounded mass of the cranium is met with. A sharp-pointed knife or a cannula and trocar should be introduced in the palm of the hand and pushed into the center of the rounded mass so as to evacuate the water. The hand is now used to press together the hitherto distended but thin and fragile walls, and the calf may be delivered in the natural way. If the enlarged head is turned backward it must still be reached and punctured, after which it must be brought up into position and the calf delivered.

If the hind feet present first, all may go well until the body and shoulders have passed out, when further progress is suddenly arrested by the great bulk of the head. If possible, the hand, armed

77431 O—51——12

with a knife or trocar, must be passed along the side of the shoulder or neck so as to reach and puncture the distended head. Failing in this, the body may be skinned up from the belly and cut in two at the shoulder or neck, after which the head can easily be reached and punctured. If in such case the forelegs have been left in the womb, they may now be brought up into the passage, and when dragged upon the collapsed head will follow.

If the distention is not sufficient to have rendered the bony walls of the cranium thin and fragile, so that they can be compressed with the hand after puncture, a special method may be necessary. A long incision should be made from behind forward in the median line of the cranium with an embryotomy knife (pl. XXI, fig. 1) or with a long embryotome (pl. XX, fig. 3). By this means the bones on the one side are completely separated from those on the other and may be made to overlap and perhaps to flatten down. If this fails they may be cut from the head all around the base of the rounded cranial swelling by means of a guarded chisel (pl. XX, fig. 8) and mallet, after which there will be no difficulty in causing them to collapse.

DROPSY OF THE ABDOMEN OF THE CALF (ASCITES)

This is less frequent than hydrocephalus, but no less difficult to deal with. With an anterior presentation the forelegs and head may come away easily enough, but no effort will advance the calf beyond the shoulders. The first thought should be dropsy of the belly, and the oiled hand introduced by the side of the chest will detect the soft and fluctuating yet tense sac of the abdomen. If there is space to allow the introduction of an embryotomy knife, the abdomen may be freely cut with it, when the fluid will escape into the womb and parturition may proceed naturally. If this cannot be effected, a long trocar and cannula may be passed between the first two ribs and straight on beneath the spine until it punctures the abdomen (pl. XVIII, fig. 2). Then the trocar is to be withdrawn and the liquid will flow through the cannula and will be hastened by traction on the forelegs. In the absence of the trocar and cannula, two or three of the first ribs may be cut from the breastbone, so that the hand may be introduced through the chest to puncture the diaphragm with an embryotomy knife and allow an escape of the water. In some slighter cases a tardy delivery may take place without puncture, the liquid bulging forward into the chest as the abdomen is compressed in the pelvic passages. With a posterior presentation the abdomen may be punctured more easily either in the flank or with a trocar and cannula through the anus.

GENERAL DROPSY OF THE CALF

This occurs from disease of some internal organ, such as the liver or kidney, and is recognized by the general puffed-up and rounded condition of the body, which pits everywhere on pressure but without crackling. If not too extreme a case, the calf may be extracted after it has been very generally punctured over the body, but usually the only resort is to extract it in pieces. (See Embryotomy, p. 178.)

SWELLING OF THE CALF WITH GAS

This is usually the result of the death and decomposition of the fetus when extraction has been delayed for a day or more after the escape of the waters. It is impossible to extract it whole, owing to its large size and the dry state of the skin of the calf, the membranes, and the wall of the womb. These dry surfaces stick with such tenacity that no attempt at traction leads to any advance of the calf out of the womb or into the passages. When the fetus is advanced the adherent womb advances with it, and when the strain is relaxed both recede to where they were at first. The condition may be helped somewhat by the free injection of oil into the womb, but it remains impossible to extract the enormously bloated body, and the only resort is to cut it in pieces and extract it by degrees. (See Embryotomy, p. 178.)

RIGID CONTRACTIONS OF MUSCLES

In the development of the calf, as in afterlife, the muscles are subject to cramps, and in certain cases given groups of muscles remain unnaturally short, so that even the bones grow in a twisted and distorted way. In one case the head and neck are drawn round to one side and cannot be straightened out, even the bones of the face and the nose being curved around to that side. In other cases the flexor muscles of the forelegs are so shortened that the knees are kept constantly bent and cannot be extended by force. The bent neck may sometimes be sufficiently straightened for extraction by cutting across the muscles on the side to which it is turned, and the bent knees by cutting the cords on the back of the shank bones just below the knees. If this fails, there remains the resort of cutting off the distorted limbs or head. (See Embryotomy, p. 178.)

TUMORS OF THE CALF (ENCLOSED OVUM)

Tumors or new growths appear on the unborn calf as on the mature animal, and by increasing the diameter of the body render its progress through the passage of the pelvis impossible. Large, fleshy tumors of the abdomen of the unborn calf are sometimes removed by cutting open the chest, removing the lungs and heart, cutting through the diaphragm with the knife, and removing the tumor piecemeal by alternate tearing and cutting until the volume of the body is sufficiently reduced to pass through. When this method has failed there still remains the method of cutting off the anterior part of the body, removing as much of the chest as possible, and cutting freely through the diaphragm; then, on pushing back the remainder of the body, the hind legs may be seized and brought into the passages and the residue thus extracted. The tumor, unless very large, will get displaced backward so as not to be an insuperable obstacle.

In many cases the apparent tumor is a blighted ovum that has grafted itself on the developing twin and from it has drawn its nourishment. Such tumors are usually sacs containing hair, skin, muscle, bone, or other natural tissues and only exceptionally do they show the distinct outline of the animal.

MONSTROSITY IN THE CALF

As a monstrous development in the calf may hinder calving, it is well to consider the different directions in which these deviations from the natural form appear. Monsters are such—

(1) From absence of parts—absence of head, legs, or other organ—arrested development.

(2) From some organ being unnaturally small, as a dwarfed head, leg, or trunk—arrested development.

(3) From unnatural division of parts—cleft lips, palate, head, trunk, or legs—abnormal growth.

(4) From the absence of natural divisions—absence of mouth, nose, eye, anus; the cloven foot of the calf or pig becomes solid, like that of the horse, for instance—confluence of parts that are rightfully separate.

(5) From the fusion of parts—both eyes replaced by central one, both nostrils merged into one central opening, etc.—confluence of parts.

(6) From unnatural position or form of parts—curved nose, neck, back, legs, etc.—lack of balance in the growth of muscles during development.

(7) From excessive growth of one or more organs—enormous size of head, double penis, superfluous digits, etc.—redundancy of growth at given points.

(8) From imperfect differentiation of the sexual organs—hermaphrodites (organs intermediate between male and female), male organs with certain feminine characters, female organs with certain well-marked male characters.

(9) From the doubling of parts or of the entire body—double monsters, doubled heads, doubled bodies, extra legs, etc.—redundant development (pl. XIX, figs. 1, 2, 3).

Causes.—The causes of monstrosities are varied. Some, such as extra digits or lack of horns, run in families, which produce them with absolute certainty when bred in the direct line, although they were originally acquired peculiarities that have merely been fixed by long habit in successive generations. The earliest horse had five toes, and even the most recent fossil horse had three toes, of which the two lateral ones are still represented in the modern animal by the two splint bones. Yet if the horse of the present day develops an extra toe it is pronounced a monstrosity. A more genuine monstrosity is the solid-hoofed pig, in which two toes have been merged into one. Another of the same kind is the solid shank bone of the calf, which consists of two bones united into one, but which are still found apart in the early fetus.

Other monstrosities seem to have begun in too close breeding, by which the powers of symmetrical development are impaired, just as the procreative power weakens under continuous breeding from the closest blood relations. A monstrosity consisting in the absence of an organ often depends on a simple lack of development, the result of disease or injury, as a young bone is permanently shortened by being broken across the soft part between the shaft and the end, the only part where increase in length can take place. As a result of the injury the soft, growing layer becomes prematurely hard and all increase in length at that end of the bone ceases. This accounts for some cases of absence of eye, leg, or other organ.

Sometimes a monstrosity is due to the enclosure of one ovum in another while the latter is still only a soft mass of cells and can easily close around the first. Here the ova have independent lives; they develop simultaneously, only the outer one, having direct connection with the womb and being furnished with abundant nourishment, advances most rapidly and perfectly, whereas the enclosed and starved ovum is dwarfed and imperfect.

In many cases of excess of parts, the extra part or member is manifestly derived from the same ovum and even the same part of the ovum, being merely the effect of a redundancy and vagary of growth. Such cases include most instances of extra digits or other organs and even of double monsters, as manifested by the fact that such extra organs grow from the normal, identical organs. Hence the extra digit is attached to the normal digit, the extra head to the one neck, the extra tail to the croup, extra teeth to the existing teeth, and even two similarly formed bodies are attached by some point common to both, as the navels, breastbones, and backs (pl. XIX, figs. 1, 2, 3). This shows that both have been derived from the same primitive layer of the embryo, which possessed the plastic power of building up a given structure or set of organs. An enclosed ovum, on the other hand, has no such identity or similarity of structure to the part with which it is connected, showing an evident primary independence of both life and the power of building tissues and organs. The power of determining extra growth along a given natural line is highly developed in the early embryo and is equally manifest in some of the mature, lower forms of animal life. Thus a newt will grow a new tail when that member has been cut off, and a starfish will develop as many new starfishes as the pieces made by cutting up the original one. This power of growth in the embryo and in the lower forms of animals is comparable to the branching out again of a tree at the places from which branches have been lopped. The presence of this vegetablelike power of growth in the embryo accounts for most double monsters.

The influence of disease in modifying growth in the early embryo—increasing, decreasing, distorting, etc.—is well illustrated in the varnishing, shaking, or otherwise disturbing the connections of eggs and thereby producing monstrosities. One can easily understand how inflammations and other causes of disturbed circulation in the womb, fetal membranes, or fetus would cause similar distortions and variations in the growing fetus. It is doubtless largely in the same way that certain mental disturbances of a very susceptible dam affect the appearance of the progeny. The monstrosities that seriously interfere with calving are mainly extra members or head, which cannot be admitted into the passages at the same time; some organ of the body attaining extra size; a blighted ovum being enclosed in the body of a more perfect one; or the body or legs so contracted or twisted that the calf must enter the passages doubled up.

Treatment.—Extraction is sometimes possible by straightening the distorted members by the force of traction; in other cases the muscles or tendons must be cut across on the side to which the body or legs are bent to allow such straightening. Thus, the muscles on the concave side of a wry neck or the cords behind the shank bones of a contracted leg may be cut to allow these parts to be brought into the passages. Methods for bringing up missing legs or head will still be needed. These are described in later paragraphs. In most cases of monstrosity by excess of overgrowth, it becomes necessary to cut off the supernumerary or overdeveloped parts, and the same general principles must be followed as laid down in Embryotomy (p. 178).

WRONG PRESENTATIONS OF THE CALF

The following is a list of abnormal presentations of the calf:

Simultaneous presentation of twins.

Anterior presentations	Forelegs		Legs curved at the knee. Flexor tendons shortened.
			Leg crossed over the back of the neck.
			Leg bent back at the knee.
			Leg bent back from the shoulder.
	Head		Head bent downward on the neck.
			Head and neck turned downward beneath the breast.
			Head turned to one side upon the side of the neck.
			Head and neck turned back on the side of the chest and abdomen.
			Head turned upward and backward on the back.
	Hind legs		Hind legs rotated outward. Toes and stifles turned outward.
			Hind legs bent forward, their feet resting in the pelvis.
	Transverse		Back of the calf turned to the right or left side.
	Inverted		Back of the calf turned to the floor of the pelvis and udder.
Posterior presentations	Hind legs		Hind leg bent on itself at the hock. Hock and buttocks present.
			Hind leg bent at the hips. Buttocks present.
	Tranverse		Back of calf turned to the right or left side.
	Inverted		Back of calf turned to the floor of the pelvis and udder.
Trunk presentations	Back and loins presented.	Position of calf vertical	Head up toward the spine, croup toward udder.
			Head down toward udder, croup toward spine.
		Position of calf transverse	Head toward the right side, croup toward the left.
			Head toward the left side, croup toward the right.
	Breast and abdomen presented.	Position of calf transverse	Head toward right side, croup toward left.
			Head toward left side, croup toward right.

These include all general presentations; others of a subsidiary nature will occur to the reader Thus, in each anterior or posterior presentation, with the back of the calf turned downward or to one side, the case may be complicated by the bending back of one or more members as a whole or at the joint just above the shank bones (knee or hock). So also in such anterior presentation the head may be turned back.

Head and forefeet presented—Back turned to one side.—The calf has a greater diameter from above down (spine to breastbone) than it has from side to side, and the same is true of the passage of the pelvis of the cow, which measures, on an average, $8\frac{7}{10}$ inches from above downward and $7\frac{9}{10}$ inches from side to side. Hence the calf passes most easily with its back upward, and when turned with its back to one side calving is always tardy and may be difficult or impossible. The obvious remedy is to rotate the calf on its own axis until its spine turns toward the spine of the cow. The operation is not difficult if the body of the calf is not yet fixed in the passages. The presenting feet are twisted over each other in the direction desired, and this is continued until the head and spine have assumed their proper place. If the body is firmly engaged in the passages the skin of the whole engaged portion should be freely lubricated with lard, and the legs and head twisted over each other as above. The legs may be twisted by an assistant when the head is manipulated by the operator, who drags on the rope turned halfway round the legs and assists in the rotation with his other hand in the passages.

Head and forefeet presented—Back turned down toward the udder.—This position (pl. XVI, fig. 6) is unnatural, and the parturition is difficult for two reasons: First, the natural curvature of the fetus is opposed to the natural curvature of the passages; and, second, the thickest part of the body of the calf (the upper) is engaged in the narrowest part of the passage of the pelvis (the lower). Yet, unless the calf is especially large and the pelvis of the cow narrow, parturition may usually be accomplished in this way spontaneously or with little assistance in the way of traction on the legs. If this cannot be accomplished, two courses are open: First, to rotate the calf as when the back is turned to one side; second, to push back the presenting forelegs and head and search for and bring up the hind legs, when the presentation will be a natural, posterior one.

Presentation of the hind feet with the back turned to one side or downward.—These are the exact counterparts of the two conditions last described, beset with similar drawbacks, and are to be dealt with on the same general principles (pl. XVII, fig. 4). With the back turned to one side the body should be rotated until the back turns toward the spine of the dam, and with the back turned down it must be extracted in that position (care being taken that the feet do not perforate the roof of the vagina) or it must be rotated on its own axis until the back turns upward, or the hind legs must be pushed back and the forelegs and head advanced, when the presentation will be a natural, anterior one.

Impaction of twins in the passage.—It is very rare to have twins enter the passages together so as to become firmly impacted. As a rule, each of the twins has its own separate membranes, and as the water bags of one will naturally enter first and be the first to burst, so the calf that occupied those membranes will be the first to enter the passage and the other will be thereby excluded. When the membranes of both have burst without either calf having become engaged in the pelvis, it becomes possible for the forelegs of one and the hind legs of the other to enter at one time, and if the straining is very violent they may become firmly impacted (pl. XVIII, fig. 1). The condition may be recognized by the fact that two of the presenting feet have their fronts turned forward, whereas the two others have their fronts turned backward. If the four feet belonged to one natural calf, they would all have the same direction. By means of this difference in direction the operator can easily select the two feet of one calf, place running nooses upon them just above the hoofs or fetlocks, and have an assistant drag on the ropes while the feet of the other calf are pushed back. In selecting one of the twins to come first, several considerations should have weight. The one that is most advanced in the passage is, of course, the first choice. Though the forefeet of one are presented, yet if the head is not in place the calf presenting its hind feet is to be chosen as being less likely to obstruct. Again, if for either calf one leg only is presented and the other missing, the one presenting two feet should be selected to come first. As soon as one calf has been advanced so as to occupy the pelvis the other will be crowded back so that it will not seriously obstruct.

Forelegs curved at the knee—Legs sprawling outward.—In this case not only are the knees somewhat bent in a curve, but the calf has a position as if it rested on its breastbone, while the legs were drawn apart and directed to the right and left. The shoulder blades being drawn outward from the chest and the elbows turned out, the muscles extending from the trunk to the leg are unduly stretched and keep the knees bent and the feet directed outward so as to press on the sides of the passages. They become retarded in their progress as compared with the more rapidly advancing head, and may bruise or even lacerate the walls of the vagina. It would seem easy to rectify this by extending the legs, but the already tense and overstretched muscles operate against extension in the present position, and it is not easy to rotate the legs so as to apply the shoulder flat against the side of the chest. Under these circumstances a repeller (pl. XX, fig. 7) may be planted in the breast and the body of the calf pushed backward into the womb, when the legs will extend easily under traction and the presentation becomes at once natural.

Forelegs curved at knee—Flexor tendons shortened.—In this case the feet will press against the floor of the pelvis though the leg has no outward direction, and the shoulder meanwhile presses against the roof of the same passage. Unless the knees can be sufficiently straightened by force, a knife must be used to cut across the cords behind the knee, when the legs may be straightened sufficiently.

Forelegs flexed at knee—Flexor tendons not shortened.—This is mostly seen in cases in which the body of the calf is in the proper position, its back being turned up toward the back of the dam, and in cows with a drooping abdomen. The feet have been supposed to catch beneath the brim of the pelvis, and being retarded while the head advances into the passages, they get bent at the knee and the nose and knees are presented (pl. XVI, fig. 2). The calf, however, is not an inanimate body advanced by the mere contraction of the womb. It moves its legs freely under the stimulus of the unwonted compression, and in moving the feet as they are advanced they slip down over the pelvic brim and finding no other firm support they bend back until, under the impulsion, they can no longer straighten out again. The knees, therefore, advance with the neck and head, but the feet remain bent back. The result is that the upper part of the leg is also flexed, and the shoulder blade and arm bone with their masses of investing muscles are carried backward and applied on the side of the chest, greatly increasing the bulk of this already bulky part. As the elbow is carried back on the side of the chest, the forearm from elbow to knee further increases the superadded masses of the shoulder and renders it difficult or impossible to drag the mass through the passages. When the forelegs are fully extended, on the contrary, the shoulder blade is extended forward on the smallest and narrowest part of the chest, the arm bone with its muscles is in great part applied against the side of the back part of the neck, and the forearm is continued forward by the side of the head so that the nose lies between the knees. In this natural presentation the presenting body of the calf forms a long wedge or cone, the increase of which is slow and gradual until it reaches the middle of the chest.

The difficulty of extending the forelegs will be in proportion to the advance of the head through the pelvic cavity. In the early stage all that is neccessary may be the following: To introduce the oiled hand, the left one for the right leg or the right one for the left, and passing the hand from the knee on to the foot, to seize the foot in the palm, bend it forcibly on the fetlock, and lift it up over the brim of the pelvis, the knee being, of course, pressed upward against the spine. As soon as the foot has been raised above the brim of the pelvis (into the passage) the leg can be straightened out with the greatest ease.

When, however, the shoulders are already engaging in the pelvis the feet cannot thus be lifted up, and to gain room a repeller (pl. XX, fig. 7) must be used to push back the body of the calf. This is an instrument with a long, straight stem, divided at the end into two short branches (2 to 3 inches long) united to the stem by hinges so that they can be brought into a line with the stem for introduction into the womb and then spread to be implanted in the breast. In the absence of a repeller a smooth, round, fork handle may be used, the prongs having been removed from the other end. A third device is to have an assistant strip his arm to the shoulder and, standing back to back with the operator, to introduce his right arm into the passages along with the operator's left (or vice versa) and push back the body of the calf while the operator seeks to bring up a leg. The repeller or staff having been planted safely in the breast of the calf, an assistant pushes on it in a direction either forward or slightly upward, so as not only to follow the natural curve of the body and favor its turning in the line of that curve within the womb, but also to carry the shoulders upward toward the spine and obtain more room for bringing up the missing feet. It is good policy, first, to put a halter (pl. XXI, figs. 4*a* and 4*b*) on the head or a noose (pl. XXI, fig. 3) on the lower jaw and a rope round each leg at the knee, so as to provide against the loss of any of these parts when the body is pushed back into the womb. This offers the further advantage that by dragging on these ropes the body can be advanced in the passage until the foot is reached, when the rope must be slackened and the repeller used to get room for bringing up the foot. If the cow is lying, the operator should first secure the foot on the upper side and then, if necessary, turn the cow on its opposite side so as to bring up the other.

In using the instruments some precautions are necessary. They must be warmed invariably before they are introduced, and they should be smeared with lard or oil to make them pass easily and without friction. The assistant who is pushing on the instrument must be warned to stop if at any time the resistance gives way. This may mean the turning of the fetus, in which case the object of repulsion has been accomplished, but much more probably it implies the displacement of the instrument from the body of the fetus, and unguarded pressure may drive it through the walls of the womb.

When the calf enters the passage with its back turned down toward the belly and udder, the bending back of the forelegs is rare, probably because the feet can find a straighter and more nearly uniform surface of resistance in the upper wall of the womb and the backbone and do not slide over a crest into an open cavity, as they do over the brim of the pelvis. The weight of the calf, too, gravitating downward, leaves more room for the straightening of the bent legs, so that the desired relief is much more easily obtained. The manipulation is the same in principle, only one must add the precaution of a steady traction on the feet in extraction, lest, owing to the adverse curvature of the fetus, the hoofs are suddenly forced through the roof of the vagina, and, perhaps, the rectum as well, during a specially severe labor pain.

When the back of the calf is turned to the right or the left side, the main difference is that in addition to straightening the legs the fetus must be rotated to turn its back upward before extraction is attempted. In this case, too, it may be difficult to bring up and straighten the lower of the two legs until the body has been rotated into its proper position. Cord the upper straightened leg and head, then rotate the body and search for the second missing leg.

Forelegs bent back from the shoulders.—This is an exaggeration of the condition just described and is much more difficult to remedy, owing to the distance and inaccessibility of the missing leg. It usually happens with the proper position of the body, the back of the calf being turned toward the back of the mother. The head is presented in the passage and may even protrude from the vulva during an active labor pain, but it starts back like a spring when the straining ceases. Examination with the oiled hands in the intervals between the pains fails to detect the missing legs (pl. XVI, fig. 1). If, however, the hand can be introduced during a pain it may be possible to reach the elbow or upper part of the foreleg. In the absence of a pain, a halter or noose on the head may be used to advance the whole body until the foreleg can be seized just below the elbow. This being firmly held and the head or body pushed back into the womb, room may be obtained for bringing up the knee. The foreleg is used as a lever, its upper part being strongly forced back while its lower part is pressed forward. If a pain supervenes the hold must be retained, and whatever gain has been made must be held if possible. Then during the next pain, by pushing back the body and continuing to operate the foreleg as a lever, a still further advance may be made. As the knee is brought up in this way, the hand is slid down from the elbow toward the knee, which is finally brought up over the brim of the pelvis and into the passage. It is now corded at the knee, and the subsequent procedure is as described in the preceding paragraphs. In a large, roomy cow with a small calf, the latter may pass with one or both forelegs bent back, but this is an exceptional case, and, as early assistance is the most successful, there should never be delay in hope of such a result.

One foreleg crossed over the back of the neck.—This is a rare obstacle to calving but one that is not altogether unknown. The hand introduced into the passage feels the head and one forefoot, and farther back, the other foot, from which the womb can be traced obliquely across the back of the neck (pl. XVI, fig. 3). The latter foot, projecting transversely, is likely to bruise or tear the vagina. If still deeply engaged in the vagina, it may be seized and pushed across to the opposite side of the neck, when the presentation will be natural.

Head bent down beneath the neck.—In this case, with drooping belly and womb allowing the brim of the pelvis to form a ridge, the advancing calf, having unduly depressed its nose, strikes it on the brim of the pelvis, and the neck advancing, the head is bent back and the poll and ears either enter the pelvis or strike against its brim. The two forefeet are presented, but they make no progress, and the oiled hand introduced can detect no head until the poll is felt at the entrance of the pelvis, between the forelegs. The two forefeet must be fixed with running nooses and dragged on moderately while the oiled hand seeks to bring up the head. The hand is slid down over the forehead and brim of the pelvis until the nose is reached, when it is passed into the mouth, the muzzle resting in the palm of the hand. The legs are now pushed upon, and in the space thus gained the muzzle is drawn up so as to enter it into the pelvis. In doing this the operator must carefully see that the mouth does not drop open so that the sharp front teeth cut through the floor of the womb. Should this danger threaten, the hand should be made to cover the lower jaw as well. The lessened security of the hold is more than compensated for by the safety of the procedure. With the nose in the pelvis, it has only to be drawn forward and the parturition is natural.

Head bent down beneath the breast.—This is an exaggerated condition of that last described. The head, arrested by the brim of the pelvis and already bent back on the neck, is pressed farther with each successive contraction until it has passed between the forelegs and lodges beneath the breastbone (pl. XVI, fig. 4). On examination, the narrow upper border of the neck is felt between the forelegs, but as a rule the head is out of reach below. Keeping the hand on the neck and dragging on the feet by the aid of ropes, the hand may touch and seize the ear, or, still better, one or two fingers may be inserted into the orbit of the eye.

Then in pushing back on the legs, with or without the aid of a repeller applied against the shoulder, space may be obtained to draw the head into a vertical position and even to slip the hand down so as to seize the nose. Should it be impossible to draw the head up with the unassisted fingers, a blunt hook (pl. XXI, fig. 6) may be inserted into the orbit, on which an assistant may drag while another pushes on the legs or repeller. Meanwhile the operator may have an opportunity of reaching and seizing the nose or of passing a blunt hook into the angle of the mouth. Success will be better assured if two hooks (pl. XXI fig. 7) are inserted into the two orbits, so as to draw up the head more evenly. In other cases a noose may be placed on the upper jaw or even around both jaws, and traction made on this and on the hooks in the orbits while the legs are pushed back and while the operator pushes back on the poll or forehead. In still more difficult cases, in which even the orbits cannot be reached, a sharp hook on the end of a straight iron rod (pl. XX, fig. 2) may be inserted over the lower jaw as far forward as it can be reached, and by dragging on this, while the body is pushed back, the head will be brought up sufficiently to allow the operator to reach the orbit or nose. If even the jaw cannot be reached, the hook may be inserted into the neck as near the head as possible and traction employed to bring the head within reach.

In all such cases the cow's head should be turned downhill, and if there is special difficulty she should be turned on her back and held there until the head is secured. In cases of long standing, with the womb closely clasping the body of the calf, relaxation may be sought by the use of chloroform or a full dose of chloral hydrate—2 ounces. The free injection of warm water into the womb will also be useful.

Head turned back on the shoulder.—With a natural, anterior presentation this may happen because of the imperfect dilation of the mouth of the womb. Under the contractions of the uterus the forefeet pass through the narrow opening into the vagina, while the nose, striking against it and unable to enter, is pressed backward into the womb and turns aside on the right or left shoulder. The broad muzzle of the calf forms an especial obstacle to entrance and favors this deviation of the head. The worst form of this deviation is the long-standing one with shortening of the muscles of the neck on that side, and oftentimes distortion of the face and neck bones.

When the head is bent on the shoulder the feet appear in the natural way but no progress is made. Examination reveals the absence of the nose from between the knees, and farther back from above and between the elbows, a smooth rounded mass in felt extending to the right or left, which further examination will identify with the neck. Following the upper border of this the hand reaches the crown of the head with the ears, and still further the eyes, or even, in a small calf, the nose.

As the bulky head of the calf cannot be extracted along with the shoulders, it becomes necessary to push the body of the fetus back and straighten out the head and neck. The cow should be laid with her head downhill and with that side up toward which the head is turned. If the pains are very violent or the womb strongly contracted on the calf, it may be best to seek relaxation by giving chloroform or 2 ounces of chloral hydrate. If the calf or the passages are dry, sweet oil may be injected, or the whole may be liberally smeared with fresh lard. In the absence of these, warm water made slightly slippery by Castile soap may be injected into the womb in quantity. Ropes with running nooses are placed on the presenting feet and the oiled hand introduced to find the head. If, now, the fingers can be passed inside the lower jawbone and the head dragged upward and toward the passage, this procedure unwinds the spiral turn given to the neck in bending back and greatly improves the chances of bringing the nose forward. If, at first, or if now, the lower jaw can be reached, a noose should be placed around it behind the incisor teeth and traction made upon this, so that the head may continue to be turned, forehead up, toward the spine and jaws down, thereby continuing to undo the screwlike curve of the neck. If, on the contrary, the nose is dragged on by a cord passing over the upper border of the neck, the screwlike twist is increased and the resistance of the bones and joints of the neck prevents any straightening of the head. As soon as the lower jaw has been seized by the hand or noose, a repeller (pl. XX, fig. 7), planted on the inside of the elbow or shoulder most distant from the head, should be used to push back the body and turn it in the womb, so that the head may be brought nearer to the outlet. In this way the head can usually be brought into position and the further course of delivery will be natural.

Sometimes, however, the lower jaw cannot be reached with the hand, and then the orbit or, less desirably, the ear may be used. The ear may be pulled by the hand, and by the aid of the repeller on the other shoulder the calf may be so turned that the lower jaw may be reached. Better still, a clamp (pl. XVIII, figs. 3 and 4) is firmly fixed on the ear and pulled by a rope, while the repeller is used on the opposite shoulder, and the hand of the operator pulls on the lower border of the neck and lifts it toward the other side. To pull on the upper border of the neck is to increase the spiral twist, whereas to raise the lower border is to undo it. If the outer orbit can be reached, the fingers may be inserted into it so as to employ traction, or a blunt finger hook (pl. XXI, fig. 8) may be used, or a hook with a rope attached, or, finally, a hook on the end of a long staff. Then, with the assistance of the repeller, the body may be so turned and the head advanced that the lower jaw may be reached.

In case neither the ears nor the orbit can be reached, a cord should be passed around the neck of the calf as near the head as possible, and traction made on that while the opposite shoulder is pushed toward the opposite side by the repeller, assisted by the hand dragging on the lower border of the neck. To aid the hand in passing a rope around the neck a cord carrier (pl. XXI, fig. 5) can be used. It fails, however, to help in the most difficult part of the operation—the passing of the cord down on the deep or farthest side of the neck—and to remedy this a cord carrier has been devised, with a ring at the end, a joint 6 or 8 inches from the end, and another ring on the handle, close to this joint (pl. XX, fig. 4). A cord is passed through both rings and a knot tied on its end, just back of the terminal ring. The instrument, straightening out, is inserted until it reaches just beyond the upper border of the neck, when, by dragging on the cord, the movable segment is bent down on the farther side of the neck and is pushed on until it can be felt at its lower border. The hand now seizes the knotted end of the cord beneath the lower border of the neck and pulls it through while the carrier is withdrawn, the cord sliding through its rings. The cord, pushed up as near to the head as possible, is furnished with a running noose by tying the knotted end round the other, or, better, the two ends are twisted around each other so as to give a firm hold on the neck without dangerously compressing the blood vessels. By pushing on the opposite shoulder with the repeller and assisting with the hand on shoulder, breastbone, or lower border of the neck, such a change of position will be obtained as will speedily bring the head within reach. Afterward, proceed in the manner previously described.

These cases are always trying, but it is rarely necessary to resort to embryotomy. When absolutely required, first remove one foreleg, and then, if still unsuccessful, the other, after which the head can easily be obtained. (See Embryotomy, p. 178.)

Head turned upward and backward.—In this case the face rests upon the spine; the forefeet appear alone in the passage but fail to advance, and on examination the rounded, inferior border of the neck can be felt, extending upward and backward beneath the spine of the dam, and if the calf is not too large the hand may reach the lower jaw or even the muzzle (pl. XVI, fig. 5). A repeller is planted in the breast and the body of the calf and pushed backward and downward to make room and bring the head nearer to the passage; or in some cases the body may be pushed back sufficiently by the use of the forelegs alone. Meanwhile the head is seized by the ear or the eye socket, or, if it can be reached, by the lower jaw, and pulled downward into position as space is obtained for it. If the hand alone is insufficient, the blunt hooks may be inserted in the orbits or in the angle of the mouth, or a noose may be placed on the lower jaw, and by traction the head will be easily advanced. In case of a large fetus, the head of which is beyond reach, even when traction is made on the legs, a rope may be passed around the neck and pulled, while the breastbone is pressed downward and backward by the repeller, and soon the change of position will bring the orbit or lower jaw within reach. With the above-described position the standing position of the cow is most favorable for success, but if the calf is placed with its back down toward the udder, and if the head is bent down under the brim of the pelvis, the best position for the cow is on her back, with her head downhill.

In neglected cases, with death and putrefaction of the fetus and dryness of the passages, it may be necessary to extract in pieces. (See Embryotomy, p. 178.)

Outward direction of the stifles—Abduction of hind legs.—As an obstacle to parturition, this is rare in cows. It is most likely to take place in cows with narrow hip bones and when the service has been made by a bull having great breadth across the quarter. The calf may take after the sire in the breadth of its quarters, and if at the same time the toes and stifles are turned excessively outward and the hocks inward the combined breadth of the hipbones above and the stifles below may be so great that the pelvis will not easily admit them. After the forefeet, head, and shoulders have all passed out through the vulva, further progress suddenly and unaccountably ceases, and some dragging on the parts already delivered does not serve to bring away the hind parts. The oiled hand introduced along the side of the calf will discover the obstacle in the stifle joints turned directly outward and projecting on each side beyond the bones that circumscribe laterally the front entrance of the pelvis. The evident need is to turn the stifles inward. This may be attempted by the hand introduced by the side of the calf, which is meanwhile rotated gently on its own axis to favor the change of position. To correct the deviation of the hind leg is, however, difficult, as the legs themselves are out of reach and cannot be used as levers to assist. If nothing can be done by pushing the body of the calf back and rotating it and by pressure by the hand in the passages, the only resort appears to be to skin the calf from the shoulder back, cut it in two as far back as can be reached, then push the buttocks well forward into the womb, bring up the hind feet, and so deliver.

Hind legs excessively bent on the body and engaged in the pelvis.—In this case the presentation is apparently a normal, anterior one; forelegs and head advance naturally and the parturition proceeds until half the chest has passed through the external passages, when suddenly progress ceases and no force will effect further advance. An examination with the oiled hand detects the presence, in the passages, of the hind feet and usually the hind legs up to above the hocks (pl. XVII, fig. 1).

The hind legs should be returned into the body of the womb. If they have not advanced too far into the pelvis, this may be done as follows: A rope with running noose is passed over each hind foot and drawn tight around the lower part of the hock. The ropes are then passed through the two rings in the small end of the rotating instrument (pl. XX, fig. 5), which is slid into the passages until it reaches the hocks, when the ropes, drawn tight, are tied around the handle of the instrument. Then in the intervals between the pains the hocks are pushed forcibly back into the womb. If by this means flexion can be effected in hocks and stifles, success will follow; the hind feet will pass into the womb and clear of the brim of the pelvis and the body may now be advanced without hindrance, the hind legs

77431 O—51——13

falling into place when the hip joints are extended. At the same time pressure on the hind legs must not be relaxed until the buttocks are engaged in the pelvis, as otherwise the feet may again get over the brim and arrest the progress of delivery.

When the hind legs are already so jammed into the pelvis that it is impossible to return them, the calf must be sacrificed to save the mother. Cords with running nooses are first put on the two hind feet. The body must be skinned from the shoulders back as far as can be reached and then cut in two, if possible, back of the last rib. The remainder of the trunk is now pushed back into the body of the womb, and by traction on the cords the hind feet are brought up into the passages and the extraction will be comparatively easy.

Hind presentation with one or both legs bent at the hock.—After the bursting of the water bags, though labor pains continue, no part of the fetus appears at the vulva unless it is the end of the tail. On examination, the buttocks are felt wedged against the spine at the entrance of the pelvis and beneath them the bent hock joints resting on the brim of the pelvis below (pl. XVII, fig. 3). The calf has been caught by the labor pains while the leg was bent beneath it and has been jammed into or against the rim of the pelvis, so that extension of the leg became impossible. With the thigh bent on the flank, the leg on the thigh, and the shank on the leg, and all at once wedged into the passage, delivery is practically impossible.

The obvious remedy is to push the croup upward and forward and extend the hind legs, and in the early stages this can usually be accomplished in the cow. A repeller (pl. XX, fig. 7) is planted across the thighs and pointed upward toward the spine of the cow and pushed forcibly in this direction during the intervals between labor pains. Meanwhile the oiled hand seizes the shank just below the hock and uses it as a lever, pushing the body back and drawing the foot forward, thus effectually seconding the action of the repeller. Soon a distinct gain is manifest, and as soon as the foot can be reached it is bent back strongly at the fetlock, held in the palm of the hand, and pulled up, while the repeller, pressing on the buttocks, assists in making room for it. In this way the foot may be brought safely and easily over the brim of the pelvis without any risk of laceration of the womb by the foot. After the foot has been lifted over the brim, the whole leg can be promptly and easily extended. If there is special difficulty in raising the foot over the brim, help may be had by traction on a rope passed around in front of the hock, and later still by a rope with a noose fastened to the pastern. In the worst cases, with the buttocks and hocks wedged deeply into the passages, it may be difficult or impossible to push the buttocks back into the abdomen, and in such case the extension of the hind leg is practically impossible without mutilation. In some roomy cows a calf may be dragged through the passages by ropes attached to the bent hocks, but even when this is possible there is great risk of laceration of the floor of the vagina by the feet. The next resort is to cut the hamstring just above the point of the hock and the tendon on the front of the leg (flexor metatarsi) just above the hock, and even the sinews behind the shank bone just below the hock. This allows the stifle and hock to move independently of each other, the one undergoing extension without entailing the extension of the other. It also allows both joints to flex completely, so that the impacted mass can pass through a narrower channel. If now, by dragging on the hocks and operating with the repeller on the buttocks, the latter can be tilted forward sufficiently to allow the extension of the stifle, the jam will be at once overcome, and the calf may be extracted with the hock bent, but the stifle extended. If even this cannot be accomplished, it may now be possible to extract the whole mass with both hocks and stifles fully bent. To attempt this, traction may be made on the rope around the hocks and on a sharp hook (pl. XX, fig. 2) passed forward between the thighs and hooked to the brim of the pelvis. Everything else failing, the leg or legs may be cut off at the hip joint and extracted, after which extraction may proceed by dragging on the remaining leg, or by hooks on the hip bones. Little is to be gained by cutting off the leg at the hock, and the stifle is less accessible than the hip, and amputation of the stifle gives much poorer results.

Hind legs bent forward from the hip.—Breech presentation.— This is an exaggeration of the condition last described, only the hocks and stifles are fully extended and the whole leg carried forward beneath the belly (pl. XVII, fig. 2). The water bags appear and burst, but nothing is presented unless possibly the tail. Examination in this case detects the outline of the buttocks, with the tail and anus at its upper part.

The remedy, as in the case last described, consists in pushing the buttock upward and forward with a repeller, the cow being kept standing and headed downhill, until the thigh bone can be reached and used as a lever. Its upper end is pushed forward and its lower end raised until, the joints becoming fully flexed, the point of the hock can be raised above the brim of the pelvis. If necessary a noose may be passed around the leg as far down toward the hock as possible and pulled on forcibly, while the hand presses forward strongly on the back of the leg above. When both hocks have been lodged above the brim of the pelvis the further procedure is as described under the last heading.

If, however, the case is advanced and the buttocks wedged firmly into the passages, it may be impossible safely to push the fetus back into the womb, and the calf must either be dragged through the passage as it is, or the legs or the pelvis must be cut off. To extract successfully with a breech presentation, the cow must be large and roomy and the calf not too large. The first step in this case is to separate the pelvic bones on the two sides by cutting from below backward, exactly in the median line below and where the thighs come together above. This may be done with a strong embryotomy knife but is most easily accomplished with the long embryotome (pl. XX, fig. 3). The form illustrated in plate XX, figure 1, with a short cutting branch jointed to the main stem, is preferred, as the short cutting piece may be folded on the main stem so that its cutting edge will be covered, and it can be introduced and extracted without danger. This is pushed forward beneath the calf's belly, and the cutting arm opened, inserted in front of the brim of the pelvis, and pulled forcibly back through the whole length of the pelvic bones. The divided edges are now made to overlap each other and the breadth of the haunch is materially reduced. One end of the cord may then be passed forward by means of a cord carrier (pl. XXI, fig. 5) on the inner side of one thigh until it can be seized at the stifle by the hand passed forward on the outer side of that thigh. This end is now pulled back through the vagina, the other end passed through the cord carrier and passed forward on the inner side of the other thigh until it can be seized at the stifle by the hand passed forward outside that thigh. This end is drawn back through the vagina like the first and is tied around the other to form a running noose. The rope is now drawn through the ring until it forms a tight loop, and encircles the belly just in front of the hind legs. On this, strong traction can be made without interfering with the full flexion of the legs on the body, and if the case is a suitable one and the body of the fetus and the passages are both well lubricated with oil or lard, a successful parturition may be accomplished. A less desirable method is to put a rope around one thigh or around each and drag on these, but manifestly the strain is not so directly on the spine, and the legs may be somewhat hampered in flexion.

This method being inapplicable, the next resort is to cut off one or both hind legs at the hip joint. Free incisions are made on the side of the haunch to expose the hip joint, and the muscles are cut away from the head of the thigh bone down to its narrow neck, around which a rope is passed and firmly fixed with a running noose. The joint is now cut into all around, and while traction is made on the cord the knife is inserted into the inner side of the joint and the round ligament severed. The cord may now be dragged on forcibly and the muscles and other parts cut through as they are drawn tense, until finally the whole member has been extracted. Traction on the rope around the other thigh will now suffice to extract, in most cases, but if it should fail the other leg may be cut off in the same manner, and then hooks inserted in front of the brim of the pelvis or in the opening in the bones of its floor will give sufficient hold for extraction. Another method is to insert a knife between the bone of the rump (sacrum) and the hipbone and sever their connections; then cut through the joint (symphysis) between the two hipbones in the median line of the floor of the pelvis, and then with a hook in the opening on the pelvic bones drag on the leg and cut the tense soft parts until the leg is freed and extracted.

Presentation of the back.—In this presentation straining may be active, but after the rupture of the water bags no progress is made, and the hand introduced will recognize the back with its row of spinous processes and the springing ribs at each side pressed against the entrance to the pelvis (pl. XVII, fig. 6). The presence or absence of the ribs will show whether it is the region of the chest or the loins. By feeling along the line of spines until the ribs are encountered, it is found that the head lies in that direction. If, on the contrary, the ribs are followed until they disappear, and a blank space is succeeded by hipbones, the tail is being approached. The head may be turned upward, downward, to the right side, or to the left.

The object must be to turn the fetus so that one extremity or the other can enter the passage, and the choice of which end to bring forward will depend on various considerations. If one end is much nearer the outlet than the other, that would naturally be selected for extraction, but if they are equidistant the choice would fall on the hind end, as having only the two legs to deal with without any risk of complication from the head. When the head is turned upward and forward it will usually be preferable to bring up the hind leg, as, owing to the drooping of the womb into the abdomen, rotation of the fetus will usually be easier in that direction, and if successful the resulting position will be a natural posterior presentation, with the back of the calf turned toward the rump of the cow. Similarly with the croup turned upward and forward, that should be pushed on forward, and if the forefeet and head can be secured it will be a natural anterior presentation, with the back of the calf turned upward toward the rump of the cow.

Warm water or oil should be injected into the womb. The turning of the calf will demand the combined action of the repeller and the hand, but in all such cases the operator has an advantage in that the body of the fetus is wholly within the body of the womb, and therefore movable with comparative ease. No part is wedged into the pelvic passages as a complication. The general principles are the same as in faulty presentation fore and hind, and no time should be lost in making the manipulations necessary to bring the feet into the pelvis, lest they get in bent or otherwise displaced and add unnecessary complications.

With a transverse direction of the calf, the head being turned to one side, the pressure must be directed laterally, so that the body will glide around on one side of the womb, and the extremities when reached must be promptly seized and brought into the passages. Sometimes struggling of a live fetus will greatly aid in rectifying the position.

Breast and abdomen presented—All four feet in the passages.—In this form the calf lies across the womb with its arched back turned forward and its belly toward the pelvis. All four feet may be extended and engaged in the passages, or one or more may be bent on themselves so as to lie in front of the pelvis. The head, too, may usually be felt on the right side or the left, and if detected it serves to identify the exact position of the fetus. The position may further be decided on by examination of the feet and legs. With the legs extended the front of the hoofs and the convex aspect of the bent pasterns and fetlocks will look toward that flank in which the head and shoulders lie. On examination still higher the smooth, even outline of the knee and its bend, looking toward the hind parts, characterize the foreleg, whereas the sharp prominence of the point of the hock and the bend on the opposite side of the joint, looking toward the head, indicate the hind leg (pl. XVII, fig. 5).

The remedy for this condition is to be sought in repelling into the womb those legs that are least eligible for extraction, and bringing into the passages the most eligible ones. The most eligible will usually be those that project farthest into the passages, indicating the nearer proximity of that end of the calf. An exception, however, may be made in favor of that extremity that will give the most natural presentation. Thus if, owing to obliquity in the position of the fetus, the hind legs promise a presentation with the back of the fetus turned down toward the udder, and the forelegs one with the back turned up toward the spine, the latter should be selected. Again, if the choice for the two extremities is evenly balanced, the hind may be chosen as offering less risk of complication, there being no head to get displaced.

The first step is to place a running noose on each of the four feet, marking those of the fore legs to distinguish them from the hind legs. If the forelegs are to be brought into the passage, a noose should also be placed on the lower jaw. Then run the ropes attached to the two feet that are to be pushed back through the ring of a cord carrier (pl. XXI, fig. 5), pass the rings down to the feet, and by the aid of the carrier push them well back into the womb and hold them there. Meanwhile, drag on the ropes attached to the other two feet to bring them into the passage or, in case of the forelegs, on the two foot ropes and the head rope. The other feet must be pushed back into the womb until the body of the calf is fully engaged in the passages. After this they can no longer find an entrance but must follow as the body escapes.

NEGLECTED AND AGGRAVATED CASES

In laying down the foregoing rules for giving assistance in critical cases of calving, it is not intimated that all cases and stages can be dealt with successfully. Often assistance is not sought for many hours or even days after labor pains, and escape of the waters makes known the danger of delay. Frequently, many misguided and injurious attempts at rendering assistance have been made, such as violent pulling when resistance is insurmountable without change of position, injuries to the vagina and womb by ill-considered but too forcibly executed attempts to change the position, repeated and long-continued contact with rough hands and rougher ropes and hooks, gashes with knives and lacerations with instruments in unskilled hands, introduction of infecting material on filthy hands and instruments, and the septic inflammations started in the now dry and tender passages and womb. Frequently death, putrefaction, and bloating of the calf in the womb render the case extremely unpromising and make it impossible to apply successfully many of the measures previously recommended. The labor pains of the cow may have practically ceased from exhaustion of the animal; the passages of the vagina may be so dry, tender, friable, red, and swollen that it requires considerable effort even to pass the oiled hand through them, and the extraction of the calf or any portion of it through such a channel seems a hopeless task; the womb may be equally dry, inflamed and swollen, so that its lining membrane or even its entire thickness is easily torn; the fetal membranes have lost their natural, unctuous, and slippery character and cling firmly to the dry walls of the womb, to the dry skin of the calf, or to the hands of the operator; the dead and putrefying calf may be so bloated with gases that the womb has been overdistended by its presence, and the two adhere so closely that the motion of the one on the other is practically impossible. In other cases reckless attempts to cut the calf in pieces have left raw surfaces with projecting bones that dangerously scratch and tear the womb and passages.

In many cases, as a last resort, it is necessary to cut the fetus to pieces (embryotomy) or, in still more serious cases, to perform a Cæsarean section (extraction through the flank).

DISSECTION OF THE UNBORN CALF (EMBRYOTOMY)

In some cases the dissection of the calf is the only feasible means of delivering it through the natural passages; and although it is especially applicable to the dead calf, it is also on occasion called for in the case of the living one. As a rule, the living calf should be preserved, if possible, but if this threatens to entail the death of the cow it is only in the case of offspring of rare value that its preservation is to be preferred. To those acquainted with the toil, fatigue, and discomfort of embryotomy, no discussion is necessary as long as there is a prospect of success from the simple and generally easier method of rectifying the faulty position of the calf. When the correction of the position is manifestly impossible, however, when distortions and monstrosities of the fetus successfully obstruct delivery, when the pelvic passages are seriously contracted by fractures and bony growths, when the passages are virtually almost closed by swelling, or when the calf is dead and excessively swollen, no other resort may be available. In many cases of distortion and displacement the dismemberment of the entire calf is unnecessary, the removal of the offending member being all that is required. It will be convenient, therefore, to describe the various suboperations one by one and in the order in which they are usually demanded.

Amputation of the foreleg.—In cutting off a foreleg the one which is presented should be selected, since it is much more easily operated on, and its complete removal from the side of the chest affords so much more space for manipulation that it often makes it easy to bring the other missing leg or the head into position. The first consideration is to skin the leg from the fetlock up and leave the skin attached to the body. The reasons for this are: (1) That the skin is the most resistant structure of the leg, and when it has been removed the entire leg can be easily detached; (2) the tough skin left from the amputated leg may be used as a cord in subsequent traction on the body of the calf; (3) the dissection and separation of the leg are far more safely accomplished under the protection of the enveloping skin than if the operator's hands and instruments were in direct contact with the walls of the passages or womb; (4) the dissection can be much more easily effected while the skin is stretched by the left hand, so as to form a comparatively firmer resistant point for the knife, than in attempting to cut the soft, yielding, and elastic tissues, which naturally offer little solid resistance but constantly recede before the cutting edge of the instrument. The preservation of the skin is therefore a cardinal principle in the amputation of all parts in which it is at all feasible.

The presenting foot is enclosed in a noose and drawn well out of the passages. Then a circular incision through the skin is made around the leg just above the fetlock. From this the skin is slit up on the inner side of the leg to the breast. Then the projecting part of the leg is skinned up to the vulva, traction being made on the foot by an assistant so as to expose as much as possible. The embryotomy knife may now be taken (pl. XXI, fig. 2), and a small hole having been cut in the free end of the detached portion of skin, that is seized by the left hand and extended while its firm connections with the deeper structures are cut through. The looser connections can be more quickly torn through with the closed fist or the tips of the four fingers held firmly together in a line, or with the spud of which there are several kinds. Much of the upper part of the leg can be skinned more speedily without the knife, but it must be used to cut across tough bands whenever these interrupt the progress. The skinning should be carried upward on the outer side of the shoulder blade to the spine, or nearly so. Then with the knife the muscles attaching the elbow and shoulder to the breastbone are cut across, together with those on the inner side of the shoulder joint and in front and behind it as far as these can be reached. Steady traction is now made on the foot, the remaining muscles attaching the shoulder blade to the trunk are torn through with a cracking noise, and the whole leg, including the shoulder blade and its investing muscles, comes away. If the shoulder blade is left the bulk of the chest is not diminished, and nothing has been gained. Before going further, it is well to see whether the additional space thus obtained in the passages will allow the missing leg or head to be brought into position. If not, the other presenting part, leg or head, is to be amputated and extracted. For the leg the procedure is a repetition of that just described.

Amputation of the head.—The head is first seized and drawn well forward, or even outside the vulva, by a rope with a running noose placed around the lower jaw just behind the incisor teeth, by a sharp hook inserted in the arch of the lower jaw behind the union of its two branches and back of the incisor teeth, or by hooks inserted in the orbits, or, finally, in case the whole head protrudes, by a halter (pl. XXI, figs. 4*a* and 4*b*).

In case the whole head protrudes, a circular incision through the skin is made just back of the ear, and the cut edge being held firmly by the left hand, the neck is skinned as far as it can be reached. Then the great ligamentous cord above the spine is cut across at the farthest available point, together with the muscles above and below the spine. Strong traction on the head will then detach it at this point and bring it away, but should there still be too much resistance the knife is inserted between the bodies of two vertebrae just behind one of the prominent points felt in the median line below, and their connecting fibrous cartilage is cut through, after which comparatively moderate pulling will bring it away. The detached neck and body at once slip back into the womb, and if the forelegs are now brought up and pulled they are advanced so far upon the chest that the transverse diameter is greatly diminished and delivery correspondingly facilitated.

If the head is still enclosed in the vagina two methods are available: (1) The removal of the lower jaw and subsequent separation of the head from the neck; (2) the skinning of the whole head and its separation from the neck.

To remove the lower jaw the skin is dissected away from it until the throat is reached. Then the muscles of the cheeks and side of the jaw (masseters) are cut through and those connecting the jaw with the neck. When traction is made on the rope around the lower jaw it will usually come away with little trouble. Should it resist, its posterior extremity on each side (behind the grinding teeth) may be cut through with bone forceps or with a guarded bone chisel (pl. XX, fig. 8). After the removal of the lower jaw the way will be open to separate the head from the neck, the knife being used to cut into the first or second joint from below or the bone forceps or chisel being employed to cut through the bones of the neck. Then traction is made on the head by means of hooks in the orbits, and the hand, armed with an embryotomy knife, is introduced to cut through the tense resisting ligament and muscles above the bones. The skin and the strong ligamentous cord attached to the poll are the essential parts to cut, as the muscles can easily be torn across. Unless there are great difficulties in the way it is well to skin the head from the eyes back, and on reaching the poll to cut through the ligament and then bring the head away by pulling.

If it is decided to remove the entire head at once, it may be skinned from the front of the eyes back to behind the lower jaw below and the poll above, then cut through the muscles and ligaments around the first joint and pull the head away, assisting, if need be, in the separation of the head by using the knife on the ligament of the joint.

If the calf is double-headed, skinning of the head must be carried backward until the point has been reached at which both heads branch from the single neck, and the separation must be made at that point. The muscles and ligaments are first to be cut through; and if the part cannot then be detached by pulling, the bodies of the vertebrae may be separated by passing the knife through the joint. The second head may now be secured by a noose around the lower jaw or hooks in the orbits and brought up into place, the body being pushed back toward the other side by a repeller, so as to provide space.

Except a double-headed calf, or in a head protruding or nearly so and one or both forelegs presented, it is rarely desirable to undertake amputation of the head. The desired space in the passages can usually be obtained by the much simpler and easier procedure of removing one or both forelegs.

Amputation of the hind legs.—This is sometimes necessary on the one extended leg when the other cannot be brought up and delivery cannot be effected; in calves having extra hind legs; when the calf is dead, putrid, and bloated with gas; and in some cases of breech presentation, as described under that head.

When the leg is extended the guiding principles are as in the case of the forelegs. The skin is cut through circularly above the fetlock and slit up to beneath the pelvic bones on the inner side of the thigh. It is then dissected from the other parts as high as it has been slit on the inner side and to above the prominence (trochanter major) on the upper end of the thigh bone on the outer side of the joint. In this procedure the hands and spud can do much, but owing to the firmer connections the knife will be more frequently required than in the case of the foreleg. The muscles are now cut through all around the hip joint, and strong traction is made by two or three men on the leg. If there is still too much resistance, a knife is inserted into the joint on the inner side and its round ligament cut through, after which extraction will be comparatively easy. This accomplished, it will often be possible to extract the fetus with the other leg turned forward into the womb. If the calf is bloated, it may be necessary to remove the other leg in the same way and even to cut open the chest and abdomen and remove their contents before extraction can be effected. In the case of extra legs, it may be possible to bring them up into the passages after the presenting hind legs have been removed. If this is not practicable, they may be detached by cutting them through at the hip joint, as described under Breech Presentation, page 173.

Another method of removing the hind leg, after having skinned it over the quarter, is to cut through the pelvic bones from before backward, in the median line below, by knife, saw, or long embryotome (pl. XX, fig. 1), and then disjoint the bones of the spine (sacrum) and the hipbone (ilium) on that side with embryotome, knife, or saw, and then drag away the entire leg, along with all the hipbones on that side. This has the advantage of obtaining more space and thereby facilitating subsequent operations. Both legs may be removed in this way, but on the removal of the second the operator is without any solid point to drag on in bringing away the remainder of the fetus.

Division across the middle of the body.—In cases of extra size, monstrosity, or distortion of one end of the body it may be necessary to cut the body in two and return the half from the passages into the womb, even after one-half has been born. The presenting members are dragged on forcibly by assistants to bring as much of the body as possible outside. Then cut through the skin around the body at some distance from the vulva, and with hand, knife, and spud detach it from the trunk as far back into the passages as can be reached. Next cut across the body at the point reached, beginning at the lower part (breast, belly) and proceeding up toward the spine. This greatly favors the separation of the backbone when reached and further allows its being extended so that it can be divided higher up. When the backbone is reached, the knife is passed between the two bones, the prominent ridges across their ends acting as guides, and by dragging and twisting the one is easily detached from the other. With an anterior presentation, the separation should be made behind the last rib if possible, whereas with a posterior presentation as many of the ribs should be brought away as can be accomplished. When one-half of the body has been removed, the remaining half is to be pushed back into the womb, the feet sought and secured with nooses, and the second half removed in one piece if possible; if not, then after the removal of the extra leg or other cause of obstruction.

Removal of the contents of chest or abdomen.—If the body of the calf sticks fast in the passages by reason of the mere dryness of its skin and of the passages, the obstacle may be removed by injecting sweet oil past the fetus into the womb through a rubber or other tube, and smearing the passages freely with lard. When the obstruction depends on excess of size of the chest or abdomen or thickening of the body from distorted spine, much advantage may be derived from the removal of the contents of these great cavities of the trunk. It has already been shown how the haunches may be narrowed by cutting the bones apart in the median line below and causing their free edges to overlap each other. The abdomen can be cut open by the embryotomy knife or the long embryotome in the median line, or at any point, and the contents pulled out with the hand, the knife being used when special resistance is encountered. If the abdomen is so firmly impacted that it cannot be dealt with in this way, one hind leg and the hipbone on the same side may be removed as described under Amputation of the Hind Legs, page 181. This will allow the introduction of the hand into the abdomen from behind, so as to pull out the contents. By introducing an embryotomy knife in the palm of the hand and cutting through the muscle of the diaphragm, the interior of the chest can be reached in the same way and the heart and lungs removed.

In dealing with an anterior presentation, when it becomes necessary to remove the contents of the chest, the usual course is to cut through the connections of the ribs with the breastbone (the costal cartilages) close to the breastbone on each side, and from the abdomen forward to the neck. Then cut through the muscles connecting the front of the breastbone with the neck and its hinder end with the belly, and pull out the entire breastbone. Having torn out the heart and lungs with the hand, make the rib cartilages on the one side overlap those on the other, to lessen the thickness of the chest, and proceed to extract the body. If it seems necessary to empty the abdomen as well, it is easy to reach it by cutting through the diaphragm, which separates it from the chest.

Delivery through the flank (*Caesarean section*).—This is sometimes necessary when the distortion and narrowing of the hipbones are such as to forbid the passage of the calf, or when inflammation has practically closed the natural passages and the progeny is more valuable than the dam; also in cases in which the cow has been fatally injured or is ill beyond possibility of recovery and yet carries a living calf. It is often a last resort after long and fruitless efforts to deliver by the natural channels, and in such cases the saving of the calf is all that can be expected. The hope of saving the dam is greatest if she is in good health and not fatigued, in cases, for example, in which the operation is resorted to on account of broken hipbones or abnormally narrow passages.

The stock owner will not attempt such a serious operation as this. Yet, if the cow has just died or is to be immediately sacrificed, no one should hesitate to resort to it in order to save the calf. If the cow is alive, it is important that she be perfectly still. Her left foreleg being bent at the knee by one person, another may seize the left horn and nose and turn the head to the right until the nose rests on the spine just above the shoulder. The cow will sink down gently on her left side without shock or struggle. One may now hold the head firmly to the ground, while a second, carrying the end of the tail from behind forward on the inside of the right thigh, pulls upon it so as to keep the right hind leg well raised from the ground. If time presses she may be operated on in this position, or if the cow is to be sacrificed this may be done by a blow on the head with an ax. Then the prompt cutting into the abdomen and womb and the extraction of the calf involve no serious difficulty.

If, however, the cow is to be preserved, her two forefeet and the lower hind one should be safely fastened together and the upper hind one drawn back. Two ounces of chloral hydrate, given by injection, should induce sleep in 20 minutes, and the operation may proceed. If the cow is to be preserved, wash the right flank and apply a solution of 4 grains of corrosive sublimate in a pint of water.

Then, with an ordinary scalpel or knife, dipped in the above-mentioned solution, make an incision from 2 inches below and in front of the outer angle of the hipbone in a direction downward and slightly forward to a distance of 12 inches. Cut through the muscles and more carefully through the transparent lining membrane of the abdomen (peritoneum), letting the point of the knife lie in the groove between the first two fingers of the left hand as they are slid down inside the membrane and with their back to the intestines. An assistant, whose hands, like those of the operator, have been dipped in the sublimate solution, may press his hands on the wound behind the knife to prevent the protrusion of the intestines. The operator now feels for and brings up to the wound the gravid womb, allowing it to bulge well through the abdominal wound, so as to keep back the bowels and prevent any escape of water into the abdomen. Assistance is given by two persons, who press the lips of the wound against the womb. Then an incision 12 inches long is made into the womb at its most prominent point, deep enough to penetrate its walls, but not so as to cut into the water bags. In cutting, carefully avoid the cotyledons, which may be felt has hard masses inside. By pressure the water bags may be made to bulge out as in natural parturition, and this projecting portion may be torn or cut to let the liquid flow down outside of the belly. The operator now plunges his hand into the womb, seizes the fore or hind legs, and quickly extracts the calf and gives it to an attendant. The womb may be drawn out, but not until all the liquid has flowed out, and the fetal membranes must be separated from the natural cotyledons, one by one, and the membranes removed. The womb is now emptied with a sponge, which has been boiled or squeezed out of a sublimate solution, and if any liquid has fallen into the abdomen it may be removed in the same way. A few stitches with carbolized catgut are now made in the wound in the womb. They need not be very close together, as the wound will diminish greatly when the womb contracts. Should the womb not contract at once it may have applied against it a sponge squeezed out of a cold sublimate solution, or it may be drawn out of the abdominal wound and exposed to the cold air until it contracts. Its contraction is necessary to prevent bleeding from its enormous network of veins. When contracted, the womb is returned into the abdomen and the abdominal wound sewed. One set of stitches, to be made at intervals of 2 inches, is passed through the entire thickness of skin and muscles and tied around two quills or little rollers resting on the skin (pl. XXVII, fig. 7). These should be of silver and may be cut at one end and pulled out after the wound has healed. The superficial stitches are put in every half inch and passed through the skin only. They, too, may be of silver, or pins may be inserted through the lips and a fine cord twisted round their ends like a figure 8 (pl. XXVII, fig.

9). The points of the pins may be snipped off with pliers. The edges may be still further held together by the application of Venice turpentine, melted so as to become firmly adherent, and covered with a layer of sterilized cotton wool. Then the whole should be supported by a bandage fixed around the loins and abdomen.

DISEASES OF THE GENITAL ORGANS

DESCRIPTION OF PLATES

PLATE XII. Fetal calf within its membranes (at midterm). The uterus is opened on the left side. In the uterus the fetus is surrounded by several membranes, known as the amnion or inner layer, the allantois or central layer, and the chorion or outer layer. The amnion is nearest the fetus and forms a closed sac around it filled with a fluid known as liquor amnii, in which the fetus floats. The allantois is composed of two layers, which form a closed sac in connection with the urachus, or the tube extending from the fetal bladder through the umbilical cord. The one layer of the allantois is spread over the outer surface of the amnion and the other over the inner surface of chorion. The allantois also contains a fluid known as the allantoi liquid. The chorion is the outer envelope or membrane of the fetus, completely enclosing the fetus with its other membranes. On the outer surface of this membrane are found the fetal placentulae or cotyledons, which, through their attachment to the maternal cotyledons, furnish the fetus with the means of sustaining life. The relation of the fetal and maternal cotyledons to each other is illustrated on the following plate.

PLATE XIII. Pregnant uterus with cotyledons.

The upper figure illustrates the uterus of the cow during pregnancy, laid open to show the cotyledons (*d*) on the internal surface of uterus (*c*). The ovary (*a*) is shown cut across, and the two halves are laid open to show the position of the discharge ovum at a′.

The lower figure illustrates the relation of the fetal and maternal parts of a cotyledon. A portion of the uterus (*A*) is shown with the maternal cotyledon (*BB*) attached to it. The fetal portion (*D*) consists of a mass of very minute, hairlike processes on the chorion (*E*), which fit into corresponding depressions or pits of the maternal portion. Each portion is abundantly supplied with blood vessels, so that a ready interchange of nutritive fluid may take place between mother and fetus.

PLATE XIV. Vessels of umbilical cord.

Figure 1. Fetal calf with a portion of the wall of the abdominal cavity of the right side and the stomach and intestines removed to illustrate the nature of the umbilical or navel cord. It consists of a tube (1–1′) into which pass the two umbilical arteries (3) carrying blood to the placenta in the uterus or womb and the umbilical vein (4) bringing the blood back and carrying it into the liver. The cord also contains the urachus (2′), which carries urine from the bladder (2) through the cord. These vessels are all obliterated at birth. 5, liver; 5′, lobe of same, known as the lobus Spigelii; 5″, gall bladder; 6, right kidney; 6′, left kidney; 6″, ureters, or the tubes conducting the urine from the kidneys to the bladder; 7, rectum, where it has

PLATE XIV. Vessels of umbilical cord—Continued.
been severed in removing the intestines; 8, uterus of the fetus, cut off at the anterior extremity; 9, aorta; 10, posterior vena cava. (From Fürstenberg-Leisering, Anatomie und Physiologie des Rindes.)

Figure 2. Blood vessels passing through the umbilical cord in a human fetus. (From Quain's Anatomy, vol. 2.) *L*, liver; *K*, kidney; *I*, intestines; *u c*, umbilical cord; *ua*, umbilical arteries. The posterior aorta coming from the heart passes backward and gives rise to the internal iliac arteries, and of these the umbilical arteries are branches. *Uv*, umbilical vein; this joins the portal vein, passes onward to the liver, breaks up into smaller vessels, which reunite in the hepatic vein; this empties into the posterior vena cava, which carries the blood back to the heart.

PLATE XV. Normal position of calf in utero. This is the most favorable position of the calf or fetus in the womb at birth, and the position in which it is most frequently found. This is known as the normal anterior position. The back of the fetus is directly toward that of the mother, the forelegs are extended back toward the vulva of the mother, and the head rests between them. The birth of the calf in this position usually takes place without artificial assistance.

PLATE XVI. Abnormal positions of calf in utero. (Figs. 1, 2, 3, and 5 from Fleming's Veterinary Obstetrics; fig. 4 after St. Cyr, from Hill's Bovine Medicine and Surgery; fig. 6 from D'Arboval Dictionaire de Médecine et de Chirurgie.)

Figure 1. Anterior presentation; one foreleg completely retained. The retained leg must be reached if possible and brought forward joint by joint and the fetus then extracted.

Figure 2. Anterior presentation; forelegs bent at knee. The legs must be extended before delivery can be accomplished.

Figure 3. Anterior presentation; foreleg crossed over neck. The leg should be grasped a little above the fetlock, raised, drawn to its proper side, and extended in genital canal.

Figure 4. Anterior presentation; downward deviation of head. The head must be brought into position seen in plate XV before delivery can take place.

Figure 5. Anterior presentation; deviation of the head upward and backward. Retropulsion is the first indication and will often bring the head into its normal position.

Figure 6. Anterior presentation; head presented with back down. The fetus should be turned by pushing back the fore parts and bringing up the hind parts to make a posterior presentation.

PLATE XVII. Abnormal positions of calf in utero. (Figs. 2 and 3 from Fleming; figs. 4, 5, and 6 from D'Arboval.)

Figure 1. Anterior presentation, with hind feet engaged in pelvis. A very serious malpresentation, in which it is generally impossible to save the fetus if delivery is far advanced. The remedy is to force back the hind feet.

Figure 2. Thigh and croup presentation, showing the fetus corded. The cord has a ring or noose at one end. The two ends of the cord are passed between the thighs, brought out at the flanks, and the plain end passed through the noose at the top of the back and brought outside the vulva. The fetus must be pushed back and an attempt made to bring the legs properly into the genital passage.

PLATE XVII. Abnormal positions of calf in utero—Continued.

Figure 3. Croup and hock presentation. The procedure in this abnormal presentation is the same as described for figure 2.

Figure 4. Posterior presentation; the fetus on its back. Turn the fetus to make a normal anterior presentation.

Figure 5. Sternoabdominal presentation. The fetus is on its side with legs crossing and presenting. The legs least eligible for extraction should be forced back into the uterus.

Figure 6. Dorsolumbar presentation; the back presenting. The fetus must be turned so that one or the other extremity can enter the passage.

PLATE XVIII. Normal positions of the calves in utero. Surgical instruments and sutures.

Figure 1. Twin pregnancy, showing the normal anterior and posterior presentations. (From Fleming.)

Figure 2. Abdominal dropsy of the fetus; normal presentation; forelegs corded. (After Armatage.) The drawing illustrates the method of puncturing the abdomen through the chest with a long trocar and cannula. The fluid is represented escaping from the cannula after the withdrawal of the trocar.

Figure 3. Tallich's short, bent, crotchet forceps. The forceps have bent and toothed jaws, which are intended to take hold of the fetus where neither cords nor hooks can be applied, as the ear, nose, or skin of cheek.

Figure 4. Clamp for ear, skin, etc.: 1–1, Blades with hooks and corresponding holes; 2, ring to close the blades; 3, stem with female screw for handle; 4, handle, which may be either straight or jointed and flexible.

PLATE XIX. Monstrosities. This plate illustrates various malformations and diseases of the fetus that act as the cause of difficult parturition.

Figures 1, 2, 3. Fetuses with portions of their bodies double. Figure 1 (from Fleming), double head, neck, and forelegs. Figure 2 from Encyclop. der Gesam. Thierheilkunde, 1886), double head, neck, forelegs, and body. Figure 3 (from Fleming), double faced.

Figure 4. Fetus with head very much enlarged. (From Fleming.) This affection is known as hydrocephalus, or dropsy of the brain, and is due to a more or less considerable quantity of fluid in the cranial cavity of the fetus.

Figure 5. Skull of the calf represented in figure 4. The roof of the skull is absent. (From Fleming.)

PLATE XX. Instruments used in difficult labor.

Figure 1. Long embryotome with joint.

Figure 2. Long, sharp hook. This instrument is about 3 feet in length, including the handle. Hooks of this kind, both blunt and sharp, are applied directly to the fetus to assist in delivery.

Figure 3. Günther's long-handled embryotome. This instrument and that represented in figure 1 are of special value in cutting through muscular tissue and in separating the legs from the trunk when the fetus cannot be removed entire. These embryotomes are usually 30 inches long but may be made either longer or shorter.

Figure 4. Jointed cord carrier, used in difficult parturition to carry a cord into regions which cannot be reached by the arm.

Figure 5. Instrument used to rotate or turn the fetus, known as a rotator.

Figure 6. Dilator of the neck of the womb, used when conception cannot take place owing to a contracted condition of the neck of the womb.

77431 O—51——14

PLATE XX. Instruments used in difficult labor—Continued.

Figure 7. Repeller. An instrument from 2 to 3 feet long, used to force the fetus forward into the womb. This operation is generally necessary when the presentation is abnormal and the fetus has advanced too far into the narrow inlet to the uterus to be moved.

Figure 8. Cartwright's bone chisel. Including the handle, this instrument is about 32 inches in length; the chisel portion is a little more than 2 inches long and 1 to 1½ inches broad. Only the middle portion is sharp, the projecting corners are blunt, and the sides rounded. This instrument is used for slitting up the skin of a leg and as a bone chisel when it is necessary to mutilitate the fetus in order to effect delivery.

PLATE XXI. Instruments used in difficult labor.

Figure 1. Embryotome, an instrument used when it is necessary to reduce the size of the fetus by cutting away certain parts before birth can be effected. This instrument may be long or short, straight or curved.

Figure 2. Also an embryotome. The blade can be made to slide out of or into the handle. The instrument can thus be introduced into or withdrawn from the genital passage without risk of injury to the cow.

Figure 3. Schaack's traction cord. This is merely a cord with a running noose at one end and a piece of wood at the other, to offer a better hold for the hand.

Figures 4*a* and 4*b*. Reuff's head collar for obtaining the head of the fetus.

Figure 5. Curved cord carrier, used in difficult parturition to carry a cord into regions that cannot be reached by the arm.

Figure 6. Blunt hook, used in difficult parturition.

Figure 7. Short hook forceps, used in difficult parturition.

Figure 8. Blunt finger hook.

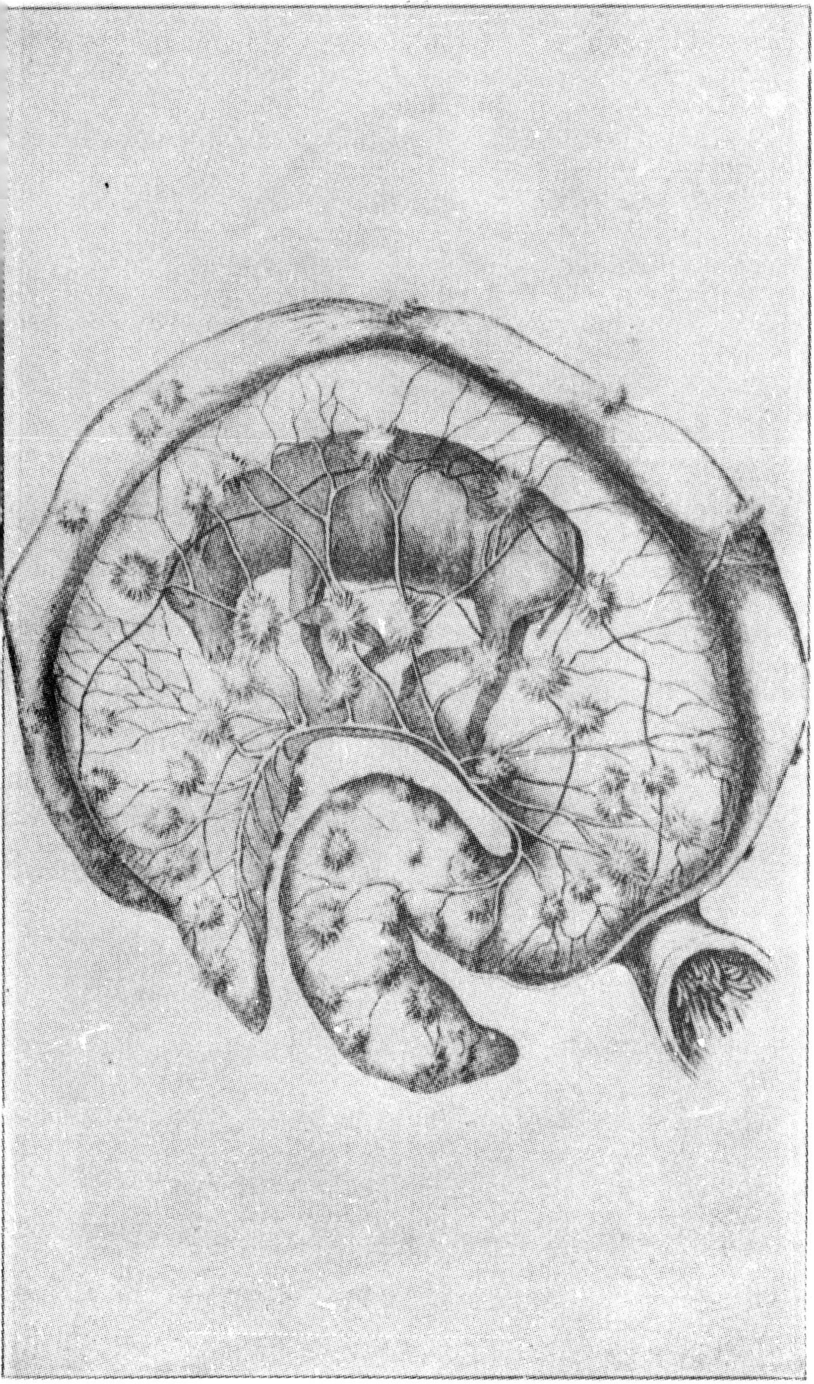

FETAL CALF WITHIN ITS MEMBRANES.

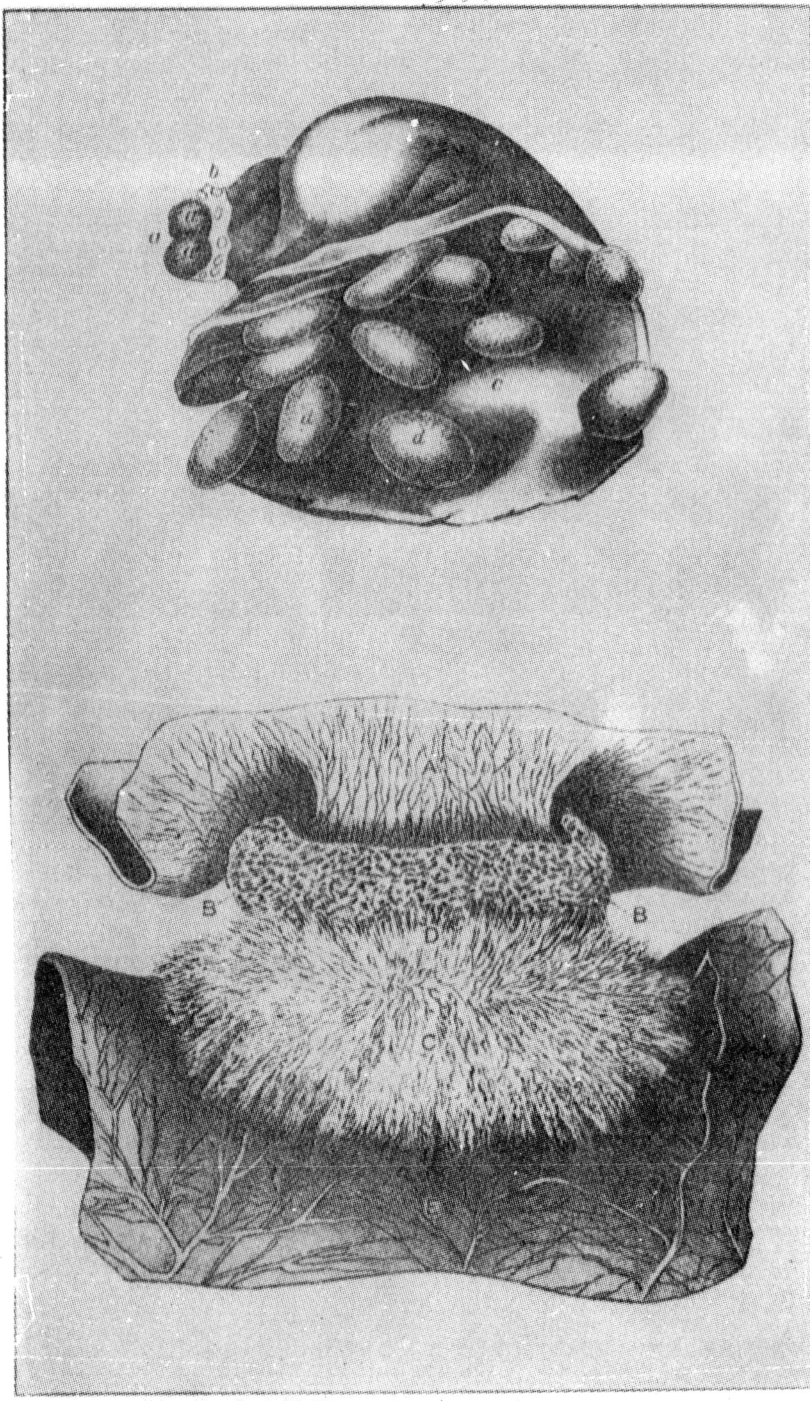

PREGNANT UTERUS WITH COTYLEDONS.

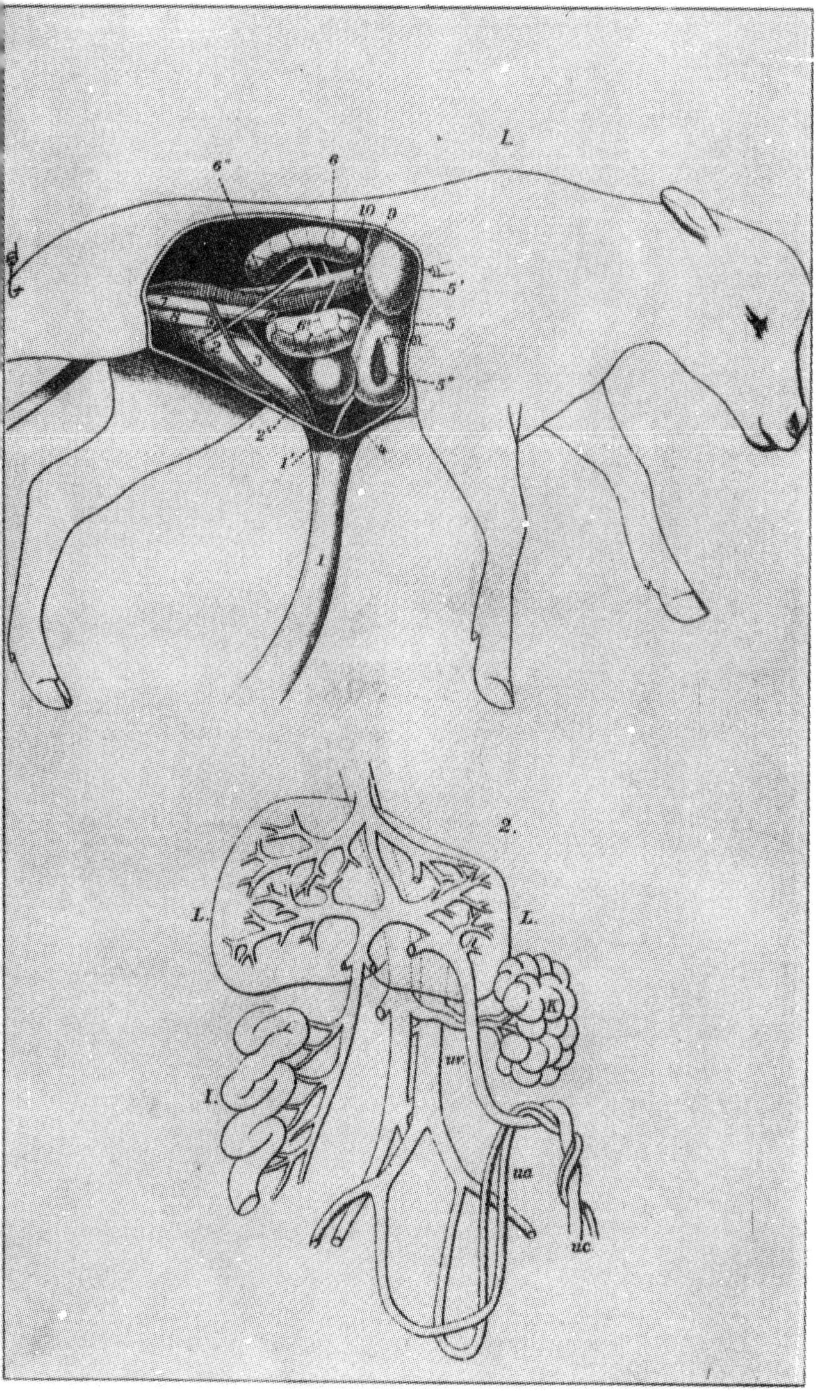

Vessels of Umbilical Cord.

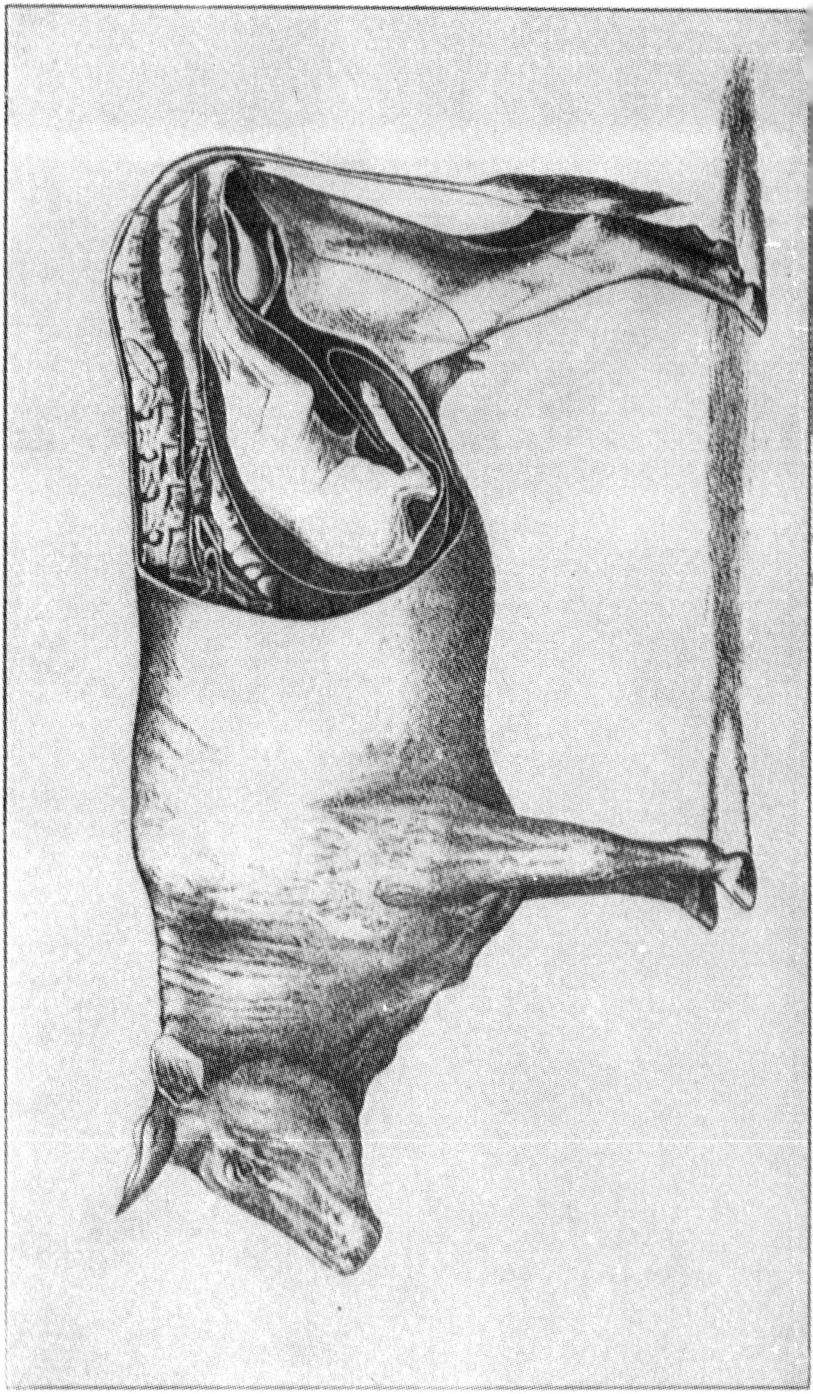

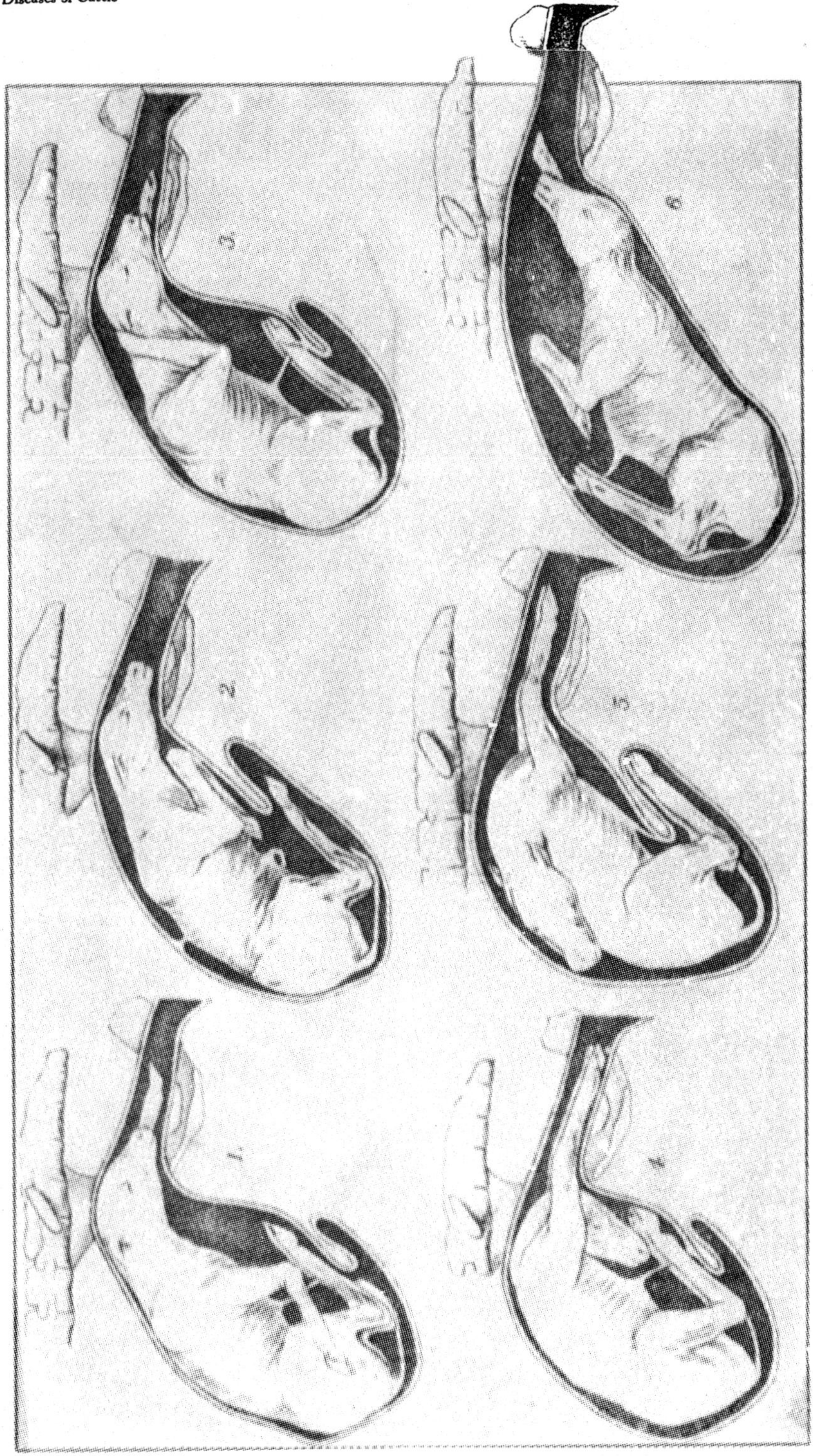

ABNORMAL POSITIONS OF CALF IN UTERO.

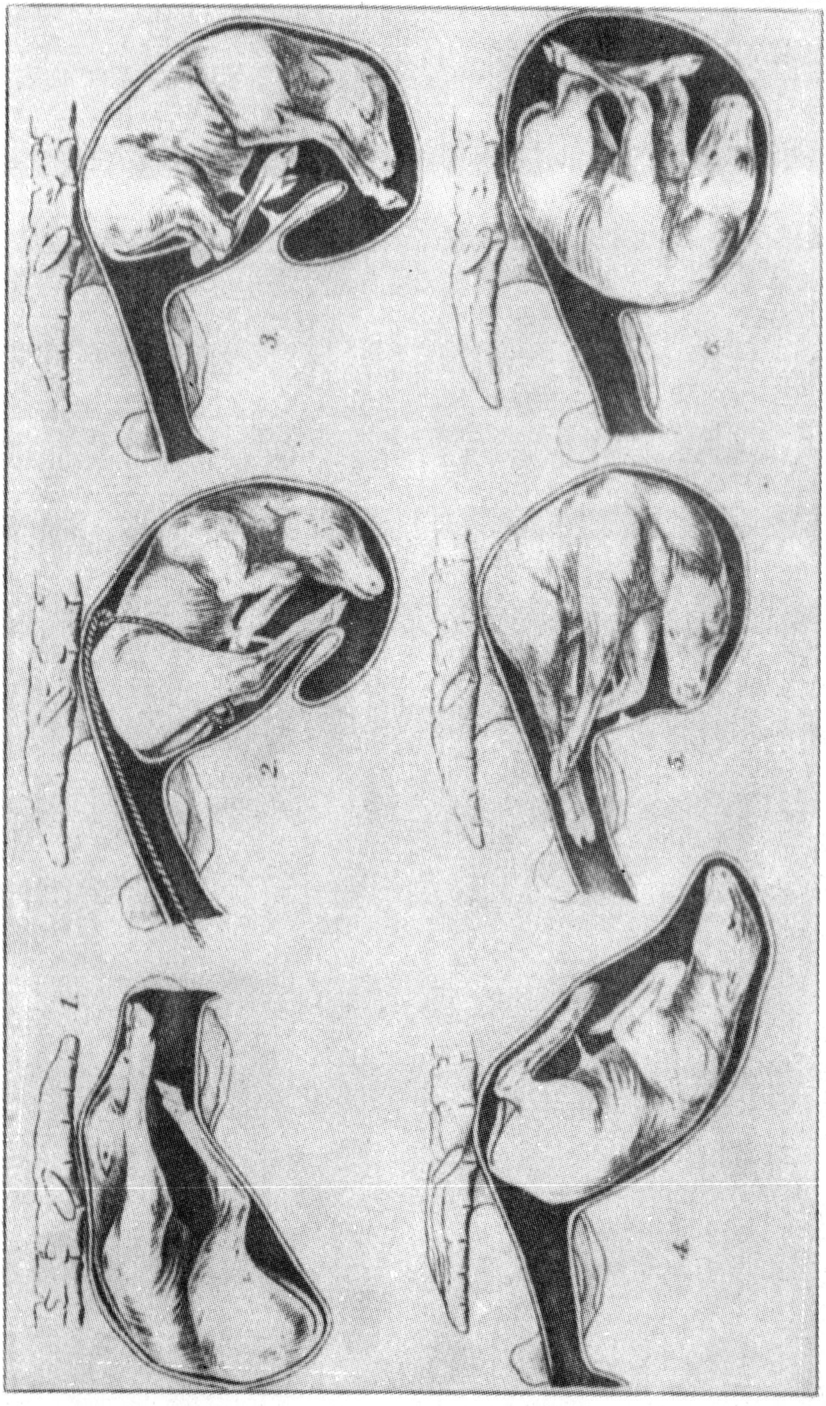

ABNORMAL POSITIONS OF CALF IN UTERO.

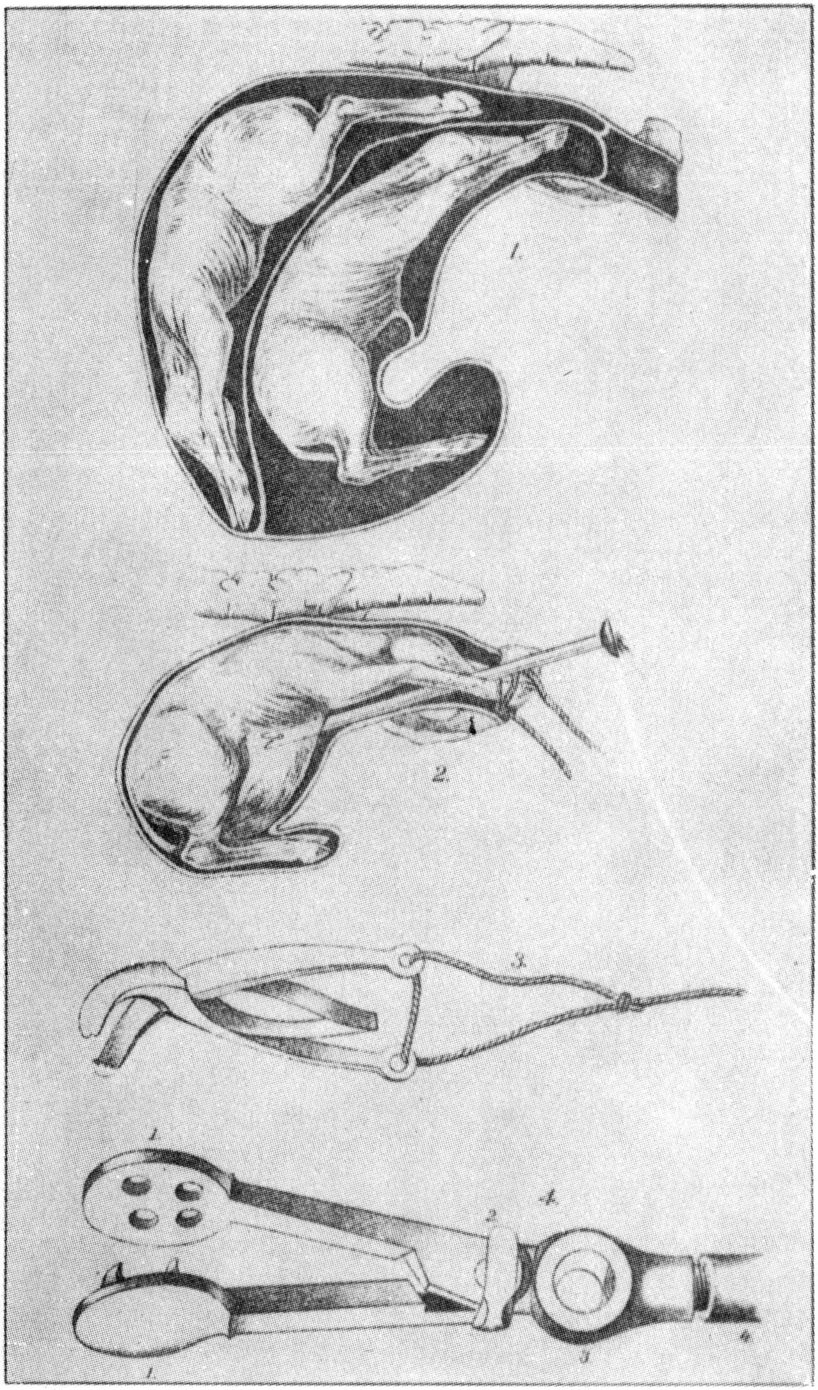

NORMAL POSITION OF CALVES IN UTERO.
SURGICAL INSTRUMENTS AND SUTURES.

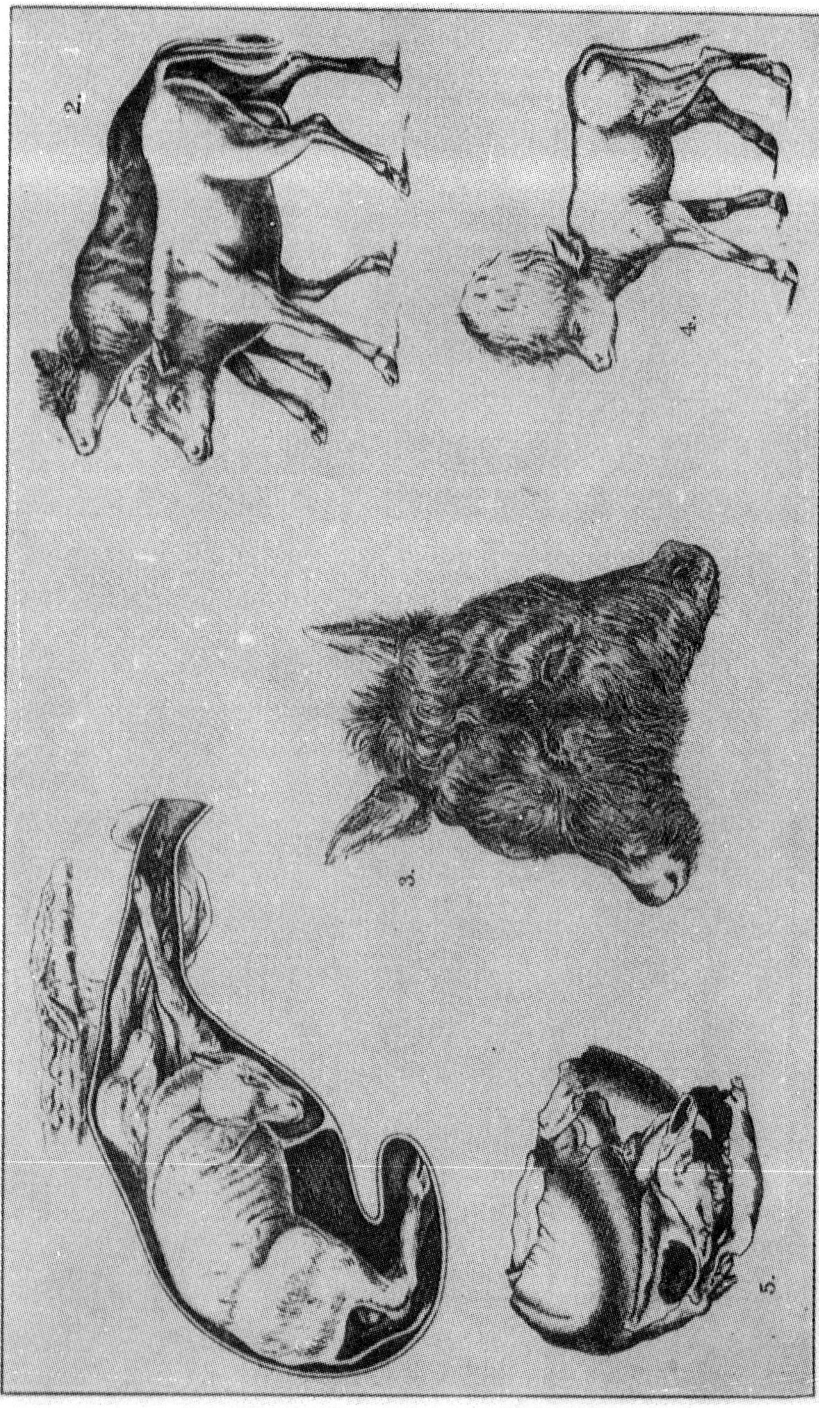
2.
4.
3.
5.

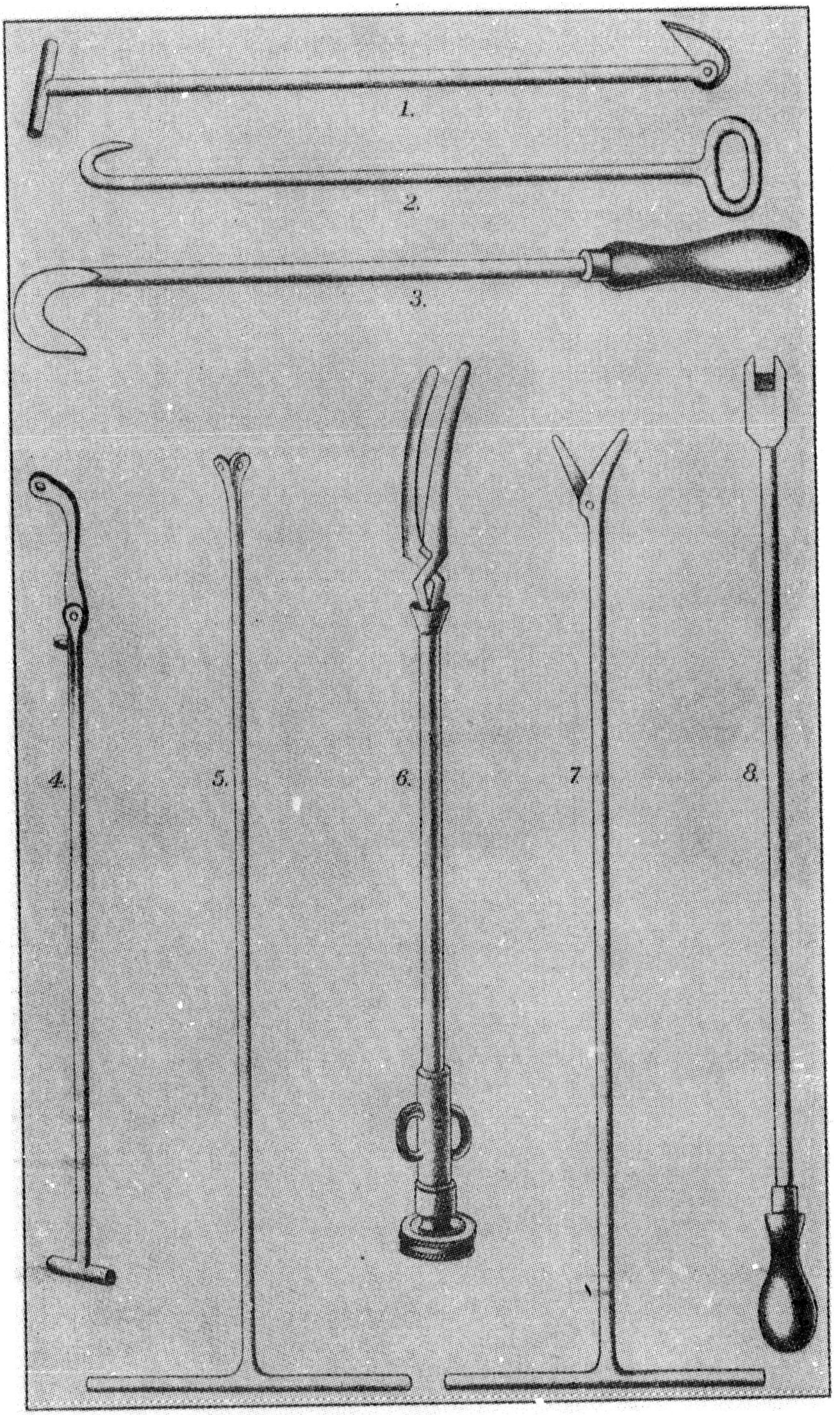

INSTRUMENTS USED IN DIFFICULT LABOR.

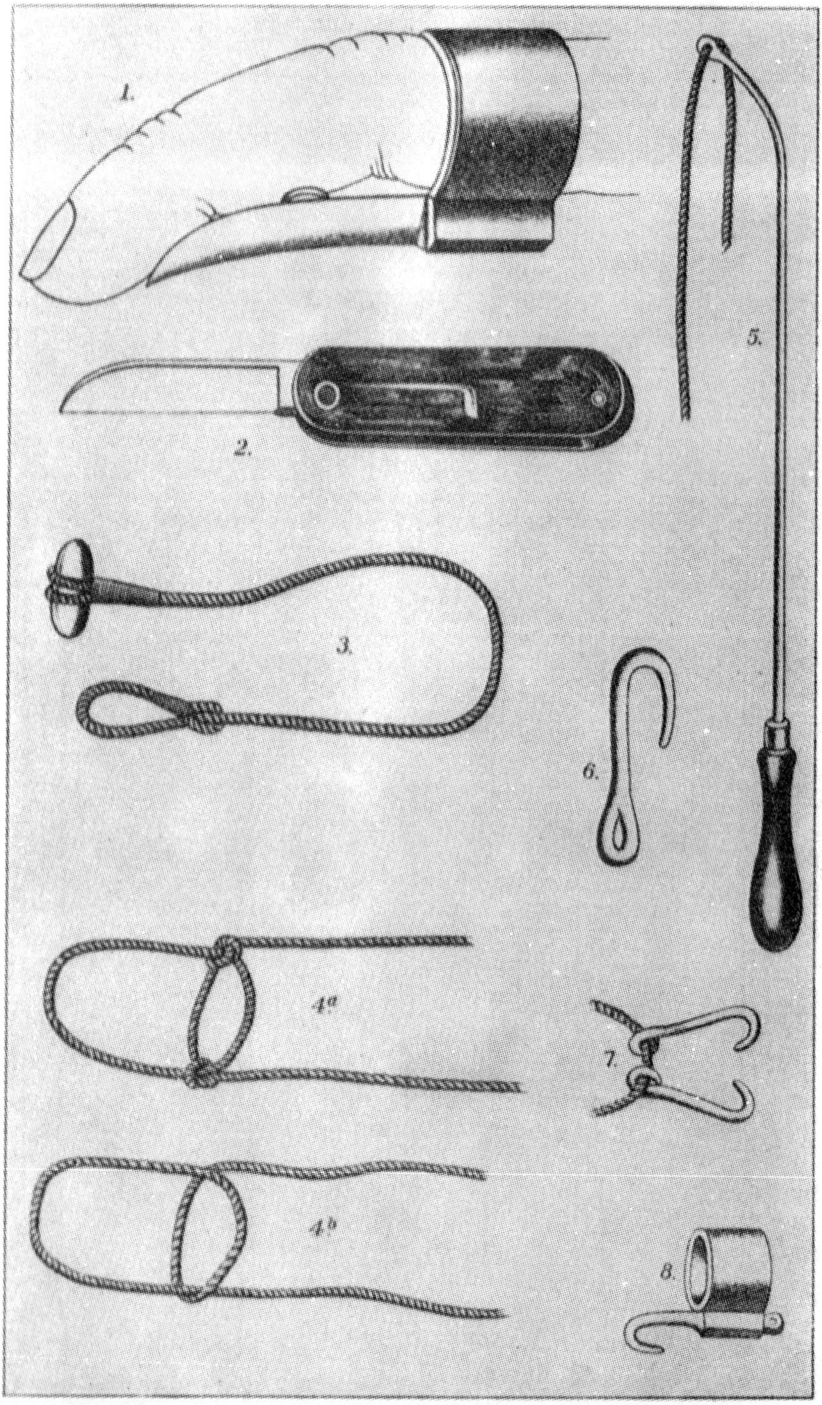

INSTRUMENTS USED IN DIFFICULT LABOR.

Diseases Following Parturition

By James Law, F. R. C. V. S.

[Revised by W. T. Miller, D. V. M., M. S., Ph. D.]

FLOODING (BLEEDING FROM THE WOMB)

Though not so common in the cow as in the human female, flooding is sufficiently frequent to demand attention. It may result from too rapid calving and a consequent failure of the womb to contract when the calf has been removed. The pregnant womb is extraordinarily rich in blood vessels, especially large and tortuous veins, which become compressed and almost obliterated under contraction but remain overfilled and often bleed into the cavity of the womb should no contraction take place. Cases have been recorded in which the labor pains had detached and expelled the fetal membranes, whereas the calf, owing to large size or wrong presentation, was detained in the womb, and the continued dilatation of the womb in the absence of the fetal membranes led to a flow of blood that accumulated in clots around the calf. Other causes are laceration of the cotyledons of the womb, or an antecedent inflammation of the placenta, and the unnatural adhesion of the membranes to the womb, which bleeds when the two are torn apart. Weakness of the womb from overdistention, as in dropsy or twins, is not without its influence. Finally, eversion of the womb (casting the withers) is an occasional cause of flooding. The trouble is only too evident when the blood flows from the external passages in drops or in a fine stream. When it is retained in the cavity of the womb, however, it may remain unsuspected until it has rendered the animal almost bloodless. The symptoms in such case are paleness of the eyes, nose, mouth, and of the lips of the vulva, a weak, rapid pulse, violent and perhaps loud beating of the heart (palpitations), sunken, staring eyes, coldness of the skin, ears, and legs, perspiration, weakness in standing, staggering gait, and finally, inability to rise, and death in convulsions. If these symptoms are seen, the oiled hand should be introduced into the womb, which will be found to be open and flaccid and contains large blood clots.

Treatment.—Treatment consists in the removal of the fetal membranes and blood clots from the womb (which will not contract while they are present), the dashing of cold water on the loins, right flank, and vulva, and if these measures fail, the injection of cold water containing a mild antiseptic into the womb through a rubber tube furnished with a funnel. In obstinate cases a good-sized sponge soaked in tincture of muriate of iron should be introduced into the womb and firmly squeezed, to bring the iron into contact with the bleeding surface. This is at once an astringent and a coagulant for the blood, besides stimulating the womb to contraction. In the absence of this agent astringents (solution of copperas, alum, tannic acid, or acetate of lead) may be introduced into the womb, and one-half-dram doses of acetate of lead may be given by the mouth, or 1 ounce powdered ergot of rye may be given in gruel. When nothing else is at hand, an injection of oil. of turpentine will sometimes promptly check the bleeding.

EVERSION OF THE WOMB (CASTING THE WITHERS)

Like flooding, this is the result of failure of the womb to contract after calving. If that organ contracts naturally, the afterbirth is expelled, the internal cavity of the womb is nearly closed, and the mouth of the organ becomes so narrow that the hand cannot be forced through. When, however, it fails to contract, the closed end of one of the horns, or divisions, may fall into its open internal cavity, and under the compression of the adjacent intestines and the straining and contraction of the abdominal walls, it is forced farther and farther, until the whole organ is turned outside in, slides back through the vagina, and hangs from the vulva. The womb can be instantly distinguished from the protruding vagina or bladder by the presence, over its whole surface, of 50 to 100 mushroomlike bodies (cotyledons), each 2 to 3 inches in diameter and attached by a narrow neck (pls. XII, XIII). When fully everted, it is further recognizable by a large, undivided body hanging from the vulva, and two horns, or divisions, which hang down toward the hocks. In imperfect eversions the body of the womb may be present with two depressions leading into the two horns. In cases of long standing the organ becomes inflamed and gorged with blood until it is as large as a bushel basket, its surface has a dark-red, bloodlike hue, and tears and bleeds on the slightest touch. Still later laceration, raw sores, and even gangrene are shown in the mass. At the moment of protrusion the general health is not altered, but soon inflammation and fever with violent and continued straining induce exhaustion, and the cow lies down and makes no attempt to rise.

Treatment.—Treatment varies somewhat, according to the degree of the eversion. In partial eversion, with the womb protruding only slightly from the vulva and the cow standing, an assistant pinches the back to prevent straining while the operator pushes his closed first into the center of the mass and carries it back through the vagina, assisting in returning the surrounding parts by the other hand. In more complete eversion, but with the womb as yet of its natural bulk and consistence and the cow standing, straining being checked by pinching the back, a sheet is held by two men to sustain the everted womb and raise it to the level of the vulva. It is now sponged clean with cold water, which is useful in driving out the blood and reducing the bulk, and finally it may be sponged with a weak solution of carbolic acid (1 dram to 1 quart of water).

The closed fist may now be planted in the rounded end of the largest horn and pushed on to turn it back within itself and carry it on through the vagina, the other hand being used meanwhile to assist in the inversion and in pushing the different masses in succession within the lips of the vulva. In case of failure, take a long linen or cotton bandage, 5 or 6 inches wide, and wind it around the protruding womb as tightly as it can be drawn, beginning at the free end and gradually covering the entire mass up to the vulva. By this means the greater part of the blood will be forced out of the organ and its bulk greatly reduced. An additional advantage is the protection given to the womb by its investing bandage while it is being pushed forward into the vagina and abdomen. In manipulating the exposed womb there is always danger of laceration, but when the organ is covered with a sheet it is almost impossible to tear it. The subsequent manipulation is, as in the other case, by pushing the blind end forward within itself with the closed fist and carrying this on through the vagina into the abdomen with the constant assistance of the other hand. Often it will be convenient to use the edge of the left hand to push the outer part of the protruding mass inside the lips of the vulva, while the right hand and arm are carrying the central portions forward through the vagina. An intelligent assistant, pushing with the palms of both hands on the outer portion of the mass, also affords material assistance. As the womb is turned within itself the wrapping bandage gradually loosens, but once the great mass has entered the passages it is easy to compel the rest to follow, and the compression by the bandage is no longer so important. When the womb is fully replaced, the bandage is left in its interior in a series of loose folds and can be easily withdrawn. It is well to move the hand from side to side to insure that the two horns of the womb are fully extended and on about the same level before withdrawing the arm and applying a truss.

When the womb has been long everted and is gorged with blood, inflamed, and friable, there is often the additional disadvantage that the animal is unable or unwilling to rise. When the animal is lying down the straining cannot be controlled so effectually, and, even in the absence of straining, the compression of the abdominal organs is so great as to prove a serious obstacle to reduction. The straining may be checked by 2 ounces of chloral hydrate or by inhalation of chloroform to produce insensibility. Then by raising the hind parts on straw bundles, the gravitation of the abdominal organs forward will lessen the resistance. If this is not successful, the cow may be turned on her back, and if return is still impossible, the hind legs may be tied together and drawn up to a beam overhead by the aid of a pulley. In this position, in place of the pressure backward of the bowels proving a hindrance, their gravitation forward is of material help to reduction. As a preparation for returning the womb, it should be sponged with ice-cold water, raised on a sheet, and wrapped in a tight bandage. Another method that is especially commendable in these inflamed conditions of the womb is to bring a piece of linen sheet, 30 by 36 inches, under the womb, with its anterior border close up to the vulva, then turn the posterior border upward and forward over the organ, and cross the two ends over this and over each other above. The ends of the sheet are steadily drawn to tighten its hold on the womb, which is thus held on the level of the vulva or above; and cold water is constantly poured on the mass. The reduction is further sought by compression of the mass with the palms applied outside the sheet. Fifteen or twenty minutes is usually sufficient to cause the return of the womb, provided straining is prevented by pinching the back, or otherwise.

In old and aggravated cases, the womb being torn, bruised, or even gangrenous, the only resort is to amputate the entire mass. This is done by tying a strong, waxed cord around the protruding mass close to the vulva, winding the cord around pieces of wood to draw it as tightly as possible, cutting off the organ below this ligature, tying a thread on any artery that may still bleed, and returning the stump well into the vagina.

Retention of the returned womb is the next point and is most easily accomplished by a rope truss. Take two ropes, each about 18 feet long and 1 inch in thickness. Double each rope at its middle, and lay the one above the other at the bend to form an ovoid of about 8 inches in its long diameter. Twist each end of the one rope twice around the other so that this ovoid will remain when they are drawn tight (pls XXII and XXIII). Tie a strap or rope around the back part of the neck and a surcingle around the body. Place the rope truss on the animal so that the ovoid ring will surround the vulva, the two ascending ropes on the right and left of the tail and the two descending ones down inside the thighs on the right and left of the udder. These descending ropes are carried forward on the sides of the body and tied to the surcingle and to the neck collar. The ascending ropes proceed forward on the middle of the back, twist over each other, and are tied to the surcingle and collar. The upper and lower ropes are drawn so tightly that the rope ring is made to press firmly all around the vulva without risk of displacement. This should be worn for several days, until the womb has closed and all risk of further eversion is at an end. Variations of this device are found in the use of a narrow triangle of iron applied around the vulva and fixed by a similar arrangement of ropes, surcingle, and collar (pl. XXIII, fig. 3), a common crupper similarly held around the vulva (pl. XXII, fig. 1), stitches through the vulva, and wire inserted through the skin on the two hips (pl. XXIII, fig. 2), so that they will cross behind the vulva; also pessaries of various kinds should be inserted into the vagina. None of these devices, however, have any advantage over the simple and comparatively painless rope truss just described. Additional precautions consist in keeping the cow in a stall higher behind than in front and seeing that the diet is slightly laxative and nonstimulating.

If the womb has been cut off, injections of a solution of a teaspoonful of carbolic acid in a quart of water should be used daily, or more frequently, until the discharge ceases.

EVERSION OF THE BLADDER

A genuine eversion of the bladder is almost unknown in the cow, owing to the extreme narrowness of its outlet. The protrusion of the bladder, however, through a laceration sustained in calving, in the floor of the vagina and its subsequent protrusion through the vulva sometimes occurs. In this case the protruding bladder contains urine; this can never be the case in a real eversion, in which the inner surface of the bladder and the openings of the ureters are both exposed outside the vulva. The presence of a bag containing water, which is connected with the floor of the vagina, will serve to identify this condition. If the position of the bladder in the vulva renders it impracticable to pass a catheter to draw off the urine, pierce the organ with a hypodermic needle or even a very small trocar and cannula, and draw off the water, when it will be found an easy matter to return the bladder to its place. The rent in the vagina can be stitched, but as there would be risk in any subsequent calving it is best to feed the animal for market.

RUPTURE OF THE BLADDER

This has been known to occur in protracted parturition when the fetus finally passed while the bladder was full. The symptoms are

77431 O—51——15

those of complete suppression of urine and tenderness of the abdomen, with a steady accumulation of liquid and fluctuation on handling its lower part. If the hand is introduced into the vagina it is felt to be hot and tender and perhaps slightly swollen along its floor. As a final test, if the lower, fluctuating part of the abdomen is punctured with a hypodermic needle, a straw-colored liquid of a urinous odor flows out. The only chance for recovery would be in opening the abdomen, evacuting the liquid, and stitching the rent in the bladder, but in such a case, and with inflammation already begun, there would be little to hope for.

RUPTURE OF THE WOMB

When the womb has been rendered friable by disease, rupture may occur in the course of labor, but much more frequently it occurs from violence sustained in attempting assistance in difficult parturition. It is also likely to occur during eversion of the organ through efforts to replace it.

If the womb is ruptured while the calf is still present, it usually bleeds freely and continuously until the fetus has been extracted, so that the womb can contract on itself and stop the bleeding. Another danger is that in case of a large rent the calf may escape into the cavity of the abdomen and parturition becomes impossible. Still another danger is that of the introduction of septic germs and the setting up of a fatal inflammation of the lining membrane of the abdomen (peritoneum). Still another is the escape of the small intestine through the rent and on through the vagina and vulva, so as to protrude externally and receive perhaps fatal injuries. In case of rupture before calving, that act should be completed as rapidly and carefully as possible, the fetal membranes removed, and the contraction of the womb sought by dashing cold water on the loins, the right flank, or the vulva. If the calf has escaped into the abdomen and cannot be brought through the natural channels, it should be extracted through the side, as in Caesarean section. If the laceration occurred during eversion of the womb, it is usually less serious because the womb contracts more readily under the stimulus of the cold air so recently applied. In case the abdomen has been laid open it is well to stitch the rent, but if not, it should be left to nature and will often heal satisfactorily so that the cow may even breed successfully in after years.

Rupture of the floor of the vagina already has been referred to as allowing the protrusion of the bladder. Laceration of the roof of this passage also occurs as the result of deviations of the hind legs and feet upward when the calf lies on its back. In some such cases the opening passes into the rectum, or the foot may even pass out through the anus, so that that opening and the vulva are laid open into one.

Simple, superficial lacerations of the vaginal walls are not usually serious and heal readily unless septic inflammation sets in, in which case the cow is likely to die. Such lacerations may be treated with soothing and antiseptic injections, such as carbolic acid, 1 dram; water, 1 quart.

The more serious injuries depend on the complications. Rupture of the interior part of the canal, close to the mouth of the womb, may lead to the introduction of infecting germs into the cavity of the abdomen or protrusion of the bowel through the rent and externally, either of which may prove fatal. If neither of these conditions occur, the wound may heal spontaneously. Rupture into the bladder may lead to nothing worse than a constant dribbling of the urine from the vulva. The cow should be fattened if she survives. Rupture into the rectum entails a constant escape of feces through the vulva, and, of course, the same condition exists when the anus as well has been torn open. In the mare, ruptures of this kind have been successfully sewed, but a cow so affected is probably best to feed for market.

CLOTS OF BLOOD IN THE WALLS OF THE VAGINA

During calving the vagina may be bruised resulting in the escape of blood beneath the mucous membrane and its coagulation into large, bulging clots. The vulva may appear swollen, and on separation of the lips the mucous membrane of the vagina is seen to be raised into irregular, rounded swellings of a dark-blue or black color, which pit on pressure of the finger. If the accumulation of blood is not extensive it may be reabsorbed, but if abundant it may lead to irritation and dangerous inflammation and should be incised with a lancet and the clots cleared out. The wounds may then be sponged twice a day with a lotion made of 1 dram of zinc sulfate, 1 dram of carbolic acid, and 1 quart of water.

RETAINED AFTERBIRTH

Of all our domestic animals, the cow is especially subject to retained afterbirth. This may be partly accounted for by the firm connections established through the 50 to 100 cotyledons (pl. XIII, fig. 2) in which the fetal membranes dovetail with the follicles of the womb. It is also most likely to occur after abortion, in which preparation has not been made by fatty degeneration for the severance of these close connections. In the occurrence of inflammation, causing the formation of new tissue between the membranes and the womb, the presence of unnaturally firm adhesions prevents the spontaneous detachment of the membranes. Again, weakened conditions of health and imperfect power of contraction are potent causes of retention, the general debility showing particularly in the inability of the womb to contract, after calving, with sufficient energy to expel the afterbirth. Hence the condition is common when animals are fed insufficient feed or feed containing little nutrient and in years or localities in which the roughage has been damaged by molds. Ergoted, smutty, or musty fodder (pl. V), by causing abortion, may be a cause of retention. Old cows are more subject than young ones, probably because of diminishing vigor. Temporary retention is sometimes due to too rapid closure of the neck of the womb after calving, causing strangulation and imprisonment of the membranes.

Symptoms.—The symptoms of retention of the afterbirth are usually only too evident, as the membranes hang from the vulva and rot away gradually, causing a very offensive odor. When the afterbirth is retained within the womb by closure of its mouth and similarly in cases in which the protruded part has rotted off, the decomposition continues and the fetid products escaping by the vulva appear in offensively smelling pools on the floor and mat together the hairs near the root of the tail. The septic materials retained in the womb cause inflammation of its lining membrane, and this, together with the absorption into the blood of the products of putrefaction, leads to ill health, emaciation, and drying up of the milk.

Treatment.—Since the afterbirth of healthy animals often is not expelled until after a few hours, owners are justified in viewing its retention with little alarm until 24 hours after the act of abortion or parturition, provided the animal appears to be normal otherwise. Retention of the afterbirth longer than 24 hours signifies that inflammation of the uterus may be present and responsible for its adherence. When the afterbirth has been retained for 2 or 3 days, putrefaction usually becomes marked. In this putrefactive process within the uterus, poisonous substances may be generated and absorbed by the animal, causing fever, loss of appetite, and other evidences of severe trouble. Invasion of the blood stream by bacteria may terminate fatally.

The afterbirth frequently can be removed before putrefaction is excessive by reaching into the uterus with the hand and separating as carefully as possible the attached areas and flushing the organ out afterwards with mild antiseptic solutions or warm salt water. A 0.5 percent Lugol's solution[1] is often used for this purpose.

[1] Lugol's solution of iodine is compounded as follows: Iodine, 5 parts; potassium iodide, 10 parts; and boiled water to make 100 parts. One part of this compound to 200 parts of boiled water makes a solution suitable for uterine irrigation. Lugol's solution may be purchased from any druggist.

Boiled water that has been cooled to body temperature and to every gallon of which 1 heaping tablespoonful of table salt has been added makes a satisfactory irrigating fluid. The flushing may be done by the use of a soft-rubber tube with a diameter of about half an inch, a funnel being attached to the tube. The fluid should not be allowed to remain in the uterus but should be siphoned out by lowering the external end of the tube when filled with the fluid.

The afterbirth can seldom be removed by hand without causing some injury to the uterine walls, a factor that renders the operation of uncertain value. A putrefactive afterbirth in contact with injured uterine walls may be more harmful and more likely to kill the animal than when in contact with an uninjured uterine surface.

A less drastic method is consequently often advisable. This method permits the afterbirth to remain attached to the uterine walls, while by introducing mild antiseptic substances into the uterus the rapid multiplication of germs is prevented until the membranes come away of themselves. Separating the pendent portion of the afterbirth from the retained part about 6 or 8 inches exterior to the vulva is a means of reducing the contamination of surroundings. A dram (1 level teaspoon) of iodoform combined with a quart of mineral or olive oil and introduced into the uterus through a rubber tube is recommended. The milk of animals so treated may have an iodoform odor for several days and therefore should not be used for food. Such irrigating fluids as those mentioned for washing out the uterus after removal of the afterbirth by hand may be used but seem to be less efficient than iodoform and oil. It is seldom advisable to introduce irrigating fluids more often than once a day or once in 2 days. Although animals have been known to retain the afterbirth as long as 10 days after a single administration of iodoform and oil, as described, they appeared to experience little discomfort or harm.

Retention of the afterbirth is a more serious condition than is often realized, since it may be followed by or induce barrenness. Because of this fact the assistance and experience of a veterinarian are highly desirable.

INFLAMMATION OF THE VAGINA (VAGINITIS)

This may occur independently of inflammation of the womb and usually as the result of bruises, lacerations, or other injuries sustained during calving. It will be shown by swelling of the lips of the vulva, which, together with their lining membrane, becomes of a dark-red or leaden hue, and the mucous discharge increases and becomes whitish or purulent, and it may be fetid. Slight cases recover spontaneously, or under warm fomentations or mild astringent injections (a teaspoonful of carbolic acid in a quart of water), but severe cases may go on to the formation of large sores (ulcers), or considerable portions of the mucous membrane may die and slough off. In all severe cases the antiseptic injections must be applied assiduously. The carbolic acid may be increased to one-half ounce to a quart, or chlorine water or hydrogen peroxide solution may be injected at least three times a day. Hyposulfite of soda, 1 ounce to a quart of water, is an excellent application.

LEUCORRHEA (MUCOPURULENT DISCHARGE FROM THE PASSAGES)

This discharge is caused by a continued or chronic inflammation of the womb or the vagina or both. The inflammation usually results from injuries sustained in calving, from irritation by putrid matters in connection with retained afterbirth, or from the use of some object in the vagina (pessary) to prevent eversion of the womb. Exposure to cold or other cause of disturbance of the health may so affect an organ as susceptible as this at the time of parturition as to cause inflammation.

Symptoms.—The main symptom is the glairy, white discharge flowing constantly or intermittently when the cow lies down, soiling the tail and matting its hairs and those of the vulva. When the lips of the vulva are drawn apart the mucous membrane appears red, with minute elevations, or pale and smooth. The health may not suffer at first, but if the discharge continues and is putrid the health fails, the milk shrinks, and flesh is lost. If the womb is involved the hand introduced into the vagina may detect the mouth of the womb slightly open and the liquid collected within its cavity. Examination with the oiled hand in the rectum may detect the outline of the womb beneath, somewhat enlarged, and fluctuating under the touch from contained fluid. In some cases heat is more frequent or intense than natural, but the animal rarely conceives when served and, if she does, is likely to abort.

Treatment.—Treatment with the injections of mild antiseptic solutions and warm salt water as recommended for retained afterbirth may be undertaken. Three drams of ferrous sulfate and one-half ounce of ground ginger may also be given in the feed daily.

INFLAMMATION OF THE WOMB (METRITIS, INFLAMMATION OF WOMB AND ABDOMEN, OR METROPERITONITIS)

Inflammation of the womb may be slight or violent, simple or associated with putrefaction of its liquid contents and general poisoning, or it may extend so that the inflammation affects the lining membrane of the whole abdominal cavity. In the last two cases the malady is a very grave one.

Causes.—The causes are largely the same as those in inflammation of the vagina. Greater importance, however, must be attached to exposed to cold and wet and to septic infection.

Symptoms.—The symptoms appear 2 or 3 days after calving, when the cow may be seen to shiver, or the hair stands erect, especially along the spine, and the horns, ears, and legs are cold. The temperature in the rectum is elevated 1° or 2°, the pulse is weak, hard, and rapid (70 to 100), appetite is lost, rumination ceases, and the milk shrinks in quantity or stops entirely, and the breathing is hurried. The hind legs may shift uneasily, the head and eyes turn to the right flank, and the animal grinds its teeth. There is redness of eyes, nose, and mouth, and usually a dark redness about the vulva. Pressure on right flank gives pain, causing moaning or grunting, and the hind legs are moved stiffly, extremely so if the general lining of the abdomen is involved. In severe cases the cow lies down and cannot be made to rise. There is usually marked thirst, the bowels are costive, and dung is passed with pain and effort. The hand inserted into the vagina perceives the increased heat, and when the neck of the womb is touched the cow winces. Examination through the rectum detects enlargement and tenderness of the womb. The discharge from the vulva is at first watery, but becomes thick, yellow, and finally red or brown, with a heavy or fetid odor. Some cases recover speedily and may be almost well in 2 days; a large proportion die within 2 days of the attack, and some merge into the chronic form, terminating in leucorrhea. The worst cases involve (1) local septic infection and ulceration, (2) gangrene of the parts, (3) general septicemia, or (4) inflammation involving the veins of the womb, which causes coagulation of the blood contained in them, and the washing out of the clots to the right side of the heart and the right lung leads to the blocking of the vessels in the latter and complicating pneumonia. Inflammation of the womb and passages after calving are always liable to these complications and consequently to a fatal issue.

Treatment.—The womb should be flushed out thoroughly with warm salt water to remove, as far as possible, the collections of fetid material. Then the organ may be irrigated with a mild antiseptic solution, such as 0.5 percent Lugol's solution, as advised for treatment of retained afterbirth. This procedure may be repeated once or twice daily for several days, but owing to the serious nature of the affection and the difficulties of judging the progress of healing, treatment should be carried out by a veterinarian. It is usually desirable to open the bowels with a drench of 1½ pounds of Glauber's salt and 1 ounce of ginger in 4 quarts of warm water, and to apply fomentation of warm water or even mustard poultices or turpentine to the right flank.

In violent attacks with high temperature and great prostration, besides the salts, agents must be given to lower the temperature and counteract septic poisoning. If the temperature rises to 106° or 107° F., direct application of cold or iced water to the surface should be made. The animal may be covered with wet sheets and cold water poured on them frequently until the temperature in the rectum is lowered to 102° F. In summer the cow may be allowed to dry spontaneously; in winter it should be rubbed dry and blanketed. Even in the absence of high temperature much good may be obtained from the soothing influence of a wet sheet covering the loins and flanks and well covered at all points by a dry one. This may be followed next day by a free application of mustard and oil of turpentine.

In this disease, even more than in difficult and protracted parturition or retained afterbirth, the attendants must carefully guard against the infection of their hands and arms from the diseased parts. The hand and arm before entering the passages should always be well smeared with petrolatum impregnated with carbolic acid.

MILK FEVER OR PARTURIENT APOPLEXY

The condition known as milk fever occurs, as a rule, immediately after calving and usually appears in the best-producing cows in the herd at the time when they have reached their full production of milk, between the ages of 5 and 9 years. It is characterized by its sudden appearance and acute course. The animal becomes paralyzed and passes into a semiconscious or unconscious condition that may terminate in death. Why this condition develops in some cows and not in others is not definitely known. However, it is known that at the time of onset of the disease there is a marked fall in the calcium or lime content of the blood and that by increasing the amount of calcium circulating in the blood a cure can be effected. Apparently such factors as heavy milk production, excessive feeding, and lack of exercise predispose the animal to such an attack.

The symptoms of milk fever are characteristic and easily recognized. Soon after, or in a few cases immediately before calving the cow may show signs of excitement and anxiety followed by constipation and colicky symptoms. The owner may notice a staggering gait and weakness, especially of the hindquarters. Eventually the cow, no longer able to stand, goes down and assumes the posture so characteristic of this disease with the hind legs extended forward and the head thrown back toward the flank. A comatose condition usually follows, during which there is danger in attempting to administer medicine by the mouth as the throat muscles are temporarily paralyzed and the material may pass into the windpipe and lungs and cause pneumonia. Pulse and respiration are weak, and the temperature is more frequently subnormal than otherwise. Unless prompt remedial measures are undertaken, death will follow within 3 days. Although the symptoms given are found in most milk fever cases, an occasional case may occur in which the usual symptoms are missing, and in addition the case may be complicated by the presence of other conditions. Veterinary advice should be obtained, therefore, in all cases of milk fever.

Treatment.—Two methods of treatment are available and appear to be equally efficient. Both accomplish the same purpose—the restoration of calcium to the blood. The newer method consists in administering calcium salts, dissolved in sterile water, to the animal either by way of a vein or under the skin. Either calcium gluconate or calcium chloride may be used, but the former is preferable, especially for injection under the skin as it is much less irritating and less likely to cause abscess formation and sloughing. As the dosage of either of these salts depends on the method of administration and also on the size of the animal, the remedy should be used only by a veterinarian. In some cases it may be necessary to repeat the treatment a second and even a third time before permanent recovery is attained. The principal advantage of this method is that no manipulation of the teats and udder is necessary, and consequently there is no danger of introducing infection into the quarters and thus causing mastitis.

The other method of treatment consists in inflating the quarters of the udder with sterile air and tying the teats with broad tapes. The udder is allowed to remain inflated for several hours after the cow has regained her feet. The treatment must be performed with the utmost regard to cleanliness. A clean cloth should be laid beneath the udder, which is then washed clean and disinfected with 5 percent carbolic acid solution.

The apparatus used for inflating the udder consists of a rubber-bellows arrangement attached to a rubber tubing, which in turn is connected with a hollow metal cylinder containing sterile cotton for the filtration of air. Another rubber tube is attached to the other end of the metal cylinder, and at the other end of this rubber tube is the metal teat catheter. The last tube and metal catheter should be thoroughly sterilized by boiling, and the hollow metal cylinder should be loosely packed with sterile cotton.

The catheter is then inserted into one of the teats of the previously cleaned udder, and the rubber bulb is operated by repeated compressions until the quarter is well inflated. Massage of the quarter during inflation will assist in filling the recesses of the gland with sterile air. The catheter is then withdrawn and the teat tied with broad tape. After inflating all four of the quarters the veterinarian will have an opportunity to attend to any complications or to administer stimulants if necessary. Medicinal treatment is usually superfluous, however, in uncomplicated cases of milk fever. Following the sterile-air treatment alone, it is no uncommon experience to find the cow on her feet in from 30 to 60 minutes and eating as though there had been no disturbance of her normal condition.

Should the first sterile-air treatment fail to give relief, the procedure should be repeated, as the air previously injected may have escaped or been absorbed. The tapes may be removed in about 5 hours, or soon after the cow regains her feet. The air should remain in the udder for about 24 hours, after which time it should be completely extracted by the manipulation used in milking. It is then safe to permit the calf to suck. An occasional case of milk fever fails to respond to this method but is immediately relieved by the use of the calcium salts. On the other hand, a few cases are not benefited by the injection of these agents but do very well following inflation of the udder.

Prevention.—Although it is impossible to foretell which animals may suffer from milk fever at the time of calving, some general measures may be used that are believed to be of assistance in warding off such an attack. When the cow is dried off prior to calving she should be placed on a light ration of bran and a little ground oats, supplemented with suitable hay and possibly some succulent roots or an occasional feed of silage or beet pulp. She should be housed in a dry, comfortable, well-ventilated stable with sanitary surroundings, properly bedded, and given sufficient and regular exercise daily up to the time of calving. Several days prior to calving she should receive a full dose of Epsom salts. Cows that are known to have had milk fever at previous calvings may be given a dose of calcium salts, in the manner previously described, immediately before calving as a possible precautionary measure.

MASTITIS (GARGET, CAKED UDDER)

Mastitis, or inflammation of the udder, is a widespread disease, particularly in dairy cattle, and is caused by the entrance of bacteria into the udder. The disease can, therefore, be carried or transmitted from diseased to healthy cows. The continued spread of mastitis in dairy herds results each year in an enormous loss to the dairyman. Milk from diseased cows does not contain the usual quantities of butterfat, milk sugar, and other elements present in milk from healthy udders. On the other hand, it may contain large numbers of bacteria, leucocytes (white blood cells), and other products resulting from the disease. Consequently, such milk is low in nutritive value and is rejected frequently because of high bacteria and leucocyte counts. In addition to losses from this source, cows affected with mastitis cannot produce the volume of milk of which they would be capable if their udders were healthy. This decrease in production, in many cases, may amount to as much as 25 percent or more and necessitates early disposal of diseased animals as unprofitable. Mastitis is, therefore, one of the chief causes for the heavy turn-over in cattle in dairy herds.

Cause.—Several kinds of bacteria are capable of producing mastitis when they have finally become established in the quarter or quarters of the udder. However, only a few are responsible for most cases of the disease. Among the varieties of bacteria occasionally found in cases of mastitis are several that may be harmful to man. At one time tuberculosis of the udder was a common cause of the disease. However, because of the progress made in the eradication of tuberculosis from cattle of this country, mastitis from this source is extremely rare. Other diseases, such as septic sore throat, which may be caused by drinking raw milk, may result from contamination of the milk after it leaves the cow or from a case of mastitis. In either instance the infection is the result of contact with a diseased handler or milker. The presence of these bacteria can be recognized only by bacteriological examination of the milk. Fortunately the occurrence of these diseases is very infrequent. Most of the varieties of bacteria found in mastitis are harmless for the consumer and when milk is properly pasteurized, practically all danger is eliminated.

The bacteria that cause mastitis are usually carried from diseased cows to the teats of healthy cows on the hands of milkers or in the teat cups of milking machines during milking. The bacteria then enter the opening in the teat, pass up the teat canal, and establish themselves in the milk cistern or lower part of the quarter. From this point they spread slowly or rapidly, depending on circumstances, to other parts of the organ. When disease-producing bacteria have thus become implanted in the udder, they remain there, as a rule, for the rest of the life of the animal.

As a result of the persistence of these bacteria in the udder, mastitis is a chronic disease in most cases. Acute cases occur from time to time in individual animals, but for the most part they are flare-ups of already-established chronic cases and should be regarded as such in the management of the disease. Because of its nature, chronic mastitis runs a somewhat obscure course and as a consequence it may become widely disseminated through the herd before its presence is recognized. Similarly, many cows affected with chronic mastitis undoubtedly are purchased to replace animals that have been sold on account of the disease. This is due to the fact that the symptoms of the disease are not outstanding and are somewhat difficult to detect.

Symptoms.—Of the symptoms associated with the disease, changes in the milk, such as the presence of flakes or clots and a watery or unusual appearance, are most frequently observed. Other symptoms may be occasional slight swellings in the udder for a day or two, a more rapid decrease in milk production than is generally expected, the so-called short milker, persistent inflammation in the udder after calving and at the end of the lactation period, and frequent high bacterial counts in the milk. The decrease in milk secretion is caused by the continued irritant effect of the bacteria that leads to hardening of the glandular tissue of the affected quarter. The resulting changes appear in the form of hard circumscribed areas or diffuse hardening of the gland, which can be detected with some experience when the empty udder is manipulated.

Unlike the chronic form of the disease, acute mastitis is readily detectable and is the form most familiar to the cattle owner. The symptoms are characteristic. The affected part is hot, tense, very hard, and tender, and the animal moves with reluctance and some difficulty because of the soreness of the udder. Milk secretion is largely or entirely suspended, and what there is of it is lumpy or stringy and in some cases appears as a straw-colored fluid, occasionally tinged with blood, containing yellowish clots. Frequently the secretion, during an attack at calving time, may contain blood from the rupture of a small blood vessel. When certain kinds of bacteria are involved in an acute attack the secretion may even be purulent and offensive. At times these common symptoms may be accompanied with a general systemic disturbance such as depression, rough coat, dull eyes, loss of appetite, suspended rumination, and possibly constipation. There may or may not be fever, and exceptionally, a dropsical condition under the skin of the abdomen.

The acute form of the disease can be caused by any factors that tend to aggravate the chronic mastitis already present, or in some cases it may result from a recent invasion of the udder by mastitis bacteria. Among the causes or combinations of causes capable of arousing the chronic condition or favoring bacterial invasion of the udder are: Exposure to cold or wet weather; sudden changes of temperature; blows, kicks, bruises, or abrasions of the udder; wounds of the teats; feeding heavily for milk production; infrequent, irregular, or incomplete milking; introduction of contaminated foreign bodies such as tubes or pieces of straw into the teat canal; indigestion; or any systematic disturbance of the animal's health. Although this form of disease occurs most frequently at calving time and at the end of the lactation period, it may appear whenever any of these conditions are present. With appropriate treatment, the acute symptoms subside in many cases, and the udder resumes its usual appearance. The milk also appears normal although the yield may not return to its previous level. However, recovery from an acute attack is more apparent than real since the bacteria responsible for the mastitis are still present in the udder and are capable of producing further attacks under favorable conditions. Finally, acute mastitis may result at times in atrophy or drying up of the quarter, the formation of abscesses, or gangrene of the udder. When any of these conditions occur, a veterinarian should be consulted as to suitable treatment.

Diagnosis.—Acute mastitis is readily diagnosed from the characteristic symptoms of the disease. Chronic mastitis, on the other hand, presents some difficulties in detection. Since detection of all diseased animals must be the first step in any program for controlling the spread of the disease, a number of methods designed for this purpose have been recommended. Some of these tests are applicable for use in the herd, whereas others can be carried out successfully only by a veterinarian or in the laboratory. Probably the most practical test for the dairyman is the strip cup. This is simply a tin cup covered with a fine wire screen or black cloth. Two or three streams of milk from each quarter are drawn onto the strainer immediately before the animal is milked. Any quarter in which abnormal milk or clots are found is affected with mastitis. However, these changes do not appear regularly in the milk of all cows having chronic mastitis. Consequently, repeated use of this test is necessary to detect every diseased animal. For greatest effectiveness, the strip cup should be used before each milking.

A second method that can be used in the dairy barn is the bromthymol-blue or "thybromol" test. This procedure requires more equipment and a great deal more experience in its interpretation than the strip-cup test. The test is carried out either with a dye solution and test tubes or with papers impregnated with this solution. A definite quantity of milk from one quarter is added to a measured quantity of dye solution in a test tube, or a few drops of milk are placed on the paper containing the dye. The color resulting from this mixture depends on the degree of acidity of the milk. Milk from healthy quarters gives a yellowish-green shade, whereas that from quarters affected with mastitis is predominantly green, or, in exceptional cases, a bright yellow. Although this test detects a somewhat larger number of diseased animals at any one time than the strip cup, it too should be used at frequent intervals to find every affected cow, although not necessarily at every milking. The changes in the milk that these tests detect are the result of bacterial activity in the quarter, but they do not reveal the kind of bacteria present. Although mastitis bacteria remain in the udder at all times in most cases, such changes may not be detected regularly in the milk. Consequently, failure to find evidence of mastitis with these tests in cows previously shown to be diseased does not mean that these animals are no longer affected. Therefore, cows that have been found to have mastitis at any time should be handled as such for the purpose of controlling the disease as long as they remain in the herd.

Treatment.—Acute attacks of mastitis will subside fairly rapidly when properly handled, and the animal will be restored to comparative usefulness although the underlying cause of the condition may remain unchanged. One of the most important points in the treatment of an acute attack of mastitis is frequent milking of the affected quarter or quarters. This should be done every hour or two until the secretion returns to normal and should be accompanied with gentle massage with downward pressure in order to work as much of the diseased material as possible into the milk cistern, from which it can be removed by gentle stripping. At the same time camphorated oil or a suitable ointment may be rubbed into the skin to facilitate the massage. The secretion should be collected in a bucket containing disinfectant and disposed of in such a manner that other animals cannot have access to it. At the beginning of the attack, applications of cold packs may assist in reducing the condition. If the affected part does not respond readily to this treatment, it is advisable to change to applications as hot as the hand will stand until the inflammation has left the part. The ration should be changed to one consisting principally of roughage, with the concentrates such as cottonseed and linseed meal eliminated. No attempt should be made to force an antiseptic fluid into the quarter unless the operation is recommended and performed by a veterinarian.

No entirely effective measures are available for the treatment and cure of all cases of chronic mastitis. Treatment is still largely in the experimental stage. The most suitable method of handling chronic mastitis in the herd seems to be prevention of spread of the disease from affected to healthy cows by a program of sanitation and segregation rather than by any attempt to cure the diseased animals. Such a program consists in early detection of infected animals by a veterinarian and the use of approved sanitary measures.

When each animal has been examined and the condition of the udder determined, those animals with marked cases of mastitis should be removed from the herd and slaughtered. Such animals are of little or no value, and they are the chief sources from which infection spreads. The remaining animals should then be divided into three groups—the healthy cows in one, those that are suspected of having the disease in another, and those with slight cases of mastitis in the third. These last cows may be retained temporarily in the herd because the trouble has not progressed to the point where the milk is unfit for use and milk production has not decreased to an unprofitable point.

It is desirable that cows of each of these groups be stabled together and assigned permanent stalls. In this way a permanent order of milking can be established and followed with little difficulty. If it is impractical to stable the three groups separately, at least the healthy group should be kept separate from the other two. Since the disease is spread during milking, the healthy cows must be milked first each time, the ones suspected of having mastitis next, and those having the disease last. When first-calf heifers are added to the milking herd, they can be safely included in the healthy group unless definite evidence of mastitis is observed at the time of calving. When animals have freshened again after division of the herd, they should be put back in the same group, provided they have not developed mastitis in the meantime. If they have become infected, they should be placed in the third group. When a milking animal (a cow that has had one or more calves) is obtained from another herd, it should be bought only after the udder has been examined or subject to such examination after 60 to 90 days if it cannot be examined at the time of purchase. Such an animal should be kept isolated during this period. If the animal is found to be healthy, it is placed in the first group; otherwise it is rejected. Any member of the healthy or suspected group that develops mastitis must be immediately placed with the diseased animals. Such an animal can usually be recognized by the secretion of abnormal milk or changes in the udder.

Udders should be thoroughly cleaned before milking. A practical method is to cut small hand towels in half and place the pieces in a suitable chlorine solution (150 to 400 parts of chlorine per million parts of water). Chlorine solutions should be kept in porcelain, enamel, glass, wood, or graniteware containers but never in galvanized iron, tin, or aluminum vessels. Remove a towel from the solution, wring out the excess fluid, and wipe the udder thoroughly, using a separate towel for each animal. This cleanses the skin and leaves it comparatively dry. After each milking the towels should be washed, boiled, and, if possible, dried in the sun. When a milking machine is used, the teat cups should be rinsed in a chlorine solution of the above strength before each cow is milked. If milking is done by hand, the milker should wash his hands in warm, soapy water or chlorine solution and dry them before milking the next animal. After milking, the teats of each animal should be dipped in fresh chlorine solution to disinfect the ends of the teats and remove any milk that remains on them. Between milkings the machine must be thoroughly cleaned and disinfected as described in Farmers' Bulletin 1315.

As any injuries to the udder cause it to be more easily attacked by mastitis bacteria, care should be taken to prevent such injuries. This may be done, in part, by providing properly constructed stalls that allow adequate space for each cow, stall partitions to prevent cows from treading on one another's teats, and a well-bedded, dry floor. The generous use of lime or superphosphate in the stable helps to keep the floor dry.

If the foregoing procedures are strictly followed, there should be little further spread of the disease to the healthy animals. Also there should be a reduction in the severity of the disease in the affected group. However, it must be emphasized that successful operation of this disease-control measure depends entirely on daily observance of all of the points mentioned. Finally, adequate veterinary supervision of the herd should be maintained at all times.

AGALACTIA OR SUPPRESSION OF MILK

The disease known as agalactia or suppression of milk is not infectious in cattle, as it is in sheep and goats. Neither is it so common. Occurring, as it usually does, at calving time, agalactia seems to be unfavorably influenced by such predisposing causes as indigestion, loss of appetite, mastitis, insufficient or unsuitable feed, plant poisoning, severe insect stings on the udder, thirst, enforced driving, fear or excitement, or the removal of the calf. Incidentally, agalactia is a symptom often seen in rabies in the cow.

Treatment.—The animal, if a heifer, should first be examined for the possibility of atresia, or imperforation of the teats. When this possibility is eliminated, attention should be directed toward determining, if possible, the contributing cause or causes, which should receive prompt attention.

The animal should be surrounded with an environment most conducive to her comfort. She should be supplied with an abundance of fresh, clean, drinking water, and have a generous allowance of a ration, preferably in the form of a warm mash, calculated to stimulate milk secretion. Milk secretion may be assisted by internal medicinal treatment. Massaging the udder with lard or an ointment may assist in bringing her to her milk. Efforts should be made to milk her twice daily, at regular milking time, even though the efforts are unrewarded. If the calf is brought to her side shortly before milking time this appeal to her maternal instinct may exert a favorable influence.

LEAKY QUARTER AND FISTULA

When a heavy-milking cow comes up to the barn with milk dripping or streaming from one or more of her quarters, the animal should be milked three or even four times daily instead of twice. Cows of only moderate production may likewise leak milk at times if their milking is long delayed or their capacity of retention is otherwise abnormally taxed. Persistent loss of milk through teat leakage, however, is not only annoying but very unprofitable for the owner.

Chronic leaking is probably due in most cases to weakness of the teat orifice, to a fistula of the teat, or to the effects of a previous operation for the relief of stricture or other teat obstruction.

Treatment.—Weakness of the teat orifice may be overcome sometimes by the local application of tincture of iodine or saturated alum solution twice daily. The common practice of stopping a leaky teat with a rubber band or tape, or inserting a plug between milkings, is inadvisable, as it only tends to aggravate the weakness of the part or to increase the size of the opening, and may cause mastitis. Flexible collodion, into which has been incorporated 1 or 2 percent of metallic iodine, may be used to seal the teat orifice twice daily, or immediately after milking.

Teat fistula, due to injuries, constitutes a common and annoying form of teat leakage. Efforts to reduce a teat fistula, however, had better be postponed, if possible, until the milking period of the animal has been terminated. The procedure, which is a surgical one, consists in scarifying the edges of the fistulous opening, bringing the lips together, and suturing them into place to establish a closure of the aperture by healing. This operation should not be attempted by one unfamiliar with the principles of surgery, however, as skill and surgical cleanliness are absolutely necessary, while at best there always remains the danger of establishing a serious infection of the gland. The aftercare consists in bathing the wound several times daily with a sterile 1-percent solution of table salt or a mild antiseptic solution.

If a cow in full flow of milk receives a barbed-wire cut or other injury to the teat that would probably develop into a fistula, the correct procedure would be to have a veterinarian suture the wound immediately rather than to await the drying off of the animal and risk the consequences of a leaky quarter. A sterile milk tube under these circumstances should always be inserted before attempting to draw milk from an injured teat.

Rudimentary extra teats should never be removed unless for a compelling reason, as such an operation is a very common cause of leaky quarters.

MILKSTONE OR CALCULUS

Milkstone or calculus is a term loosely applied to concretions in the udder. Some stones are formed by coagulated casein and may be an indirect result of udder inflammation, whereas others are simply accumulations of lime salts from the milk that may sometimes be distinguished by the occasional discovery of gritty particles in the bottom of the milk pail or on the strainer cloth.

77431 O—51——16

Treatment.—After a prolonged, gentle massaging of the teat extremity with a belladonna ointment, the concretions, if not very large, may be passed with the aid of a sterile spring teat dilator. In case the stones cannot be removed in this way it may be necessary to remove them by means of an opening in the side of the teat. This operation should not be undertaken by the layman, as the danger of seriously infecting the udder by insanitary procedure cannot be overestimated, as well as the extreme likelihood of leaving a fistulous, leaky teat. Unless the concretions are sufficiently large to constitute an obstruction, their surgical removal, even by a veterinarian, had better be postponed until the cow has been dried off.

BLOODY MILK

Bloody milk is a symptom of any of the following conditions: Mastitis, mechanical injury to the udder, or tuberculous infection of the udder. The operation of milking also may aggravate a tendency to hemorrhage if the udder is injured or inflamed.

Treatment.—The cause should be determined if possible and the proper remedial measures applied. The following general treatment may be sufficient to afford relief in mild cases:

Milk out the udder completely at least four times daily, at regular intervals; bathe the udder with cold water, then dry and apply camphorated oil to the quarter with gentle massage; avoid an excessively rich diet; encourage the animal to utilize as bulky a ration as is consistent with her milk production; administer an occasional dose of Epsom salts (about 1 pound) as needed, also one-half ounce of saltpeter once daily. Should the hemorrhage persist, treatment by a veterinarian is advisable.

Redness of milk that does not appear until several hours after milking is probably due to contamination of the milk with some one of the chromogenic (color-producing) organisms. The thorough sterilization of utensils and the proper care and cleanliness in handling the milk should prevent this occurrence.

ROPY MILK

Milk is sometimes ropy, stringy, or slimy. What is known as ropy milk is due to bacterial infection after the milk is drawn. To eliminate this condition the cause should be found and removed and all utensils cleaned and sterilized to prevent further contamination.

At times stringy or slimy milk is procured from the udder and is usually caused by either injury or mastitis. Such milk should be boiled or treated to kill any bacteria and then discarded. Likewise, the utensils into which the milk is drawn should be thoroughly cleansed and disinfected or sterilized. The animals should also be treated.

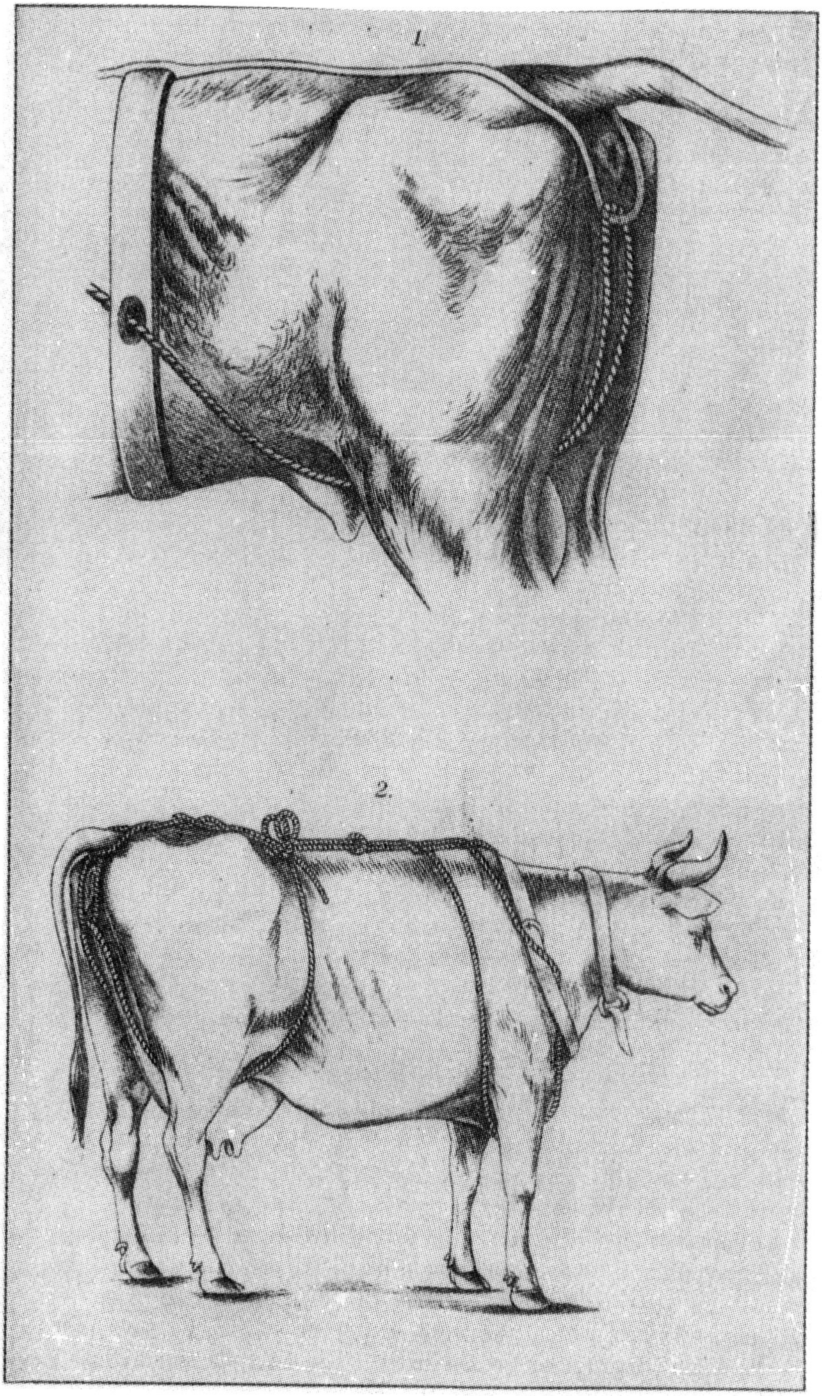

SUPPORTS FOR PROLAPSED UTERUS.

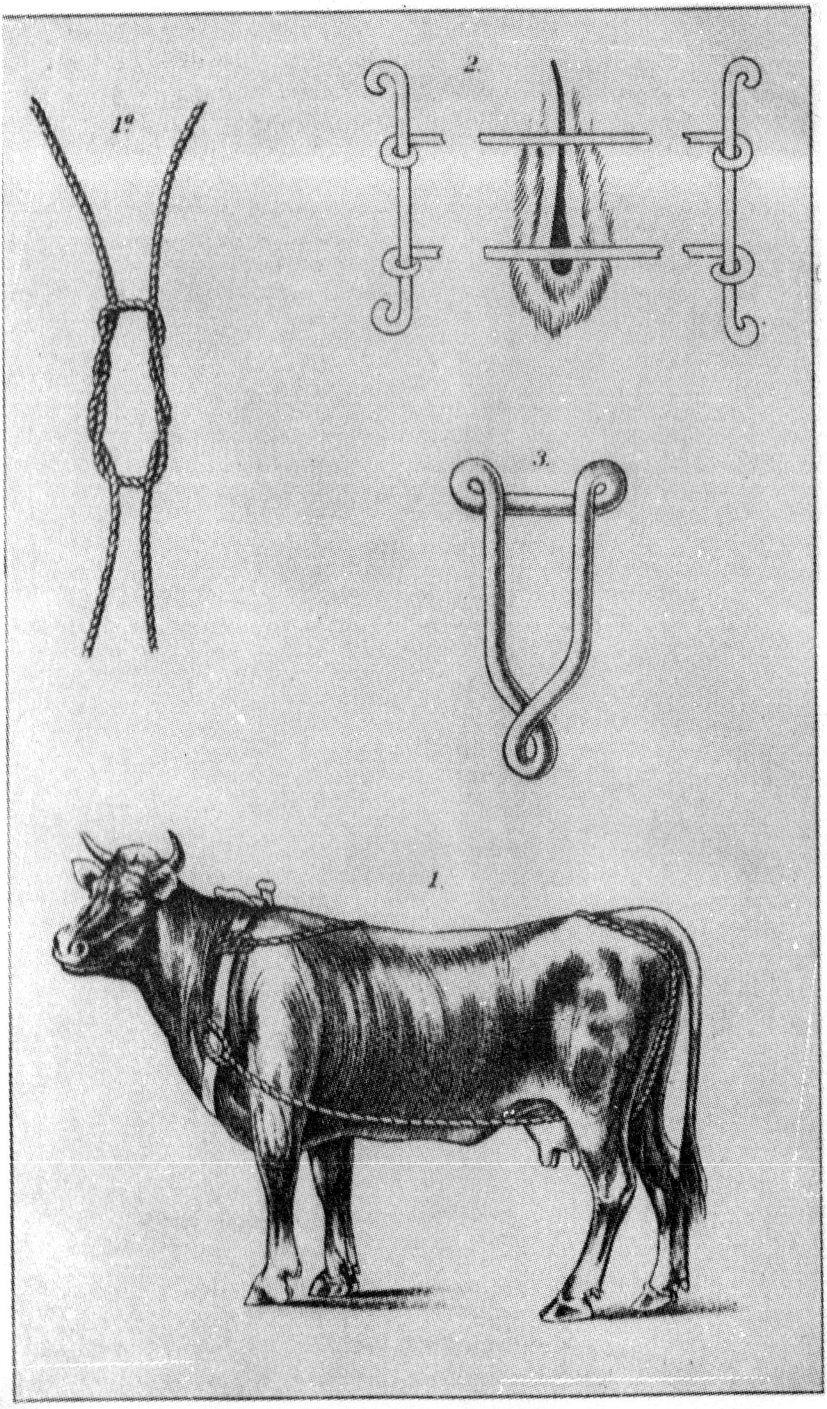

SUPPORTS FOR PROLAPSED UTERUS.

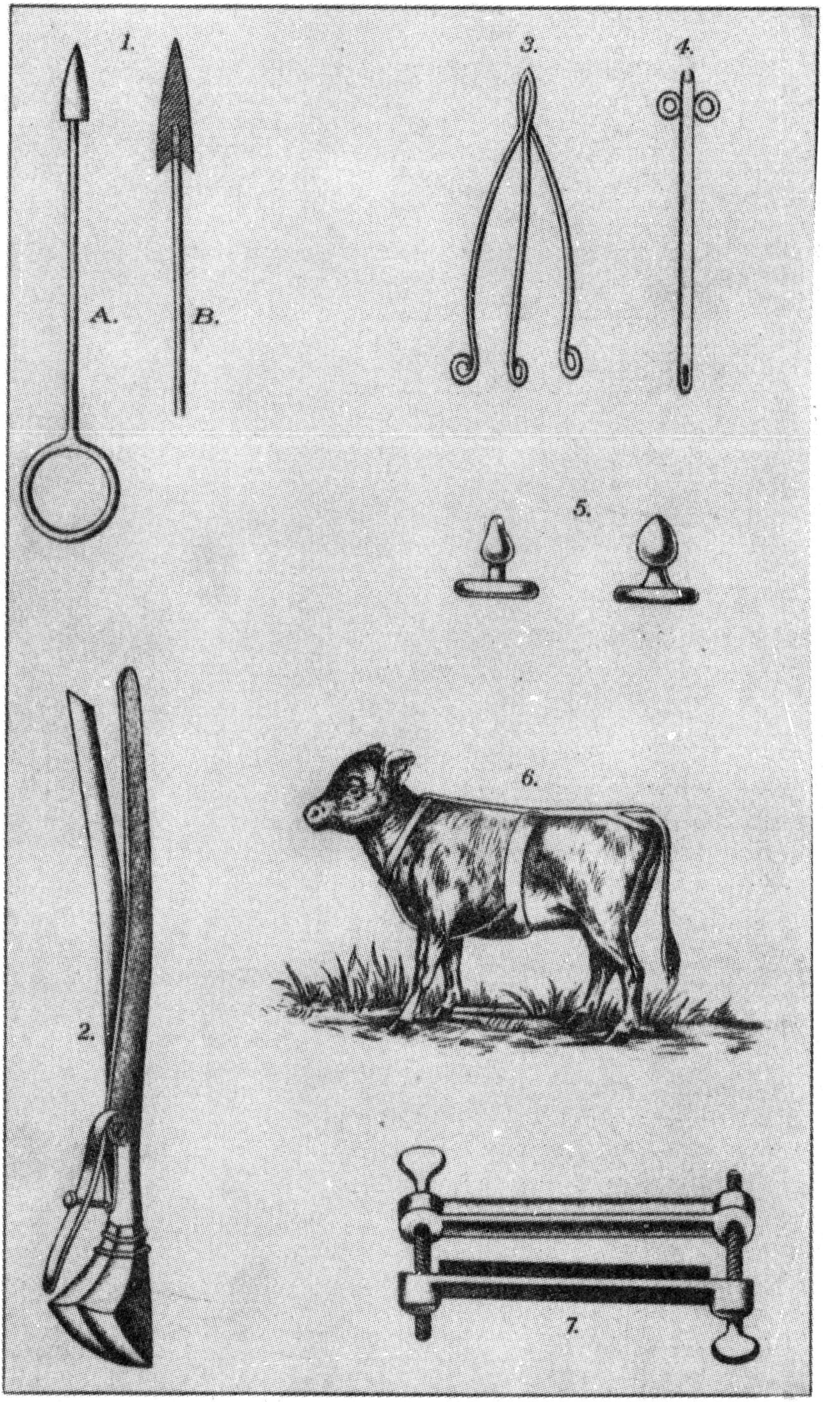

INSTRUMENTS USED IN DISEASES FOLLOWING PARTURITION.

DISEASES FOLLOWING PARTURITION

DESCRIPTION OF PLATES

PLATES XXII, XXIII. Supports for prolapsed uterus. These illustrations show various appliances used in prolapse or inversion of the uterus. The uterus should first be returned to its proper situation and then some apparatus applied to prevent a recurrence of the inversion or protrustion.

PLATE XXII:

Figure 1. Crupper, strap truss. (From Hill's Bovine Medicine and Surgery.)

Figure 2. Renault's rope truss. The rope for this truss should be 25 to 30 feet long and about the thickness of the little finger.

PLATE XXIII:

Figure 1. Cow to which Delwart's rope truss has been applied.

Figure 1*a* shows the loop of Delwart's truss.

Figure 2 Zundel's labial sutures. These consist of two wires passed through the lips of the vulva in a horizontal direction, and two additional wires passed through the loops at the ends of the horizontal wires in order to hold them in place.

Figure 3. Iron truss for holding the vagina or uterus in place after calving. The cords are passed through the eyes at the corners of the triangular iron; the base of the triangle fits under the tail. The truss is 5 to 7 inches long and about 2½ inches wide.

PLATE XXIV. Instruments used in diseases following parturition.

Figure 1. Lüthi's perforating sound, for opening the milk canal through the teat when this has become occluded: A, The sound, one-half natural size; B, section of head of sound, natural size, showing cutting edge.

Figure 2. Bistouri caché. A blade hidden in its sheath that by pressure of the finger may be made to protrude a certain distance. This distance is regulated by the screw near the handle. The instrument is used to open the milk canal when closed up. It is introduced into the milk canal with its blade in the sheath and withdrawn with the blade protruding.

Figure 3. Spring teat dilator, about one-half natural size, for dilating the milk canal.

Figure 4. Ring teat syphon, for withdrawing milk when the teat is sore or injured.

Figure 5. Gutta-percha bougie, for dilating the opening of the teat.

Figure 6. Truss applied to calf for umbilical or navel hernia. (From Fleming's Veterinary Obstetrics.)

Figure 7. Armatage's iron clamp for umbilical or navel hernia. When this clamp is applied care must be taken not to include a portion of the bowel.

Diseases of Young Calves

By James Law, F. R. C. V. S.

Revised by Chester Dale, D. V. M., M. A.

SUSPENDED BREATHING

The moment the circulation through the navel string is stopped the blood of the calf begins to become overcharged with carbon dioxide (CO_2), and unless breathing is speedily established death follows promptly. Fortunately the desire to breathe, roused by the circulation of the venous blood and the reflex action from the wet and chilling skin, usually starts the contractions of the diaphragm at once and life is insured. Among the obstacles to breathing are suffocation before or during birth from compression of the navel cord and the arrest of its circulation; the detachment of the fetal membranes from the womb before the calf is born; a too free communication between the two auricles (foramen ovale) of the heart by which the nonaerated blood has mixed too abundantly with the aerated and induced debility and profound weakness; a condition of ill health and debility of the calf as a result of semistarvation, or disease of the cow; fainting in the debilitated calf when calving has been difficult and prolonged; the birth of the calf with its head enveloped in the fetal membranes, so that it is unable to breathe; and the presence of tenacious phlegm in the mouth and nose, acting in the same manner.

Besides the importance of proper care and feeding of the cow as a preventive measure, attention should be given at once to relieve the newborn calf of its investing membrane and of any mucus that has collected in mouth or nostrils. Wiping out the nose deeply with a finger or feather excites to sneezing, hence to breathing. Blowing into the nose has a similar effect. Sucking the nostril through a tube applied to it is even more effective. Slapping the chest with the palm of the hand or with a towel dipped in cold water, compression and relaxation alternately of the walls of the chest, may start the action, and ammonia or even tobacco smoke blown into the nose may suffice. Every second is precious, however, and if possible the lungs should be dilated by forcibly introducing air from a bellows or from the human lungs. As the air is blown in through bellows or a tube the upper end of the windpipe must be pressed back against the gullet, as otherwise the air will go to the stomach. In a large dairy a piece of elastic tubing one-third of an inch in inside diameter should be kept at hand for sucking and blowing in such cases.

BLEEDING FROM THE NAVEL

This may occur in two conditions—when the cord is cut off too close to the navel and left untied and when it tears off at the navel (pl. XIV). It may bleed also when torn across naturally, if it is sucked by the dam or another calf. In an animal with little coagulability of the blood it will flow under almost any circumstance. When any cord is left it is always safe to tie it, and it is only when it is swollen and may possibly contain a loop of the bowel that there is danger in doing so. By pressing upward any bulky contents such danger is avoided. If the cord is torn or cut too close to be tied, bleeding may be checked by applying alum, copperas, or for a fraction of a second the end of an iron rod at a dull-red heat. If much blood has been lost it may be advisable to transfuse several ounces of blood or of a physiological salt solution.

URINE DISCHARGED THROUGH THE NAVEL

Before birth the urine passes from the bladder by a special tube through the navel and navel cord into the outer water bag (allantois) (pl. XII). This closes at birth, and the tube shrinks into a fine cord up to the bladder. It is only in the bull calf that it is likely to remain open, doubtless because of the long, narrow channel through which the urine must otherwise escape. The urethra, too, is sometimes abnormally narrow, or even closed, in the male. If part of the cord remains, it should be tied and the whole allowed to wither naturally. If the cord has been removed, and the tube (urachus) protrudes and discharges the urine, the tube alone must be tied. If there is nothing pendent the urachus must be seized, covered by the skin, and a curved needle being passed through the skin and above the duct, it may be tied along with this skin. A blister, causing swelling of the skin, will often close the orifice as will the hot iron. If the urethra of the male is closed it can rarely be remedied.

INFLAMMATION OF THE URACHUS (NAVEL URINE DUCT)

This may originate in direct, mechanical injury to the navel in calving or shortly after, with or without the lodgment of irritant or septic matter on its lacerated or cut end. The mere contact with healthy urine, hitherto harmless, can now be looked on as becoming suddenly irritating. The affection is usually marked by the presence of redness and swelling at the posterior part of the navel and the escape of urine and a few drops of whitish, serous pus from the orifice of the urachus. In those cases in which urine is not discharged a tender swelling, like a thick cord extending upward and backward from the navel into the abdomen, may be identified. The navel enlargement may be considerable, but it is solid, does not gurgle on handling, and cannot be done away with by pressing it back into the abdomen, as in a case of hernia.

In cases at first closed the pus may burst out later, coming from the back part of the navel and the swelling extending backward. In other cases whitish pus may pass with the urine by the ordinary channel, showing that it has opened back into the bladder. In other cases the umbilical veins become involved, in which case the swelling extends forward as well as backward. Thus the disease may result in destructive disorders of the liver, lungs, and, above all, of the joints.

The disease may usually be warded off or rendered simple and comparatively harmless by applying antiseptics to the navel string at birth. For this purpose tincture of iodine may be used.

ABSCESS OF THE NAVEL

As the result of irritation at calving or by the withered cord, or by licking with the rough tongue of the cow, inflammation may attack the loose connective tissue of the navel to the exclusion of the urachus and veins, and lead to the formation of pus. In this case a firm swelling as large as the fist appears, which softens in the center and may finally burst and discharge. The opening, however, is usually small and may close prematurely, so that abscess after abscess is formed. It is distinguished from hernia by the fact that it cannot be returned into the abdomen, and from inflammation of the veins and urachus by the absence of swellings forward and backward along the lines of these canals.

Tretament consists in an early opening of the abscess by a free incision and the injection twice a day of an astringent antiseptic solution.

INFLAMMATION OF THE NAVEL VEINS (UMBILICAL PHLEBITIS)

In this affection of the navel the inflammation may begin directly from mechanical injury, as in either of the two forms just described, but on this are inoculated infective microbes, derived from a retained and putrefying afterbirth, an abortion, a metritis, a fetid discharge from the womb, an unhealthy open sore, overcrowding, filthy floor or bedding, or an offensive accumulation of manure, solid or liquid. As the microbes vary in different cases, given outbreaks will differ materially in their nature. One is purulent infection with the tendency to secondary abscesses in the joints, liver, and lungs; another is from a septic germ and is associated with fetid discharge from the navel and general, putrid, blood poisoning. In determining the causes of the disease, the debility of the calf, when the mother has been underfed or badly housed or when either she or the fetus has been diseased, must not be overlooked.

Symptoms.—The symptoms vary. With the chain-form germs (streptococci) the navel becomes intensely red, with a very firm painful swelling, ending abruptly at the edges in sound skin and extending forward along the umbilical veins. The secondary diseases are circumscribed, black engorgements (infarctions) or abscesses of the liver, lungs, kidneys, bowels, or other internal organs, and sometimes disease of the joints.

With the ordinary pus-producing germs (*Staphylococcus pyogenes aureus* and *Streptococcus pyogenes*) the local inflammation in the navel causes a hot, painful swelling, which rapidly advances to the formation of pus, and the raw, exposed surface, at first bright red, becomes dark red or black, soft, friable, and pultaceous. If the pus is white, creamy, and comparatively inoffensive in odor, the secondary formations in internal organs and joints are mainly of the same purulent character (secondary abscesses).

If, on the other hand, the discharge is very offensive and the pus more serous, watery, or bloody, there is reason to suspect the presence of some of the septic bacteria, and the results on the general system are a high fever and softening of the liver and spleen and no tendency to abscess of the internal organs. Diarrhea is a common symptom, and death ensues early, the blood after death being found unclotted.

Complicated cases are common, and in all alike the umbilical veins usually remain open and can be explored by a probe passed at first upward and then forward toward the liver.

Prevention.—Apply tincture of iodine to the navel string at birth.

Local treatment.—This consists in the application of antiseptics to the parts.

If complications have extended to the liver or other internal organs or the joints, other treatment will be necessary. In acute cases of general infection an early fatal result is to be expected.

PYEMIC AND SEPTICEMIC INFLAMMATION OF JOINTS IN CALVES (JOINT ILL)

This occurs in young calves within the first month after birth. It persists in the joints when once attacked and is usually connected with disease of the navel. Joint ill attacks the structures outside as well as inside the joints and, above all, the ends of the bones and tends to the destruction and crumbling of their tissue and even to the formation of open sores, through which the fragile bones are exposed. The microbes from the unhealthy and infected wound in the navel pass into the system through the veins, or lymphatics, and form colonies and local inflammations and abscesses in and around the joints.

Symptoms.—The symptoms are the swelling of one or more joints, which are very hot and tender. The calf is stiff and lame, lies down constantly, and does not care to suckle. There is very high fever. accelerated breathing and pulse, and swelling and purulent discharge (often fetid) from the navel. There may be added symptoms of disease of the liver, lungs, heart, or bowels. The important point is to determine the condition of the navel in all such cases of diseased and swollen joints beginning the first month of life, and in all cases of general stiffness, for besides the diseases of the internal organs abscesses may be formed among the muscles of the trunk, though the joints appear sound. Calves thus afflicted, if they do not speedily die, tend to become emaciated and die later in a state of weakness and exhaustion.

Prevention.—Prevention must consist in keeping the buildings as sanitary as possible and in treating the navel as recommended for Inflammation of the Navel Veins.

Treatment.—Treatment is, in the main, antiseptic. In the milder forms of the disease, the joints may be painted daily with tincture of iodine. Swellings containing pus may be opened, drainage established, and the parts treated antiseptically.

UMBILICAL HERNIA (BREACH AT THE NAVEL)

This may exist at birth from imperfect closure of the muscles around the opening; it may even extend backward for a distance from the two sides failing to come together. Apart from this, the trouble rarely appears after the calf has been on solid feed for some time as the paunch then extends down to the right immediately over the navel and thus forms an internal pad, preventing the protrusion of intestine.

Symptoms.—The symptoms of umbilical hernia are a soft swelling at the navel, usually a gurgling of the contents of the swelling when handled, and the ability to return the entire swelling into the abdomen by pressure. The only exception is when the walls of the sac have become greatly thickened. These, of course, will remain as a swelling after the bowel has been returned; and when a permanent adhesion has developed between the protruding bowel and the sac, it is impossible to return it fully without first severing that connection. In the diseases of the navel hitherto considered, the swellings have no gurgling contents and cannot be returned completely into the abdomen.

Treatment.—Treatment is not always necessary. A small hernia the size of an egg in a newborn calf usually disappears of itself as the animal changes its diet to solid feed and has the paunch fully developed as an internal pad.

In other cases apply a leather pad 8 inches square attached around the body by two elastic bands connected with its four corners, and an elastic band passing from its front border to a collar encircling the neck, and two other elastic bands from the neck collar along the two sides of the body to the two bands passing up over the back (pl. XXIV, fig. 6).

The application of a clamp like those used in castration is a most effective method, but great care must be taken to see that all the contents of the sac are returned so that none may be enclosed in the clamp (pl. XXIV, fig 7).

Surgical procedures by a competent operator are often advisable.

DROPSY OF THE NAVEL

A sac formed at the navel, containing liquid accumulated because of sucking by other calves, is unsightly and sometimes injurious. After assurances that it is simply a dropsical collection, it may be deeply punctured at various points with a large-sized lancet or knife, fomented with hot water, and then daily treated with an astringent antiseptic solution.

BLUE DISEASE (CYANOSIS)

This condition appearing in the calf at birth is due to the orifice between the two auricles of the heart (foramen ovale) remaining open too much and allowing the nonaerated (venous) blood to mix with the aerated (arterial) blood. It is beyond the reach of treatment. It is recognized by the blueness of the eyes, nose, mouth, and other mucous membranes, the coldness of the surface, and the extreme sensitiveness to cold.

CONSTIPATION

At birth the bowels of the calf contain the meconium, a tenacious, gluey, brownish-yellow material largely derived from the liver, which must be expelled before they can begin their functions normally. The first milk of the cow (colostrum), rich in albumin and salts, is nature's laxative to expel this offensive material and should never be withheld from the calf. If, for lack of colostrum, from subsequent dry feeding of the cow or from any other cause, the calf is costive, strains violently without passage, lies down and rises as in colic, and fails in appetite, no time should be lost in giving relief by an ounce dose of castor oil, assisting its action by injections of soapsuds or oil. Whatever meconium is within reach of the finger should be carefully removed. It is also important to give the cow a laxative diet.

INDIGESTION

This may occur from many causes, as costiveness; a too liberal supply of milk; too rich milk; furnishing a very young calf milk from a cow long after calving; allowing a calf to suck the first milk of a cow that has been hunted, driven hard, shipped, or otherwise violently excited; allowing the calf too long time between meals, so that impelled by hunger it quickly overloads and clogs the stomach; feeding from the pail milk that has been held over in unwashed and unscalded buckets, so that it is fermented and spoiled; feeding the milk of cows kept on unwholesome feed; keeping the calves in cold, damp, dark, filthy, or bad-smelling pens; feeding the calves on artificial mixtures containing too much starchy matter; or giving the calves too much artificial feed that may be appropriate in smaller quantity. The licking of hair from themselves or others and its formation into balls in the stomach will cause obstinate indigestion in the calf.

Symptoms.—The symptoms are dullness, indisposition to move, uneasiness, eructations of gas from the stomach, sour breath, entire loss of appetite, lying down and rising as if in pain, fullness of the abdomen, which gives a drumlike sound when tapped with the fingers.

The costiveness may be marked at first, but soon it gives place to diarrhea, by which the offensive matters may be carried off and health restored. In other cases it becomes aggravated, merges into inflammation of the bowels, fever sets in, and the calf gradually sinks.

Prevention.—Prevention consists in avoiding the causes enumerated or any others that may be detected.

Treatment.—Treatment consists in first clearing away the irritant present in the bowels. For this purpose 1 or 2 ounces of castor oil may be given, and if the sour eructations are marked a tablespoonful of limewater may be given and repeated 2 or 3 times a day. If the disorder continues after the removal of the irritant, a large tablespoonful of rennet, or 30 grains of pepsin, may be given at each meal along with a teaspoonful of tincture of gentian. Any return of constipation must be treated by injections of warm water and soap.

ACUTE CONTAGIOUS SCOURING IN THE NEWBORN (WHITE SCOURS)

White scours is an infectious disease usually occurring sometime during the first few days of life; it is characterized by weakness, prostration, lack of appetite, and a light-colored diarrhea. When the disease becomes established in a stable, it attacks almost every calf born in the building unless rigid enforcement of preventive measures is practiced.

The germ generally associated with the disease is the colon bacillus. However, other germs may sometimes be responsible for the trouble. The colon bacilli are widely distributed, being normally present in the intestines of animals, where they multiply and are expelled with the feces. Ordinarily these bacteria are relatively harmless but in some manner attain a virulence capable of producing disease in newborn calves.

Symptoms.—The most intense symptoms of white scours are profuse, yellowish white, and very offensive bowel discharges. These are accompanied with great dullness, weakness, and prostration, sunken eyes, retracted belly, short, hurried breathing, and very low temperature. The calf lies on its side with the head resting on the ground, lethargic and unconscious to all around it. As a rule death ensues within 24 to 36 hours.

Prevention.—Control of the disease has been accomplished by adopting a regular plan of feeding and using certain sanitary measures.

For controlling the disease several plans of care, feeding, and other sanitary measures have been proposed. The following preventive measures suggested by Professor Udall of Cornell University have proved to be very successful when carried out systematically:

1. The cow should freshen in a clean parturition stall. Such stalls are valuable in the control of all acute infections incident to parturition. On large breeding farms and in purebred herds they are an economic necessity. But regardless of the circumstances of birth the offspring should receive colostral milk at the earliest possible moment. In practice it has been observed that if a normal calf remains with the dam for 12 hours it obtains sufficient colostrum and does not obtain too much milk. The modern dairy cow gives more milk than is needed by any single calf. When a newborn calf with a ravenous appetite becomes gorged with milk all the circumstances for the development of a colon septicemia are favorable—the stomach is overloaded, the intestines contain meconium, and the digestive tract is not yet able to function actively.

Some authors attach importance to washing and disinfection of the external genitals and douching the vagina previous to birth, and to receiving the newborn calf on a sterile sheet. These precautions are difficult to apply and are entirely unnecessary. It is, however, highly desirable that an experienced attendant be present at the time of birth to exert traction when the presentation is normal and the delivery slow because of an oversized fetus, to prevent the cow from lying with the rear end against the wall during expulsive efforts, to disinfect the navel immediately after birth, and, when necessary, to assist the newborn calf in obtaining the colostral milk shortly after birth. Prompt assistance is often necessary to secure a live calf from a posterior presentation. Failure to provide such assistance may result either in death at delivery or a weakened calf that succumbs within the first week.

Disinfect the navel by placing it in a 2-ounce wide-mouthed bottle half filled with tincture of iodine. With the mouth of the bottle pressed against the abdomen invert it and hold in this position for at least 5 minutes; in this manner the region of the navel is thoroughly saturated. Do not use the same iodine more than once.

2. At the end of 12 hours the calf is muzzled and all feed is withheld for the next 24 hours. At the end of the fasting period the meconium has passed, the stomach and bowels are relatively empty, and the animal has not suffered any discomfort. When the fasting period ends at night a pint each of milk and lime water warmed to body temperature are fed.

3. The regular feeding day begins on the morning of the third day 36 hours after birth. Thus a calf born in the morning would remain with the dam until night and be fasted until the following night, when it would be fed a pint each of milk and lime water. A calf born in the evening would remain with the dam during the night and be fasted from the morning of the second to the morning of the third day. The quantity of milk allowed on the third day, the first regular feeding day, is about 6 percent of the weight of the calf, using the dam's milk. For the Guernsey breed, with a birth weight of 65 to 70 pounds, this is 4 pounds. It is preferably divided into three feedings, to each of which is added a pint of lime water. The mixture is heated to 100° F. and fed in a sterilized pail. The quantity of lime water added to each feed is never more than 1 pint. A daily increase of 8 ounces of milk for the first 3 weeks will constitute a suitable addition. At the end of the first week the calf may receive 8 to 12 percent of its body weight of milk daily. During the first week, take the calf's temperature before the noon feed. If it is 103° or more, give an enema and 3 ounces of liquid petrolatum and withhold feed until the temperature is normal and the calf ravenously hungry.

Housing conditions should protect calves against extreme cold, sudden changes in temperature, and cold drafts from open doors. They should be kept dry, warm, and clean. If the calf barn is large and the control of temperature is imperfect, small blankets made of heavy sacking may be used; these are either sewed or tied to fit the body closely and are worn for about 2 weeks. A suitable temperature in calf barns is 55° to 60° F. Individual pens may be desirable for the first few days, but small tightly boarded pens are difficult to ventilate and they predispose to unthriftiness and pneumonia after the first 2 weeks. Where muzzles are used, the dangers from mingling are greatly reduced, and calves thrive best when kept muzzled and on a milk diet for the first 30 days.

Some dairy farmers raise calves on nurse cows but this method has not proved to be generally successful. The use of a nurse cow for a newborn, sick calf is often fatal to the calf as well as a danger to the udder of the cow. On the other hand calves that become unthrifty and develop scours from overeating roughage at 4 to 6 weeks of age, may improve rapidly when placed on a nurse cow.

Weak and undersized calves need to be fed often and kept on a decidedly restricted diet until they become strong and vigorous. The early fasting period should be omitted. It is helpful to supplement the low milk diet with olive oil (4 ounces daily). If the newborn calf is unable to rise and suckle, it may receive 8 ounces of the dam's milk three to five times daily. Prompt administration of the dam's blood (50 to 100 cubic centimeters subcutaneously) often results in marked improvement in these cases. It should be given as soon as possible after birth. In herds where the calves are commonly born weak or sick the mortality is high under any circumstances, and preventive measures involve a survey of the breeding and nutritional condition of the entire herd.

Losses from white scours may be reduced by allowing the cows to freshen at pasture or in open fields, and excluding the calf from the barn for at least 10 days.

It is obvious that not all of these directions are suitable for average conditions, but where losses among valuable animals are heavy, extreme measures may be necessary.

Treatment.—The sick calf may be given a large dose of castor oil, 4 to 6 ounces. Coffee may be given as a stimulant, and the strength of the calf may be preserved by giving raw eggs in pasteurized milk. Limewater may be given at frequent intervals. Decoctions of linseed, barley, or oats are sometimes given.

The administration of calf-scour serum or the use of 50 to 100 cubic centimeters of the dam's blood administered subcutaneously may aid materially in overcoming the disease. Recent experiments indicate that a hyperimmune homologous serum is of value as a preventive. This serum is prepared by hyperimmunizing cattle with colon germs from calves that have died of the disease. It is used only in herds from which these calves came. Calves are injected intravenously with the serum, and the first injection is given preferably within 12 hours after birth. So far the limited use of this type of serum has been mostly in large dairy herds and good results have been reported. However, the owner should remember that the most important means of combating this condition is to prevent primary infection of the new-born calf. This can be accomplished only through extreme care and strict sanitary measures, as previously outlined.

OTHER AILMENTS OF THE CALF

Among these are several congenital imperfections, such as imperforate anus, vulva, or prepuce, which may be recognized by the inability of the animal to pass dung or urine in spite of straining, and the formation of swellings in the anus, vulva, or sheath. Each must be carefully incised with the knife taking care not to injure the muscles that circumscribe the respective openings. Another imperfection is tongue-tie, in which the thin, flacid, mucous membrane passing from the median line of the lower surface of the tongue binds the latter too closely to the floor of the mouth and renders the tongue unfit for taking in feed in afterlife. This must be cut with knife or scissors to give the tongue a reasonable degree of liberty.

77431 O—51——17

Aphtha, or thrush, is another trouble of the suckling calf, showing itself as a white, curdy elevation on the tongue, lips, cheeks, or gums, and when detached leaving a raw, red, angry surface. It is due to the growth of a vegetable parasite long recognized as the *Oïdium albicans* (*Saccharomyces albicans*). Local antiseptic treatment, if persistent, is usually effective.

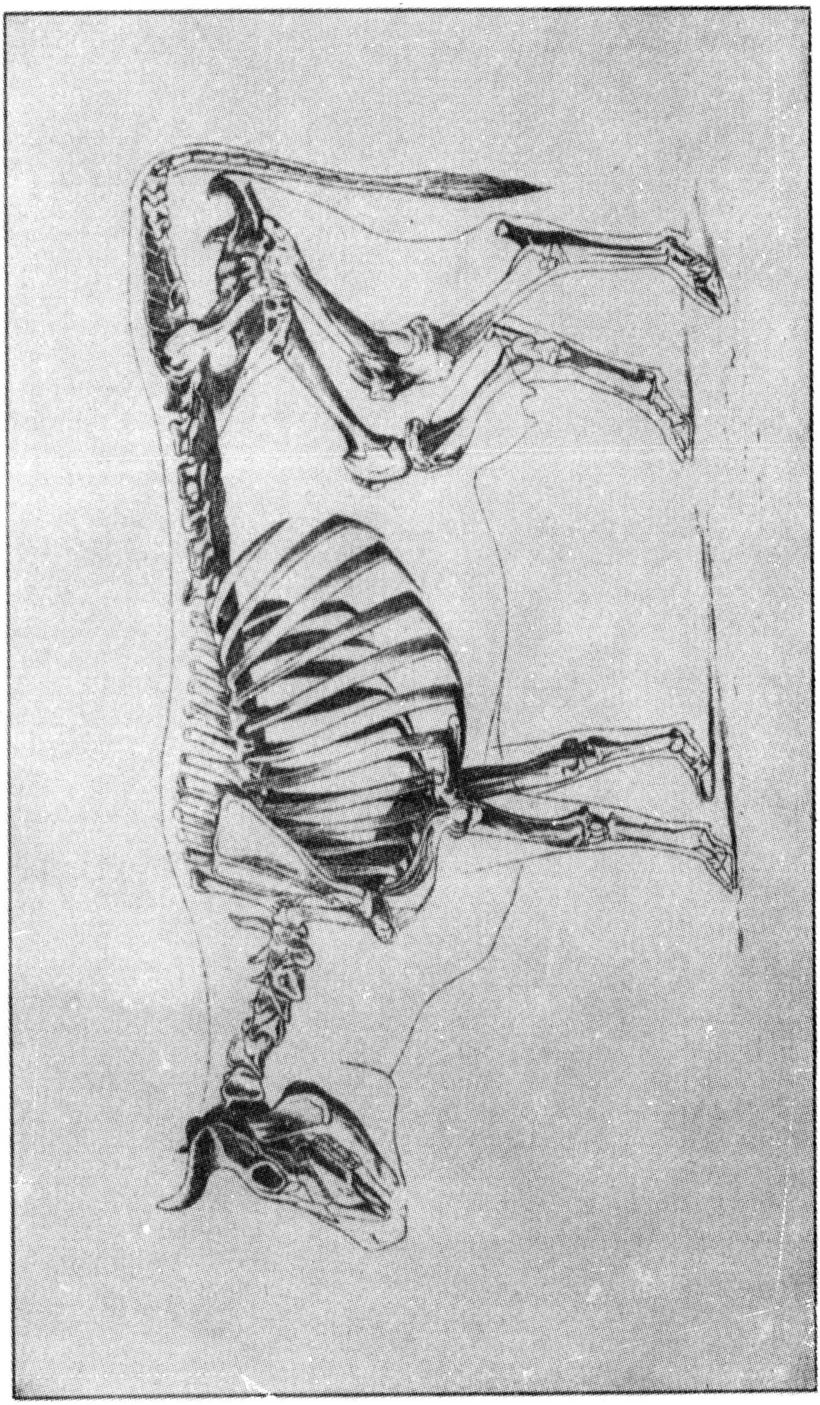

SKELETON OF THE COW.

Bones: Diseases and Accidents

By V. T. Atkinson, V. S.

[Revised by John R. Mohler, A. M., V. M. D., D. Sc.]

Some knowledge of the skeleton is advisable to facilitate the study of diseases of bones and the accidental injuries to which they are exposed. The skeleton of the adult bovine animal is made up of the following number of bones:

Spinal column	45	
Head	28	
Chest	27	
Shoulder	2—	1 on each side.
Arm	2—	1 on each side.
Forearm	4—	2 on each side.
Forefoot	40—	20 on each side.
Pelvis	2—	1 on each side.
Thigh	2—	1 on each side.
Leg	6—	3 on each side.
Hind foot	38—	19 on each side.
Total	196	

Without attempting to burden the reader with the technical names and a scientific classification of each, it appears desirable to describe some of the characteristics of forms in general and of a few classes into which they may be divided, leaving the special study of individual bones to the illustrations of the skeleton (pl. XXV), which will serve better than a great deal of writing to fix in the mind of the reader the location, relation, and function of each one. In early fetal life the place of bone is supplied by temporary cartilage, which gradually changes to bone. Bones are composed of a form of dense connective tissue impregnated with lime salts and contain two elementary constituents—the organic or animal and the inorganic or earthy. In young animals the former predominates; with increasing years the relative proportions of the two change, so that when advanced age is reached the proportion of inorganic far exceeds the organic. The gradual change with advancing years from organic to inorganic has the effect of rendering the bone harder and more brittle, and though it is stronger, the reparative process is slower when injury occurs.

The bones are nourished in two ways: (1) From the outside through their covering, called the periosteum—the thin, strong membrane that covers every part of the bone except the articular surface of the joints; and (2) from within through the minute branches of blood vessels that pass into the bones through holes (foramina) on their surface and are distributed in the soft structure (medulla) of the inside. The structure of the bone is divided into two parts—the compact or hard material of the outside, which gives strength and is more abundant in the shafts of long bones, and the cancellated, softer tissue of the inside, which affords accommodation to the blood vessels necessary for the nourishment of that part of the structure.

In shape, bones are divided into three classes—long, flat, and short. The long bones are the ribs and those mostly found in the legs; the flat bones are found in the head, the shoulder, and the pelvis; the short bones occur in the spinal column and in the lower portions of the legs.

With this introduction, which seems almost indispensable, consideration is now given to diseases of the bones, for they undergo disease processes like any other living tissue. Treatment of bones that are diseased or that have been injured through accident should, however, be left to a competent veterinarian as he is better able than the stockman to deal with conditions that arise.

OSTEITIS

Inflammation of the compact structure of bones (osteitis) may be either acute or chronic and may involve the whole extent of the bone affected or may be confined to only a portion of it. This inflammation results from injury, such as concussion, laceration, or a crushing bruise; also from specific influences, as in actinomycosis (lumpy jaw) or cases of foot rot. The latter affection frequently involves the bones, and for this reason the pastern is the most frequent seat of osteitis. There is dull pain on pressure and a painful swelling of bone when pus is present. Suppuration may involve the overlying soft tissues, causing an abscess, which may finally break through the skin. The inflammatory condition sometimes assumes an ulcerated form (caries) or from interrupted nutrition of the part deprived of the blood necessary to its nourishment may cause death of a large section of bone (necrosis); this dead fragment (sequestrum), becoming separated from the main portion of bone, acts as a foreign body.

Treatment.—This consists in resting the affected part and in giving vent at the earliest possible moment to whatever pus may be present. Free drainage should then be maintained. Apply antiseptic dressings and pack with tampons of cotton soaked in antiseptic solutions. A laxative to keep the bowels moving freely is the only internal treatment necessary.

PERIOSTITIS

This disease is an inflammation of the external covering of bone (periosteum) and is usually produced by wounds, pressure, or crushing the part. The periosteum is well supplied with sensitive nerve endings and when inflamed is very sensitive to pressure and may cause lameness. This condition is often difficult to determine, and even an acute observer may fail to locate the point of its existence. There are three forms of periostitis—aseptic, purulent, and fibrous.

Aseptic periostitis.—When this disease becomes chronic, it causes such a bony enlargement (exostosis) as is seen in the callous formation following the fracture of a bone. The formation of such a tumor or enlargement on the surface of a bone is likely to occur in any part of the bone covered with periosteum, and when found near a joint involving two or more bones it is likely to result in their union (ankylosis).

Applications of cold water to check the inflammatory processes is recommended for the first few days in aseptic periostitis, followed by hot fomentations to hasten resorption of fluids. Massage may then be given with camphor ointment, mercurial ointment, soap liniment, or Lugol's solution. In the chronic form, point firing or a biniodide-of-mercury blister may be beneficial.

Purulent periostitis.—This form follows wounds that reach the periosteum and become infected, as observed in compound fractures, or it may result from advancing purulent conditions in neighboring structures, as in foot rot. It may also occur in the course of an infectious disease, when small abscesses are formed under the periosteum (sub-periosteal abscess). It may lead to necrosis of the bone or a fistulous tract from the bone to the surface. There is usually much pain and fever, and the odor from the wound is offensive.

In this form of periostitis the periosteum should be freely incised, followed either by continuous irrigation or frequent injection of the wound with antiseptic solutions.

Fibrous periostitis.—This form of the disease consists in the thickening of the outer layer of the periosteum from the inflammation reaching it from neighboring structures. This newly formed fibrous tissue may become ossified or may transmit the inflammation to the deeper bony structures. It is frequently seen in cases in which there has been an intense inflammation of the skin close to an underlying bone.

The treatment should be the same as that recommended for aseptic periostitis.

OSTEOMYELITIS

This term refers to an inflammation of the bone marrow, which is most commonly seen following the bacterial infection of a compound fracture and usually results in pus formation. The bone is melted away and pus escapes from the bone under the periosteum, involving the soft tissues. It is principally confined to the long bones and seldom affects more than one.

Treatment.—The bone should be opened for the purpose of curetting out the diseased portion of the marrow cavity and removing all the necrotic pieces of bone. This should be undertaken only by a competent veterinarian. The aftertreatment may consist in tamponing the wound with pledgets of iodoform gauze or a mixture of iodoform (1 part) and glycerin (4 parts). The wound in the soft tissue should be kept open until the cavity in the bone has filled with granulation tissue.

RICKETS

This disease is an affection of young, growing bones and mostly involves the ribs and long bones of the legs. It consists in a failure of the organism to deposit lime salts in bone, and for that reason the bones do not ossify so rapidly as they should. The cartilaginous ends of the bones grow rapidly, but ossification does not keep pace with it. The bones become long and their ends bend at the joints, the legs become crooked, and the joints are large and irregular. All the bones affected with this disease are thicker than normal, and the gait of the animal is stiff and painful. A row of bony enlargements may be found where the ribs articulate with the cartilages connecting them with the breastbone and is called the "beaded line." A catarrhal condition of the digestive tract is usually observed. The disease may result from an inherited weakness of constitution, poor hygienic surroundings, or improper diet. The correct formation of bone is believed to be somewhat influenced by heredity, but a lack of minerals, sunlight, or vitamin D, which is found abundantly in most milk, clovers, and alfalfa, is the direct cause of the disease. Calves and foals are less frequently affected with rickets than dogs and pigs.

Treatment.—The affected animal should have nourishing feed containing a proper quantity of minerals, especially calcium and phosphorus. Outdoor exercise and plenty of fresh air are indispensable. Limewater should be given once daily either alone or added to the milk for very young calves, and ground bonemeal mixed with the feed of older animals. Calcium phosphate, 1 dram, given twice daily to a 2-month-old calf, and proportionately increased for older animals, may prove efficacious in this disease. When there is plenty of sunlight, this treatment may be sufficient. However, most animals are benefited by administration of such preparations as cod-liver or salmon oil, which contains large quantities of vitamin D. In some cases the long bones of the legs are too weak at birth to support the weight of the animal, and temporary splints, carefully padded and wrapped on with some soft bandages, become necessary.

OSTEOMALACIA (CREEPS)

This is a condition of bone brittleness or softening of bone found usually in adult life. The affected bones, usually of the legs and pelvis, become enlarged. The bone substance loses its compactness and becomes soft, but at times the bones may become brittle as a result of which fractures may occur. This disease is seen in milk cows during heavy lactation or in the later stages of pregnancy, and the greater the yield of milk the more rapid the progress of the disease. Heifers with their first calves are frequently affected, as these animals require a considerable quantity of minerals for their own growth and for the nourishment of their offspring. Mature as well as young animals require for proper development not only that bone-forming minerals, chiefly calcium and phosphorus, be present in their rations in adequate quantities but also in proper proportion. Certain sections of the United States are known to grow forage that does not have the proper balance between these elements, and it is here that the disease is most frequently encountered.

Symptoms.—In marked cases there are gradual emaciation and symptoms of gastrointestinal catarrh, with depraved appetite, the animal eating bones, manure, decayed wood, dirt, leather, and other such products. Muscular weakness is prominent, together with muscle tremors, which simulate chills, but are not accompanied with any rise of temperature. The animal has a stiff, laborious gait; there is pain and swelling of the joints and constant shifting of the weight from one leg to another. The restricted movements of the joints are frequently accompanied with a crackling sound, which has caused the name of "creeps" to be applied to the disease. The coat is dull and rough and the skin dry and hidebound. The animal is subject to frequent sprains or fracture of bones without apparent cause, as in lying down or turning around, and when such fractures occur they are difficult to unite. The upper bones of the legs, the haunch bone, and the middle bones of the spinal column are principally involved. The disease occurs on old, worn-out soil poor in lime, and has also been observed to follow a dry season.

Treatment.—An attempt must be made to supply the lacking mineral elements in the feed. Feed rich in minerals may be given, such as beans, cowpeas, alfalfa, clover, oats, cottonseed meal, or wheat bran. Cottonseed meal is one of the best feeds for this purpose, but it should be fed carefully, as too large quantities of it are injurious to cows. A good quality of bonemeal free from odors may be placed in a clean box, which should be accessible to the cattle at all times. Should there be difficulty in inducing the animals to eat the bonemeal, a small quantity of salt may be added at first. Later, only the bonemeal should be placed before them.

SPRAINS

The most common accident occurring to bones and joints is a sprain of the ligaments uniting the bones or the tendons uniting the muscles and bones. A sprain is the result of a sudden forcing of a joint in an unnatural direction, or, if in a natural direction, beyond the power of the ligament or tendon to restrain it properly, so that part of the fibers of either are ruptured. When such an accident occurs pain is immediately inflicted, varying in degree with the extent of the injury, which is soon followed by swelling with more or less heat and tenderness. If the seat of the injury is in any of the legs, lameness is likely to result. Of the causes of sprain, slipping on ice or a wet floor, playing, and fighting with another animal are the most common.

Sprain of the shoulder joint.—This is likely to occur from any of the causes just mentioned or from the animal slipping suddenly into a rut or hole. When such an accident occurs, sudden lameness will result. The animal drags the leg when walking and carries it in a circular direction, outward and forward at each step. The leg should be carefully examined; pressure over the joint causes the animal to evince pain. If the person making the examination is in doubt it is well to make a comparison between the shoulders by pressing first on one and then the other.

After such an accident the animal should be tied so as to limit as far as possible the use of the injured joint. Soft feed should be given to keep the bowels acting freely.

During the first 3 days the treatment should consist of cold-water irrigation to check the inflammation and relieve the pain. Hot fomentations may then be applied to hasten the absorption of the inflammatory fluids. When the pain has somewhat abated, equal parts of mercurial ointment and green soap may be rubbed into the swollen tissue. Should lameness continue after the tenth day, good results will be obtained from the application of a blister. The animal's head should be carefully tied until the third day, to prevent its licking the blister. The blistered surface should then be smeared with lard or petrolatum every other day until the scabs fall off. Gentle exercise should be allowed after the fourth or fifth day from the application of the blister. If the lameness still remains, the blister may be repeated in 3 weeks or a month.

Sprain of the fetlock.—This may occur from misstep when the animal is moving rapidly, and the twisting or wrenching of the foot is sufficient to rupture partially the ligaments that bind the bones together at that part. Such an accident also frequently occurs by the foot getting fastened in a hole in the floor; the wrenching is the result of the animal's attempt to liberate it. Lameness, followed by swelling of the joint and pain when it is handled or when the animal moves the joint, and heat, are the more noticeable symptoms. If the sprain is very severe, the animal occasionally does not bear its weight on the affected leg.

The most important consideration in the treatment of this affection is rest, which is best enforced by keeping the animal in the stall and placing strong, muslin bandages about the inflamed joint. As in the sprain of the shoulder, cold water in the form of douches, continuous irrigation with hose or soaking tub, or finely chopped ice poultices are recommended for the first 3 days. Following this apply a Priessnitz bandage[1] moderately tight about the joint, which not only conduces to rest but also favors absorption. Massage with stimulating liniments, such as soap or camphor liniments, may later be applied to the affected parts.

If the lameness has not disappeared by the tenth day, the blister advised for the sprain of the shoulder should be applied and the same precautions observed with regard to tying the animal's head and subsequent smearing with petrolatum. When a blister is applied in this locality, the back part of the heel should be first filled with lard or petrolatum, and care taken to prevent any of the blistering preparation from coming in contact with the skin of that part. If this precaution is not observed, scratches may ensue and be troublesome.

Sprain of the hip.—This is likely to result from the animal's slipping in such way as to spread the hind feet wide apart. The patient becomes stiff in the hind legs or lame in one hind leg, walking with a a straddling gait and swinging the leg outward as it is carried forward. Tenderness may occasionally be detected on pressure, but owing to the heavy covering of muscles outside the joint this test is not always reliable.

In acute cases give rest and cold local applications. After the fourth or fifth day the blister mentioned for sprain of the shoulder may be applied with advantage, and if this proves insufficient firing

---

[1] A Priessnitz bandage is a dressing that combines the three properties of keeping a part warm, moist, and subjecting it to uniform pressure. It consists of three layers of material. The inner layer is composed of absorbent cotton or some other material that is capable of holding moisture. This is soaked in water and wrapped around the part. The second layer consists of a substance that is impervious to moisture, as oiled silk or oiled paper, and is applied about the inner layer to prevent evaporation. The third, or outside, layer is composed of a flannel or woolen bandage to prevent the radiation of heat and thus keep the moist inner layer at the temperature of the body.

may be undertaken, but this operation should be performed by a veterinarian.

Sprain of the back.—Sprain of the back, particularly in the region of the loins, is not an uncommon accident among cattle. It is likely to occur from the animal's slipping with both hind feet sidewise so as to twist the back, or from slipping violently backward so that great stress is thrown on the loins. The patient moves with difficulty, using the hind parts in a guarded manner, as if afraid of causing severe pain. Occasionally, if the sprain is severe, the animal rises with difficulty. Pressure on the back in the immediate region of the loins causes pain. Such cases may be mistaken for paralysis. In severe cases, during the early stages of the injury, although the nerve supply is not interfered with, the injury to the muscles and resulting pain is so great that the condition is almost equal to paralysis, although likely to be attended with more favorable results. Hot applications, such as blankets wrung out of hot water and changed often, may afford relief during the earlier stages. Afterwards the blister mentioned for sprain of the shoulder may be applied with advantage.

FRACTURES (BROKEN BONES)

Bones may be accidentally broken in many ways and from different causes. Fractures in general are likely to result from external force suddenly and violently applied, either directly to the part or at a distance, the force being transmitted through the stronger bones until it expends itself by breaking a weaker one remote from the seat of the injury. Occasionally violent contraction of muscles is sufficient to break a bone. Certain bones, those of the legs in particular, owing to their exposed position, are more likely to fracture than others. Owing to certain predisposing causes, such as age, habit, or hereditary constitutional weakness, the bones of some animals are more easily fractured than those of others. The bones of an animal advanced in years are more subject to fracture because of the preponderance of inorganic matter rendering them more brittle. They are also occasionally rendered liable to fracture by a previously existing diseased condition. Fractures are divided into four classes—partial, simple, compound, and comminuted.

Partial fractures.—Partial fractures are those that are likely to occur in a young animal, in which the preponderance of animal matter or the semicartilaginous condition of the bone makes it tough, so that even when considerable force is applied the bone bends and breaks on the side opposite that to which the force was applied, after the manner in which a green stick bends and breaks.

Simple fractures.—A simple fracture is one in which the bone is severed in two parts, transversely, longitudinally, or obliquely, without serious injury to the adjoining structures.

Compound fractures.—A compound fracture is one in which an open wound permits the air to communicate with the ends of the broken bones.

Comminuted fractures.—A comminuted fracture is one in which the bone is shattered or divided into a number of fragments.

Complicated fractures.—A complicated fracture is one in which other structures surrounding the bones are injured.

General symptoms of fracture.—When a fracture of one or more of the large bones of a leg occurs, symptoms are well marked. After the accident the animal refuses to touch the foot to the ground and, if compelled to move, does so with great pain and reluctance. There is more or less shortening of the leg with trembling of the muscles in the vicinity of the injury. There are also deformity and increased mobility, so that, instead of the natural joints of the leg and the natural, muscular control of their motion, a new joint, over which the animal has no control, is formed where the fracture occurred. The leg, shortened by the ends of the bones being forced past one another from the muscular contraction that invariably takes place, hangs dependent from the body. As a result, it swings in an awkward and unnatural manner, permitting the toe and foot to assume positions in their relations to other parts of the body that otherwise would be impossible. If the fractured bone is so situated that the parts may be moved one upon another, a grating sound, known as crepitus, will be heard.

General treatment of fractures.—When a fracture occurs, the advisability of attempting treatment must first be determined. If the animal is young, valuable, and of reasonably quiet temperament, and the fracture is not too great in extent, the chances of recovery are fair. On the other hand, if the animal is of little value, irritable, advanced in years, and the fracture is a serious compound or comminuted one, the wiser course would generally be to put the creature out of its misery.

If treatment is to be attempted, no time should be lost in restoring the parts as nearly as possible to their natural position and retaining them there. If the ends of the bones have been drawn one past the other, they should be drawn out by firm and continuous tension, until they again assume the position in which they were before the accident. All this can better be done before the swelling (which is sure to result) takes place. If the swelling has occurred before the injury is noticed, do not attempt to treat it, but proceed at once to treat the fracture as though the swelling were not present, for no step can be taken toward recovery until the ends of the bone have been restored to their proper position. When that is done and proper appliances have been used to prevent them from being again misplaced, the swelling, which is the result of irritation, will be relieved. In selecting the appliances to be used in the treatment of fracture, the judgment and ingenuity of the operator are of much importance. Splints, made of wood shaped to fit the leg and padded with soft material where they come in contact with bony prominences and held in position by means of bandages, is the oldest method, and with some is still most popular. The fracture pads used in human surgery and for sale in medical supply houses, are very convenient. After being dipped in water they may be molded to fit the leg and be retained by means of bandages. Heavy sole leather is also used after being soaked in warm water and molded to the shape of the leg and holes cut in it to fit over any sharp irregularities in the natural shape of the bones. Gutta-percha sheets also are satisfactory. They are prepared and used in the same way as the leather.

Another and perhaps the simplest of all methods is the application of a plaster of paris bandage, which is made as follows: Strips of thin cheesecloth 3 inches wide and 8 or 9 feet long are laid flat on a board and on them is spread a layer of plaster of paris about one-eighth of an inch thick; then, beginning at one end, roll carefully so as to gather the plaster in between the layers of the bandage. The cloth should be thin and the plaster of paris fresh and active. After preparing 4 or 5 of such bandages the operator is ready to dress the fracture. After the parts have been brought into position, this should be done by covering all that part of the leg to which the plaster of paris bandage is to be applied with a single layer of the dry bandage, letting it extend both above and below the part to which the plaster bandage is to be applied and including under the folds of the dry bandage at each end a layer of absorbent cotton, which is intended to form a pad to prevent the ends of the plaster bandage from chafing the skin beneath. When this is done one of the plaster bandages should be placed in a vessel of water and allowed to remain till the air bubbles have ceased to rise from it, which will generally indicate that it is soaked through. Then, take it in the hand, wind it carefully around and around the leg, unrolling the bandage as it is wound around the limb, and occasionally smoothing down the plaster of paris. Should it form roughly or in ridges, the hand may be dipped in water to impart increased moisture to it. When the winding of one bandage is about finished, place another in the water, so that the winding operation may be continued without delay. The bandages should be applied till the cast is from one-half to three-quarters of an inch thick. Then gently restrain the animal for one-half or three-quarters of an hour till the plaster is hardened. Any of the appliances used should be so manipulated as to prevent absolutely any motion of the detached parts. If the fracture is near a joint, it is generally best to include the joint in the appliance. The part of the limb below the bandage should be carefully and firmly wrapped with an ordinary cotton bandage all the way from the plaster bandage down to the hoof. This last bandage will tend to prevent swelling, which is likely to occur, the result of the dependent position in which the animal is forced by nature to keep the injured limb.

When plaster of paris bandages are applied to a compound fracture, the injured part may be previously dressed with a small, thick pad of cotton immediately over the wound. In applying the bandage the operator may, with a little care, so arrange it as to keep the folds of the bandages off the cotton, or have only a thin layer over it, which may be easily cut out and the cotton removed, leaving a convenient opening through which to dress the wound without removing the bandage. The ends of the bandage or other appliance should be carefully watched to see that the skin does not become chafed, particularly at the lower end. If the bandage should become weak or broken at any part, it may be strengthened without removal by applying other bandages immediately over it. If swelling has taken place before the bandage has been applied, there is likely to be some loosening as it disappears, and even without the swelling there may be a tendency of the bandage to slide downward. This may be overcome by fastening it to a suspender attached to a surcingle or passed over the body and attached to the opposite leg. If the looseness cannot be overcome in this way, the space may be filled by pouring in a thin paste of plaster of paris. A better method, however, is to remove the bandage and apply another. Owing to the hardness of the bandage it will be removed with some difficulty. A deep grove should be cut down completely through it on the opposite sides. This may be done with a chisel and a small hammer if the bandage is carefully held by an assistant so that the concussion of the blows is not transmitted to the injured bones. The patient should have a roomy stall and should be tied by the head to prevent any attempts to move around. In some cases slings have been used. Ordinarily, however, they are not satisfactory with cattle, and if applied should be for only a few days at a time and to lessen the animal's disposition to lie down rather than to prevent it. When they are used continuously, the pressure on the abdomen may interfere with digestion and the general health of the animal.

Modes of union.—The animal should be kept as quiet as possible and given such feed as will have a tendency to keep the bowels slightly relaxed. The success of the operation depends chiefly on the skill of the operator, but not alone in the selection and use of the appliances, for much attention must be given to subsequent management. The patients are restless, and a single awkward motion may undo the work of weeks so far as the union of the parts of the bone is concerned. Union takes place in the same way and, if the conditions are favorable, with greater rapidity than in the human being. The injury that caused the fracture is almost sure to have extended to some of the adjacent tissues, and even though the fracture may be of the simplest type there is almost sure to be considerable hemorrhage around the ends of the broken bone. This, however, is unimportant if the skin remains intact, unless a very large vessel should be injured, or the fracture should open some of the important cavities of the body, in which case a fatal hemorrhage may result. If, on the other hand, the fracture is compound the external opening furnishes a fertile field for the lodgment of disease-producing germs.

Unless great care is taken in such cases, a suppurative process is likely to be established that will seriously interfere with, if not entirely arrest, the process of union between the bones; or it may become so serious as to endanger the general health of the animal and even be attended with fatal results. This last danger is greater if the injury has occurred to the bones of the arm or thigh. In such cases, owing to the dense covering of fascia that ensheathes the muscular covering, pus is likely to be imprisoned and later saturate the whole structure, not only endangering the leg, but, by absorption, may set up blood poisoning and seriously interfere with the general health of the patient, even to causing death. In order to prevent such complication as far as possible the wound should be carefully cleansed with a mild solution of carbolic acid, then dusted over with iodoform before the bandages are applied, and cleansed and dressed daily in the same way. After dressing, always cover with absorbent cotton. In the early process of union an exudation of lymph takes place, which is at first fluid. It gradually becomes thicker and firmer till it forms a callus, known as the external or ensheathing callus, in the shape of a ring or ferrule surrounding the detached portions of the bone. Occasionally this callus forms only at the ends of the bones and fills the spaces between them, when it is known as the intermediate callus. The process of union may be divided into five stages. In the first stage, including the first 8 days, the detached portions of the bone and the sharp projections that are not sufficiently nourished are absorbed. The blood that escaped into the surrounding tissues, the result of the injury, is gradually absorbed, and the effused lymph, which ultimately constitutes the temporary cartilage, takes its place. In the second stage, from the tenth to the twentieth day, the tumor or callus is formed, and fibrocartilage is developed inside and around the exposed end of the bone. In the third stage, extending from the twentieth to the fortieth or fiftieth day, according to the age and strength of the animal, the fibrocartilaginous structure undergoes a change and is gradually converted into bone, forming a ferrule on the outside and a plug on the inside, which serve to hold the part in position. In the fourth stage, extending to about the sixth month, the whole of the new structure is converted into bone. In the fifth stage, extending to the end of the first year, the callus is absorbed, being no longer necessary, and the connection between the cavities of the two bones is again established.

Common complications.—The process of union just described is healthy and normal. Diseased conditions may at any time supervene during the treatment and render the operation unsuccessful. In a compound fracture, in which the open wound communicates with the ends of the bones, a septic condition is likely to arise that may become so serious as to endanger the animal's life. Under such circumstances amputation is not uncommonly resorted to, particularly in valuable animals. Even in the simplest form of fracture, if the splints or bandages are improperly applied and the fractured bone is left so loosely guarded that the broken ends move one upon another, the formation of the calluses previously described is likely to be interfered with, and in place of a strong, rigid, and healthy union a formation of elastic cartilage is the result. This false structure unites the broken ends of the bones in such a way that they move one upon another, depriving the bone of its stability and usefulness. When once the healthy process of union is interrupted in the manner just described, it is again established with great difficulty. It no longer does any good to continue the restraining power; in fact, the change of the temporary cartilage into bone is more likely to be reestablished if the parts move violently upon each other for a short time so as to set up and renew the process of inflammation. Then if the restraint is again applied there is some chance of union. In order to avoid this danger as far as possible, care should be taken that the bandage fits closely and that it is kept on till a perfect union has taken place. It is impossible to say at just what time the splints or bandages can safely be removed. In a young and healthy animal of quiet temperament, if the parts have been firmly held in position throughout the whole time, from 30 to 40 days may be regarded as reasonably safe. Under more unfavorable conditions as to age, vitality, and restraint, the period would better be extended to 60 days, if the general condition of the animal is such as to permit of so long a continuance. After the appliance has been removed the animal should be allowed to stand quiet for a few days, then be given very gentle exercise, gradually increased for a week or 10 days, by which

77431 O—51——18

time the patient will be so far recovered as to be placed on pasture. It should, however, be alone for a time, to avoid any chance of injury from fighting or other accidents that association with other animals might involve.

SPECIAL FRACTURES

Fracture of the horns.—Of the special fractures likely to occur, that of the horn is perhaps the most common. It is always the result of violent mechanical means, such as blows, injury occurring while fighting, or from the animal's getting its head locked in some manner while feeding from a rack. When it occurs there are two ways in which the injury may affect the animal. First and most common, the horny crust is likely to be stripped from the bony projection that is covers. Second, the crust and bone may both be broken or bent down, in which case the fracture occurs at the root of the horn and involves part of the bones of the head in the immediate vicinity. In the first case, if the horny covering is knocked off, little attention is necessary. The animal may be relieved from suffering if the stump is smeared with pine tar and wrapped in cloth. If the core is much lacerated, perhaps it would be better to amputate. The necessity for such operation must be determined by the condition of the injury and to some extent by the owner's ideas on the subject. When the operation is performed, it should be done with a sharp, fine-toothed saw and by sawing the horn off close enough to include a little of the skin and hair around its base. The practice of dehorning has become popular in many parts of the country. It is a simple operation, and, although attended with some immediate suffering, does not produce serious constitutional disturbance. The advisability of performing the operation on all cattle is a question of expediency and must be justified by the expectation of benefit on the part of the feeder. If the horn should be broken so that the core and crust are bent out of shape without the detachment of one from the other, it may be restored to its normal position and retained there by means of a splint made to fit across the back of the head, so as to be laced to both horns. The sound horn holds the broken one in position. Such a splint may be fastened on by means of either a wire or cord and allowed to remain 6 weeks or 2 months.

If both the horn and core have been broken off, bleeding is usually severe and should be checked by astringents, such as alum, or by pressure. After the hemorrhage has ceased, the exposed portion of the fracture should be covered with pine tar, with or without a bandage. An imperfect growth of horn will in due time cover the exposed bone.

Fractures of the bones of the face.—These occasionally occur, and when over the cavities of the nose they produce depression, disfigurement, and impeded respiration, owing to the lessening of the caliber of the nasal passages.

When this accident occurs, the depressed bone should be gently forced back in place by introducing the finger into the nostril. However, if the fracture is too far up, a probe may be passed and the parts retained by placing immediately over it a plaster of thin leather or strong canvas smeared with tar, extending out to the sound surroundings. Care should be taken to embed the hair over the fractured portion in the tar of the plaster, so that it will be firmly held and prevented from again becoming depressed. If only one nostril is involved, the depressed portion may be held in position by packing that nostril with absorbent cotton. This practice, however, has the objection of giving the animal great discomfort and in some cases a disposition to aggravate the injury.

Fracture of the skull (cranium).—Fractures of the bones forming the cavity in which the brain is situated are, owing to their strength, comparatively rare among cattle. Such an accident results only from external violence, and it is hardly possible that it occurs without some fragment of the broken bone pressing on the brain so as to cause coma or other severe nervous derangement or even death.

If the animal survives the first shock, efforts should be directed toward relieving the pressure, which may be done by making an opening in the bone (trephining) and with a hook drawing the depressed part outward. Interference is not so likely to be attended with good results as to be warranted in all cases. The effects of a very severe shock that may not have produced a fracture, although the symptoms are alarming, will in many cases pass off, leaving the animal in a better condition than if an operation had been performed.

Fracture of the lower jaw.—This occasionally occurs and is more likely to result from the kick of a horse than from any other cause. The front part of the jaw may be split or shattered in any direction in which the force may have been applied. Bloody discharges from the mouth and failure to eat or ruminate are symptoms most likely to attract attention.

The treatment is simple and consists in first removing detached pieces of bone, then drawing the parts together and retaining them by means of pieces of copper wire fastened around the teeth, and feeding the animal on sloppy feed until recovery takes place. The wound should be dressed once or twice a day with a 3-percent solution of carbolic acid, forced gently in with a syringe, so as to remove any feed that may have become impacted and interfere with the healing process.

Fracture of the vertebra (spinal column).—This is not so common among cattle as among other animals. If the fracture is through the body of the bone, there may be pressure on or laceration of the spinal cord, causing paralysis of all parts posterior to the seat of injury. Fractures of the prominences on a vertebra occasionally occur without interfering with the canal in which the spinal cord is situated. Such accidents are likely to pass unnoticed, for, although the animal may suffer considerable pain, it may not be manifested in such a way as to attract attention, and the deep covering of muscles serves effectually to conceal the injury. When the fracture occurs in the upper part of the neck, paralysis of the muscles used in respiration results, and death from asphyxia very shortly ensues. The more common accident is to the loins, and when a fracture of the body of a vertebra occurs in this region so as to produce pressure on the spinal cord, paralysis of the hind legs and quarters is the result. Diagnosis of such an accident is more difficult than in any other fracture. The parts cannot be moved one upon another so that crepitus is noticeable. The heavy coating of muscles conceals irregularities of shape, which otherwise may attract attention. About the only reliable symptom is paralysis of the parts posterior to the injury. Careful examination may reveal the seat of the injury. If it was the result of a blow, there may be some abrasion of the skin. The diagnosis is important only as an aid in determining the proper course to pursue.

If paralysis is present and a depression or irregularity of the spinal column is so apparent as to leave no doubt of the existence of a fracture, the only alternative is to destroy the animal, for there can be no hope of recovery. If, on the other hand, paralysis is incomplete and there is no depression or irregularity of the spinal column or other evidence of fracture, the patient should be made as comfortable as possible by being placed in a well-bedded box-stall and a few days permitted to elapse before the case is abandoned. The symptoms last described may possibly be the result of a severe strain of the muscles of the loins, in which case an improvement will soon be noticeable.

Fractures of the pelvis.—The pelvis, or bony framework that gives shape to the posterior part of the body, is liable to fracture in many ways. A common one is by a separation of the two bones that constitute the whole pelvis along the bottom and center line (symphysis pubis). In early life the two bones are separate and distinct. The union between them, which is at first cartilaginous, undergoes a change and is converted into bone, so that in adult life the whole pelvis is practically one bone. The point on which the two bones are united is weaker than the adjoining parts of the bone. When an animal slips violently and spreads the legs wide apart, the weaker materials give way and the bones are divided. If the accident is noticed when it occurs, it is likely to throw light on the nature of the injury. The animal will immediately become stiff behind, and spread the legs apart. Further examination may be made by introducing the hand, previously carefully oiled, into the rectum or vagina and pressing down along the central line, which will cause the patient to evince acute pain. In this case no appliance can be used to advantage. The animal should be tied in a stall until the parts become reunited and the lameness disappears.

Fracture of the posterior parts of the bone (ischium) that forms the point of the buttocks occasionally occurs. The buttock on the injured side will be less prominent than on the other. Careful manipulation will generally move the parts so that crepitus may be recognized. If the fracture is through the posterior part of the bone, it is unimportant and deserves no more attention than placing the animal in such position as to insure it against subsequent injury until the bones are united. Some distortion may result but not enough to warrant interference.

Fracture through the body of the bone on a line with the hip joint (acetabulum) occasionally, though rarely, occurs, and is nearly always associated with dislocation of the hip joint and the forcing of the head of the upper bone of the leg (femur) upward, far out of its place. The violent contraction of the powerful muscles of the hip renders it impossible to reduce the dislocation, and even if it were possible the fractured pelvis could not be held in position, so that the case becomes at once hopeless. It may be recognized by the animal's standing on three legs, the leg on the injured side seeming shorter than its fellow and hanging pendulous, the muscles of the hip violently contracted and hard to the touch. The animal evinces great pain when the leg is moved. There is likely to be some apparent distortion in the relations between the point of the hip and the point of the buttock. This will be more readily noticed by comparing the injured side with the other. The parts may be moved so as to produce crepitus. The examination may be completed by introducing the oiled hand into the vagina or rectum, when the two sides of the pelvis will reveal well-marked differences.

Fracture of the point of the hip.—The anterior and external part of the pelvis (ilium), commonly known as the point of the hip, is liable to fracture, which stock owners describe as "hipping," or being "hipped," or having the hip "knocked down." This accident may be the result of crowding while passing through a narrow door, of falling violently on the point of the hip, or from a violent blow directed downward and forward against it. The lesion generally extends across the flat surface of the bone from its outer and posterior edge forward and inward. Distortion is likely to be the only noticeable symptom. The detached portion varies in size in different cases and with it the resulting deformity. The animal is slightly lame, but this symptom soon disappears. The detached portion of the bone is drawn downward and away from the main part by the action of the muscles below, which are so powerful as to render return impossible. The bones therefore remain permanently separated and union takes place by fibrous callus. The animal suffers little inconvenience and for practical use may be as serviceable as before the accident, though the distorted appearance depreciates its value.

Fracture of the ribs.—Such an occurrence can take place only as the result of a direct injury, as from blows or crowding. The posterior ribs, being more exposed, are more likely to fracture. Pain in moving, slight swelling over the seat of injury, and difficult breathing are obvious symptoms. If the fracture is complete, crepitation may be occasionally noticed by placing the hand flat over the injured part and carefully observing the motion as the chest contracts and expands during respiration. This symptom is more noticeable when the animal coughs. Unless the point of the broken bone penetrates the cavity of the chest, the fracture is usually unimportant and calls for no treatment other than quiet. If the breathing is very labored and attended with much pain, motion may be limited by applying a wide bandage firmly around the chest. The animal should receive a restricted quantity of feed and water for a few days, the stomach being kept as nearly empty as possible. Sloppy feed should be given to encourage, as much as possible, free action of the diaphram in breathing.

Fracture of bones of the legs.—On this subject much has been said in the preceding remarks on general fractures. As a rule, fracture through one of the large bones of the shoulder (scapula) or thigh (femur) is very difficult to manage. The powerful contraction of the muscles and the changing shape of the leg resulting from their action render it impossible to retain the detached parts of the bone in proper position. Therefore, though union should take place, there is almost sure to be considerable deformity and more or less lameness. Fracture of the arm (humerus) or leg (tibia) is likely to be attended with better results. The muscular covering is not so thick, the sheath in which they are held is more tense, and the change in the shape of the leg from muscular action not so noticeable, the muscular force not so great, all of which facilitate replacing the dislodged ends and retaining them.

Fracture of the knee (carpus) and hock (tarsus).—This seldom occurs except from a very violent injury and is generally associated with other injury and serious complications. Displacement does not generally occur to any considerable extent. The treatment consists in holding the leg perfectly quiet in a natural position, which may be done by the application of long, wooden splints retained by bandages, or a plaster of paris bandage.

Fracture below the knee.—Fracture of the long bone below the knee (metacarpus) and hock (metatarsus) is relatively common. In young animals of quiet temperament the treatment of simple fractures here is likely to be attended with good results. On the other hand, a compound fracture in this region becomes a serious matter. The structures that surround the bones are so thin that a small degree of sloughing will expose parts of the bones and is likely to lead to serious complications and probably fatal results.

Fractures of bones below the fetlock.—These fractures are comparatively unimportant unless associated with other serious injury. The parts can generally be held in position without much difficulty, and union generally takes place rapidly.

Appliances.—Of the appliances used in the treatment of the fracture of limbs above the knee, splints made of wood or iron strips and bandages are likely to serve best. Below the knee, plaster of paris bandages are preferable. Although some authorities disapprove of the use of this type of bandage, it has many advantages over any of the other appliances when used alone, and in many ways it may be uesd with advantage in combination with others.

DISLOCATIONS

Luxation, or displacement without fracture of the bones forming a joint, is comparatively rare among cattle. It most frequently occurs in the stifle joint, where dislocation of the kneepan (patella) takes place. A glance at the skeleton (pl. XXV) will show the relations better than they can be described. It will be observed that the small, irregularly shaped bone (patella) plays on the anterior rounded part of the lower edge of the thigh bone (femur) and between it and the upper end of the shank bone (tibia). The outer ridge on the lower end of the thigh bone is less prominent than the inner one, so that displacement, when it does take place, is by slipping outward. Such an accident may occur from direct injury or external force, as a blow, or from slipping. When it occurs the symptoms produced are somewhat alarming. The animal is unable to draw the leg forward and either stands with it thrown back with the toe pointing downward, or, if it should succeed in getting its weight upon it, holds it firmly on the ground, fearing to move it. Examination of the outside of the joint will disclose the situation of the patella outside its proper place. If the operator is not familiar with the normal appearance of the joint, it is well to make a comparison between the injured and the sound one. If compelled to move, the animal does so with great difficulty, jerking the leg that it is unable to bring forward, hopping with the other, and partially dragging the injured one.

Treatment.—The treatment is simple. A rope 20 feet long should be applied around the fetlock of the affected leg, passed forward between the front legs and up over the opposite side of the neck, back over the withers, and wrapped once behind the elbow around that portion of the rope that passes between the front legs. The leg is then drawn away from the body and forcibly pushed forward by an assistant, while another person tightens up the slack in the rope until the affected leg is off the ground in front of the supporting leg. The rope is then drawn taut and the assistant grasps the tail and pulls the cow toward the affected side. The animal makes a lurch to keep from falling, contracts the muscles, and the patella slips into place with a sharp click, and the animal walks off as if nothing had happened. If the animal resists this method of handling, it may suffice to manipulate the dislocated kneepan by shoving it inward and forward with the heel of the hand while the affected leg is drawn well forward. Unless some precaution is taken the accident is likely to recur, as the ligaments have been stretched by the dislocation till they no longer hold the bone with that firmness necessary to retain it. The animal should be tied and the foot fastened forward, so that the patient can just stand on its comfortably, by means of a rope or strap around the fetlock carried forward between the front legs, around the neck, and tied on the breast.

Should this accident occur more than once it is a good practice to apply a blister around the joint, as recommended for sprain of the shoulder, and observe the precautions as to restraint and subsequent treatment there recommended. With this one exception dislocations in cattle occuring independently of other complications are rare.

Dislocation with fracture may occur in any of the joints, and if one is suspected or discovered, examination should always be made for the other before treatment is applied. When a fracture occurs near a joint the force sufficient to rend the bone is likely to be partly exerted on the immediate tissues, and when the bone gives way the structures of the joints may be seriously injured. Occasionally the injury to the joint becomes the most important complication in the treatment of a fracture. In order clearly to understand the reason for this some information is necessary on the structure of the joints.

The bones constituting the skeleton of the animal body are united in such a manner as to admit of more or less motion one upon another. In some of the more simple joints the bones are held together by the dense structures around them and admit of little or no movement, as the bones of the head. In other joints the bones are bound together by dense, cartilaginous structures and admit of only limited motion, such as union of the small bones at the back part of the knee and hock (metacarpal and metatarsal). In the more nearly perfect form of joint the power of motion becomes complete and the structures are more complex. The substance of the bone on its articular surface is not covered with periosteum but is sheathed in a dense, thin layer of cartilage, shaped to fit the other surfaces with which it comes in contact (articular). This layer is thickest toward its center when covering bony eminences, and is elastic, of a pearly whiteness, and resisting, though soft enough to be easily cut. The bones forming an articulation are bound together by numerous ligaments attached to bony prominences. The whole joint is sealed in by a band or ribbonlike ligament (capsular ligament) extending around the joint and attached at the outer edge of the articular surface, uniting the bones and hermetically sealing the cavities of the articulation. This structure and the articular surface of the bone are covered by a thin, delicate membrane, known as the synovial membrane, which secretes the joint oil (synovia). This fluid is viscid and colorless, or slightly yellow, and although it does not possess a large quantity of fat, its character somewhat resembles oil, and it serves the same purpose in lubricating the joints that oil does to the friction surface of an engine. The tissues of the joint when used in a natural way are able to withstand the effect of great exertion. When unnaturally used, however, as they are very delicate and complex, they are liable to inflammatory and other changes of a serious nature. The synovial membrane and, in fact, the whole structure of the joint are susceptible to injury and serious inflammatory derangement, and the capsular ligament is likely to be distended from excessive secretion of synovia. The latter process may be almost noninflammatory and attended with little inconvenience or importance other than a blemish to the animal, which in cattle is not serious. It may occur on the back part of the leg above the fetlock or on the inner and fore part of the hock, corresponding in its location to windgalls and bog spavin of the horse. Continuous support by bandages will generally force reabsorption, and as the leg is not subjected to violent action, as in the horse, the affection is not so likely to recur.

RHEUMATISM

Symptoms accompanying inflammation of the joints, muscles, connective tissue, and heart have long been referred to as rheumatism. It is doubtful whether there is a specific disease that can rightfully be so named. Hidden infections in various parts of the body, septic inflammation of such organs as the womb, bladder, stomach, and intestines, and general intoxication due to alimentary disturbance, are some of the conditions in which the so-called rheumatism may develop. Since the affection is in reality a symptom or symptom-complex that may be observed in many diseases, it is obvious that a determination of the location and nature of the cause must be made before any rational treatment can be undertaken.

Surgical Operations

By William Dickson and William Herbert Lowe, D. V. S.

[Revised by William M. Mohler, D.V. M.]

Surgery is both a science and an art. The success of surgical operations depends on the judgment, skill, and dexterity, as well as on the knowledge, of the operator. The same fundamental principles underlie and govern animal and human surgery, although their applications have a wide range and are very different in many essential particulars. Hygiene and sanitation are essential to the best results in veterinary as well as in human surgery.

Asepsis is an ideal condition which, although not always possible in animal surgery, is highly important in connection with the mechanical details of all surgical operations in proportion to their nature and seriousness.

Aseptic surgery is the performance of operations with sterile instruments, the hands of the operator and the site of operation being as nearly sterile as possible, and the wound treated during operation with sterile solutions and protected with sterile bandage material after the operation. In other words, it is the preservation of the highest degree of cleanliness in connection with operations.

Local or general anesthesia should be resorted to in painful and serious surgical operations, as operations on all living creatures should be performed humanely and all unnecessary pain and suffering avoided. Anesthesia is necessary where absolute immobility of the patient is essential and where entire muscular relaxation is indispensable. The anesthetic condition is also favorable for the adjustment of displaced organs.

Large animals have to be cast and secured before an anesthetic is administered. For complete anesthesia, inhalations of chloroform are generally employed; sometimes of both ether and chloroform. The quantity of chloroform required to produce insensibility to external impressions varies in different cases and must be regulated, as well as the admixture of air, by a competent assistant.

If the probability of the success of an operation is remote and the animal is in healthy physical condition, so that its flesh is good for human food, it is more advisable to butcher the animal than to attempt a surgical operation that offers little encouragement to the owner. The best judgment must be exercised in determining a matter of this kind, for no animal suffering from inflammation or that is feverish is fit for human food.

All cases of major operative surgery require the skill and dexterity of the experienced veterinary surgeon, and no one else should attempt such an operation, for unnecessary suffering must be prevented. Nevertheless, the more knowledge and understanding an owner of animals has of the principles of surgical operations and manipulations, the better for all concerned. In the first place, such an owner will appreciate more fully the skill of the qualified veterinarian, and, in the second place, he will be better prepared and equipped to render assistance to a suffering animal when no practitioner is accessible and in cases of emergency. There are, moreover, minor operations, some of which can hardly be classed as surgical, that the stockman and farmer should be able to perform himself.

In the performance of any operation on an animal of the size and strength of the bull or cow, the first consideration is to secure the animal in such a manner as to preclude its injuring either itself or those taking any part in the operation. The nature and time likely to be occupied by an operation must, of course, largely determine the method to be adopted.

Most of the operations with which the present chapter is concerned are usually performed on the animal in a standing position.

A bull should always be held by a staff attached to the ring in his nose. To secure the cow in a standing position, grasp the nose, the finger and thumb being introduced into the nostrils, and press against the cartilage that makes a division between them. If she has horns, grasp one of them with the disengaged hand. If this is insufficient the animal should be secured to a post, along the side of a fence, or put into a stanchion. An excellent method of restraint is to tie a long rope in a slip noose over the horns, pass it around the chest just behind the forelegs, taking a half hitch on itself, taking another half hitch in front of the hind limbs, passing the free end under the tail, bringing it forward and making it fast either to the head or one of the hitches. The head should be raised to the level of the back before the final knot is tied to render it too serious and painful a matter for her to repeat the first attempt she makes to lower it. Should the nature or extent of the operation be likely to take considerable time, it is invariably the best plan to throw the animal. In the bovine this is easily done, either by horse hobbles, should they be at hand, or by a simple rope. If horse hobbles are used, they should be fastened on the leg just above the fetlocks (ankle joints), as in that position they are less likely to come off than if placed around the pastern.

Of the many ways of applying the rope for this purpose the following two are the best and simplest:

(1) Take a long, strong rope (one that has been used a few times is more flexible), double it, and at 2 or 3 feet from the doubled end, according to the size of the animal, make a knot and pass the collar thus formed over the animal's head, allowing it to rest on what would be the collar place in a horse. Now, pass the ends of the rope between the forelegs, carry one around each hind leg just above the fetlock joint, from outside in, under itself once, and bring the free ends forward, passing each through the collar loop on its own side and bringing the slack back toward and beyond the hind quarters (pl. XXVI, fig. 2). Two or three men should then take hold of each rope and at a given signal pull. The animal's hind legs being drawn forward, the balance is lost, and if the animal does not fall or lie down it can be readily pushed over on its side and secured in the desired position.

(2) The three half hitches. Take a rope 30 or more feet long, make a slip noose at the end and pass it over the animal's horns, leaving the knot in the loop between the horns. If the animal has no horns, attach the rope to the halter. Then pass the rope backward along the neck to the withers, just in front of which take a half hitch on it, passing it along the back, take one half hitch just behind the forelegs and a second in front of the hind legs around the flank (pl. XXVI, fig. 1). The free end of the rope is taken hold of by one or two assistants while another holds the animal's head. By pulling firmly on the rope, or inducing the animal to make a step or two forward while steady traction is made on the rope, the beast will lie down, when its feet can be secured in the way most convenient for the operator.

There are numerous other methods, involving more or less complete restraint, which may be equally efficacious, but one or the other of the ways indicated will be found to meet fully all ordinary cases.

RINGING THE BULL

This is usually and ought always to be done before the calf has attained sufficient weight or strength to make his restraint a matter of serious difficulty. An ordinary halter is usually all that is required, the strap being secured to a tree or post. A jointed copper ring is ordinarily used.

The common method of punching a round piece out of the nasal septum for the introduction of the ring is open to objection, as portions of the fine nervous filaments are destroyed. The sensibility of the parts is thus lessened and the object of ringing to some extent defeated. The insertion of the ring by means of a trocar and cannula is preferable, as the method is not open to this objection.

A little instrument, which has been used in veterinary practice for some time and which can be made by any worker in metal, consists of a steel point riveted into a short cannula made to fit on one end of the ring while open (pl. XXVII, fig. 11). When attached to the ring it is easily and quickly passed through the septum, the half of the ring following as a matter of course. It can then be removed and the ends of the ring brought together and fastened by means of the screw for that purpose.

DEHORNING

In cattle in the wild state, the utility of the horns as weapons of offense and defense is apparent, but in domesticated cattle horns constitute a menace to the safety of their companions. Horned cattle frequently inflict painful and serious injuries to others. Deaths as a result of such injuries are not unusual. Dehorning is therefore advisable as a matter of general safety.

On farms where breeding is conducted, the most desirable method is to prevent the horns from growing on the young calves. This action results in a more symmetrical appearance of the poll and eliminates the dangers from the presence of horns on the young cattle prior to their removal at a later age. A calf should be treated not later than 1 week after it is born—preferably when it is from 3 to 5 days old. The agent to be used may be either caustic soda or potash in the form of sticks about the thickness of an ordinary lead pencil. These caustics must be handled with care, as they dissolve the cuticle and may make the hands or fingers sore. The preparation of the calf first consists in clipping the hair from the parts, washing clean with soap or warm water, and thoroughly drying with a cloth or towel. The stick of caustic should be wrapped in a piece of paper to protect the hands and fingers, leaving one end of the stick uncovered. Moisten the uncovered end slightly and rub it on the horn buttons or little points that may be felt on the calf's head—first on one, then on the other—two or three times, allowing the caustic to dry after each application. Apply the caustic to the horn button only, for if it is brought in contact with the surrounding skin it will cause pain. Too much moisture on the stick of caustic allows the application to spread to the surrounding skin. After treatment keep the calf protected from rain, as water on the head after application of the caustic will cause it to run down over the face.

Dehorning of adult animals is usually performed after the age of 2 years, when there is less probability of the horns again growing. The horns should be severed from the head from a quarter to a half inch below where the skin joins the base of the horn, cutting from the back to the front if a saw is used. If the horn is not cut close enough to the head, an irregular, gnarly growth of horn is likely to follow.

Before attempting to dehorn the animal, it should be securely controlled by ropes in a stanchion or by casting. On the range the cattle are usually controlled by casting or by placing them in a "squeezer" connected with a corral. A clean, sharp meat saw or a miter saw with a rigid back may be used. Various types of dehorning shears or clippers are in general use. One type of dehorner has a stationary knife edge with its cutting edge shaped like a very wide V, and opposing this, another knife of similar shape moving in a slide, so that the cutting edges act on the horn from all four sides at once, all the edges passing the center at the same time. Another type has a movable knife, with one oblique or one curved edge, and the cutting is done in one direction only. The power for cutting with these instruments is supplied by pulling together two long handles which, in order to transmit a greater force, are generally so constructed that they act through the medium of a series of cogs. In dehorning with these instruments the cutting edges should be slipped down over the horn and the knives closed, so that their edges set firmly against the horn in such position that the cut will be made in the right place and in the right direction. The handles should then be drawn together with a quick, firm, strong pull so that the horn will be completely severed by the first act and without twisting.

When possible, dehorning should be performed in cool weather when flies are not troublesome. The loss of blood from the operation is not sufficient, as a rule, to be of consequence, and if care is taken to prevent substances from getting into the openings left after the removal of the horns, it is not necessary to apply any dressing. Pine tar or a mixture of pine tar and tannic acid may be applied, particularly if the weather is warm. In recent years local anesthetics have been used to a considerable extent in preparing the animal for the dehorning operation. Such agents tend to desensitize the area of operation and reduce hemorrhage.

TRACHEOTOMY

This operation consists in making an opening in the trachea, or windpipe. It is necessary whenever there is an obstruction from any cause in the upper part of the respiratory tract that threatens the death of the animal by asphyxia (suffocation). The mode of procedure is as follows: Have an assistant extend the animal's head as far as possible to make the trachea tense and prominent; make a longitudinal incision about 2 to 2½ inches long through the skin and deeper tissues and trachea at the most prominent part of the trachea, which is about the middle or upper third, and then insert the tracheotomy tube. The latter should be removed once or twice daily and cleansed, and the wound dressed antiseptically. To ascertain when it is time to discontinue the use of the tube and to allow the wound to close, the hand should be held over the opening, which will require the animal to use its natural passages in breathing. Observe whether it is performed in a natural manner, and if so, remove the tube and allow the wound to close. Often the operation has to be performed in great haste without the proper instruments and under great disadvantages, the operator having to cut down quickly, open the trachea and spread the parts, using some instrument improvised by him at the time. This operation only gives the animal relief in breathing, and therefore the proper remedial treatment should be adopted at the onset of the attack and continued until the cause (the disease) has been overcome.

RUMENOTOMY

The opening of the paunch, or rumen, in cattle and the removal of a part or the whole of the ingesta through the opening is termed "rumenotomy." The operation should be performed in severe cases only, where the rumen is excessively overloaded and distended. The animal is placed with its right side against a wall and firmly held in position by strong assistants. The incision is made in the same place that the trocar is inserted for puncturing that organ in cases of bloat. The opening is increased in size until the operator's hand can be inserted into the rumen. Before any of the contents are removed from that organ a linen cloth should be placed from the outer wound into the rumen to prevent any of the ingesta from getting into the abdominal cavity. Some practitioners, after removing a portion of the contents of the rumen, introduce such medicine as may be needed before closing the wound. Clean the wound and close the opening in the rumen with uninterrupted (pl. XXVII, fig. 8) carbolized catgut sutures. Next close the external wound, consisting of the integument, muscle, and peritoneum, with stout, interrupted (pl. XXVII, fig. 6) metallic sutures. No feed should be given for several hours after the operation, and then gruels only. (See Distention of Rumen or Paunch with Feed, p 18.)

TREATMENT OF ABSCESSES

An abscess may be detected, if situated externally, by heat, pain, redness, and swelling in the early stages, and, if further developed, by the fluctuation that is present. When any of these symptoms are absent, the suppuration should be encouraged by hot fomentations and poultices. Care must be taken that the abscess is not opened too soon, or to some extent it may cause it to scatter, and the escape of pus will be lessened. The time to open an abscess is just before it is ready to break and should be done with a sharp lance, a crucial incision sometimes being necessary. The cavity should be syringed out with an antiseptic solution. To prevent the wound from closing too rapidly, it should be packed with sterile gauze.

WOUNDS

For the purposes of the present work wounds may be divided into three classes: (1) Incised, (2) punctured, and (3) lacerated or contused. In any wound all that the most suitable applications can accomplish are, in the first place, to prevent the access of poisonous germs in the animal's surroundings, such as the soil and the manure, and, in the second place, when the process of repair is for some reason temporarily inactive or altogether arrested, to incite that curative inflammation that is the invariable method by which the cure is effected.

INCISED WOUNDS

This type of wound has clean-cut edges and may be either superficial or deep. In wounds of all descriptions there is necessarily more or less bleeding, and this is especially likely to be the case in incised wounds, particularly when they penetrate to a considerable depth, or when they are inflicted on a part where blood vessels of any considerable size approach the surface. To arrest the hemorrhage must therefore be the first consideration. If the hemorrhage is slight, a generous use of cold water is all that is necessary, but if one or more vessels of any size have been wounded or entirely severed, they should be taken up and ligated. If the blood flows continuously, and is dark in color, it proceeds from a vein, but if bright-colored and jerky in its flow, it is arterial.

The taking up of an artery simply means the tying of the bleeding vessel, which should be accomplished as follows: To discover the bleeding artery take a piece of clean absorbent cotton, dip it in cold water, and by gentle pressure on the wound clear it of the accumulated blood. The jet of fresh blood reveals the end of the vessel, which is readily recognized by its whitish-yellow or buff color. It should be seized with a forceps or pincers and slightly drawn clear of the surrounding tissues. Now take the thread and place the middle of it under the artery, take up the ends, tie one simple knot tightly, pressing the thread down with the forefinger so as not to include the forceps, then a second one over it and cut off the ends. The bleeding being arrested, the operator can now carefully clean and inspect the wound, taking care to remove all blood and foreign matter and clip

77431 O—51——19

the hair around the edges before stitching it. If the wound is superficial, the lips may be brought together by a series of independent stitches (pl. XXVII, fig. 6) about one-half to three-fourths of an inch apart. The stitches should not be drawn tightly; it is sufficient to bring the edges of the wound in apposition.

If the wound is deep, the needle should be introduced perpendicularly at as great a distance from the lip of the wound as the depth it is to be inserted, to give the thread sufficient hold. All the stitches should be as nearly as possible at equal distances from the border of the wound, to prevent unequal strain, and the knots should be made at the side, not over the wound (pl. XXVII, fig. 6). When the wound is large and deep, care should be taken to have an opening in the lowest part to allow for the escape of the discharges.

In deep wounds that run crosswise of a leg or muscle it is often advisable to use what is technically known as the quilled suture, which is most readily understood by reference to plate XXVII, figure 7. With this method a curved needle with an eye in the point and a strong double thread should be used. The needle thus threaded is introduced perpendicularly at least an inch from the wound on one side, carried across below and brought out the same distance from the border of the cut on the opposite side, the thread being seized and held in position while the needle is withdrawn, leaving a loop of thread protruding on one side and two loose ends on the other side of each stitch. When stitches have been made, take a light piece of wood about the size of a lead pencil, corresponding in length to the size of the wound or slightly longer, insert it through each of the loops, and draw up the free ends of the threads, which should in turn be tied securely on a similar piece of wood on that side.

PUNCTURED WOUNDS

Owing to the uncertainty of their depth and the structures they may involve, punctured wounds are by far the most dangerous and difficult to treat. Not only is the extent of the damage hidden from view, but the very character of the injury, as can be readily understood, implies at least the possibility of deep-seated inflammation and consequent discharge of pus, which, when formed, is kept pent up until it has accumulated to such an extent that it burrows by simple gravity, as no other exit is possible. In this way foreign matter, such as a broken piece of the stake or snag, or whatever caused the wound, may be carried to an indefinite depth, or the cavity of a joint may be invaded and very serious, if not fatal, consequences occur.

The danger is especially marked when the injury is inflicted on parts liable to frequent and extensive motion, but all punctured wounds should receive unusual care, as no judgment can be accurately formed from the external appearance of the wound. Although a probe can ascertain the depth, it throws little light on the extent or exact nature of the internal injury. For this reason all punctured wounds should be carefully searched by means of a probe or some substitute devised for the occasion, such as a piece of wire with a smooth blunt end or a piece of hard wood shaped for the purpose. Stitching of punctured wounds is not admissible. After the opening of the wound and its surroundings are thoroughly cleansed, tincture of iodine should be injected directly into the wound.

If a punctured wound is not deep, and when the bruising and laceration are slight, it is possible for healing to take place by adhesion. The process of repair by this method is far superior to that by granulation, which is referred to later. With this object in view, the animal should be kept as quiet as possible. A dose of physic, such as a pound of Glauber's or Epsom salts, should be administered as a drench, and an application of warm antiseptic fomentation or poultices, when this is practicable, made frequently to the surface of the wound.

In wounds of this description the process of repair may be complicated by the appearance of exuberant granulations, known as proud flesh, which are an overgrowth of new tissue—granulation tissue; but these should not be interfered with unless they continue after the acute stage of inflammation has been subdued. If, after this, they persist, they may be treated with a 10-percent solution of copper sulfate (bluestone) or silver nitrate (lunar caustic) in water.

CONTUSED OR LACERATED WOUNDS

These wounds are usually caused by a blow with some blunt instrument or by falls. The seriousness depends largely on the depth of the injury, and treatment should be directed to allaying the inflammation and preventing the consequent tendency to sloughing. To this end soothing applications, such as antiseptic fomentations and poultices, are advisable.

Barbed-wire cuts.—These wounds are specified simply because in some sections of the country there is a fixed idea that there is a specific poison in barbed wire, causing injuries that require treatment differing from that which is applicable to ordinary wounds. Barbed-wire cuts differ from ordinary wounds only in the parts being often lacerated and torn, and the treatment for wounds of that description should be as described later in this section.

METHODS OF HEALING

Technically methods of healing may be divided into a number of distinct processes but practically into two only, namely, by primary union, or adhesion, and by granulation. As suppuration is not so likely to occur in cattle as in horses, healing by the former and more speedy process is much more common in the first-named species, particularly in clean-cut or incised wounds, provided they have been stitched within 12 hours from the time the injury that caused them was inflicted, that they have been kept antiseptically clean, and that the patient by some means has been kept fairly quiet. This latter stipulation is probably hardest to comply with. Quiet is an important factor in the process of repair among the lower animals.

The second method of healing, namely, by granulation, which is, however, the manner in which most wounds in animals heal, takes much longer. In punctured wounds of any depth healing necessarily takes place in this way only, and the treatment should be directed largely to alleviating pain and moderating inflammation.

AFTERTREATMENT AND DRESSING OF WOUNDS

The dressing of wounds is one of the most important branches of veterinary surgery, and one of the most constant difficulties that the practicing veterinarian has to contend with lies in the lack of cooperation on the part of owners in the care and attention in the aftertreatment of wounds.

In summarizing the treatment of wounds, the following recommendations should be observed: Wounds must be cleansed and kept clean by the use of antiseptic solutions that do not produce irritation, and applying the solutions with a syringe or with clean pieces of absorbent cotton. Bleeding should be stopped before the closing of the wound by sutures or bandages. An opening at the bottom of all wounds, except small superficial wounds, should be provided as a drainage outlet for the escape of wound secretions or pus if it should form. The edges of wounds and the muscles involved in the wound should be kept as quiet as possible during the process of healing. Every wound should be protected by a sterile or antiseptic dressing whenever it is possible to retain a dressing in place. Dressings should be changed when they have become drenched with wound secretions or pus or have become disarranged or too loose, permitting dirt to enter between them and the skin. If swelling appears beyond the edges of a bandage, it is an indication that it is too tight and it should then be removed and again applied. The hands of the operator and all instruments and dressings coming in contact with a wound at any time should be as clean as possible by the use of antiseptics.

CASTRATION

Castration consists in the removal of the essential organs of generation and is performed on both the male and the female. In the male the organs removed are the testicles and in the female the ovaries.

CASTRATION OF THE MALE

Castration in the male is performed for several purposes. It may be necessary, as in certain diseased conditions of the testicles and in strangulated hernia, but the usual object of the operation is to enhance the general value of the animal for beef purposes. The operation will improve the quality of the flesh and cause an added development of the most valuable portions of the dressed carcass.

The operation on the male may be either the uncovered or the covered. In the former the incision is made down to the testicle proper, and in the latter the cut is made through the scrotum or the outside covering and through the dartos, or the next coat, care being taken to cut no deeper tissues or coats. The age at which the operation is performed varies, but usually it is performed between the second and third months. If done in early life, there is less danger of complications, the organs being in a latent condition and not fully developed. There are many different methods of operating, only the principal ones being mentioned. In the uncovered operation a good free incision should be made, exposing the testicle completely. It may be removed by simply cutting it off. The only danger of doing this is that hemorrhage is likely to follow. To obviate this, before the division of the spermatic cord it should be twisted several times in the following manner: Take hold of the cord with the left hand, having it between the thumb and the index finger. Twist the free portion several times with the right hand, all the time being careful to push with the left hand toward the body of the animal. In this way the danger of injury to the cord during the animal's struggles will be overcome. There will be no hemorrhage, or very little, if it has been done properly. This is the most simple manner of torsion. Forceps and other instruments are made to perform the operation in this manner. Another method involving clamps, although extensively used on the horse, is not practiced to so great an extent on the bovine. It is a very old method and is considered very safe. Clamps, however, have been largely supplanted by the emasculator, a type of pincers, which crushes the cord through the unbroken skin. This instrument is used successfully on both young and adult animals and has the advantage of permitting a bloodless operation, leaving no open wound.

The methods described apply only to the animal in a normal condition. Before the operation is made, everything should be examined to see that it is as it should be. If otherwise a special operative procedure will be necessary. Regardless of the mode of operation adopted, the principal precautions to be taken in order to attain success as as follows: First, thorough cleanliness under strict aseptic and antiseptic precautions; second, a free and boldly made incision; third, the avoidance of undue pulling or tension on the spermatic cord; fourth, free drainage, which can be maintained provided the original incision has been properly made.

Castration of the male is not ordinarily a serious operation, and when properly performed there is little danger from complications. Although the danger is slight, the complications which may arise are sometimes of a serious nature. Hemorrhage, either primary or secondary, tetanus (or lockjaw), abscesses, hernia (or rupture), gangrene, and peritonitis are the most serious complications that follow castration. Whichever complication arises will require its own special treatment, and will be dealt with fully under another heading. Generally speaking, the animal, after being castrated, should either be regularly exercised or be allowed freedom so that it can exercise itself. Sudden temperature changes are dangerous. The animal should be fed moderately on feeds that are easily digested.

CASTRATION OF THE FEMALE

The operation of ovariotomy (spaying) may be performed on account of diseased conditions, but the chief object of the operation is to make the animal more profitable to its owner by lessening the lacteal secretion and also improving the physical condition from the point of view of beef production. When the cow is spayed, it does away with all trouble attending estrum, or heat, gestation, and parturition with its accidents and ailments. The operation should be performed by a competent veterinarian and under such anesthetic as he may select.

The operation on the female should be performed when the heifer is in her prime and in moderate condition, not too plethoric and not in heat or pregnant. This operation may be performed in one of two ways—by the flank or by the vagina—each operation having its special advantages. In the flank operation the animal may be operated on either while standing or while lying down. If standing, she should be placed against a wall or partition and her head held by a strong assistant. The legs also must be secured to prevent the animal from kicking. A vertical incision should be made in the left flank, about the middle of the upper portion, care being taken not to make the opening too far down, in order to avoid the division of the circumflex artery that traverses that region. The operator should now make an opening through the peritoneum, which is best done with the fingers. Next the hand and arm should be introduced into the abdominal cavity and the hand directed backward toward the pelvis, searching for the horns of the uterus; if followed up the ovaries will easily be found. They should then be drawn outward and may be removed either by the

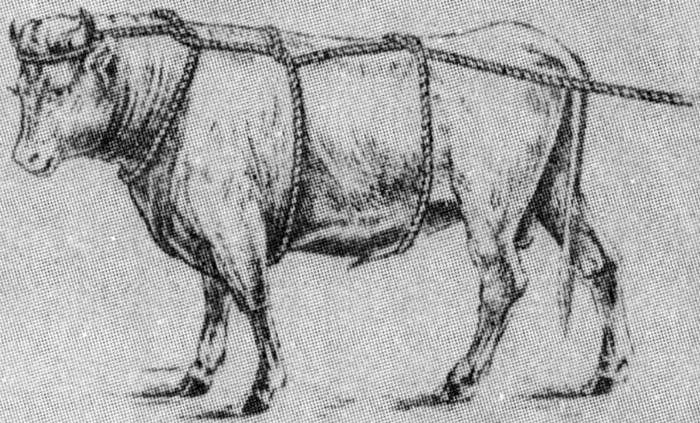

1.

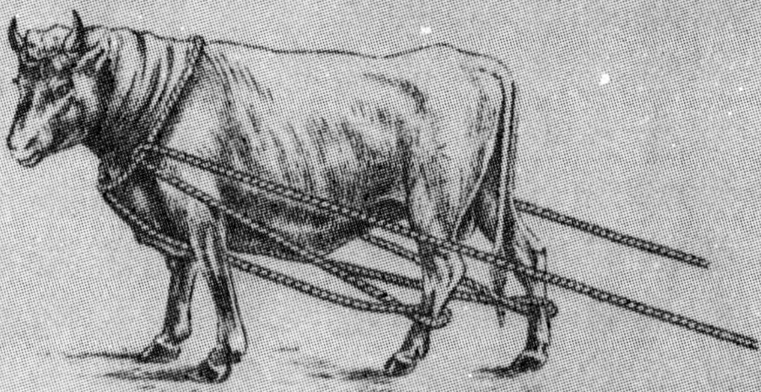

2.

DEVICES FOR CASTING CATTLE.

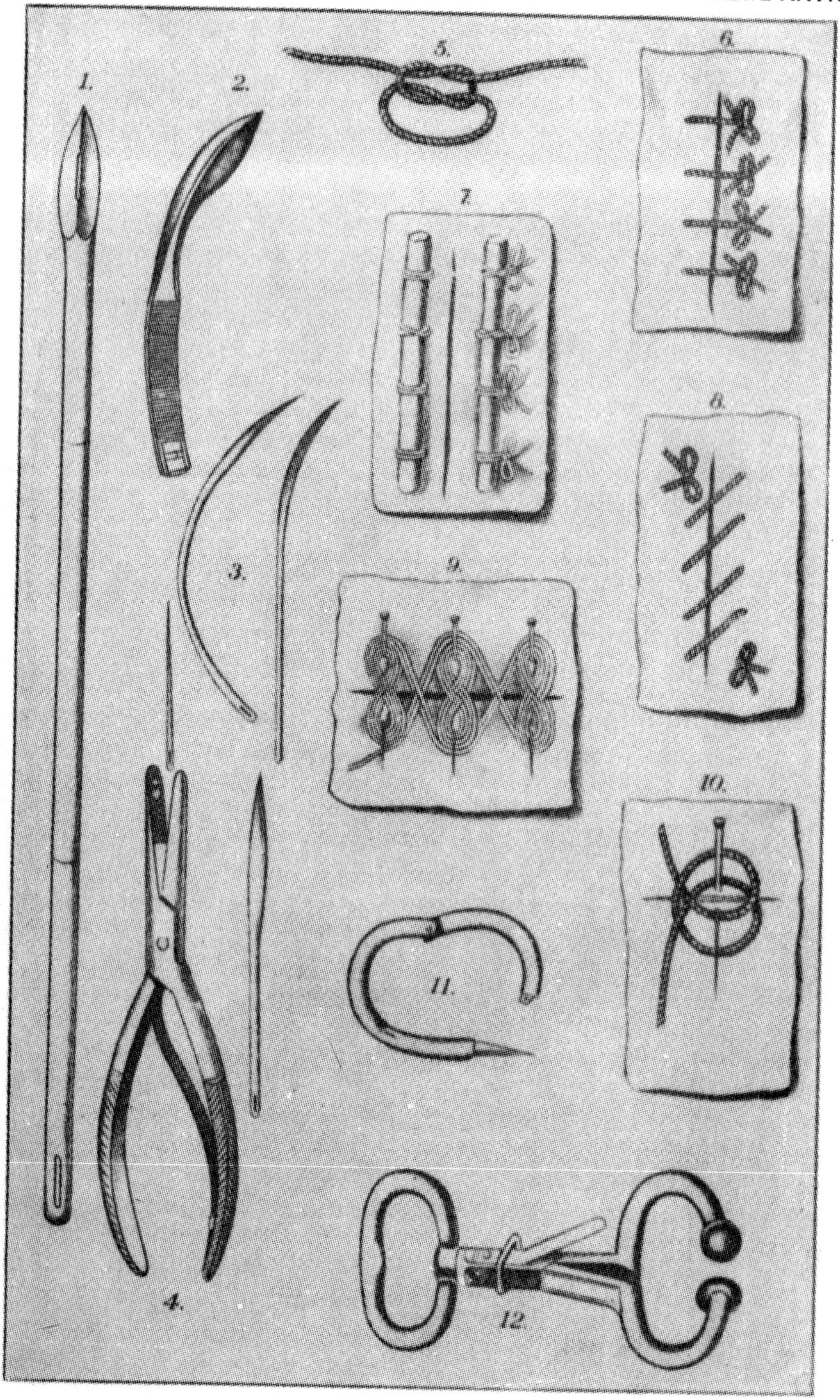

SURGICAL INSTRUMENTS AND SUTURES.

écraseur or by torsion. Closing and suturing the wound will complete the operation. An adhesive plaster bandage can be beneficially applied.

The operation by the vagina is more complicated and requires special and expensive instruments. The mode of procedure in brief is as follows: A speculum is introduced into the vagina, and an incision is made into the superior wall of that passage about 2 inches from the neck of the uterus, cutting from below upward and from before backward. An incision that should not exceed 3½ inches in length should be made. The next step is to get possession of the ovaries. They are situated in a fold of the broad ligament and should be drawn carefully through the incision into the vagina. Now take the long-handled scissors, specially made for this purpose, with which the thick border of the broad ligament is divided. The torsion forceps are introduced and applied to the broad ligament above the ovary. The left hand is then introduced, and the thumb and the index finger grasp the broad ligament above the forceps. With the right hand torsion is applied and the ovary removed. The other ovary may be removed in the same manner.

What has been said with regard to complications and aftertreatment in the case of the male also applies to the female.

OTHER SURGICAL OPERATIONS

Descriptions of other surgical operations not given in this chapter may be found in other parts of this work by reference to the index.

SURGICAL OPERATIONS

DESCRIPTION OF PLATES

PLATE XXVI. Devices for casting cattle. (From Fleming.)

Figure 1. Reuff's method.

Figure 2. Miles' method.

PLATE XXVII. Surgical instruments and sutures. (After Reynders and Fleming.)

Figures 1 and 2. Seton needles.

Figure 3. Various forms of surgical needles.

Figure 4. Suture forceps or needle holder, for passing needles through thick and dense tissues.

Figure 5. Knot properly tied.

Figures 6, 7, 8, 9, 10. Various forms of sutures. Fig. 6, interrupted suture; 7, quilled suture; 8, uninterrupted suture; 9, twisted suture, made by passing suture pins through the parts to be held together and winding the thread about them so as to represent the figure 8; 10, single-pin suture.

Figure 11. Appliance for ringing the bull, one-fourth natural size.

Figure 12. Nose clamp, with spring and keeper.

Tumors Affecting Cattle

By John R. Mohler, A. M., V. M. D., D. Sc.

Chief, Bureau of Animal Industry

[*Synonyms:* New growth, neoplasm, neoformation, pseudoplasm, swelling, and hyperplasia.]

Definition.—Tumors [1] are abnormal masses of tissue, noninflammatory and independent in character, arising, without obvious cause, from cells of preexistent tissue, possessing no physiologic function, and characteristically unrestrained in growth and structure. The term "tumor" is applied in such cases because they produce local enlargement.

They are noninflammatory; that is, the process of inflammation is not directly the cause or accompaniment of them. An inflammatory new growth tends to disappear on the subsidence of the inflammatory process, whereas spontaneous disappearance of a tumor is comparatively rare.

Tumors are independent. For instance, their nutrition bears no relation to the nutrition of the body. A lipoma, or fatty tumor, in the subcutaneous tissue, may continue to increase to huge bulk while the body is steadily emaciating. Again, the tissues of the aged gradually undergo atrophy, yet cancers arise at this time and grow rapidly.

Tumors are unrestrained in growth and structure. In the development of an animal we know at what period of its existence the mass of tissue called liver will develop—what its site, structure, and size will be. We know that it will remain only in that locality, and not, as it were, colonize throughout the system. With tumors it is different; there are no laws by which we can forecast the time, place, nature, or size of development of them. There is no cartilage in the kidney or parotid gland, yet a chondroma, or cartilage tumor, may

[1] The term "tumor" literally means a swelling, and thus has been applied to the prominence caused by an overdistended bladder, to the enlargement of pregnancy, to the swelling produced by an abscess, to the overgrowth of tissue (hyperplasia) associated with injury and consequent inflammation, and to numerous other phases of tissue enlargement directly connected with recognized disease processes. For this reason it is becoming more common for scientists to apply the word "neoplasm" to the new growths described in this chapter. Because of the still popular use of the word "tumor," it is retained in this chapter for the designation of those new growths to which the sevenfold characterization of the descriptive definition applies.

develop in either. Even when a new growth of tissue is begun as a result of an injury and consequent inflammation—as. for instance, proud flesh—there is a limitation of its size, but the controlling influences that govern the size of an organ or normal mass of tissue and limit the extent of an inflammatory overgrowth are all absent in the case of tumors. They are unrestrained, lawless.

Metastasis expresses the lawlessness of tumors in regard to their being limited to the original site of development. Small particles of tumors enter the blood vessels or lymph streams and are carried to distant parts of the body, where they lodge and begin new tumor formations. Expansion by colonization in this manner is a rule with many tumors, and, since they exercise no function of use to the organism, this dissemination of actively growing particles becomes a menace to the system by numerically increasing the body's burden, opening new channels of drain on the system, and adding new centers for the absorption of putrefactive materials when the secondary tumors shall have degenerated. This is what makes metastasis such an important element in the malignancy of tumors.

Tumors possess no physiological function. They are absolutely useless. Fibrous tumors bind no parts of the organism together; bony tumors add nothing to the supporting framework of the body; the tissue of fatty tumors never serves as a storehouse of feed and energy; the cells of an adenoma, or gland tumor, furnish no secretion; a tumor composed of muscle tissue produces no increase to the strength of the individual—its muscle cells are not contractile.

Tumors arise from cells of preexistent tissue. Tumor tissue is not a new variety. Whatever the structure of a tumor, its counterpart is found among the tissues of the body. The lawlessness of the tumor, however, shows itself in more or less departure from the normal type. This departure is usually a reversion to a more elementary or embryonic stage; therefore, the tumor tissues may be said to be structurally immature.

Tumors arise without obvious cause, and, with a few exceptions, there is no information concerning the specific cause of tumor formation. (See Papilloma, p. 267.) Various theories have been advanced from time to time, but none have been applicable to more than a limited number of cases. The most important theories are mentioned briefly.

(1) *The theory of tumor diathesis.*—Bilroth taught that tumors are caused by a peculiar predisposition consisting of a diseased state of the fluids of the body. This constitutional taint may be acquired, but, having been acquired, is also hereditary. This theory is known also as the hereditary hypothesis, but although heredity appears to play some role in the causation of certain neoplasms, its application is too limited to make it of value.

(2) *The mechanical or irritant theory.*—Virchow assumed that tumors arise as the result of previous irritation of the part. This has been noticed particularly in the case of certain cancers. They frequently develop on the edges of old ulcers and thus depend apparently on chronic irritation. Cancer of the lip in pipe smokers is a case in point. Cancerous tumors of the skin often develop on the arms of workers in paraffin, tar, or soot, the chemical irritation of these substances being the cause. On the contrary, the proportion of those thus affected among the exposed is very small. Therefore, if the real cause were in the irritation vastly more cases would occur.

(3) *The theory of nervous influence.*—That is based on the observed fact that (*a*) tumors occur more frequently in man and the higher animals than in the lower animals, in which the nervous system is not so highly developed; (*b*) certain formations seem to be directly connected with nerve distribution, whereas others have been associated with alternations in neighboring nerve trunks.

(4) *The embryonal theory.*—This is known also as Cohnheim's hypothesis. In early fetal life there occurs a production of cells in excess of those required for the construction of the various parts of the body, so that a certain number of them are left over in the fully developed tissue or become misplaced during the sorting of cells for future development of tissues and organs. These cells lie dormant until favorable conditions arise or until a sufficient stimulus is applied, when, released from their inactivity, they begin to reproduce and grow. Not being normally related to their site, they lack the controlling and limiting influences of the part, and, their embryonic character enduing them with a most potent proliferating power, they develop in a lawless and unrestrained manner. There are tumors whose existence can be explained only on these grounds. Still, this theory falls far short of answering the question as to the origin of all tumors.

(5) *The parasitic theory.*—This is not only one of the latest, but, merely as a hypothesis, it is the most attractive and plausible of all. The serious objections to it, however, are the almost uniform failure that has met the attempts to transplant these tumors from one animal to another and the absence of any constant variety of organism in them. Several forms of parasites have been found in certain tumors, but nothing definite has been shown with reference to the relation they bear to the causation of the neoplasm.

CLASSIFICATION OF TUMORS

In Senn's work on tumors the following occurs: "A uniform system of classification of tumors is one of the great wants of modern pathology, and all attempts in this direction have proved failures."

It would be folly, therefore, to burden the pages of a work of this kind with one or several of the proposed systems that have, admittedly, at some important point, failed of their purpose. Since the value of this chapter depends chiefly on its practical character, which in turn is measured by its aid in diagnosis, prognosis, and treatment, the old but important clinical division is here adopted.

Tumors are either malignant or benign. The essential difference between the two classes is that whereas *benign tumors depend for their ill effects entirely on their situation, malignant neoplasms wherever located primarily inevitably destroy life by metastusis, or ability to spread to other tissues.* The clinical features of each group are in many cases sufficiently marked to distinguish them.

MALIGNANT TUMORS

(1) These are invariably pernicious and from the beginning tend to destroy life.

(2) The cellular element predominates; therefore, they grow rapidly.

(3) Possessing no capsule, they infiltrate surrounding tissues.

(4) They invade adjacent lymph glands.

(5) They recur even after apparently complete removal.

(6) They manifest metastasis; that is, they become disseminated in different organs.

(7) Their presence results in a progressive emaciation.

BENIGN TUMORS

(1) These in and of themselves do not tend to produce death.

(2) As the cellular element is not likely to predominate, they grow slowly.

(3) They are encapsulated and, when diffuse, do not infiltrate surrounding tissues.

(4) They do not invade adjacent lympth glands.

(5) They do not recur after complete removal.

(6) They do not manifest metastasis.

Benign tumors, though harmless, may, by the accident of their location, indirectly produce death. Mere pressure on the brain substance of an otherwise innocent tumor, compression of the blood supply for vital organs, growth in such manner as to cause obstruction in the alimentary tract or pressure on nerves, may cause death, or, prior to death, so combine the effects of anemia (deficiency of blood), starvation, and pain, with its consequent restlessness, as to produce a veritable cachexia (condition of general ill health).

On the other hand, a malignant tumor in its primary growth may so implicate a vital organ as to destroy life before metastasis can occur or even before cachexia can develop. Thus, to the untrained observer, environment may so operate as to cause these two classes of new growths to simulate each other. The boundary lines may seem to overlap. It is here that the microscope, as the court of last appeal, adjudicates positively in the diagnosis between these two clearly marked divisions.

It may almost be asserted that a true classification of tumors cannot be made until we know more about their cause. The arrangement here presented is offered to meet the practical needs of the veterinarian, student, and farmer rather than of the pathologist.

We may roughly divide the tissues of the body into structural and lining tissues. The structural tissues are composed of the tissues of special function and simple connective tissues. The lining or covering tissues, both internal and external, are known as epithelium.

Section A of the following tabulation contains the true tumors or proper neoplasms.

Section B includes the cysts, some of which are true tumors, whereas others are false ones, but the latter are added because of their gross resemblance to the true and the consequent necessity of considering them at the same time.

TUMORS AND CYSTS

A.—Tumors

BENIGN

I.—Tumors composed of tissues resembling those of special function

1. Type of muscle tissue ———— Myoma.
2. Type of nerve tissue ———— Neuroma.
3. Type of vascular tissue ———— Angioma.
4. Type of gland tissue ———— Adenoma.

II.—Tumors composed of fully developed connective tissue

1. Type of fibrous tissue ———— Fibroma.
2. Type of adipose, or fat, tissue ———— Lipoma.
3. Type of cartilage tissue ———— Chondroma.
4. Type of osseous, or bone, tissue ———— Osteoma.
5. Type of neuroglia, or nerve, sheath ———— Glioma.
6. Type of mucoid, or mucous, tissue ———— Myxoma.

MALIGNANT

III.—Tumors composed of embryonic or immature connective tissues

1. Type of immature connective tissue ———— Sarcoma.
2. Type of endothelial tissue ———— Endothelioma.

IV.—*Tumors in which epithelial elements predominate*

1. Type of various epithelial cells and associated tissues........ Carcinoma.

B.—Cysts

I.—*Cysts that develop in preexisting cavities*

1........ Retention cysts.
2........ Proliferation cysts.

II.—*Cysts that are of congenital origin and are true tumors*

1........ Dermoid cysts.

III.—*Cysts that originate independently as the result of pathological changes and are nontumorous*

1. Cysts formed by the softening and disintegration of lesions........ Softening cysts.
2. Cysts formed around parasites........ Parasitic cysts.
3. Cysts formed by an outpouring of blood and lymph into the tissue spaces with subsequent encapsulation of the fluid........ Extravasation cysts.

The principle of naming tumors is simple. The Greek word "oma" (plural "omata") means tumor. This word "oma" is added to the stem of the word ordinarily used to designate the kind of tissue of which the tumor is composed. Thus a tumor formed of fibrous tissue is a fibroma. The only exception to this is in the naming of the two large classes of malignant neoplasms. There the names were formed from the fleshlike appearance of the one and the crablike proliferations of the other—namely, sarcoma (sarks=flesh), carcinoma (karkinos=crab).

DIAGNOSIS OF TUMORS

In the diagnosis of tumors note is taken of (1) clinical history and (2) examination of the tumor.

(1) *Clinical history.*—Circumstances connected with the origin of the tumor and its rapidity of growth may point to an inflammatory swelling rather than a tumor. The location of the tumor at its commencement is important, as, for instance, in diagnosing between lipoma and carcinoma, the former being more or less movable under the skin, whereas carcinoma develops in the skin. Although tenderness on pressure may be caused by compression of a sensitive nerve by a tumor or by tumors of the nerve or nerve sheaths, as a rule this symptom is indicative of inflammatory swelling rather than of the existence of a tumor.

(2) *Direct examination of the tumor.*—In the application of this diagnosis the trained observer will note color, size, shape, and surface structure, transmission of light, movableness, consistence, resistance, pulsation, and crepitation. Percussion, auscultation, and exploration are also available methods. Finally, microscopic examination of the growing portions of the tumor by a pathologist will be most satisfactory.

GENERAL TREATMENT OF TUMORS

For a benign tumor treatment is required only when it damages the animal's value or for sake of appearance. When it is possible. the removal of the tumor by an operation is indicated. If the tumor has a small, constricted base, remove by torsion, ligation, or with an écraseur. Ligation following the incision of the skin with a knife avoids the pain of pressing on the sensitive nerves of the skin and is suitable for tumors of broad base and small bodies. A firing iron, such as is used in line or feather firing, may also be used in removing tumors with small attachments. This not only stops the bleeding but forms a firm scab, under which healing may occur rapidly. Tumors that cannot be removed by the above methods may be treated with acids or caustics, such as sulfuric acid, hydrochloric acid, caustic potash, arsenic, silver nitrate, or chromic acid, but it is difficult to limit the action of these drugs. The injection, into the tumor, of such chemicals as aniline dyes, alcohol, acetic acid, citric acid, or ergotin is of doubtful value, as is also the injection of the germs of erysipelas—thought by some to be a specific. Certain tumor formations, such as actinomycosis and botryomycosis, being due to specific organisms, may be treated successfully by the internal administration of potassium iodide, together with the injection into the tumor or the painting of its surface with either Lugol's solution or the tincture of iodine. The most reliable means of treating tumors is by extirpation with cutting instruments, or regular operative procedure. The after treatment is the same as for any ordinary wound of similar size.

DESCRIPTION OF INDIVIDUAL TUMORS

Although a full list of the tumors that may be found in bovines has been given in the table, there are a number that warrant a detailed description. This is given on the following pages for the most important of them.

MYOMA

These tumors simulate the type of muscle. They are sharply circumscribed and, as a rule, are very hard, a condition due usually to combination with fibroma, and are then known as fibromyoma. In fact, the clinical differentiation between myoma and fibroma is almost impossible. Myomas are found in the uterus, vagina, stomach, intestines, gullet, and bladder of a bovine animal. They grow very large, but, as a rule, are benign. Treatment should consist in their removal.

NEUROFIBROMA

A true neuroma built up of nerve fibers and nerve cells is infrequent in cattle. False neuromas, or neurofibromas, are knotty, spreading tumors of the size of a large potato, which are developed within the nerve sheaths and composed of nerve fibers and connective-tissue bands interlaced. The commingling of these varied fibers is often so intricate that separation is practically impossible. This tumor is most frequently found on the shoulder of cattle. Treatment is surgical.

ANGIOMA

The angiomas are tumors composed mainly of blood vessels or blood spaces and are observed on the skin of man, where they are called birthmarks or mother marks. Cavernous angiomas are seen in cattle and affect the liver and the mucous membrane of the nasal septum. In the liver they appear as smooth, flat, nonprojecting tumors of a dark-red or purple color and of about the size of a silver 10-cent piece. The tumors are somewhat softer in consistence than the adjoining liver substance into which they are gradually fused. These tumors are frequently observed by meat inspectors in livers of slaughtered cattle. Treatment of angioma is unnecessary.

ADENOMA

The structure of this tumor simulates the type of gland tissue. It is rarely seen in cattle except in combination with cancer or sarcoma A growth that occurs more frequently in bovines, especially in new-born calves, and that in some instances bears a striking resemblance to an adenoma is the so-called goiter.

GOITER (STRUMA)

This is a noninflammatory enlargement or a hyperplasia of the thyroid gland. Although goiter cannot be definitely classed among tumors, yet, owing to its resemblance to the latter, it is discussed under this heading. Simple goiter as it occurs in cattle is caused by a deficiency of iodine in the diet and is most prevalent in districts where there is a lack of this element in the soil and in the drinking water. A goiter may consist of (1) simple enlargement of the follicles that are filled with albuminous matter (follicular goiter); (2) an increase of connective tissues between the follicles, causing the swelling to be

77431 O—51——20

dense and resistant (fibrous goiter); (3) a great increase in size of one or more follicles, forming a cyst (cystic goiter); (4) great dilatation of the blood vessels in the gland accompanied with pulsation with each heart beat (vascular goiter).

Symptoms.—Goiter may be observed at the side of the throat, reaching the size of a fist or even larger, or it may hang down below the windpipe. In cattle the two thyroid glands are close together, and when the disease affects both, there may be but one uniform swelling in front of the windpipe below the angle of the jaw. This swelling may be hard, soft, or doughy in consistence, and with each beat of the heart it may pulsate like an artery. It may cause labored breathing by pressure on the windpipe, and death may result from pressure on this structure, on the gullet, or on the adjoining large vessels. This is the condition known as big neck in newborn calves.

Treatment.—In young animals treatment is usually satisfactory and consists in giving the animal a complete change of feed and plenty of exercise in the open air. If the condition appears to be enzootic in the district, remove the animal to another location when possible. Iodine, either in the form of ointment or tincture, should be applied to the swelling. Injections of iodine solution, 5 grains of iodine in 1 dram of 25-percent alcohol, may also be made into the substance of the gland. When the swelling that follows this injection has subsided it may be repeated. Potassium iodide should be given internally in 1½-dram doses twice daily for a cow, or in 20-grain doses twice a day for a calf. Extirpation of all but a small section of the enlarged gland may be accomplished successfully by a competent veterinarian, but if the gland should be entirely removed, myxedema and death follow.

Since it is definitely known that goiter in newborn calves is due to low iodine assimilation, the disease may be prevented readily by the administration of iodine salts to cows during the last 3 months of pregnancy. The iodine may be given in the form of potassium iodide, 1 grain daily on the feed or in the drinking water. In districts in which goiter is prevalent, it is suggested that iodized salt be substituted for the regular stock salt.

FIBROMA

Fibromas are tumors made up chiefly of connective tissue and are usually confined to the skin and subcutaneous tissue. Indurative fibromas of the skin appear as tumors of gelatinous connective tissue or as firm, white vascular connective-tissue growths, which are more or less sharply outlined, move readily over the underlying tissues in company with the skin, and are due to mechanical injuries, perforating wounds, repeated abrasions, or the invasion of pus cocci or botryomyces into the tissues.

These tumors in cattle are frequently found on the dewlap as solid lumps, hard as stone to the touch, lying loosely between the layers of skin, and gradually losing themselves in the softer tissues of the neck above, or as smooth, hard tumors of glistening white substance with interlacing lines of softer tissue. They may be found also in the region of the knee or at the elbow. The skin over the growths, in accordance with the originating cause, will be chafed, covered with scabs, or even ulcerated and accompanied with collateral edema.

These connective-tissue tumors grow slowly but reach enormous size. They sometimes follow injuries to the region of the throat and form there as hard, firm growth, even reaching the size of a child's head.

A fibroma on the larynx is not an infrequent occurrence in cattle. These tumors are always sharply outlined and have a roughened surface. They may be differentiated from actinomycotic tumors (see chapter on Infectious Diseases of Cattle, p. 315) in the same location by their firm, fibrous structure and by the absence of pus from the interior.

A tumor is sometimes seen on the muzzle of cattle, which assumes a diameter equaling the width of the muzzle. It is a voluminous connective-tissue formation known as fibroma diffusum.

Another form is sometimes observed on the tongue. It grows on a broad, spreading base, and becomes very hard. It is almost lacking in blood vessels, although the few that are present are plainly in view, and in consequence is poorly supplied with fluids. It is smooth, white or whitish yellow in color, is sharply limited from the normal substance of the tongue, may be covered with mucous membrane on which prominent papillae are located or only by a thin, delicate layer of epithelium, and is usually found in the middle part of the tongue, where it may reach the size of two fists.

Pedunculate or stemmed fibrous tumors frequently grow on or near the extremity of the tails of cows. They apparently result from a wound, such as tying the tail fast while milking or shaving it too closely while trimming for show purposes, and usually contain bloody or gelatinous material within, or, again, they may be largely edematous throughout.

Treatment.—The treatment of large fibromas is surgical and consists in the removal of the tumor, followed by suturing of the wound. Small external tumors may be painted with zinc chloride, chromic acid, or a concentrated solution of bichloride of mercury.

PAPILLOMA (WART)

When fibromas develop from the lining or covering tissues they frequently form papillary growths, more or less thickly covered with epithelium, and are then called papillomas, or warts.

Papillomas consist of villouslike projections, resulting from a proliferation of the outer layer (epithelium) of the skin or mucous membrane. These growths are also called angle berries and may assume a variety of forms. Sometimes there is a preponderance of epidermis in the formation, and the tumor then appears as a hard, dense, insensitive, clublike growth, or wart. Again the swelling is chiefly in the derma or true skin and results in what is known as a flesh wart (verruca carnea). In other cases the growth of papillar bodies projects in great cauliflowerlike tumors with deeply furrowed and lobulated surfaces, over which a covering of epidermis may or may not be present. These are usually much softer and are well supplied with blood vessels. It is not uncommon for them to be pedunculate or stemmed, and in this case considerable rotary motion or twisting is possible. Their color is cloudy gray or grayish red, with white bands of connective tissue radiating from the center. Their consistence varies. Upon their surfaces and within their clefts and fissures they undergo retrogressive changes, softening, bleeding, or ulcerations.

A favorite location for the papilloma in cattle is the udder and teats, where they may develop in such numbers as to cover the entire surface and make the animal troublesome to milk. The sides of the head, neck, and shoulders also afford satisfactory conditions for their growth and are frequently seen to be affected by them.

Cause.—Common warts in cattle have been shown by experiments to be infectious. The infective constituent is what is known as a filtrable virus, meaning that it will pass through an earthen, germ-retaining filter. By experimental skin inoculations with wart material, these growths can be produced with a fair degree of regularity in healthy cattle less than 1 year of age. Under ordinary circumstances infection is thought to take place through injuries to the skin when the injured part comes in contact with warty animals, rubbing posts, fences, buildings, or any structure with which an affected animal has come in contact.

Treatment.—Warts may be removed with scissors, twisted off with the fingers, or ligatured by means of a rubber band or horsehair. The roots should then be cauterized with tincture of iron, glacial acetic acid, or lunar caustic. Acids should never be used in removing warts about the eyes or in the mouth. Papillomas of the eyelids sometimes change to cancers and should be removed by taking out a wedge-shaped section of the eyelid. Young cattle should be given arsenic internally in the form of Fowler's solution, 1 tablespoonful twice a day for a 6-month-old calf.

Prevention.—Preventive measures consist in removing all warty cattle from the herd, particularly affected calves and yearlings, and in cleaning and disinfecting all exposed stables, pens, chutes, and rubbing posts.

In dairy herds, cows having warts on their teats and udders should be milked last and the milkers should wash and disinfect their hands thoroughly after each milking to prevent the possible spread of the virus from one animal to another. The essential point in preventing and controlling these growths is to keep in mind that they are infectious or "catching."

POLYPS

Polyps are usually fibromas or myxomas and occur on the mucous membrane of the nasal passages or genital tract. They grow on a narrow stem, bleed readily when injured, and often contain a center of thin, limpid fluid. A bloody discharge sometimes comes from the affected nostril, but this is not always easy to detect in cattle, owing to the pliancy of their tongues and to their habit of licking an irritated nostril. Usually these tumors grow downward and may project from the nostril, causing snoring sounds and uneasy breathing. They may occasionally force themselves backward into the throat, where they interfere seriously with respiration, the patient being obliged to breathe with an effort and even forced to cough in order to dislodge temporarily the obstruction from the larynx. Such tumors, when near the nostril, may easily be removed by the use of forceps or a sterilized loop made of bailing wire. Serious bleeding is not likely to follow their removal, but an astringent wash, such as a solution of the perchloride of iron, if applied to the cut surface, will be very beneficial. In case the tumor is not within easy reach, the services of a competent veterinarian should be obtained to perform the necessary operation.

LIPOMA

This is a tumor consisting chiefly of fat cells. The growth is irregularly rounded and distinctly lobulated, very soft, and almost fluctuating. It is insensitive, grows slowly, and is always enclosed in a distinct fibrous capsule, from which it can be shelled out easily. It may become very large and often hangs pendulous from a long, elastic pedicle. In cattle this tumor may be found in the subcutaneous tissues, especially of the back and shoulders, uterus, and intestines, and in the last position it may cause strangulation, or "gut tie," by winding around a loop of the intestine.

Treatment.—When found on the skin the tumor may be readily removed with a knife or by a ligature. Caustics or other methods of cauterization produce wounds that heal slowly. This method, therefore, cannot be recommended in the treatment of this tumor.

CHONDROMA

This tumor formation is composed of cartilage cells. It is a rounded and often unevenly nodular and sharply described tumor. It is hard, dense, elastic, and painless and develops principally where normal cartilage cells are found. It is rare in cattle but has been found in the subcutaneous tissues and nasal cavites.

Treatment.—Extirpation.

OSTEOMA (BONY TUMOR)

Bones may occasionally grow in such a profuse and irregular manner that the product, or osteophyte, assumes the character of a tumor. The bone tissue may possess either spongy or compact properties and may grow either from the periphery of the bone or within its interior. These tumors most frequently appear about the head of the animal, either on the jawbones, within the nasal passages, or in connection with the horns. They are usually of bony hardness, painless, benign, and sharply outlined.

Treatment.—Treatment consists in either removing them through proper surgical procedure, or preventing their further development by counterirritation with blisters or firing iron.

MYXOMA

Characteristic myxomas are mucoid tumors that originate chiefly from the mucous membrane and are found especially within the nasal passages and uteri of cattle. They may reach the size of three fists, are smooth or velvetlike, or may be lobulated, broad at the base, and consist of a glassy-looking mass of connective tissue, which usually is a distinctive yellowish color. Being homogeneous and elastic, the moist, jellylike tissue composing the tumor may easily be destroyed or crushed. When cut through, these tumors soon collapse from the loss of their fluids. They sometimes enclose elliptical cavities filled with slimy, gelatinous masses.

Treatment.—Extirpation.

SARCOMA

This is a malignant tumor of the type of embryonal tissue, and consists of several varieties, such as the round cell, spindle cell, giant cell, alveolar, and melanosarcoma. They grow by preference in connective tissue and are quite vascular. Sarcomas appear either as single or multiple nodules, varying in size from a hempseed to a hazelnut, or as a moderate number of tumors of the size of hens' eggs. Their surface, at first smooth, later becomes lumpy and tuberous from internal degeneration. Secondary nodules may appear near the primary tumor. The outer skin is not involved so soon as in cancer, nor does ulceration follow so rapidly. Sarcoma is the most frequent and dangerous tumor that is found in cattle. It occurs in young animals and is found on the serous membranes, in the glandular organs, and on the outer skin, especially of the neck and shoulders—in fact, in nearly every tissue and in almost every part of the body. This tumor is often found in places exposed to traumatisms and at seats of scars or of irritations from pressure and inflammation.

Treatment.—Treatment should consist in early and complete removal of the entire tumor. Operations of this character should always be performed by a competent veterinarian.

CANCER (CARCINOMA)

Cancers are tumors of epithelial tissues and are malignant. There are several varieties of cancers, such as hard, soft, and colloid, but only those growing on the surface are mentioned here. These malignant tumors of the superficial organs develop primarily from the epidermis or from the glands of the skin. They appear secondarily as spreading infections from milk glands, thyroids, anal glands, or as embolisms. In such cases their character depends wholly on the kind of cancer from which they have sprung. The infiltrating cancer begins as an elevation of the skin, which progresses until it becomes rough and nodular. The surface later becomes attacked, and an ulcer results whose edges are outlined by a hard, firm zone.

The ulcerations may remain limited by cicatricial tissue, but it is more likely that the infiltration and destruction of tissue will spread out wider and deeper until a so-called rodent ulcer is formed. One of the most frequent sites of cancer in cattle is in the eye.

Such growths, formerly called fungus hematodes, are now more commonly referred to as cancer eye. They also occur on the skin, on the genitals, in the stomach, and within the organs.

In cancer eye, the growth begins most frequently at the inner corner of the eye as a papillary elevation, or as small nodules that become fused. They grow larger and become papillomatous, with superficial ulcerations and a tendency toward hemorrhage. In some cases the eye is displaced by the growing tumor or is attacked by the cancer cells and entirely destroyed. The tumor may spread to the lungs, or other tissues or organs and eventually cause the death of the animal.

Cancerous growths on the external genitals and the anus usually have a rough, irregular surface from which there is a constant sloughing of decomposed tissue accompanied with a penetrating disagreeable odor.

The diagnosis of cancer may be made clinically by noting the simultaneous infection of the lymph glands that surround the primary lesion. Deeply burrowing and infiltrating forms that appear as lumps and ulcerations cause marked disfiguration of the affected part. The surface becomes a soft, greasy mass; later it cracks open and from the fissures blood-colored pus exudes, being continually formed by the moist degeneration of the tissues beneath. At first the general health of the animal does not appear to be affected, but later the cancer nodules spread to important organs and give rise to marasmus and progressive emaciation. Cancer is not a frequent tumor of cows. Fröhner states that of 75 cases of tumors in cattle that came under his observation 2, or 2.6 percent, were found to be cancers, whereas 20, or 26.6 percent, were sarcomas.

Treatment.—Treatment consists in the early and complete removal of the tumor. This has been most successful in such superficial cancers as those of the eye, penis, anus, testicle, vulva, and sheath. If the disease has advanced too far, this treatment may not prove efficacious, owing to the great malignancy of the cancer and its tendency to recur. In such cases the animal may be slaughtered, but the flesh should be used for food only after inspection by a competent veterinarian.

DESCRIPTION OF CYSTS

Cysts may be true or false tumors and consist of a capsule containing a fluid or semisolid content. Among the most important cysts, which have been referred to briefly in a previous table, the following are probably the most noteworthy, owing to the frequency with which they are found in bovines:

SOFTENING CYSTS

Softening cysts result from the degenerative liquefaction of normal or diseased tissues, especially of tumors of different kinds, followed by the encapsulation of the fluid.

PARASITIC CYSTS

Parasitic or foreign-body cysts result from the inflammatory reaction induced by such parasites as the echinococcus (hydatid cyst) or by the presence of various kinds of foreign bodies.

EXTRAVASATION CYSTS

Extravasation cysts are caused by injuries that rupture blood vessels, followed by an increase of fibrous tissue forming a capsule about the fluid. The hygromata in front of the knee in cattle, so-called tumor of the knee, and serous cysts belong to this variety.

Hygromata, or tumors of the knee.—These consist of the simplest form of a collection of serous fluid mixed with fibrin within a distended bursa. The walls surrounding the fluid become firm, smooth, and dense.

Outwardly the tumor appears to be fluctuating, though tense, whereas the skin that covers it may be normal, denuded of hair, or covered with hard epidermal scales, possibly half an inch in thickness, forming a hard, horny plate. The cavity that contains the fluid may be the size of a hen's egg, an apple, or a child's head. Its walls are formed by the diseased secreting membrane of the bursal sac and are readily detachable from the subcutis of the skin. The internal surface is often uneven or supplied with projections or tufted growths that support a fibrous network within the tumor.

Tumors of the knee may also assume a granular type, as the result of chronic inflammation or following operative or spontaneous evacuation of pus from the part. They are either firmly connected with the skin or are detachable from it, and when laid open disclose a whitish red, porklike tissue surrounding a central nucleus of pus, or a fistulous tract leading to the outer surface. They are caused by the chronic inflammation resulting from bruises received by cattle in lying down and in rising or they may be due to falls on uneven, hard ground.

Treatment for hygromata is as follows: When the swelling first appears, cold water should be applied, followed later by bandaging with cloths wrung out of warm water. If the swelling is soft, it should be punctured at the lowest point, and afterwards the cavity should be syringed with Lugol's solution. If the tumor is hard and nonfluctuating, a mercurial blister may cause absorption and thus avoid further injury to the part.

Serous cysts.—These swellings are another variety of extravasation cysts and are caused by such injuries as butting, running against hard objects, and shipping bruises, which are followed by an outpouring of blood and lymph into the tissue spaces. These cysts develop rapidly and may reach the size of a man's head or be even larger. They are soft, edematous, and hot at first and contain a serous or blood-tinged fluid. Later, partially organized clots and shreds of a fibrinous nature and of a gelatinous consistence are formed within, and the temperature of the swelling is reduced. They appear on the surface of the body, especially on the belly and flank of cattle.

Treatment of serous cysts consists in opening the cyst at the most pendant point with a sharp knife. The cavity should be washed out twice daily with a 5-percent solution of carbolic acid, and drainage encouraged by keeping the incision open.

DERMOID CYSTS

These cysts have a wall that is almost an exact duplicate of the structure of the skin and frequently contain epidermal structures, such as hair and teeth, which, in the development of the embryo, have been misplaced. Thus in an ovary or testicle there may be found a dermoid cyst, containing a tooth or a ball of hair. Dental cysts are included in this class.

Dental cysts.—Occasionally the teeth of cattle, instead of developing normally within strong supporting alveolae, remain enclosed within a cystic membrane, which assumes a tumorlike character. One tooth may be included alone in the cyst or a number may be enclosed together. However this may be, the malformation progresses, especially if confined to the incisor teeth, until the remaining teeth that began to develop normally are crowded out of position and rendered useless. The tumor may reach the size of a man's fist. It appears to be fleshy and dents upon pressure, but it may also appear, on closer examination, to contain irregular sections of thin bone. The outer surface is always smooth, and no indication of purulence, softening, or scab formation is ever exhibited. On being laid open with the knife, the tumor is seen to be surrounded by a firm, smooth membrane that limits it completely from the adjoining tissues. It is filled with material that possesses partly edematous, partly fleshy, and partly bony properties. It is supposed that this mass is composed of rudiments of the jawbone or of the alveolar walls which, becoming spongy, lose themselves in the soft, fleshy mass contained within the capsule of the tumor. Occasionally the tumor is hollow and the cavity extends back into the body of the lower jaw for a considerable distance.

Tumors of this kind, being of congenital origin, are naturally observed most frequently in young cattle, but they may continue to expand for several months after the birth of the calf, even until they become troublesome and unsightly.

Treatment for dental cysts consists in the complete extirpation of the cyst and the destruction of the lining pouch by curetting.

RETENTION CYSTS

Retention cysts arise from the retention of normal secretions, owing to obstruction of a duct leading from a gland. The mucous cysts found in the mouth, udder, and vestibule of cows are samples of this form.

Mucous cysts.—Saclike pendulous tumors, caused by retention of the secretions from the mucous glands, sometimes develop in the mouth, nose, pharynx, and vulva of cattle. These are of sizes varying from those of peas to pigeon eggs, are roundish and translucent, and surrounded by a delicate, vascular membrane. They contain a siruplike substance more or less thick and transparent and whitish yellow in color.

Treatment consists in the puncturing of the swelling, if accessible, and the destruction of the cyst walls by the injection of Lugol's solution.

PROLIFERATION CYSTS

These are found especially in the ovaries of cows, called cystic ovaries, and may produce nymphomania (chronic bulling).

The treatment recommended in this case is the manual rupture of the cysts, per rectum; puncture of the cysts with an ovarian scalpel; or the removal of the diseased ovaries by a competent veterinarian.

Diseases of the Skin

By M. R. Trumbower, D. V. S.

[Revised by John R. Mohler, A. M., V. M. D., D. Sc.]

GENERAL DISCUSSION

The skin consists of two parts—a superficial layer, the epidermis, or cuticle, and the deep, or true, skin, the dermis, cutis vera, or corium.

The epidermis, cuticle, or scraf skin, is an epithelial structure, forming a protective covering to the corium. It varies in thickness, is quite insensible and nonvascular, and consists of a sheet of cells.

The epidermis is divided into a firm, transparent, superficial layer and a deep, soft layer. The latter is the rete mucosum, the cells of which contain the pigment that gives color to the skin. The deep surface of the epidermis is accurately molded on the papillary layer of the true skin, and, when removed by maceration, has depressions that correspond to the elevations on the dermis. From the cuticle, tubular prolongations pass into the sebaceous and sudorific glands; thus the entire surface of the body is enclosed by the cuticle.

The dermis, or true skin, is vascular and highly sensitive, as it contains the tactile ends of the nerves of touch. It is covered by epidermis and attached to the underlying parts by a layer of areolar tissue, which usually contains fat. The cutis consists of a fibroareolar tissue and vessels of supply. It is divided into two layers, the deep, or true, corium and the upper, or papillary. The corium consists of strong interlacing fibrous bands, chiefly white; its meshes are larger and more open toward the attached surface, giving lodgment to the sweat glands and fat. The papillary, or superficial layer is formed of a series of small conical eminences or papillae, which are highly sensitive and consist of a homogeneous, transparent tissue. The blood vessels form dense capillary plexuses in the corium, terminating by loops in the papillae. The papillary nerves run in a waving manner and usually terminate in loops.

Hair is an appendage of the skin and forms its external covering. It is a special modification of epidemis, has the same essential structure, and consists of a root, shaft, and point. The root has a bulbous extremity, is lighter and softer than the stem, and is lodged in a recess or hair follicle, which may either be in the corium or subcutaneous areolae. The follicle is dilated at the bottom to correspond to the root bulb, and the ducts of one of more sebaceous glands open into it. At the bottom of each follicle is a conical, vascular papilla, similar in every respect to those on the surface of the dermis; this papilla fits into a corresponding depression in the root of the hair. The shaft consists of a center, or medulla, a surrounding fibrous portion, and an external coating, or cortex. The medulla consists of cells containing pigment or fat, is opaque, and deeply colored. All kinds of hair do not have this medulla. The fibrous portion occupies the bulk of the stem, and the cortex is merely a single layer of thin, flat, shinglelike scales.

The sebaceous glands, lodged in the corium, are most abundant in parts exposed to friction. They generally open into the hair follicles, occasionally on the surface of the body. Each gland consists of a small duct that terminates in a lobulated recess. These lobules vary and, as is the duct, are lined with epithelium. They are filled with sebaceous matter which, as it is secreted, is detached into the sacs. They are very plentiful between the dewclaws of cattle.

The sudorific glands, or sweat glands, are situated in the subcutaneous areolar tissue, surrounded by a quantity of fat. They are small, round, reddish bodies, each of which consists of one or more fine tubes coiled into a ball, the free end of the tube being continued up through the true skin and cuticle and opening on the surface. Each sweat gland is supplied with a cluster of capillary blood vessels that vary in size, being very large when perspiration is excessive. The contents of the smaller ones are fluid, and of the larger, semifluid.

The skin may be regarded as an organ supplementary in its action to the lungs and kidneys, since by its secretion it is capable of removing a considerable quantity of water from the blood. It also removes small quantities of carbon dioxide, salts, and in certain instances during suppression of the renal secretions a small quantity of urea. The skin is also the chief organ for the regulation of animal heat, by or through conduction, radiation, and evaporation of water, permitting of loss of heat, while it also, through other mechanisms, is able to regulate the heat lost. The hair furnishes protection against extreme and sudden variations of temperature by reason of the fact that hairs are poor conductors of heat and enclose between them a still layer of air, itself a nonconductor. The hairs are also furnished with an apparatus by which the loss of heat may be regulated; thus, in cold weather, through the contraction of unstriped muscular fibers of the skin, the hairs become erect and the external coat becomes thicker. Cold, too, acts as a stimulus to the growth of hair, and in consequence the coat is thicker in winter than in summer. The hairs also furnish protection against wet, as they are always more or less oily from the secretion of sebaceous glands and thus shed water. Through their elasticity they furnish mechanical protection, and through the thickness of the coat, to a certain degree, resist the attacks of insects. Finally, the hairs assist the sense of touch.

The sweat glands are constantly discharging a watery secretion in the form of insensible perspiration, and by their influence act as regulators of the temperature of the body; hence, in warm weather, the secretion of the skin is increased, which tends to prevent overheating. Sweating, in addition to regulating heat, is also an active agent in removing effete material from the blood; therefore, this secretion cannot be checked without danger. If the skin is covered with an impermeable coating of grease or tar, death results from blood poisoning, due to the retention of materials destined to be excreted by the skin.

All secretion poured out by the skin is modified not only by the condition of the atmosphere but also by the character and quantity of the feed, by the amount of exercise, and especially by the quantity of fluid taken.

The sebaceous secretion lubricates the skin and hairs. It consists of soft, fatty material suspended in water and is characterized by an odor peculiar to the animal by which it is secreted.

No attempt to classify the various diseases of the skin is made here, for in a work of this kind it would tend to confuse the reader.

We shall first consider a class of diseases that are of an inflammatory type; next, those caused by faulty secretion and abnormal growth; then, diseases of parasitic origin; lastly, local injuries of the skin.

PRURITUS (ITCHING)

Pruritus is not a disease, only a sensation, and therefore a symptom. It is one of the symptoms accompanying most of the diseases which are considered in this chapter. It is, then, a functional affection produced by slight irritation from without or by an internal cause acting on the sensory nerves of the skin. Nothing characteristic is seen except the secondary lesions produced mechanically by scratching or rubbing.

There are various forms of itching, the result of specific skin diseases, in which pruritus is a secondary symptom. In such cases it should not be regarded as an independent affection.

Causes.—Many causes may induce pruritus. The most common one is dirt on the skin, resulting from insufficient care. If the ceiling of the stable is open, so that dust and straw may fall, the skin is irritated and pruritus may result. It also occurs in some forms of indigestion. The parts of the body most exposed to this condition are the croup, the back, the top of the neck, and the root of the tail.

Another cause is found in affections of the liver and of the kidneys, when an increase of effete material must be thrown off by the skin. Morbid materials circulating in the blood may produce a tickling or smarting sensation of the skin in their passage from the blood to the free surface of the skin. Certain irritating substances when eaten may be excreted by the skin, and coming thus in direct contact with the sensory nerves produce itching, or they may cause distinct inflammation of the skin. In another class of cases the pruritus may be ascribable to an atrophy, contraction, or hardening of the skin, when the nerves become irritated by the pressure. These conditions may be so slightly marked in the thick skin such as that of cattle, that they cannot be recognized. Cattle frequently rub themselves as soon as they pass from the stable into the open air—changing from a warm to a cold atmosphere. Again, one does all its rubbing in the stall. It may be impossible to find lice. These conditions are generally attributable to high feeding and to too close confinement. They may be associated with inflammatory irritation or not; certainly it is impossible to discover any morbid changes in the skin. There is to some extent a delightful sensation produced by rubbing, and it may partly become a habit of pleasure.

Treatment.—The most effective treatment is a change of feed, plenty of exercise, and in most cases the administration of an active cathartic—1 to 1½ pounds of Epsom salts, a handful of common salt, a tablespoonful of ginger or pepper, mixed with 2 quarts of water, all of which is to be given at one dose. For an external application, when the skin is abraded or thickened from rubbing, a solution of borax, 4 ounces to the quart of water, may be used. Carbolic acid, ½ ounce to a quart of water, will give relief in some cases.

INFLAMMATORY DISEASES OF THE SKIN

ERYTHEMA

This is the simplest form of inflammation of the skin. It consists in an increased redness, which may occur in patches or involve considerable surface. The red coloration disappears when pressed by the finger but soon returns after the pressure is removed. There is seldom much swelling of the affected part, though often there is a glutinous discharge that dries and mats the hair or forms a thin scale on the skin. In simple erythema the epidermis alone is affected; when it becomes chronic, fissures form and extend into the corium, or true skin.

Causes.—Simple erythema, consisting of an inflammatory irritation, is seen in very young calves in which the navels leak. The discharge being urine, it causes an irritation of the surrounding skin. Chafing, which is another form of erythema, is occasionally seen on the udders of cows from rubbing by the legs; chafing between the legs is not uncommon among fat steers. Chronic erythema is found in the form of chapped teats of cows and chapped lips in suckling calves. Chapped teats may be caused by any irritation, such as sudden chilling after the sucking of the calf, "wet milking" by the attendant, damp or filthy conditions in the stable, wet bedding, overstocking, exposure of tender skin to sun rays in summer, or freezing in winter. Some cows are peculiarly subject to sore teats. The skin is first rough and inclined to scale, and later wrinkles are formed. These fissures, when neglected in the early stage of formation, become deep, very painful, often bleeding at the slightest touch, and when milked in that condition cause the animal to become a kicker. Occasionally the lower portions of the legs become irritated and chapped when cattle are fed in a muddy or wet yard in winter, or if they are compelled to wade through water in frosty weather. Another form of erythema occurs in young cattle highly fed and closely stabled for a long winter. The erythema appears in patches, and as it is most common near the end of the winter it is known as the "spring eruption" or "spring itch."

Treatment.—Favorable conditions, such as dry quarters and bedding, cleanliness of the udder, and "dry milking" are essential. Wash the udder with warm soapy water and then paint the chapped surface once daily with compound tincture of benzoin or a mixture of 1 part of tincture of iodine and 4 parts of glycerin. It may be advisable to anoint the teats with petrolatum before milking, so that the milk may be drawn with the least pain to the animal.

URTICARIA (NETTLE RASH, OR SURFEIT)

This is a mild, inflammatory affection of the skin, characterized by sudden development of patches of various sizes, from that of a nickel to one as large as the hand. The patches of raised skin are marked by an abrupt border and are irregular in form. All the swelling may disappear in a few hours, or it may go away in one place and reappear on another part of the body. It is always accompanied with a great desire to rub the affected part. In its simplest type, as just described, it is never followed by any serous exudation or eruptions, unless the surface of the skin becomes abraded from scratching or rubbing.

Causes.—Digestive derangements caused by overloading the stomach when the animal is turned out to graze in the spring, certain feed constituents, high feeding of fattening stock, functional derangement of the kidneys, spinal and other nervous affections, are the most common sources of nettle rash.

The disease consists in paralysis of the nerve ends that control the volume of the capillary vessels in certain areas of skin, thus permitting the vessels to expand, their contents in part to exude, and thus produce a soft, circumscribed swelling.

Treatment.—Administer a full dose of Epsom salts. Give soft, easily digested feed, and wash the affected parts with a solution of sodium bicarbonate (common baking soda), 8 ounces to the gallon of water twice a day, or diluted glycerin may be applied to the skin.

ECZEMA

Eczema is a noncontagious inflammation of the skin, characterized by any or all of the results of inflammation at once or in succession, such as erythema, vesicles, or pustules, accompanied with more or less infiltration and itching, terminating in a watery discharge, with the formation of crusts or in scaling off. The disease may run an acute course and then disappear, or it may become chronic; therefore, two varieties are recognized, vesicular (or pustular) and chronic eczema.

Causes.—Eczema is not so common among cattle as in horses and in dogs, in which it is the most common of all skin diseases. Among cattle it is occasionally observed under systems of bad hygiene, filthiness, lousiness, overcrowding, overfeeding, excessively damp or too warm stables. It develops now and then in cattle that are fed such sour substances, as distillery byproducts or garbage. Localized eczema may be caused by irritant substances applied to the skin such as turpentine, ammonia, the essential oils, mustard, and Spanish-fly ointment. Occasionally an eruption with vesiculation of the skin has been induced by the excessive use of mercurial preparations for the destruction of lice. Eczema may arise from local irritation to the skin or from an autointoxication. Cattle fed the refuse from potato-starch factories develop a most obstinate and widespread eczema, beginning on the legs.

Symptoms.—In accordance with the variety of symptoms during the progress of the disease, eczema may be divided into different stages or periods: (1) Swelling and increased heat of the skin; the formation of vesicles, which are circumscribed, rounded elevations of the epidermis, varying from the size of a pinhead to that of a split pea and containing a clear, watery fluid; (2) exudation of a watery, glutinous fluid, formation of crusts, and sometimes suppuration, or the formation of vesicles containing pus (pustules); (3) scaling off (desquamation), with redness, and thickening of the skin. From the beginning of the disease the animal commences to rub the affected parts; hence the various stages may not always be easily recognized,

77431 O—51——21

as the rubbing produces more or less abrasion, thus leaving the skin raw—sometimes bleeding. Neither do these symptoms always occur in regular succession, for in some cases the exudation is most prominent, being very profuse, and spreads the disorder over a large surface. In other cases the formation of incrustations, or rawness of the skin, is the most striking feature. The disease may be limited to certain small areas, or it may be diffused over the greater part of the body; the vesicles, or pustules, may be scattered in small clusters, or a large number run together. The chronic form is really only a prolongation of the disease, successive crops of pustules appearing on various portions of the body and frequently invading fresh sections of the skin, whereas the older surfaces form scabs, or crusts, upon the raw, indurated skin.

In long standing cases the skin breaks and forms fissures, especially on portions of the body that bend—the neck and legs. Thus the disease may be prolonged indefinitely. When eczema reaches its latest period, either acute or chronic, scaling off of the affected parts is the most prominent feature. The formation and shedding of these successive crops of scales constitute the character of the disease frequently called psoriasis.

Treatment.—The treatment of eczema is often anything but pleasant. There is no one method that is always successful, no matter how early it is begun or how small an area is involved. An endeavor should be made to remove the cause by giving attention to the general health of the animal and to its environment. Feeding should be moderate in quantity and not too stimulating in character—green feed, bran mashes, ground oats, clean hay, plenty of salt. If the animal has been fed too high, give an active purgative—Epsom salts preferred—once a week, if necessary.

If the animal is in poor condition and debilitated, increase the ration furnishing nutritious and readily digested feed. If the animal is lousy, the parasite must be destroyed before the eczema can be cured. The external treatment varies with the character of the lesions; no irritating application is to be made while the disease is in its acute vesicular, or pustular, stage, and, in the chronic stage, active stimulants must be used. Much washing is harmful, yet crusts and scales should be removed in order to obtain satisfactory results from the external applications. Both objects, however, can be attained by judiciously combining the curative agents with such substances as will at the same time cleanse the parts.

In the vesicular stage, when the skin is feverish and the epidermis peeling off, thus exposing the exuding dermis, an application of boric-acid solution, 2 drams of the acid to 8 ounces of water, often relieves the smarting or itching and also checks the exudation and dries the surface. If this fails to have the desired effect, compound cresol, 1 ounce to 2 quarts of water, should be used as a wash. Either of these washes may be used several times a day until incrustation is well established. Then compound solution of cresol, 1 ounce to 2 quarts of sweet oil, or the benzoated oxide of zinc ointment, applied thoroughly once a day to the affected surfaces will be efficacious. When the eczema is not the result of an external irritant, it takes usually from 1 to 2 weeks to heal.

In chronic eczema, when there is a succession of scabs or scales, indolent sores, or fissures, the white-precipitate ointment mixed with equal parts of petrolatum or fresh lard, may be applied every second day. Care should be taken to protect the parts so that the animal cannot lick off the ointment.

Administrations of appropriate medicinal agents prescribed by a competent veterinarian are indicated. An alkali given internally, such as 2 ounces of sodium bicarbonate twice daily, may be beneficial.

PUSTULES (IMPETIGO)

Impetigo is an inflammatory disease of the skin, characterized by the formation of distinct pustules, about the size of a pea or a bean, without itching. The pustules develop from the papular layer of the skin and contain a yellowish-white pus. After reaching maturity they remain stationary for a few days, then they disappear by absorption and dry up into crusts, which later drop off, leaving on the skin a red spot that soon disappears. Occasionally the crusts remain firmly adherent for a long time, or they may be raised and loosened by the formation of pus underneath. The dry crusts usually have a brown or black appearance.

Causes.—Impetigo affects suckling calves, in which the disease appears upon the lips, nostrils, and face. It is attributed to some irritant substance contained in the mother's milk. Impetigo also occurs among grazing animals, regardless of age, and it especially attacks animals with white hair and skin. The mouth, face, and limbs become covered with pustules, which may rupture in a few hours, followed by rapid and successive incrustations; the scabs frequently coalesce, covering a large surface; pus may form under them, and thus the whole thickness of the skin become involved in the morbid process. This form of the disease is attributed to the local irritant properties of such plants in the pasture as St. Johnswort (*Hypericum perforatum*), smartweed (*Polygonum hydropiper*), vetches, and honeydew. Buckwheat, at the time the seeds become ripe, as well as bedding with buckwheat straw, is said to have caused it.

Treatment.—Suckling calves should be removed from the mother, and a purgative given to the latter to divert the poisonous substance secreted with the milk. When the more formidable disease among grazing cattle appears, the pasturage should be changed and the affected parts of the animal thoroughly anointed once a day with sweet oil containing 2 drams of carbolic acid to the pint. This should be continued until the crusts soften and begin to drop off, then the parts may be cleansed thoroughly with warm water and soap. Subsequently the white-precipitate ointment or carbolized petrolatum should be applied daily until the parts are healed.

PEMPHIGUS (WATER BLISTERS)

This is an inflammatory disease of the skin, characterized by successive formations of rounded, irregularly shaped water blisters, varying from the size of a pea to that of a hen's egg.

Causes.—Obscure.

Symptoms.—The formation of a blister is preceded by a congestion or swelling of the skin. Yellowish-colored water collects beneath the cuticle, and raises the latter from its bed in the form of a blister. The blisters appear in a succession of crops; as soon as one crop disappears another forms. They usually occur in clusters, each one being distinct, or they may coalesce. Each crop usually runs its course in a week. The disease is attended with itching or burning sensations that cause the animal to rub, thereby frequently producing excoriations and formation of crust on the affected region.

Treatment.—The blisters should be opened as soon as formed to allow the escape of the serum, followed by a wash composed of chloride of zinc, 1 dram to 15 ounces of water. When there is any formation of crusts, carbolized petrolatum should be applied.

FURUNCULUS (BOILS)

This is an acute affection of the skin, usually involving its whole thickness, characterized by the formation of one or more abscesses, originating generally in a sebaceous gland, sweat gland, or hair follicle. They usually terminate by absorption or by the formation of a central core, which sloughs out, leaving a deep, round cavity that soon heals.

Causes.—These are the result of an impoverished state of the blood, of kidney diseases, or of local friction or contusions, with the entrance of pus cocci through the damaged skin or through a hair follicle or a sebaceous gland.

Symptoms.—Boils in cattle usually appear singly, not in clusters; they may attain the size of a hen's egg. The abscess begins as a small round nodule, painful on pressure and gradually increases in size until the central portion of the skin gives way to internal pressure and the core is released and expelled. Constitutional symptoms are generally absent, unless the boils occur in considerable numbers or by their size involve a great deal of tissue.

Treatment.—Poulticing to ripen the abscess is the best treatment, but if this cannot be done, apply camphorated oil 2 or 3 times a day until the core is formed. As soon as the central or most prominent part becomes soft, the abscess should be opened to release the core. Then use carbolized petrolatum once a day until the healing is completed. If the animal is in poor condition, the ration should be increased. If the animal manifests a feverish condition of the system, give half an ounce of saltpeter twice a day several days or a week.

FAULTY SECRETIONS AND ABNORMAL GROWTHS OF THE SKIN

PITYRIASIS (SEBORRHEA, DANDRUFF, OR SCURF)

This is a condition characterized by an excessive secretion of sebaceous matter that forms on the skin in small crusts or scales.

Causes.—It is ascribable to a functional derangement of the sebaceous glands, usually accompanied with dryness and loss of pliancy of the skin. The animal is hidebound, as it is commonly termed, thin in flesh, inclined to rub, and frequently lousy. The condition is observed most often toward the spring of the year. Animals that are continually housed, and the skins of which receive no cleaning, generally have a coat filled with fine scales composed of epithelium from the epidermis and dried sebaceous matter.

Symptoms.—Pityriasis may affect the greater portion of the body, though usually only certain parts are affected, such as the ears, neck, and rump. The skin becomes scurfy, the hairy coat filled with bran-like gray or whitish scales.

Treatment.—Nutritious feed, such as linseed meal, bran, ground oats, and clean hay should be given. In the spring the disease generally disappears after the animal is turned out to pasture. When lice are present they should be destroyed.

ELEPHANTIASIS (SCLERODERMA)

This condition consists in a chronic thickening of the skin, which may affect one or more legs or involve the entire covering. It is characterized by recurrent attacks of swelling of the skin and subcutaneous areolar tissue. After each attack the affected parts remain infiltrated to a larger extent than before, until finally the skin may attain a thickness of an inch and become wrinkled and fissured. In cattle this disease is confined to hot climates. The predisposing cause is unknown.

EDEMA (ANASARCA OF THE SKIN)

This is a dropsical condition of the skin and subcutaneous areolar tissue, characterized by pitting under pressure, the fingers leaving a dent that remains a short time.

Causes.—Edema generally results from a weakened state of the system arising from previous disease. It may also depend on a functional derangement of the kidneys, on weak circulation, or obstruction to the flow of blood through the lungs. In debilitated animals and in some animals highly infested with parasites, there is swelling of the dewlap or of the fold of skin between the jaws.

Symptoms.—Painless swelling of a leg, udder, lower surface of abdomen, or lower jaw becomes apparent. This may increase in dimensions for several days or may attain its maximum in less than 24 hours. Unless it is complicated with some acute disease of a specific character, there is not much, if any, constitutional disturbance. The deep layer of the skin is infiltrated with serum, which gives it the characteristic condition of pitting under pressure.

Treatment.—When the cause can be ascertained and removed, the edema should disappear. When no direct specific cause can be discovered and the animal is debilitated, give a general tonic. If, on the contrary, the animal is in good flesh, give a purgative. External applications are useless.

Edema may be distinguished from erysipelas or anthrax by the absence of pain and fever.

DERMOID AND SEBACEOUS CYSTS (WENS)

A dermoid cyst is formed by an involution of the skin with a growth of hair on the inner wall of the sac. It may become embedded deeply in the subcutaneous tissues or may just penetrate the thickness of the skin, where it is movable and painless. These cysts are generally found within the ear or at its base, although they may form on any part of the body. Usually they have a small opening, from which a thick, cheesy matter can be squeezed out. The rational treatment is to dissect them out.

Sebaceous cysts are not unlike dermoid cysts. They are formed by a dilatation of the hair follicle and sebaceous duct within the skin and contain a gray or yellowish sebaceous mass. The tumor may attain the size of a cherry stone or a walnut. Generally they are round, movable, and painless, soft or doughy in consistence, and covered with skin and hair. They develop slowly. The best treatment is to dissect out the sac with the entire contents.

VERRUCA (WARTS)

Warts on cattle, particularly calves and yearlings, are common. They are found on many parts of the body, but their location depends somewhat on the age of the animal. In cows warts usually occur on the udder or teats, whereas in cattle less than 1 year of age they are most frequent on various parts of the head, as on the ears, around the eyes and mouth, and on the sides of the neck and shoulders. Warts on young cattle may spread from the original location to different parts of the body and may eventually cover large areas of the skin.

Occasionally warts, particularly on young cattle, become large and pendulous. As a result they sap the strength and stunt the growth of the animals. Their chief damage, however, is observed in calfskins and cattle hides after tanning. The tanned hides have roughened and weak spots where the warts occurred on the skin and frequently contain numerous pits or holes in places, such as the shoulders, where the skin was thickly studded with warts. These defects give a moth-eaten appearance to the finished leather. As a consequence, the parts affected are considered worthless.

The reduction in the value of hides, because of warts, usually varies from a few percent to 25 percent and sometimes more, depending on the extent of skin areas affected. Cattle buyers make discounts for warty animals purchased in the markets.

Since a considerable number of animals are affected with warts and the hides of many of them are greatly reduced in value, the yearly loss from a leather standpoint is doubtless large, though no definite figures are available.

Warts vary greatly in shape and size. They may be thin, long, and club shaped, an inch or more in length, and occur singly or in clusters; or they may become large cauliflowerlike tumors several inches in diameter and in extreme cases may weigh several pounds. Occasionally they occur as broad, slightly elevated masses.

Warts may be either hard or soft. The large cauliflowerlike growths are usually soft and show a tendency to bleed and slough, and frequently they give off offensive odors.

Cause.—Common warts in cattle have been shown by experiments to be infectious. The infective constituent is a filtrable virus, meaning that it will pass through an earthen, germ-retaining filter. By experimental skin inoculations with wart material, these growths can be produced with a fair degree of regularity in healthy cattle less than 1 year of age. Under ordinary circumstances infection is thought to take place through injuries to the skin when the injured part comes in contact with warty animals, rubbing posts, fences, buildings, or any structure with which an affected animal has come in contact.

Treatment.—Warts may occasionally disappear without treatment of any kind, especially as animals become older. Most cases, however, require definite and systematic treatment.

Warts that are small at the place of attachment may be removed by either clipping them off with sterile scissors or tying a sterile thread or slender cord tightly around the wart near the base. In the latter method the warts will slough off in a few days. The stumps of the warts should be touched with either glacial acetic acid or tincture of iodine. Tying off is recommended also for warts that because of their size, are likely to contain a number of blood vessels that would result in more or less bleeding if the warts were removed by cutting. Treat the roots or base of such warts also with either glacial acetic acid or silver nitrate. The removal of extremely large warts by surgical means should be performed by a veterinary surgeon.

Before warts become excessively large they may be destroyed by daily applications of glacial acetic acid or tincture of iodine. Before applying acetic acid, protect the healthy skin immediately surrounding the warts by thoroughly greasing with petrolatum or lard. Be careful not to grease the warts as that would protect them also from the acid. Small warts, as on the udders of cows, will sometimes disappear if kept soft by daily applications of sweet oil or castor oil.

If warts are numerous and cover large areas of the body, it may be advisable to give internal treatment also. The usual internal treatment for various skin disorders, including warts, it arsenic in the form of Fowler's solution. The dose is 1 tablespoonful twice daily to cattle 6 to 12 months of age. This method should be considered, however, only an indirect method of treatment. Arsenic treatment should be administered only under the supervision of a competent veterinarian. As arsenic may pass into the milk, Fowler's solution should not be given to milking cows.

Prevention.—Preventive measures consist in removing all warty cattle from the herd, particularly affected calves and yearlings, and in cleaning and disinfecting all exposed stables, pens, chutes, and rubbing posts.

In dairy herds, cows having warts on their teats and udders should be milked last and the milkers should be careful to wash and disinfect their hands thoroughly after each milking to prevent the possible spread of the virus from one animal to another. The essential point in preventing and controlling these growths is to keep in mind that they are infectious or "catching."

KELIS

Kelis is an irregularly shaped, flat tumor of the skin resulting from hypertrophy—increased growth of the fibrous tissue of the corium, producing absorption of the papillary layer.

Causes.—It may arise spontaneously or follow a scar after an injury.

Symptoms.—Kelis generally appears below the knee or hock and may occur singly or in numbers. There are no constitutional symptoms. Its growth is very slow and seldom causes any inconvenience.

It appears as a flattened, irregular, or spreading growth within the substance of the skin, is hard to the touch, and is especially characterized by divergent branches or roots, resembling the claws of a crab; hence the name. Occasionally some part of it may soften and result in an abscess. It may grow several inches in length and encircle the whole leg.

Treatment.—So long as it causes the animal no inconvenience it is best not to meddle with it; when it does, the animal should be fattened for beef as the meat is perfectly harmless to the consumer.

PARASITIC DISEASES OF THE SKIN

RINGWORM (TINEA TONSURANS AND TINEA FAVOSA)

Ringworm is an affection of the skin caused by a vegetable parasite.

The form known as tinea tonsurans is produced by the presence of a minute or microscopic fungus, *Trichophyton tonsurans*, which affects the hair and the epidermic layer of the skin and is highly contagious, being readily transmitted from one animal to another. This fungus consists of spores and filaments. The spores, being the most numerous, are round and seldom vary much in size. They are abundant in the hair follicle. The filaments are articulated, waving, and contain granules. This disease produces changes in the root and shaft of the hair, rendering it brittle and easily broken off.

This disease becomes manifest by the formation of circular patches on the skin, which soon becomes denuded of hair. The cuticular layer of the skin is slightly inflamed, and vesication with exudation occurs, followed by the formation of scaly, brittle crusts. The patches are silvery gray when incrusted and are mostly confined to the head and neck. It is a common disease among young cattle in the winter and spring. Early in the development of the patches the hairs split, twist, and break off close to the skin. This disease is attended with more or less itching. It is communicable to man.

Tinea favosa comes from another fungus, *Achorion schoenleinii* This enters the hair follicles and involves the cuticle surrounding it. Small crusts form that increase in diameter and thickness and then become elevated at their margin, forming a cup-shaped scab. the favus cup, which gives the disease its distinctive character. The number of these cups varies from a few to many hundreds. The hairs involved become brittle and broken, fall off with the crusts, leaving small bald patches. The crusts are of a pale or sulfur, yellow color at first. As they grow older they turn darker or to a brown color. This form of ringworm has a peculiar odor, resembling that of mice or musty straw. It is occasionally communicated to cattle by man, mice, or cats, all being subject to it.

Treatment.—Remove all crusts by washing with soap and water, then apply acetic acid, sulfur ointment, tincture of iodine or nitrate of mercury ointment once a day. Cleanse the stable and whitewash it to destroy the spores scattered by the crusts.

OTHER PARASITES AND PARASITIC DISEASES OF THE SKIN

For discussion of mange, itch, scab, lousiness, warbles (grub in the skin) buffalo gnats, hornfly, ticks, flies, and other parasites or parasitic diseases, see the chapter on Parasites of Cattle, page 449.

WOUNDS OF THE SKIN

SNAKE BITES AND VENOMOUS STINGS

[See discussion of these subjects in chapter on Poisons and Poisoning]

BURNS AND SCALDS

These are rare accidents among cattle, yet in cases of fire they may occur. The application of heat, whether dry or moist, unless sufficient instantly to destroy the life of a part, is always followed by the development of vesicles or blisters, which contain a thin, watery fluid. The blisters may be isolated and not large, or one blister may cover a very large surface. When the burn is severe the skin may be wholly devitalized, or the injury may extend into the deeper structures of the skin. Then sloughs will occur, followed by a contraction of the parts in healing; if on a leg, this may make the animal stiff. When the burn or scald is severe, the resulting pain is great and the constitutional disturbance very marked.

Treatment.—In mild, superficial burns, the affected area may be covered with a moderately warm starch paste or a simple boric acid ointment (1 dram of boric acid to 3 ounces of petrolatum) and the dressing repeated the next day. Usually this is sufficient, but in more severe burns it is advisable to swab the affected parts gently with a one-half percent aqueous tannic acid solution and cover with a light gauze bandage. This treatment may be repeated several times, and after a few days it is well to treat the affected area with antiseptic applications to prevent infection. A saturated solution of picric acid may be used in place of the tannic acid solution. When the severe inflammation subsides and healing begins, care should be taken to keep the wound clean and dressed frequently with antiseptics. If none of these drugs are available, the wound may be treated with bandages soaked in strong tea (which contains tannic acid) and allowed to cool.

Frostbite on any portion of the body may be treated as recommended in the article on diseases of the ears.

EMPHYSEMA (AIR OR GAS UNDER THE SKIN)

Emphysema of the skin is not a true disease of the skin, but it is mentioned as a pathological condition. It is characterized by a distention of the skin with air or gas contained in the subcutaneous areolar tissue. It may depend on a septic condition of the blood, as in anthrax or blackleg, or air may be forced under the skin about the head, neck, and shoulders, as a result of rupture of the windpipe. It occurs in the region of the chest and shoulders from penetrating wounds of the chest and lung and occasionally follows puncture of the rumen when the escaping gas is retained under the skin.

Symptoms.—The skin is enormously distended over a greater or less portion of the body; thus any region of the body may lose its natural contour and appear like a monstrosity. There is a peculiar crackling beneath the skin when the hand is passed over it, and on tapping it with the fingers a resonant, drumlike sound is heard.

Treatment.—Puncture the distended skin with a clean, broad-bladed knife and press the air out. Further treatment must be directed with a view to the removal of the cause.

Diseases of the Foot

By M. R. Trumbower, D. V. S.

[Revised by Maurice S. Shahan, D. V. M.]

LAMINITIS (FOUNDER)

The term "laminitis" denotes an inflammation of the sensitive, highly vascular structures within the wall of the hoof. Owing to the simplicity of the structure of the foot of the cow as compared with that of the horse, this disease is rarely seen in an acute form, but a mild form, commonly called "foot soreness," is not of infrequent occurrence.

Causes.—Laminitis in cattle is usually due to the digestive disorders that may follow overfeeding, especially with grains, or the consumption of feeds of poor quality, or it may develop after long drives over hard, rough, or stony roads. Other factors such as overheating, continued standing on hard footing without exercise, especially in particularly heavy animals, septic inflammations in some other part of the body, and toxic conditions may be responsible.

Symptoms.—Because of pain, affected animals shift the weight of the body from side to side, often stand fixed as though "nailed to the spot," or may lie down much of the time, in which case it is very difficult to get them to their feet. The feet are unnaturally hot, and frequently there is some swelling above the hoof. Pressure on the hoof with blacksmith's hoof pincers causes pain and flinching. The general body temperature is increased and the breathing accelerated. The animal usually refuses feed but often shows extreme thirst. When it is made to move, excessive tenderness of the feet becomes manifest, as is shown by reluctance to walk and by the very short, hesitating step. Founder affects the hindfeet as well as the forefeet although the latter are more often involved. Severe, protracted, or untreated cases may develop suppuration and may slough one or more claws.

Treatment.—In addition to treatment for the direct cause of the condition, cold packs should be applied to the feet, or if the animal can be made to stand in a pond or stream of water having a soft bottom, the inflamation is often relieved without the necessity of any additional treatment. It may be well, however, to give a purgative in cases of digestive origin. For this purpose, 1 to 1½ pounds of

Epsom salts, given in a drench, may be appropriate, though quicker acting drugs are often preferred. In some cases, purgatives are contra-indicated. The overloaded stomach may be emptied by lavage through a stomach tube or by operation (rumenotomy).

FOOT SORENESS

Cattle that have been stabled or pastured on soft ground and are driven over stony roads soon wear down the soles of their feet and become lame from foot soreness. When the soreness is excessive it may develop into an active inflammation of all the sensitive structures of the foot, laminitis, or into a local bruise commonly called a "corn." Draft oxen, as well as large beef-type bulls on rough, rocky ranges, may require shoeing for protection to the feet.

Treatment.—This consists in rest, poulticing the feet with moistened clay, followed by astringent washes.

If the pain and heat last several days, it is probable that pus has formed beneath the wall of the hoof. It is then advisable to have the animal stand for several hours daily in a tub containing an antiseptic solution, or to poultice the foot with a warm flaxseed poultice containing 2½ to 3 percent of compound solution of cresol. When not under antiseptic treatment the foot may be dressed with pine tar and cotton and bandaged with bagging, and the animal should be kept in dry, clean quarters. It may be necessary to cut through the hoof wall to allow the accumulated pus to escape.

LOSS OF HOOF

Cattle sometimes become fastened between planks or otherwise and pull off the wall of one or both claws in the effort to extricate themselves. The claws of one or more feet may be shed as the result of ergotism or acute laminitis, or foot rot, or other suppurative conditions. In alkali disease (selenium poisoning), which occurs in certain sections of the United States, a sloughing of the hoof may take place.

Treatment.—Particularly if the hoof is torn from the foot through accident there is great pain, and the animal should be placed in a clean, bedded stall and the injured foot washed in a mild antiseptic solution. The hoof will grow rapidly if the injury is not too extensive and the foot is kept clean and protected. After the initial inflammation has subsided the tissues may be covered with a thick coating of pine tar, then with a layer of oakum or absorbent cotton, another coat of tar, and finally a bandage closely and firmly applied. This may remain without disturbance until the new growing wall becomes sufficiently strong to sustain the pressure and weight of the animal. If, however, at any time oozing or bad odor indicates that pus is forming under this dressing, the bandage should be removed and the suppurating surface freshly cleansed and dressed. This may have to be repeated every few days and should be continued as long as there is any pus formation. If the loss of hoof is due to suppurative laminitis, the parts denuded of the horny covering must be thoroughly cleansed and treated with nonirritant antiseptics. Then apply a moderately thick layer of absorbent cotton and over this apply the tar and bandage. After this the antiseptic solution may be poured in daily at the top of the dressing. It will thus soak in and saturate the dressing and inflamed tissue. It may become necessary to remove all the dressing at daily or longer intervals to give the parts a fresh cleaning, and then to reapply it.

FOOT ROT (FOUL FOOT)

A variety of causes may produce inflammation of the foot between the claws, in the fibrous cushion at the junction of the hair and the hoof at the heel, or more rarely at the hair line on the outside of the foot. Bruises caused by rocks, sticks, or other objects, the softening or ulceration of the skin that may follow continued exposure to very wet corrals or pastures, as well as impaction and hardening of soil in the interdigital space, and wedged-in foreign objects are some of the causes of access to the tissues by pyogenic and necrosis-producing micro-organisms. An overgrown claw often abrades the skin, creating an entrance for the myriads of bacteria that occur in stable filth. Under some conditions, several cattle in the same herd or, less often, numbers of animals within a certain district are affected at the same time, an occurrence which has led some persons to think that foot rot is a specific, contagious disease. The use of new corrals, with fresh unpacked soil, during protracted rainy seasons sometimes results in as many cases of this disease as muddy, filthy corrals that have been in use for years. Foot rot usually affects but one foot, frequently one of the hind feet. The complicating infections following lesions of the feet in vesicular stomatitis may closely resemble some stages of foot rot. For this and other reasons mentioned later, a competent veterinarian should be called whenever lameness spreads in a herd.

Symptoms.—The animal is observed to limp. Examination of the foot shows redness, heat, and swelling above the hoof and of the soft parts between the claws. The swelling frequently spreads the claws apart to a considerable extent, or the inflammation may have advanced to softening and sloughing of the interdigital tissues. If the disease is neglected at this stage, deep abscesses may form and the pus burrow under the horny wall, or the joint within the hoof may become inflamed and the articular attachments destroyed, in which case the treatment will be difficult and recovery will be very tedious.

Treatment.—Whenever possible, new or thoroughly cleaned and disinfected dry quarters should be provided for all the animals not visibly affected. Once or twice daily they may be compelled to walk through a shallow trough containing dry air-slaked lime or a 10-percent solution of copper sulfate, which may be placed at the stable door, a gate, or other convenient place. The affected animals should be isolated in clean quarters and diligently attended.

In the earlier stages of the disease, before pus burrows beneath the horny covering, a thorough cleansing and an application of antiseptic, clean stabling, and laxative food will usually remedy the evil. If deep sloughing or suppuration has taken place all necrotic tissue should be surgically removed. This may involve removal of a part of the hoof wall, resection of the sole, or in still more advanced cases, amputation of the affected toe, all of which operations should be undertaken only by a veterinarian. Almost any good antiseptic is applicable in treating the feet if the deep-seated lesions are completely exposed to its action. Fresh chlorinated lime in a ½- to 1-percent solution or a 10- to 30-percent solution of copper sulfate is commonly used. Sometimes warm poulticing with flaxseed meal or bran to which 2 to 3 percent of compound solution of cresol, or other coal-tar antiseptic has been added, is beneficial in relieving excessive fever and pain.

Prevention.—Close attention to drainage and general cleanliness materially assists in preventing this disease. Dry, sanitary corrals and stables and general hygienic conditions are not conducive to foot rot. Overgrown hoofs should not be permitted. If the disease already exists on the premises, the isolation of affected animals and the prophylactic use of air-slaked lime or copper sulfate solution often prevent its development in normal animals.

FISSURE OF THE WALL (SPLIT HOOF)

This is rarely seen among cattle. It may occur in weak walled hoofs of heavy-bodied cattle, caused by stepping on an uneven surface, especially when the point of the toe is grown out long. Working oxen are probably most likely to suffer from this kind of injury. The point of the toe may be broken and the hoof wall split almost up to the hair.

Treatment.—The divided sections may be brought together and held in place by drilling a small hole from one side into and through the other, commencing half an inch back of the fissure on each side. A light horseshoe nail should then be driven through the hole and clinched. Pare the injured claw as short as it will bear. If infection has gained access to the deep, sensitive tissues, surgical measures and antiseptic treatment are necessary.

INTERDIGITAL FIBROMA

Hard, nodular, fibrous tumors sometimes grow in the cleft of the foot and cause inconvenience, lameness, or ulceration of the contiguous parts.

Treatment.—Such growths usually require surgical treatment. After the growth is removed, the wound requires frequent antiseptic dressing.

DEFORMITIES

Deformities in the feet of cattle usually consist in overgrowth of horny wall, generally from want of wear in animals that are stabled. The hoof may turn inward, outward, or upward and may give rise to lameness, inability to walk, foot rot, and similar ailments. Bulls and dairy cows that are continually stabled frequently have misshapen feet from want of proper wear or an occasional trimming, and this deformity may eventually lead to permanent injury. A common symptom of so-called alkali disease is an overgrown, deeply ringed, hoof wall.

Treatment.—Cut away the excess growth of horny wall with saw, knife, chisel, or rasp, until the foot assumes its natural form.

PRICKS AND WOUNDS

If an animal receives a penetrating wound from nails or other sharp objects, the orifice of the wound should be promptly enlarged and tincture of iodine or other good antiseptic injected immediately into the depths of the wound and the foot covered by a protective dressing. Although cattle are not particularly susceptible to tetanus, antitoxin should be administered for the prevention of that disease in those regions where the disease prevails. If the injury is not discovered or treated before pus formation within the hoof has taken place, drainage and antiseptic treatment, with or without poulticing, are advisable if the loss of the hoof or foot is to be prevented or systemic infections are to be avoided.

Superficial wounds made by barbed wire, glass, or other objects should be properly cleansed and treated with an antiseptic.

If a joint or tendon sheath is penetrated by a wound, the dangers are great and a veterinarian should be in attendance.

Occasionally an animal gets caught by the foot in a crevice and sustains severe bruising, wrenching, or fracture of some part of the foot. In such cases cold-water packs to the injured foot are of service until the fever and swelling disappear. Afterward the animal should rest until the usefulness of the foot is restored. Sometimes such an accident, causing fracture, renders necessary the application of bandages or amputation.

Diseases of the Eye and Its Appendages

By M. R. Trumbower, D. V. S.

[Revised by Gilbert T. Creech, D. V. S.]

DESCRIPTION

For the sake of gaining a clear comprehension of the diseases of the eye it becomes necessary to review the anatomy of this important organ. The essential organ of vision, or globe of the eye, will be first described, then its receptacle or orbital cavity, the muscles that move it, the protective membranes, or eyelids, the membrana nictitans, or accessory eyelids, and, lastly, the lachrymal apparatus.

The globe or ball of the eye is almost spherical in form. On closer inspection, however, it appears to be made up of two combined portions from spheres of different sizes. The posterior portion forms about five-sixths of the ball and the anterior portion the remaining sixth. The latter portion has a greater convexity than the former.

The eyeball consists of concentrically arranged coats and of refracting media enclosed in them. The coats are three in number, namely: (1) An external, protective tunic, made up of the sclera and cornea; (2) a middle, vascular and pigmentary tunic, the choroid; (3) an internal, nervous layer, the retina. The sclera is the white, opaque part of the outer tunic, of which it forms about the posterior five-sixths, being coextensive with the larger sphere already mentioned. The cornea forms the remaining one-sixth of the outer tunic, being coextensive with the segment of the smaller sphere. It is distinguished from the sclera by being colorless and transparent. The choroid coat may be recognized as the thin, pigmented layer subjacent to the sclera. It does not line the cornea but terminates behind the line of junction of that coat with the sclera by a thickened edge—the ciliary processes. At the line of junction of the sclera and cornea the iris passes across the interior of the eye. This (which may be viewed as a dependency of the choroid) is a muscular curtain perforated by an aperture termed the "pupil." The retina will be recognized as a delicate, glassy layer, lining the greater part of the choroid.

The refracting media of the eye are three in number, namely: (1)

77431 O—51——22

The aqueous humor, a watery fluid enclosed in a chamber behind the cornea; (2) the crystalline lens and its capsule, a transparent, soft solid of a biconvex form behind the iris; (3) the vitreous humor, a transparent material with a consistence like thin jelly, occupying as much of the interior of the eye as is subjacent to the choroid.

The sclera is a strong, opaque, fibrous membrane, which in great measure, maintains the form of the eyeball and protects the more delicate structures within it. The portion covered by the ocular conjunctiva is commonly known as the white of the eye. In form it is bell-shaped, and the optic nerve pierces it behind like a handle, the perforation being a little to its inner side. In front, the rim of the bell becomes continuous with the cornea. The outer surface of the membrane receives the insertion of the muscles of the eyeball. The coat is thickest over the posterior part of the eyeball and is thinnest a little behind its junction with the cornea.

The cornea is the anterior transparent portion of the outer coat of the eyeball. It may be viewed as a part of the sclera specially modified to permit the passage of light into the interior of the eye. Its outline is elliptical, nearly circular, and its greatest diameter is transverse. At its periphery it joins the sclera by continuity of tissue, and as the edge of the cornea is slightly beveled and has the fibrous sclera carried for a little distance forward on its outward surface, the cornea is generally said to be fitted into the sclera like a watch glass into its rim. The venous sinuses, referred to as the canal of Schlemm in the human, run circularly around the eyeball near the line of junction of the sclera and cornea. The anterior surface of the cornea is exquisitely smooth and is kept moist by the lachrymal secretions. Its posterior surface forms the anterior boundary of the chamber in which the aqueous humor is contained. The cornea is of uniform thickness and is of a dense, almost horny, consistence. Except for a few capillary loops of blood vessels at its margin, the cornea is without vessels. Its structure is comprised of five distinct layers.

The aqueous humor occupies a chamber that is bounded in front by the posterior surface of the cornea and behind by the capsule and suspensory ligament of the lens and by the ends of the ciliary processes. It is across this chamber that the iris extends. The aqueous humor is composed of a watery fluid, with a small proportion of common salt in solution.

The iris is a circular, muscular, pigmented membrane that is visible through the cornea and in the central portion of which can be seen an elliptical opening, the pupil, by variations in the size of which the amount of light transmitted to the retina is regulated. It varies somewhat in color but is most frequently of a yellowish-brown tint. Its anterior face is bathed by the aqueous humor. The greater part of the posterior surface is in contact with the capsule of the lens and glides on it during the movements of the iris. The circumferential border is attached within the sclerocorneal junction. The inner border circumscribes the pupil, which varies in outline according to its size. When much contracted, the pupil is a very elongated ellipse, the long axis of which is in the line joining the nasal and temporal angles of the eyelids. It contains muscular tissue, which, by contracting or relaxing, lessens or dilates the pupillary opening.

The choroid coat is a bell-shaped, dark membrane that lines the sclera. Its outer surface has a shaggy appearance, caused by the lamina fusca sclerae, which unites the two coats. Between the two the ciliary vessels and nerves pass forward. Behind, it is pierced by the optic nerve; in front, it is continued as the ciliary processes, which form, as it were, the rim of the bell. The ciliary processes form a fringe around the slightly inverted rim of the choroid.

The retina is the most delicate of the coats of the eyeball. It is formed by the expansion of the optic nerve on the inner surface of the choroid, and, like that coat, it is bell-shaped. Its inner surface is molded on the vitreous humor. The nervous structures of the retina terminate at a wavy line, the ora serrata, behind the ciliary processes. Ten distinct layers are described as composing the thickness of the retina.

The lens is situated behind the pupil and is contained within a capsule of its own.

The capsule is a close-fitting, firm, transparent membrane. The anterior surface forms the posterior boundary of the cavity containing the aqueous humor, and the iris in its movement glides on it. The posterior surface is in contact with the vitreous humor.

The vitreous humor occupies four-fifths of the interior of the eyeball. It is globular in form, with a depression in front for the lodgment of the lens. It is colorless, transparent, and of a consistence like thin jelly. It is enveloped by a delicate capsule—the hyaloid membrane—which is connected in front with the suspensory ligament of the lens and ends by joining the capsule behind the lens.

The orbital cavity, at the side of the head, is circumscribed by a bony margin; posteriorly, however, there are no bony walls, and the cavity is often confounded with the depression above and behind the orbit—the temporal fossa. A fibrous membrane completes this cavity and keeps it distinct from the temporal fossa. This membrane—the ocular sheath or periorbita—is attached posteriorly around the opening in the back of the orbital cavity (the orbital hiatus) and anteriorly to its inner face; then it becomes prolonged beyond the margin to form the fibrous membrane of the eyelids. When complete, the orbital cavity has the form of a regular hollow cone, open at its base and closed at the apex. The opening of this cone is directed forward, downward, and outward. Independently of the globe of the eye, this cavity lodges the muscles that move it, the membrana nictitans, and the lachrymal gland.

The muscles of the eye are seven in number—one retractor, four straight, and two oblique. The retractor oculi envelops the optic nerve between the brain and the ball of the eye and is attached to the external face of the sclerotic tunic. When this muscle contracts, it draws the globe back into the orbit, away from the light. The superior, inferior, external, and internal recti or straight muscles are attached to the back part of the orbital sheath and spread forward in four bundles over the globe of the eye, where they are inserted by a fibrous expansion into the sclera at the margin of the cornea. When they act singly, they turn the globe either upward, downward, inward, or outward. The great oblique, by its action, pivots the eye inward and upward in the orbit. The small oblique turns the eye outward and downward.

The eyelids are two movable curtains, superior and inferior, which cover and protect the eye in front. They are attached to the circumference of the orbit and have a convex external face, formed by the skin, and a concave internal face, molded on the anterior surface of the eye, and are lined by the conjunctiva, which is reflected above and below on the eyeball. The border of each lid is slightly beveled on the inner side and shows the openings of the Meibomian glands. These glands secrete an unctuous fluid, which is thrown out on the border of the lids, the function of which is to facilitate their movements and enable them to retain the tears in the ocular cavity. The eyelid is composed of a fibrous inner membrane ending in a stiff arch near the border, a muscle to close the lid, another to open it, the skin externally, and the conjunctival mucous membrane internally. The border of each lid is covered and protected by long hairs to prevent floating particles of matter in the atmosphere from gaining entrance to the eye.

The membrana nictitans, also named the third eyelid, winking eyelid, haw, etc., is placed at the inner angle of the eye, whence it extends over the eyeball to relieve it from foreign bodies that may fall upon it. It has for its framework a fibro-cartilage, irregular in shape, thick, nearly prismatic at its base, and thin anteriorly where it is covered by the conjunctiva; behind, it is loosely attached to a fatty cushion.

The lachrymal gland is between the orbital process and the upper part of the eyeball. It secretes the tears for lubricating the anterior surface of the eye. This fluid escapes upon the organ at the outer angle of the lids and is carried between them and the eyeball toward the inner angle.

The caruncula lacrymalis is a small round body, frequently entirely or partially black, situated in the inner angle of the eye, and is designed to direct the tears toward the puncta lacrimalia.

The puncta lacrymalia are two little openings, one in each eyelid a short distance from the inner corner, which admit the tears into the lachrymal ducts leading to the lachrymal canal, whence they are emptied into the nasal passages.

CONJUNCTIVITIS (SIMPLE OPHTHALMIA)

This is an inflammation of the conjunctiva, or mucous membrane of the eyeball and lids; in severe cases the deeper coats of the eye are involved and seriously complicate the attack.

Causes.—It may result from a bruise of the eyelid; from the introduction of foreign matters into the eye, such as chaff, hayseed, dust, and gnats; from exposure to cold; and from poisonous or irritating vapors arising from filthiness of stable. Dust, cinders, or sand blown into the eyes during transportation frequently cause conjunctivitis.

Symptoms.—There are a profuse flow of tears, closure of the eyelids from intolerance of light, retraction of the eyeball and corresponding protrusion of the haw, disinclination to move, diminution of milk secretion, etc. On parting the lids the lining membrane is found to be congested with an excess of blood, giving it a red and swollen appearance; the sclera, or white of the eye, is bloodshot and the cornea may be cloudy. If the disease advances, keratitis results, with its unfavorable symptoms.

Treatment.—Careful examination should be made to discover particles of chaff or other foreign bodies that may have lodged in the eye, and when discovered they should be promptly removed. This may be accomplished by flushing the eye with warm water by means of a syringe, or, if the foreign substance is adherent to the eyeball or lid, it may be scooped out with the handle of a teaspoon or some other blunt instrument. To relieve the congestion and local irritation, a wash composed of boric acid in freshly boiled water, 20 grains to the ounce, or acetate of zinc, 5 grains to the ounce of pure soft water, may be used. A few drops of this should be placed in the eye with a camel-hair pencil or soft feather three or four times daily. The animal should be placed in a cool, darkened stable; then a cloth folded into several thicknesses should be fastened to the horns in such manner as to reach below the eyes. The cloth should be kept wet with cold water during the day and removed at night. If there are much fever and constitutional disturbance, it is advisable to administer, as a drench, 1 pound of Epsom salts dissolved in 1 quart of water.

INFECTIOUS CATARRHAL CONJUNCTIVITIS (SPECIFIC OPHTHALMIA, SO-CALLED PINK EYE)

This generally appears in an enzootic or epizootic form and affects a considerable number of animals in the herd. The manner in which the disease spreads through the herd indicates that the disease is of a contagious nature, although this has not been definitely determined. It may continue in a herd for a season or for several years and affect all newly purchased animals. It is seldom seen in the winter months. It affects old and young animals alike.

Symptoms.—This form of catarrhal conjunctivitis is characterized chiefly by a mucopurulent discharge from the eyes, an intense degree of inflammation of the mucous membrane, accompanied with swelling of the eyelids and an early opacity of the cornea. The flow of tears is mixed with pus, sometimes streaked with blood, and the skin of the face is kept moist and soiled. The eyes are kept continually closed. The implication of the cornea in the disease frequently blinds the animal for a time, and occasionally suppurative keratitis, ulcers of the cornea, or staphyloma supervene. The attack is marked from the onset by fever, partial loss of appetite, partial loss of milk, suspended rumination, and the tendency to remain apart from the herd.

Treatment.—The animal should be housed in a cool, dark stable, supplied with plenty of fresh water to drink and soft succulent feed. Administer, as a drench, 1 pound of Epsom salts—if a very large animal, use 1½ pounds—dissolved in 2 or 3 pints of warm water. Treatment should begin in the early stage of the disease. In most cases the condition should yield to applications of a 1-percent solution of silver nitrate, which should be fresh at the time of using, applied to the eyes every day with a soft swab made of cotton until there is noticeable improvement in the condition, and then every second or third day until the inflammation subsides entirely.

If ulceration of the cornea or well-marked, deep-seated keratitis develops, the treatment recommended for those conditions should be adopted.

Prevention.—Whenever this affection appears in a herd, all the unaffected animals should be separated from the herd and moved to fields or quarters that have not been previously occupied by affected animals. The water supply should be changed also, especially if the cattle have been obtaining it from a stagnant pond.

KERATITIS (CORNEITIS)

This is an inflammation of the cornea proper, although the sclera at the corneal border becomes involved to some extent. It may be divided into diffuse or nonsuppurative and suppurative.

Causes.—The cornea constitutes the most prominent portion of the eyeball; hence, it is subject to a variety of injuries—scratches, pricks, contusions, lacerations, etc. Inflammation of the cornea may be due also to the extension of catarrhal conjunctivitis or intraocular disease, and it may occur occasionally without any perceptible cause.

Symptoms.—Diffuse or nonsuppurative keratitis is characterized by an exudation into an opacity of the cornea. The swelling of the anterior part of the eyeball may be of an irregular form, in points resembling small bladders, or it may commence at the periphery of the cornea by an abrupt thickening, which gradually diminishes as it approaches the center. If the whole cornea is affected, it has a uniform gray or grayish-white appearance. The flow of tears is not so marked as in conjunctivitis, nor is the suffering so acute, though both conditions often exist together. Both eyes usually become affected, unless the disease is caused by an external injury.

In favorable cases the exudate within the cornea begins to disappear within a week or 10 days, the eye becomes clearer and regains its transparency, until it eventually is fully restored. In unfavorable cases blood vessels form and are seen to traverse the affected part from periphery to center, vision becomes entirely lost, and permanent opacity (albugo or leucoma) remains. When it arises from constitutional causes recurrence is frequent and leaves the corneal membrane more cloudy after each attack, until the sight is permanently lost.

Suppurative keratitis may be a sequel of diffuse keratitis; more commonly, however, it becomes manifest abruptly by a raised swelling on or near the center of the cornea that very soon assumes a yellow, turbid color, and the periphery of the swelling fades into an opaque ring. Suppurative keratitis is seldom noticed for the first day or two—not until distinct pus formation has occurred. When it is the result of diffuse keratitis, ulceration and the escape of the contained pus are inevitable; otherwise the pus may be absorbed. When the deeper membranes covering the anterior chamber of the eye become involved, the contents of this chamber may be evacuated and the sight permanently lost.

Treatment.—Place the animal in a darkened stable, give green or sloppy feed, and administer 4 ounces of Glauber's salt (sodium sulfate) dissolved in a quart of water once a day. If the animal is debilitated a tablespoonful of tonic powder should be mixed with the feed three times a day. This may be composed of equal parts by weight of powdered copperas (ferrous sulfate), gentian, and ginger. As an application for the eye, a solution of silver nitrate, 3 grains per ounce of soft water may be used several times a day. If ulceration occurs, it is well to dust powdered calomel into the eye twice daily, or apply to the eyelids a salve of yellow oxide of mercury, 5 percent in lanolin. Some of this may go on to the cornea and beneath the lids. Apply twice daily. (See the following section: Ulcers of the Cornea.)

To remove opacity, after the inflammation has subsided apply a few drops of the following solution twice a day: Potassium iodide, 15 grains; tincture of sanguinaria, 20 drops; distilled water, 2 ounces; mix.

ULCERS OF THE CORNEA

An ulcer may be due to erosion or to the bursting of a small abscess, which may have formed beneath the delicate layer of the conjunctiva extended over the cornea, or, in the very substance of the cornea itself, after violent keratitis, or catarrhal conjunctivitis. At other times it is produced by bruises, scratches, or other direct injury of the cornea.

Symptoms.—The ulcer is generally at first of a pale-gray color, with its edges high and irregular, discharges an acrid, watery substance instead of pus, and has a tendency to spread widely and deeply. If it spreads superficially upon the cornea, the transparency of this membrane is lost; if it proceeds deeply and penetrates the anterior chamber of the aqueous humor, this fluid escapes, the iris may prolapse, and the lens and the vitreous humor become expelled, thus producing destruction of the whole organ.

Treatment.—It is of the greatest importance, as soon as an ulcer appears upon the cornea, to prevent its growing larger. The corroding process must be converted into a healthy one. For this purpose nothing is more reliable than the use of solid silver nitrate. A stick of this medicine should be scraped to a point; the animal's head should be firmly secured; an assistant should part the lids; if necessary, the haw must be secured within the corner of the eye and then all parts of the ulcer should be lightly touched with the silver nitrate. After waiting a few minutes the eye should be thoroughly washed out with a very weak solution of common salt. This operation generally has to be repeated at the end of 3 or 4 days. If healthy action succeeds, the ulcer assumes a delicate fleshy tint, and the former redness around the ulcer disappears as it heals.

In superficial abrasions of the cornea, where there is no distinct excavation, this caustic treatment is not needed. The eye should be bathed several times a day with zinc sulfate, 30 grains to half a pint of soft water, and protected against exposure to cold air and sunlight. Excessive ulceration sometimes assumes the form of fungous excrescence upon the cornea and appears to derive its nourishment from loops of blood vessels of the conjunctiva. Under these circumstances the fungoid mass must be cut away and the wound cauterized with silver nitrate, or the eye will soon be destroyed. When ulcers of the cornea appear indolent, with a tendency to slough, in addition to the treatment already prescribed, tonic powders of copperas (ferrous sulfate), gentian, and ginger, equal parts by weight, should be given twice a day, mixed with the feed; dose, one tablespoonful.

STAPHYLOMA

This is a disease of the eyeball, in which the cornea loses its transparency, rises above the level of the eye, and even projects beyond the eyelids in the form of an elongated, whitish, or pearl-colored tumor, which is sometimes smooth, at other times uneven.

Causes.—Inflammation is the only known cause, although it may not occur immediately; it frequently follows catarrhal conjunctivitis and keratitis.

Treatment.—In a few cases restoration of sight may be effected by puncturing the projecting tumor and treating it afterwards with silver nitrate in the same manner as prescribed for ulceration of the cornea. In some cases spontaneous rupture has occurred, and healing takes place without any treatment.

CATARACT

In cataract the crystalline lens loses its transparency, the power of refraction is lost and the animal cannot see.

Causes.—Cataract generally arises from a diminution (atrophy) or other change in the nutrition of the lens; it may occur as a result of inflammation of the deep structures of the eye. Cataract may be simple or complicated with amaurosis, adhesions, etc.

Symptoms.—The disease is recognized by the whiteness or loss of transparency of the lens, although the pupil dilates and contracts. Sight may be totally lost; however, evidence is usually manifested that the animal distinguishes light when brought out of a darkened stable. For the most part the formation of cataract takes place slowly, although in a few cases it originates very quickly.

Treatment.—There is only one method for the treatment of cataract—a surgical operation for the removal of the lens; but this is not advisable, for the sight cannot be restored perfectly, and objects would be seen imperfectly.

AMAUROSIS

This is a paralysis of the nerve of sight or the expansion of the retina.

Causes.—This is the result of concussion from a blow on the forehead, fracture of bone over the eye (causing downward pressure), rheumatic inflammation of the optic nerve, or extension of deep inflammation of the eye involving the retina. It sometimes occurs as the result of excessive loss of blood, or of great debility.

Symptoms.—In this eye condition blindness is seldom suspected until indicated by the animal's gait and action. Generally both eyes are affected. The eyeball remains clear, and the pupil is permanently dilated. No response to light is manifested.

Treatment.—If the disease is caused by debility, loss of blood, or associated with rheumatism, general blood tonics may be given in the feed, namely, powdered ferrous sulfate, 1 dram; gentian, 2 drams; nux vomica, one-half dram; to be given twice a day.

CORNEAL DERMATOMA (HAIRY TUMOR ON THE EYEBALL)

In a few instances this has been seen as a congenital growth. The tumor arises from the cornea or the sclera covered by its respective membrane, with a growth of hair upon its surface. The tumor may be prominent or flattened and is dark in color; the hair may protrude between the eyelids, giving the animal the appearance of having a double eyelid.

Treatment.—A surgical operation by a skilled operator is necessary for the removal of such a tumor.

STRABISMUS (SQUINTING)

This is a rare affection among cattle. Strabismus may be either single or double—affecting one eye or both. It is caused by a paralysis or a weakening of one of the straight muscles of the eyeball. Generally it is a congenital defect, and the squinting is toward the nose (strabismus convergens). It is best not to attempt to remedy the defect, as the risk in an operation is greater than the chances of success warrant.

PTERYGIUM

This term is applied to a flesh-colored membrane, triangular in form, which most frequently grows from the inner angle of the eye and extends over the cornea, thus interfering with vision. It may grow from the outer angle or even from either the superior or inferior hemisphere of the eyeball. The figure is invariably that of a triangle, with its base on the white of the eye and its apex more or less advanced over the cornea toward its center.

The distinguishing characteristics are the constancy of the triangular form and the facility with which the whole of it may be taken hold of with a pair of forceps and raised into a fold on the cornea. Every other kind of excrescence attached to this membrane continues firmly adherent to it and cannot be folded and raised from the surface of the cornea in any manner whatever.

Treatment.—Raise the fold and cut it away from all points of attachment.

TRICHIASIS (INVERSION OF THE EYELASHES)

In the simplest form of trichiasis the eyelashes bend inwardly and touch the eyeball, causing irritation and simple conjunctivitis. It may be associated also with entropion.

Treatment.—The offending eyelashes should be cut off or pulled out. In case the natural growth of the eyelashes is directed inward, an operation similar to that for entropion is necessary.

ENTROPION (INVERSION OF THE EYELID)

In inversion of the eyelid the eyelashes soon irritate the anterior face of the cornea and produce more or less inflammation and opacity. The inversion may be due to the growth of a tumor within or without the lid, to abscess, laceration, or injury, causing the lid to lose its natural conformity to the eyeball, ulcerations, etc. Surgical interference in either case is necessary to restore the lid to its natural direction.

ECTROPION (EVERSION OF THE EYELID)

This condition results in injury to the eye by permitting dust or other foreign substances to enter the eye and interferes with the natural removal of such material.

Treatment.—A delicate surgical operation—the removal of an elliptic section of the palpebral conjunctiva—may remedy the defect.

TUMORS OF THE EYELID

Occasionally tumors form on or within the substance of the eyelid. These growths may be of a fibroid nature and arise from the follicles of the hair as sebaceous tumors or may be in the form of an abscess. In debilitating diseases the lids sometimes become swollen and puffy, a condition that may be mistaken for a tumor. This condition generally disappears with the improvement of the health of the animal. Warts not uncommonly appear on or about the eyelids of cattle.

Treatment.—The removal of a tumor in the vicinity of so delicate an organ as the eye should be attempted only by a competent veterinarian.

LACERATION OF THE EYELID

This accident is not uncommon where cattle are kept in pastures that are fenced with barbed wire. An animal may be caught under the eyelid by the horn of another or the laceration may occur in the stable by means of a projecting nail or splinter of wood.

Treatment.—The edges of the wound should be brought together closely and correctly by means of pins passed through nearly the whole thickness of the lid and extending through each lip of the torn part; then a waxed silk or linen thread must be wound over each end of the pin, crossing the torn line in the form of the figure 8 (pl. XXVII, fig. 9). The pins should be placed about three-eighths of an inch apart. The projecting ends of the pins should be cut off close to the ligature and the wound kept anointed with petrolatum to which 2 percent of compound solution of cresol has been added. In place of a pin suture, silver wire, catgut, or strong linen thread may be used as in making an ordinary suture (pl. XXVII, figs. 6, 7, and 8).

FOREIGN BODIES IN THE EYE

Splinters of wood, hedge thorns, pieces of cornstalk or leaves, stems of hay or straw, twigs of trees, or weeds may penetrate the eye, break off, and remain, causing inflammation, blindness, abscess, etc. These substances may penetrate the eyeball, but more frequently they glance off and enter between the eye and the ocular sheath.

Treatment.—Their removal often becomes difficult from the fact that the organ is so sensitive and the retracting power so strong as to necessitate casting the animal, or even the administration of sufficient chloroform to render it completely insensible. The removal, however, is of paramount importance, and the aftertreatment depends on the extent and location of the injury—cold-water compress over the injured eye, the application of mild astringent and cooling washes, such as acetate or zinc sulfate, 5 grains to the ounce of water. When there is extreme suffering from pain, a solution of atropine or morphine, 5 grains to the ounce of water, may be dropped into the eye and alternated with the cooling wash several times a day. When abscesses form within the orbit a free opening must be maintained for the discharge of pus. In deep penetrating wounds of the eye there is a tendency to the formation of a fungous growth, which often necessitates the removal of the whole eyeball.

ORBITAL AND PERIORBITAL ABSCESS

Orbital abscess may form outside the globe and within the orbital sheath, as the result of a previous wound of the parts or fracture of the bony orbit, etc. Periorbital abscess commences outside the ocular sheath, beneath the periosteal membrane covering the bone, and is usually the result of a diseased or fractured bone of the orbital cavity.

Symptoms.—Orbital abscess is manifested by a pushing forward of the eyeball (exophthalmos), and a swelling of the conjunctiva and eyelids. The bulging out of the eye is in proportion to the size of the abscess; the movement of the eye is fixed, owing to the painfulness of any voluntary movement of the eyeball. Periorbital abscess generally pushes the eye to one side; otherwise the symptoms are similar to the foregoing. The pain generally is very great; paralysis of the nerve of sight may occur, and death may be caused by the abscess's extending to the brain.

Treatment.—The treatment for either orbital or periorbital abscess is the same as that for abscess in any other part of the body—a free opening for the escape of imprisoned pus. This should be made as soon as the nature of the disease is recognized. Afterward antiseptic injections may be needed to stimulate healthy granulation and to prevent septic infection of the ocular membranes. For this purpose a saturated solution of boric acid may be used. When the fever is high, Glauber's salt (sulfate of soda) may be given in 4-ounce doses once a day. The animal should be kept in a darkened stable on soft or green feed.

FRACTURE OF THE ORBIT

This accident occasionally occurs among belligerent animals or as the result of blows delivered by brutal attendants. The orbital process above the eye may be entirely crushed in, pressing down upon the eyeball. In such an event the depressed bone should be elevated into its proper place, and if it fails to unite it may have to be removed with saw or chisel. The margin of the orbit may be crushed at any point and cause periorbital abscess, or necrosis may result from the presence of a splinter of bone or the excessive destruction of bone. In all cases of fracture the animal should be kept by itself until the injured part heals.

NECROSIS OF THE BONY ORBIT

As the result of fracture of the margin of the orbit a part of the injured bone may become necrosed (dead), and periostitis and periorbital abscess will follow as a consequence. This condition at first resembles an ordinary abscess, but an examination with a probe after the abscess is open shows that the bone is rough and brittle at the point of bone involvement. The discharge has a peculiar, fetid odor and is often mixed with blood.

Treatment.—The affected bone must be laid bare and all diseased portions removed by scraping or, if necessary, with saw or chisel. Extent of injury or size of wound necessary to be inflicted, should be disregarded. A large portion of the bony orbit may be removed without serious danger to the eye, provided the eyeball itself has not been affected by the diseased condition involved in the original injury.

TUMORS OF THE ORBIT

A fungoid or cancerous tumor of the eyeball or related tissues occasionally appears, which was formerly designated fungus haematodes. This may arise without any appreciable cause or as the result of a wound. It frequently originates from some portion of the eyeball as a small, red mass, eventually bursts through, and pushes its way outside the orbit as a large, dark-red mass, bleeding at the slightest touch. It has a peculiar, fetid odor and early in its appearance destroys sight and involves all the contents of the orbit, not infrequently the bony wall itself. (See "Cancer" under general description of tumors, page 271.)

Unless the tumor is totally removed in its early stage of growth, together with the eyeball, the disease will eventually spread to other tissues and organs and cause emaciation and death of the animal. The removal of the eyeball should not be undertaken by anyone unacquainted with the anatomical structures involved in such an operation. When the operation is performed early enough the result is generally satisfactory.

Bony tumors of the orbit, the result of bruises, fractures, etc., are occasionally present in cattle. They may encroach on the contents of the orbit and cause paralysis of the optic nerve—the condition known as amaurosis—or by pressure on the posterior surface of the eyeball force it forward, or produce atrophy (shrinking). They may displace the eye in any direction, with or without disturbing vision.

Fibrous tumors growing within the orbit produce symptoms similar to those of bony tumors.

Treatment.—When the outlines of the tumor, whether fungoid, bony, or fibrous, can be detected, an operation for its removal should be undertaken as soon as the sight of the eye is disturbed in any manner. This and all other delicate operations pertaining to the eye should be performed only by a competent veterinarian.

DISLOCATION OF THE EYEBALL

The eyeball may be torn out of its socket by the horns of another animal, or it may be crowded out with the blunt end of a club, cane, or probe in the hands of a brutal attendant.

Treatment.—When the optic nerve is not lacerated and the retractor muscles at the back of the eye are intact, an attempt at reduction is advisable. This, however, must follow very soon after the injury—before swelling takes place. Divide the outer corner of the eyelid to enlarge the orifice, then by pressure with the fingers of both hands placed on the sides of the eye the ball may be put into its place. Apply a firm compress over the injured eye and keep it constantly wet with cold water containing 1 dram of sugar of lead to each quart.

If the attempt at reduction proves unsuccessful the artery at the back of the eye should be ligated, and then the whole mass cut off as deep within the orbit as possible. The orbital cavity, after being washed out with a 3-percent solution of carbolic acid or compound solution of cresol, should be packed daily with fresh absorbent cotton.

INFLAMMATION AND ENLARGEMENT OF THE HAW

The haw, or membrana nictitans, is subject to inflammation and swelling from the extension of conjunctivitis or to direct injury by foreign substances. It has a red, swollen appearance, and there is considerable pain and a profuse flow of tears. The application of a cooling lotion, such as is recommended for conjunctivitis, will soon reduce the swelling and restore it to its normal function.

There is, however, a tendency for an inflammation of this membrane to take on a chronic character, which may eventually result in a permanent enlargement, resembling a tumor. When it attains sufficient size to obstruct the sight, its removal through surgical means may be necessary. The eye is afterward treated with simple, cooling lotions.

Diseases of the Ear

By M. R. Trumbower, D. V. S.

[Revised by Gilbert T. Creech, D. V. S.]

Diseases of the ears of cattle are not common, for the reasons probably that these animals are not subjected to the brutality of drivers so much as horses and that the horns to a great extent protect them from external violence.

OTITIS (INFLAMMATION OF THE INTERNAL EAR)

Inflammation of the deep part of the ear is often difficult to recognize in cattle. It may be caused by disease of bone in that region, from blows inflicted by drivers, or from injury by other cattle. Occasionally the ear becomes involved in actinomycosis (lumpy jaw), or the inflammation may be the result of a tuberculous affection.

Symptoms.—The animal holds its head to one side or shakes it, while the ear itself is held immovable. The movement of the jaws in eating usually gives rise to a manifestation of pain; the base of the ear may be feverish and swollen and very sensitive to the touch. If the inflammation has advanced to a suppurative stage, offensive matter flows from the ear.

Treatment.—At first, treatment should consist in applying hot fomentations to reduce pain and fever, followed by the application of a sharp blister below the ear. If there is a discharge from the ear, it should be thoroughly washed out by injecting warm soapsuds, 1 part of liquid soap to 5 parts of water. Dry boric acid may then be placed in the ear, or the parts may be swabbed with a mixture of 1 part tincture of iodine and 3 parts of glycerin.

ABSCESS

Abscesses, caused by contusions, sometimes form about the base of the ear, either inside or outside. A serous cyst is found occasionally between the cartilage and the skin on the base of the ear, which may be from a similar cause.

Treatment.—With the knife make a free incision into the most prominent part of the abscess or cyst, then, with a syringe, wash out the sac with carbolized water. If the abscess recurs, open it again, wash it out, and inject tincture of iodine, or fill it with iodoform.

FUNGOUS GROWTHS

As a result of laceration or wound of any kind, fungous growths, characterized by a raw, bleeding, granulating surface, with a tendency to become pendulous, may develop on the ear.

The whole tumor or diseased structure should be cut away and the wound treated daily with an antiseptic dressing.

FOREIGN BODIES IN THE EAR

Bugs have been known to gain entrance into the ears of animals. Acorns may get into the ears of cows that have been roaming in woods; also pieces of wood from a stanchion may be lodged accidentally in the ear.

Symptoms.—There is usually a continuous uneasiness or frequent shaking of the head, occasionally the manifestation of exceedingly great pain. The animal may rub its head and ear against trees or other objects in an endeavor to dislodge the offending body.

Treatment.—A careful examination reveals the cause, which may be removed with a pair of forceps or scraped out with a hairpin or piece of wire bent at one end. If much inflammation exists, the ear may be swollen so that the foreign substance is hidden from sight; then a probe may be inserted to feel for the object, which, when found, should be removed, even if it is necessary to split the ear at the base. Afterward treat the ear frequently with warm water fomentations and the injection of soapy water or oil and water.

SCURFY EARS

Cattle are subject to scurfy ears, which may be due to a generally morbid condition of the skin or may be confined to the ears alone. The affected animal shows an inclination to rub the ear; thick scales, which sometimes have the appearance of hard, dry, horny scales, of scurf collect on it. This condition is caused chiefly by a faulty secretion of the sebaceous glands of the ear. Thoroughly clean the ear with a stiff brush, then anoint it, so far as affected, with 4 parts of petrolatum to 1 part of white precipitate ointment. If the scurfiness of the ears is only a part of a general scurfiness of the skin, the condition of the animal needs attention. (See Pityriasis, p. 285.)

FROSTBITE

It is not uncommon for young cattle that are poorly nourished and exposed outdoors to storms and extreme cold to suffer frostbite of the ear, which may constitute actual freezing of the part.

Symptoms.—Frostbite presents naturally every degree of severity from the mere chilling of the tip of the ear to positive freezing and death of a portion. In a day or two after the freezing has occurred the ear becomes swollen and very painful; the dead part remains

77431 O—51——23

cold and begins to shrivel; a line of separation then forms between the inflamed and the dead or dying portion, and finally the piece destroyed drops off, leaving a raw, healing surface. When the ear is only slightly affected by the cold, peeling off of superficial skin takes place, accompanied with some pain and itching.

Treatment.—A good liniment for frozen ears is a mixture of turpentine, ammonia, and chloroform, 1 part of each, added to 6 parts of sweet oil. Rub this on the ear several times a day. It will relieve pain and stimulate the circulation and thus favor a recovery of the injured structures.

LACERATIONS OF THE EAR

Aggressive dogs are the most frequent cause of lacerated ears, generally leaving a torn, ragged edge and bruised cartilage.

If the wound is extensive, a trimming of the ragged edges is necessary. The edges should then be fastened together with silver wire, catgut, or strong, thick, linen thread, a deep hold being taken. Pine tar should then be applied.

DISEASE OF THE CARTILAGE AND NECROSIS

Occasionally the cartilages of the ear become affected, usually the result of a deep bruise; pus forms under the skin and may discharge from any part of the ear more or less distant from the seat of the disease. When the cartilage has been extensively injured, pieces of it may become dead (necrosed) and dissolve, to be carried away with the pus, or there may be extensive sloughing and the formation of numerous, running sores. In the disease of the cartilage there is seldom much swelling or great pain. The discharge is usually very offensive and occasionally streaked with blood. Whenever there is a long-continued, persistent discharge from one or more openings in the ear, disease of the cartilage may be suspected.

Treatment.—The sinus formed by the passage of pus should be probed and searched to the bottom for the presence of a foreign substance or the evidence of decaying cartilage. When the probe touches necrosed cartilage it will feel like a piece of dry leather or partially softened wood. A counter opening must then be made at this place, and all diseased cartilage cut away with the knife. The subsequent treatment consists in keeping the artificial wound open for the discharge of pus, and the injection of zinc chloride, 5 grains to the ounce of water, once or twice a day, until the wound is healed.

ENCHONDROMA OF THE EAR

This is an excessive growth of cartilage at the base of the ear in the form of a hard, painless tumor, firmly attached to the movable ear. The only recourse for its removal is the knife in the hands of a competent veterinarian.

Infectious Diseases of Cattle

Revised by John R. Mohler, A. M., V. M. D., D. Sc.

Chief, Bureau of Animal Industry[1]

GENERAL INTRODUCTION

The importance, to the farmer and stock raiser, of a general knowledge of the nature of infectious diseases must be evident to all who have charge of farm animals. The growing facilities for intercourse between various sections of a country, and between different countries, tend to cause a wide distribution of the infectious diseases once restricted to a definite locality. Not only the animals themselves, but the cars, trucks, vessels, or other conveyances in which they are carried may become agents for the dissemination of disease. Specialization in agriculture, which leads to the maintenance of large herds of cattle, sheep, and hogs, tends to make infectious diseases more common and more dangerous. New animals are being continually introduced, which may be the carriers of disease from other herds, and when disease is once brought into a large herd the losses may become very high, because it is difficult to check it after it has once obtained a foothold.

These considerations make it plain that only the most careful supervision by intelligent men who understand the nature of infectious diseases and their causes in a general way can prevent their occurrence. Furthermore, the knowledge concerning many diseases is incomplete and probably will be for some time to come. The suggestions and recommendations offered by investigators, therefore, may not always be correct and may require frequent modification as information becomes more comprehensive and exact.

An infectious disease may be defined as any malady caused by the introduction, into the body, of minute organisms of a vegetable or animal nature that have the power of indefinite multiplication and of setting free certain peculiar poisons that are chiefly responsible for the morbid changes.

[1] The original text of this section was prepared by Drs. D. E. Salmon and Theobald Smith both deceased. In preparing the present text, the author acknowledges the assistance of Drs. A. B. Crawford, G. T. Creech, C. N. Dale, G. Dikmans, L. T. Giltner, E. Lash, W. T. Miller, Wm. M. Mohler, O. [illegible] Osteen, H. W. Schoening, M. S. Shahan, B. T. Simms, and C. D. Stein.

This definition might include diseases caused by certain animal parasites that multiply in the digestive tract but whose progeny is limited to a single generation. By common consent the term "infectious" is restricted to those diseases caused by the invasion and multiplication of certain very minute organisms included under the general classes of bacteria, fungi, protozoa, and filtrable viruses. Most of the diseases of cattle for which a definite cause has been traced are due to bacteria, but as will be seen in this discussion many are caused by the so-called filtrable viruses. Among the bacterial diseases are tuberculosis, anthrax, blackleg, and tetanus (lockjaw). Some diseases, such as cattle-tick fever and anaplasmosis, are traceable to protozoa, whereas others, such as actinomycosis and aspergillosis, are caused by fungi.

Bacteria are minute, one-celled organisms of a plantlike character. Their form is very simple, as may be seen from an inspection of the various species depicted on plate XXVIII. The description of these is given on page 317. Their magnification there will give the reader some idea of their minute size. They multiply in two ways. The bacterium elongates and then divides in the middle to form 2 daughter cells. These go through the same process at once, and thus 4 cells are produced. The division of these leads to 8, the division of 8 to 16, and so on indefinitely. The rapidity with which this multiplication takes place depends on the nature of the bacterium and on the conditions under which it is living. The bacillus of tuberculosis multiplies very slowly, whereas that of anthrax does so with great rapidity, assuming that both organisms are in the most favorable condition. Another mode of reproduction limited to certain classes of bacteria consists in the formation of a spore within the body of the bacterium. Spore formation usually takes place when the conditions pertaining to the growth of the bacteria become unfavorable. The spores are much more resistant to destructive agents than the bacteria that produced them. The anthrax spore may live several years in a dried state, but the anthrax bacillus perishes in a few days under like conditions. This matter is referred to again under the subject of disinfection.

Protozoa are one-celled, microscopic forms of animal life. One that produces cattle-tick fever is pictured on plate XLV, figures 4 and 5. These protozoa have a more complex life history than bacteria. Furthermore, with few exceptions, notably certain trypanosomes, they cannot be grown in artificial media. Therefore, their thorough investigation is exceedingly difficult.

A filtrable virus is an infectious agent that will pass through the pores of a filter capable of holding back ordinary bacteria. Viruses also differ from bacteria as a class in that they are usually

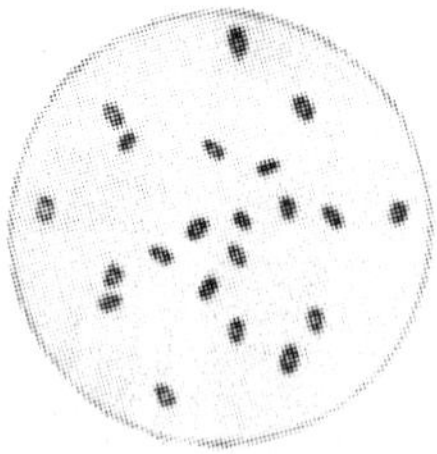

Fig. 1

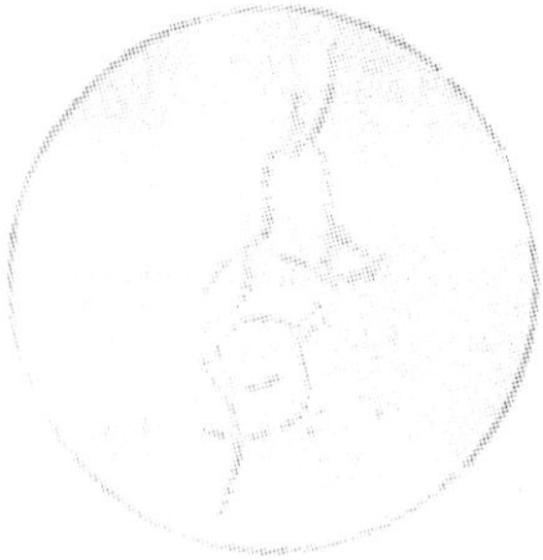

Fig. 3

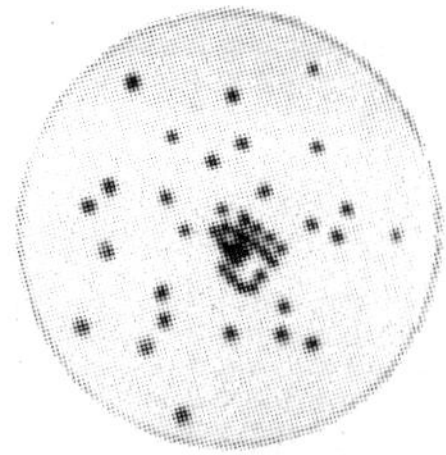

Fig. 2

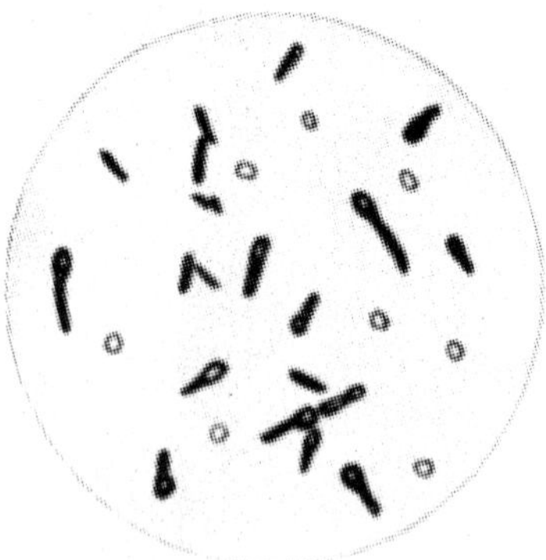

Fig. 4

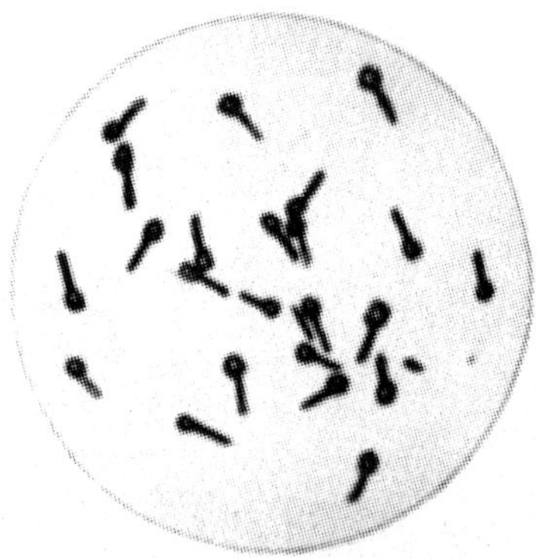

Fig. 5

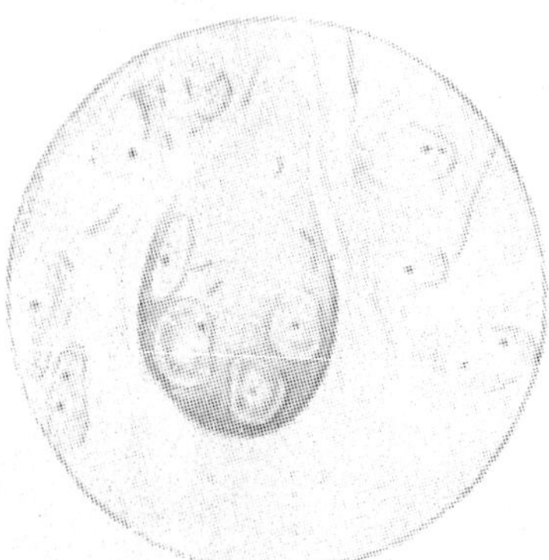

Fig. 6

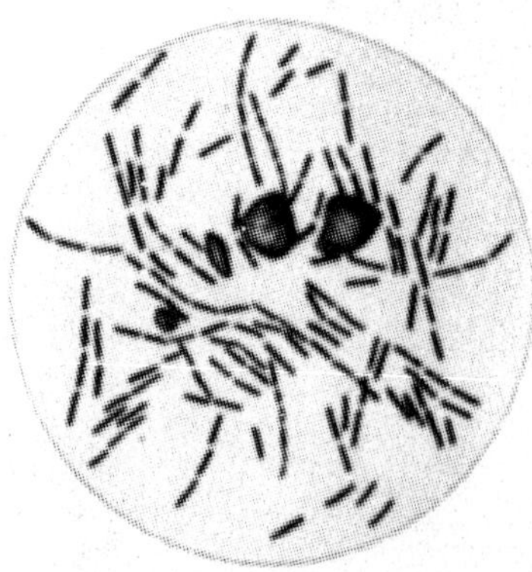

Fig. 7

HAINES DEL.

VARIOUS BACTERIA WHICH PRODUCE DISEASE IN CATTLE.

invisible, even with the modern microscope, and, further, because special methods are required for their culture, most of them not yet having been grown artificially. Examples of cattle disease attributed to this form of infection are foot-and-mouth disease, rinderpest, cowpox, and vesicular stomatitis.

The differences in the symptoms and lesions of the various infectious diseases are due to differences in the respective organisms causing them as well as to variations in the tissue that each particular infection invades. Similarly, the great differences observed in the sources from which animals become infected and the manner in which infection takes place are due to differences in the life history of these minute organisms. Much discussion has taken place in late years concerning the precise meaning of the words "infection" and "contagion."

VARIOUS BACTERIA THAT PRODUCE DISEASE IN CATTLE

DESCRIPTION OF PLATE XXVIII

The bacteria on this plate are partly from tissues, partly from cultures, and stained artificially with aniline colors (fuchsin or methylene blue). Figures 6 and 7 are copied from Fränkel's and Pfeiffer's atlas. All but figure 7 are magnified 1,000 times; figure 7 is magnified 500 times.

Figure 1. Bacteria from pneumonia in cattle. These are also the cause of hemorrhagic septicemia and are closely related to swine-plague bacteria. These bacteria were drawn from a piece of spleen pulp (rabbit).

Figure 2. Micrococci (staphylococcus) that produce inflammation and suppuration, also pyemia.

Figure 3. Micrococci (streptococcus) that produce inflammation of the lining membranes of the abdomen, thorax, heart, brain, and joints. Frequently associated with the bacteria in abscesses.

Figure 4. Bacilli of blackleg. The pale oval bodies as well as the light spots in one end of the bacilli represent spores.

Figure 5. Bacilli that produce tetanus or lockjaw. The light spot in the enlarged end of each rod represents a spore.

Figure 6. Bacilli of tuberculosis. Microscopic sections of a pearly nodule from the lining membrane of the chest cavity. The bacilli are stained red and appear as small straight rods within the cells of the nodule or tubercle.

Figure 7. Bacilli of anthrax. Bacilli from the spleen of a mouse inoculated with a culture. The bacilli were obtained from the blood of a cow that died of anthrax in Mississippi. The bacilli appear as rods stained blue. The round bodies are blood corpuscles, also stained artificially.

These words, however, are now wholly inadequate to express the complex processes of infection, and each kind of bacterium, filtrable virus, or protozoon has its own peculiar way of invading the animal body There are, however, a few broad distinctions that may be expressed with the help of these terms. Infection, as formerly stated, refers at present in a comprehensive way to all micro-organisms capable of setting up disease in the body. Some infections are transmitted directly from one animal to another, and the diseases produced may be called contagious. Among these are foot-and-mouth disease, rabies, cowpox, aud tuberculosis. Again, certain organisms are perhaps never directly transmitted from one animal to another but may come from the soil. Among these are tetanus, blackleg, anthrax to a large extent, and perhaps actinomycosis in part. There is a third class of infectious diseases, the specific bacteria of which are transmitted from one animal to another as in the contagious diseases, but the bacteria under certain favorable conditions, may find food enough in the soil and in the surroundings of animals to multiply to some extent after they have left the sick animal and before they gain entrance into a healthy one.

This general classification is subject to change if other characteristics are taken into consideration. Thus tuberculosis, because of its insidious beginning and slow course, would not by many be considered contagious in the sense that foot-and-mouth disease is; yet, in either case, the bacillus or virus must come from preexisting disease.

Again, all the diseases that seem to come from the soil and from pastures are in one sense contagious in that the virus may be taken from a sick animal and inoculated directly, with positive results, into a healthy animal. Other illustrations may be cited that show that these old terms are not in themselves satisfactory. So many conditions enter into the process of infection that no single classification will give a sufficiently correct or comprehensive idea of it. These statements will be easily understood if the different infectious diseases in the following pages are studied with reference to the way or ways in which each disease may be contracted.

Infectious diseases have, as a general rule, a period of incubation, which comprises the time elapsing between the exposure to the infection and the actual appearance of the disease. This period varies with the malady. The most common symptom of this class of diseases is fever. The severity of the fever is measured by the temperature of the animal; this is readily and accurately ascertainable by the clinical thermometer. (See pl. III, fig. 1.) The other symptoms are variable and depend on the particular organ or organs most implicated. Loss of appetite, cessation of rumination and milk secretion, and general dullness are symptoms almost invariably present in most acute infectious diseases.

During the course of infectious diseases, secondary diseases or complications may arise that are largely caused by bacteria other than those producing the original malady. These complications are often so severe as to become fatal. In general, they are due to unclean surroundings, and hence cleanliness may become an important aid to recovery.

The treatment of infectious diseases is given under each malady so far as this is allowable or advisable. These diseases are not, as a rule, amenable to treatment. When the symptoms have once appeared the disease is likely to run its course in spite of treatment, and if it is one from which animals usually recover, all that can be done is to give them the most favorable surroundings. Many infectious diseases lead sooner or later to death, treatment is useless so far as the sick animals are concerned, and it may be worse than useless for those not yet infected. Young calves obtain passive immunity against disease from their dams through the colostrum, or first milk, according to recent investigations. After the ingestion of colostrum an antitoxin appears in the blood of the young animal, thus rendering it immune, sometimes for considerable periods, to certain infections that might otherwise cause illness or death. All animals suffering with infectious diseases are more or less directly a menace to others. They represent for the time being factories of disease germs, and they are giving them off more or less abundantly during the period of disease. They may infect others directly or they may scatter the germs or virus about, and the surroundings may become a future source of infection for healthy animals. This leads to the subject of prevention as a most important point. In this place only a few general remarks will suffice to bring the subject before the reader.

The most important preventive measure is to keep disease away from a herd or farm. To do this not only should all sick or suspicious animals be avoided, but every reliable test for the detection of disease that is available to the skilled veterinarian should be applied to cattle intended to be added to a so-called clean herd. A grave form of disease may be introduced by apparently mild or trivial cases brought in from without. It is generally conceded that continual change and movement of animals are the most potent means by which infectious diseases are disseminated.

With some cattle diseases, such as anthrax, blackleg, rinderpest, and pleuropneumonia, preventive inoculation is resorted to in some countries. This may be desirable when certain other diseases have become established in any locality so that eradication is impossible. It should not be practiced in territories where a given disease may still be extirpated by ordinary precautions. Preventive inoculation is applicable to only a few maladies, and therefore its aid in the control of diseases is limited.

When an infectious disease has gained a foothold in a herd, the course to be pursued will depend on the nature of the malady. A good general rule is to kill diseased animals, especially when the disease is likely to run a chronic course, as in tuberculosis. The next important step is to separate the well from the sick by placing the former on fresh ground. This is rarely practicable; hence the destruction or removal of the sick, with thorough disinfection of the infected locality, is the next thing to be done. As to the disinfectants to be used, special directions are given under the various diseases, to which the reader is referred. Here we shall simply call attention briefly to the general subject.

DISINFECTION AND DISINFECTANTS

Disinfection consists in the use of certain substances that possess the power to destroy bacteria or their spores, or both. The efficacy of disinfectants largely depends on the mode of application and the kind of material to which they are applied; therefore some knowledge of disinfectants and of their limitations is necessary to obtain the desired results. In this discussion no attempt is made to cover the entire field but rather to indicate briefly the properties and uses of some of the disinfectants that are commonly used about the farm.

The cheapest and most available disinfectants for animal diseases are ordinary freshly slaked lime or unslaked in powder, chlorinated lime, carbolic acid, formaldehyde, compound cresol solution, lye, and sodium orthophenylphenate.

Lime.—Ordinary quicklime is one of the best and cheapest disinfectants. It is not commonly applied in the form of quicklime but as a thick mixture with water known as milk of lime. The lime is first slaked by adding 1 pint of water to 2 pounds of quicklime. Considerable heat is generated by this mixture, owing to a chemical union of the lime and the water, which forms the hydrate of lime, or water-slaked lime. The development of heat and the crumbling of the hard lumps of quicklime are indications that the lime is of good quality and that it will make a satisfactory milk of lime.

The milk of lime is obtained by adding 4 parts of water to 1 part of the slaked lime and mixing thoroughly. Lime that has been exposed to the air for a long time becomes air-slaked, that is, it takes up moisture and carbonic acid from the air and is converted into carbonate of lime, which is like marble and almost totally worthless as a disinfectant. After quicklime has been slaked with water, the slaked lime and any stock solution of milk of lime that may have been prepared should be kept in tightly closed containers to prevent deterioration, which will result from the action of the air. Whitewash is prepared by adding water to milk of lime until a mixture of suitable density is obtained.

Quicklime may be scattered about yards and lots, and the milk of lime is a good disinfectant for sickroom discharges. It should be added to urine or excreta in liberal quantity and allowed to remain in contact with these discharges for 2 hours before they are disposed of. Whitewashing of fences, pens, and the interior of outhouses serves to render them more sanitary as well as more attractive in appearance. Lime is well suited for use about dairy barns on account of the lack of any odor. It is preferable to chlorinated lime for that reason.

The advantages of lime as a disinfectant consist in its ready availability and cheapness. It is not, however, a reliable disinfectant against the most resistant forms of germ life, such as the spores of the anthrax bacillus.

Chlorinated lime.—This substance is commonly known also as bleaching powder or chloride of lime. It is a white powder that gives off the disagreeable odor of chlorine. It should be kept in hermetically sealed containers, as exposure to the air causes it to deteriorate rapidly. The efficacy of chlorinated lime largely depends on the quantity of available chlorine that it contains. The United States Pharmacopoeia requires that at least 30 percent of chlorine should be present in available form.

Although chlorinated lime is a powerful disinfectant, its potency is immediately and greatly reduced when it is brought into contact with organic matter. This is due to the fact that the available chlorine combines quickly with the organic matter and is thus diverted from its desired action on the germs. For the disinfection of sickroom discharges, manure, etc., it should be applied liberally to make allowance for the chlorine that will be used up by the organic matter. Besides being a good disinfectant, chlorinated lime is a powerful deodorant.

Chlorinated lime is only partly soluble; therefore, in preparing it for use it is well first to rub it up well with a little water so as to break up the lumps and finally dilute to the desired volume. For general household and farm use, 6 ounces of chlorinated lime should be mixed with 1 gallon of water.

Crude carbolic acid.—This product is a dark, oily fluid that is obtained during the distillation of coal tar and usually contains little or no true carbolic acid. It has been widely used in this country as a household and farm disinfectant. Essentially, crude carbolic acid is a mixture of oils and "tar acids." There is little to be said in favor of the use of crude carbolic acid as a disinfectant. Its composition is generally uncertain and it possesses no advantage over other disinfectants, which, considering their power and their ready availability, are to be preferred.

Carbolic acid (phenol).—This product in its pure form, at ordinary temperatures, is in the shape of long, white crystals. For convenience it is frequently dispensed in liquid form by the addition of 10 percent of water. A 5-percent solution of carbolic acid is sometimes used as a disinfectant. The advantages of carbolic acid are: It is reasonably effective for destroying most of the common bacteria; its action is not greatly hindered by organic matter; in a 5-percent solution it does not materially injure metals or fabrics after contact for 1 hour or less; it is readily available at all drug stores. The disadvantages are: It is not effective against all forms of bacteria; it is expensive; it is very poisonous; the strong odor is absorbed by milk.

Bichloride of mercury.—This substance, known also as corrosive sublimate and mercuric chloride, is used in a solution in water, commonly in strength of 1 to 1,000, though solutions of double that strength may be employed. Although possessing great germicidal power, it has the disadvantages of being a violent poison, of corroding metals, and of uniting with albuminous substances, such as excreta and blood, and thus forming inert compounds. Unlike the coal-tar products, it leaves no odor in the stable, which is an advantage in connection with the production of milk. On the other hand, a solution of this chemical is poisonous to animals and to man and its use for general stable disinfection is questionable. If used, it should be handled with the utmost care, and feed boxes or water troughs to which it has been applied must be washed thoroughly with clear water before animals again have access to them.

Formaldehyde.—An aqueous solution containing approximately 40 percent of formaldehyde (formalin) has in recent years become a more or less popular disinfectant. Formaldehyde is used in either liquid or gaseous form. In the former a 40-percent solution is mixed with the water in the proportion of 6 ounces to 1 gallon, and the resulting solution is applied directly to surfaces or substances that are to be disinfected.

Formaldehyde gas is in most cases impracticable for stable disinfection. When, however, a stable can be made almost airtight and the animals removed, it is very serviceable as it penetrates every crevice. Several methods are used in disinfecting with formaldehyde gas. Probably one of the most practicable is to liberate the gas by means of the chemical reaction that takes place when a formaldehyde solution is poured upon permanganate of potassium. For each 1,000 cubic feet of air space, 16⅔ ounces of crystallized or powered permanganate of potassium is placed in a wide pan; 20 ounces of a 40-percent formaltehyde solution is then poured upon it and the room immediately closed for 12 hours or longer. This method is efficient only when it is possible to seal tightly the rooms or compartments to be disinfected and when their temperature is not below 50° F.

Compound cresol solution (*liquor cresolis compositus*).—This product, now recognized by the United States Pharmacopoeia as an official preparation, is composed of equal parts of cresol (U. S. P.) and linseed-oil-potash soap. In a 3- to 4-percent solution it is an efficient disinfectant against all ordinary diseases and has the advantage of mixing readily with water. The chief objection to its use, however, is the strong odor that it is likely to impart to milk. This greatly affects its usefulness in dairy barns.

Saponified cresol solution as prepared by various manufacturers is sometimes used as a substitute for compound cresol solution (U. S. P.). Under regulations of the Department of Agriculture, only such preparations of saponified cresol solution as meet certain requirements are permitted for official disinfection of cars, boats, other vehicles, premises, etc. A list of such permitted disinfectants is furnished by the Bureau of Animal Industry Washington, D. C., on request.

Lye.—Ordinary lye, through its content of sodium hydroxide, is an effective disinfectant against foot-and-mouth disease in countries where it exists. It is effective against filtrable viruses in general and destroys most bacteria. The lye should contain approximately 94 percent, by weight, of sodium hydroxide, and for general disinfection should be used in the proportion of 1 pound to 5½ gallons of water. Care should be taken to dissolve the lye completely and to have the solution well mixed before using. As exposure to air will affect the efficiency of lye as a disinfectant, it should be taken from tight containers, and the solution should be newly prepared.

Lye has certain disadvantages that should not be overlooked. It is not effective against the germs of tuberculosis. In concentrated form it is a caustic poison. Livestock should not have access to lye or to solutions of it. Serious results may follow breathing the dust or the introduction of any of the solution into the eyes. The caustic properties of lye cause injury to painted or varnished surfaces and fabrics. These are characteristics that should not be overlooked when considering its use as a disinfectant.

Sodium orthophenylphenate.—This substance has proved to be a valuable disinfectant and, like compound cresol solution, is effective against the germs of tuberculosis. It has an advantage over saponified cresol solution in being free from objectionable odor. It is readily soluble in water and is in the form of a grayish, brownish, or white powder, which must necessarily be kept in a close container in order to prevent deterioration. It is not highly poisonous. As the solution is not effective at a low temperature, it becomes necessary to apply it hot in order to insure satisfactory results. Sodium orthophenylphenate preparations under specific named brands are permitted in official disinfection in tuberculosis-eradication work.

When it is desired to apply a disinfectant to the stable or barnyard, a preliminary cleaning up of all debris and litter is advisable, together with the scraping of the floor, mangers, and walls of the stable with hoes, also the removal of all dust and filth. This should be followed by the burning of all such accumulations, inasmuch as this material likewise contains the infectious principle and is best destroyed by heat. Heat may be applied to the surface of the affected pen or barnyard by means of a special burner, which consists of a tank, pump, hose, and nozzle for spraying with oil. The latter is ejected in the form of spray, which when ignited gives a very hot and effective flame to be applied to the infected ground. Where such burning is impracticable the surface soil of the yard and surroundings should be removed to a depth of 5 or 6 inches and then placed in a heap and thoroughly mixed with air-slaked lime. The fresh surface of the soil thus exposed may then be sprinkled with the disinfectant.

In addition to these artificial substances there are several natural sanitary agents of great importance as destroyers of virus. These are cleanliness, ventilation, drying, and sunshine. All virus, except such as may live in the soil, is killed sooner or later by drying and sunshine, and the importance of these factors in the daily life of animals need not be emphasized here. Finally, all sanitary measures that contribute to the healthfulness of animal surroundings are directly or indirectly unfavorable to disease germs, and all carelessness in the keeping of animals may be regarded as an ally of these destructive organisms.

CONTAGIOUS PLEUROPNEUMONIA

[Pls. XXIX–XXXII]

Definition and history.—This disease has been eradicated from the United States, and it is not probable that it will ever be seen in this country again. However, as much interest was manifested in it for a number of years, and as it must be identified if it ever occurs here again, the subject is treated at greater length than would otherwise be necessary.

Contagious pleuropneumonia of cattle is a specific, epizootic disease that affects bovine animals and from which other species are exempt. When the disease results from exposure in the usual manner, it is characterized by an inflammation of the lungs and pleurae, which is generally extensive and which has a tendency to invade portions of these organs not primarily affected and to cause death of the diseased portion of the lung. This disease is frequently called lung plague, which corresponds to its German name "Lungenseuche." In French it is spoken of as the "péripneumonie contagieuse."

The history of contagious pleuropneumonia of cattle cannot be traced with any certainty to a period earlier than the beginning of the eighteenth century. No doubt it existed and ravaged the herds of Europe for many years and perhaps centuries before that time, but veterinary knowledge was so limited that the descriptions of the symptoms and post mortem appearance are too vague and too limited to admit of the identification of the maladies to which they refer. It has been supposed by some writers that certain passages in the writings of Aristotle, Livy, and Virgil show the existence of pleuropneumonia at the time that their works were composed, but their references are too indefinite to be seriously accepted as indicating this rather than some other disease.

It seems evident that as early as 1713 and 1714 pleuropneumonia existed in Swabia and several Cantons of Switzerland. There are even clearer accounts of its prevalence in Switzerland in 1732, 1743, and 1765. In 1769 a disease called murie was investigated in Franche-Comté by Bourgelat, which undoubtedly was identical with the pleuropneumonia of today. From that period there are frequent and well-authenticated accounts of its existence in various parts of Europe. From 1790 to 1812 it was spread throughout a large portion of the Continent of Europe by the cattle driven for the subsistence of the armies, which marched and countermarched in all directions. It was generally prevalent in Italy in 1800. It appears to have been unknown, however, in the Department of the Nord, France, until 1826, but from 1820 to 1840 it penetrated into most parts of that country. During the same period it was introduced into and spread over Belgium and Holland.

This contagion is said to have been carried to Ireland from Holland in 1839 and is reported as existing in England in 1842. The disease was brought to the United States several different times. Probably its first introduction was by means of a diseased cow sold in Brooklyn, N. Y., in 1843. It came to New Jersey by importing affected animals in 1847. Massachusetts was infected in the same way in 1859.

The Union of South Africa was infected by a bull brought from the Netherlands in 1854. The Union authorities. however, were successful in getting rid of the disease about 1917. It is declared to exist, however, in certain regions of Africa north of the Union, including Egypt and the Sudan. Australia received the contagion by means of a cow imported from England in 1858 and continues to have areas of infection, especially in Queensland and South Australia It is reported as existing in the Union of Soviet Socialist Republics. Just how extensive the disease may be in other portions of Asia, including China and India, cannot be stated. Japan, a progressive country in matters relating to veterinary science and control, still harbors contagious pleuropneumonia.

Countries of Europe formerly infected have generally succeeded in eradicating the disease, and the extent of the affection in Europe is now limited.

In the United States, Massachusetts eradicated pleuropneumonia during the period from 1860 to 1866. New York and New Jersey made an attempt to eradicate it in 1879 but were not successful. Late in 1883 the contagion was carried to Ohio, probably by Jersey cattle purchased in the vicinity of Baltimore, Md., to which place it had extended before 1868. From the herd then infected it was spread by the sale of cattle during 1884 to a limited number of herds in Illinois, to one herd in Missouri, and to two in Kentucky. The alarm caused among the stock owners of the United States by this widespread dissemination of a disease so much dreaded led to the adoption of active measures for its control and eradication. By cooperation between the United States Department of Agriculture and the authorities of the affected States, it was possible to prevent the further spread of the contagion and to eradicate it after a few months' delay.

In 1886 pleuropneumonia was discovered in some of the large distillery stables of Chicago and among cows on neighboring lots. This led to renewed efforts for the complete eradication of this disease from the country. Congress in 1887 enlarged the appropriation available for this purpose and gave more extended authority. During the same year the disease was stamped out of Chicago and has not since appeared in any district west of the Allegheny Mountains.

The work of eradication was at the same time commenced in all the infected States. Before the end of 1889 Pennsylvania, Delaware, Maryland, the District of Columbia, and Virginia had been freed from the disease. More difficulties, however, were encountered in New York and New Jersey, on account of the larger territory infected and the density of the population. The long struggle was successful, however, and the last animal in which the disease appeared in the State of New York was slaughtered early in 1891, and the last one affected in New Jersey met the same fate early in the spring of 1892.

During these same years a supreme effort was made to stamp out this lung plague from Great Britain. From the official reports it appears that the number of infected districts and of diseased animals had rapidly diminished, but it was not until 1898 that the infection was finally eradicated.

Some other infected countries, though they maintain a veterinary sanitary service, are not making satisfactory progress in eradicating the disease. This is due partly to delays in carrying out the provisions of the laws and partly to mistaken ideas as to the measures that are necessary to accomplish the object. The United States was the last of the countries, having old infected districts, that undertook to stamp out this contagion, and, except Holland, it was the first to reach success.

Cause.—This is a contagious disease and arises only by contagion from a previously affected animal; consequently it can never be seen in the United States except as the result of importing affected animals from the countries in which it exists. When thoroughly stamped out it does not reappear; and if imported animals continue to be properly inspected and quarantined, there is every reason to believe that pleuropneumonia will never again be seen in this country.

The cause of the disease is a very minute micro-organism known as *Asterococcus mycoides*, which is readily destroyed by heat but which may survive for months in frozen tissues. There is no evidence that the virus can propagate itself outside the animal body except by specially designed methods of culture.

Some investigators and writers are of the opinion that the disease can be contracted only by an animal coming near enough to a living diseased one to receive the contagion directly from it. They hold that the contagion is exhaled with the air from the affected lungs, and that it must be almost immediately inspired by another animal in order to produce the disease. Some experimental attempts to infect animals by placing them in stables where diseased animals have been, and by placing the diseased lungs of slaughtered animals in their feeding troughs, have failed, and, consequently, apparently confirm this view.

On the other hand, it is known that the serum from affected lungs retains its virulence and may be used successfully for inoculation weeks or months after the death of the animal from which it was taken. This is particularly the case when this liquid is hermetically sealed in glass tubes. Some investigators state that they have successfully infected cattle by placing, in the nostrils, sponges or pledgets of cotton saturated with such serum. According to the best evidence obtainable, cattle have also been infected from the clothing of attendants, from horns used in drenching, and from smelling about wagons that have been used to transport affected carcasses. In the work of eradicating pleuropneumonia from the United States, many stables were found in which the disease appeared and reappeared after the slaughter of affected herds, and in spite of any precautions that were adopted. These were always old stables, with woodwork in a decaying condition and with floors underlaid with filth that could not be thoroughly removed or disinfected. In every one of these cases the destruction of the stables, the burning of the lumber of which it was constructed, the removal of the accumulations beneath the floors, and thorough disinfection, prevented the recurrence of the plague in new stables built on the same premises. This experience conclusively shows that under certain conditions, at least, stables may retain the infection for a considerable time, and that when they are restocked the disease may break out again from such infection.

As a rule, however, the disease is acquired by a healthy animal being near an affected one and receiving the contagion direct. Affected animals may give off the contagion in the early stages of the disease before the symptoms are apparent to the observer; also, they may retain this infectious character, if they survive the attack, for 6 months and probably for a year after all symptoms of the disease have disappeared.

Incubation.—The time that elapses between exposure to the contagion of pleuropneumonia and the first appearance of the symptoms of this disease varies greatly with different individuals and with different outbreaks of the disease. Ordinarily the symptoms of disease make their appearance within 3 to 6 weeks after exposure; they may be observed, however, within 2 weeks or they may not become apparent until nearly or quite 3 months. The long period of incubation and the great length of time that an animal may disseminate the contagion after apparent recovery are the factors which give the plague that insidious character so often spoken of and which greatly increase the difficulties of eradication.

Symptoms.—The symptoms are such as would be expected with inflammation of the lungs and pleurae, but they vary considerably, according to the type that the disease manifests. If the attack is acute, as is frequently seen in hot weather, the symptoms appear suddenly; breathing becomes rapid and difficult, the animal grunts or moans with each expiration, the shoulders stand out from the chest, the head is extended on the neck, the back is arched, the temperature is 104° to 107° F., the milk secretion is suspended, there is no appetite, rumination is stopped, the animal may bloat and later be affected with a severe diarrhea. Such cases are generally fatal in 7 to 20 days.

CONTAGIOUS PLEUROPNEUMONIA

DESCRIPTION OF PLATES

PLATE XXIX. Upper or dorsal surface of normal healthy lungs of a cow, reduced to one-twelfth of the natural size: *a*, *a′*, the right and left principal lobes. These are the largest and are situated posteriorly, resting upon the diaphragm; *b*, *b′*, the ventral lobes, situated between the principal lobes; and *c*, *c′*, *c″* the most anterior, or cephalic, lobes. The right anterior is divided into two lobes (*c*, *c′*), the left is single (*c″*); *d*, trachea, or windpipe.

In most of the lungs that were examined and that were affected with contagious pleuropneumonia, the principal lobes (*a*, *a′*) were primarily affected.

PLATE XXX. Bronchopneumonia. The ventral or middle lobe of the right lung affected with collapse and beginning bronchopneumonia. The light yellowish portions represent healthy lung tissue; the red represents the disease. It will be noticed that the lines between the lobules are quite faint, indicating little or no inflammation of the connective tissue between the lobules. The healthy lung tissue is seen to be raised above the level of the diseased portion. In contagious pleuropneumonia, the exact reverse is the case, the diseased portions being very much larger than the healthy.

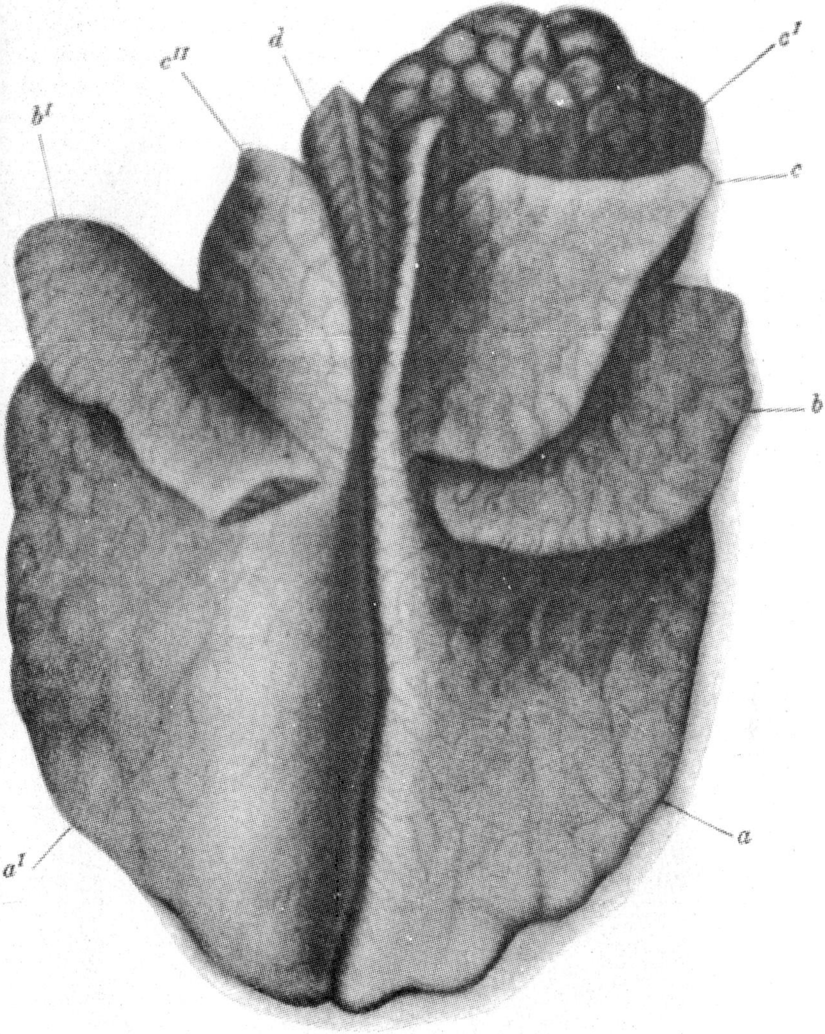

HAINES DEL.

UPPER OR DORSAL SURFACE OF NORMAL HEALTHY LUNGS OF A COW.
(One-twelfth natural size.)

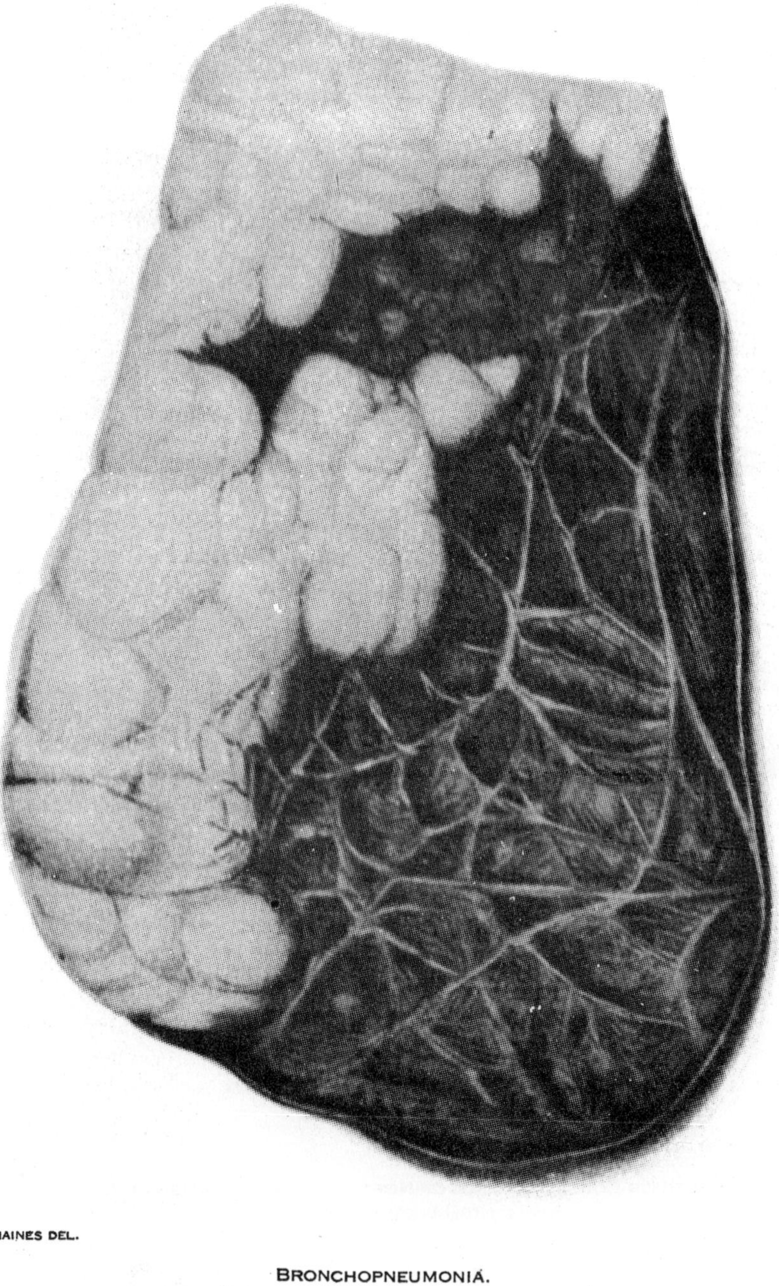

HAINES DEL.

BRONCHOPNEUMONIA.

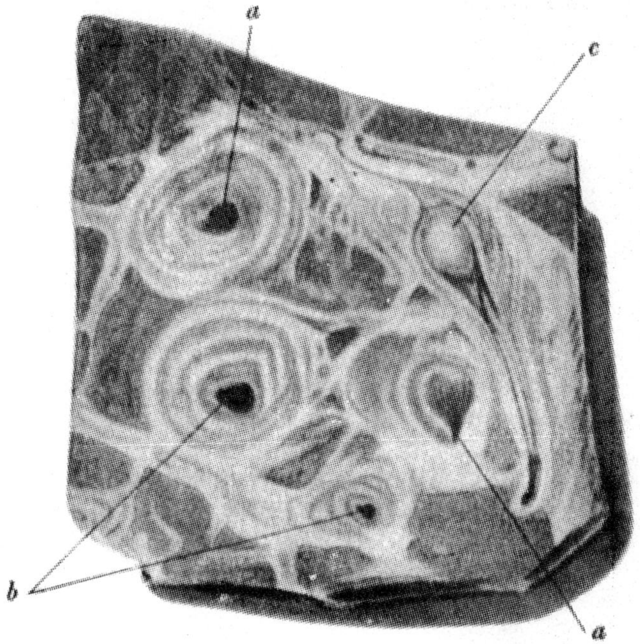

FIGURE 1

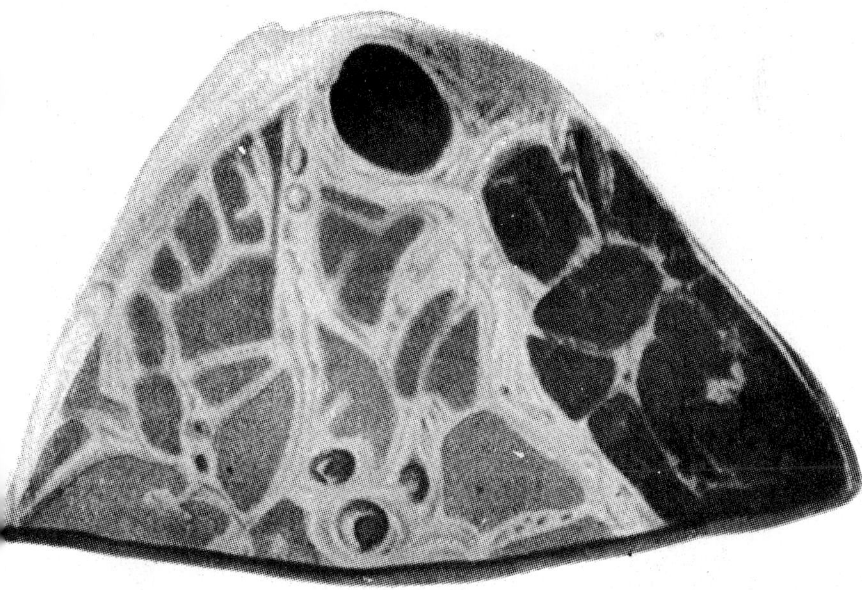

HAINES DEL.

FIGURE 2

CONTAGIOUS PLEUROPNEUMONIA.

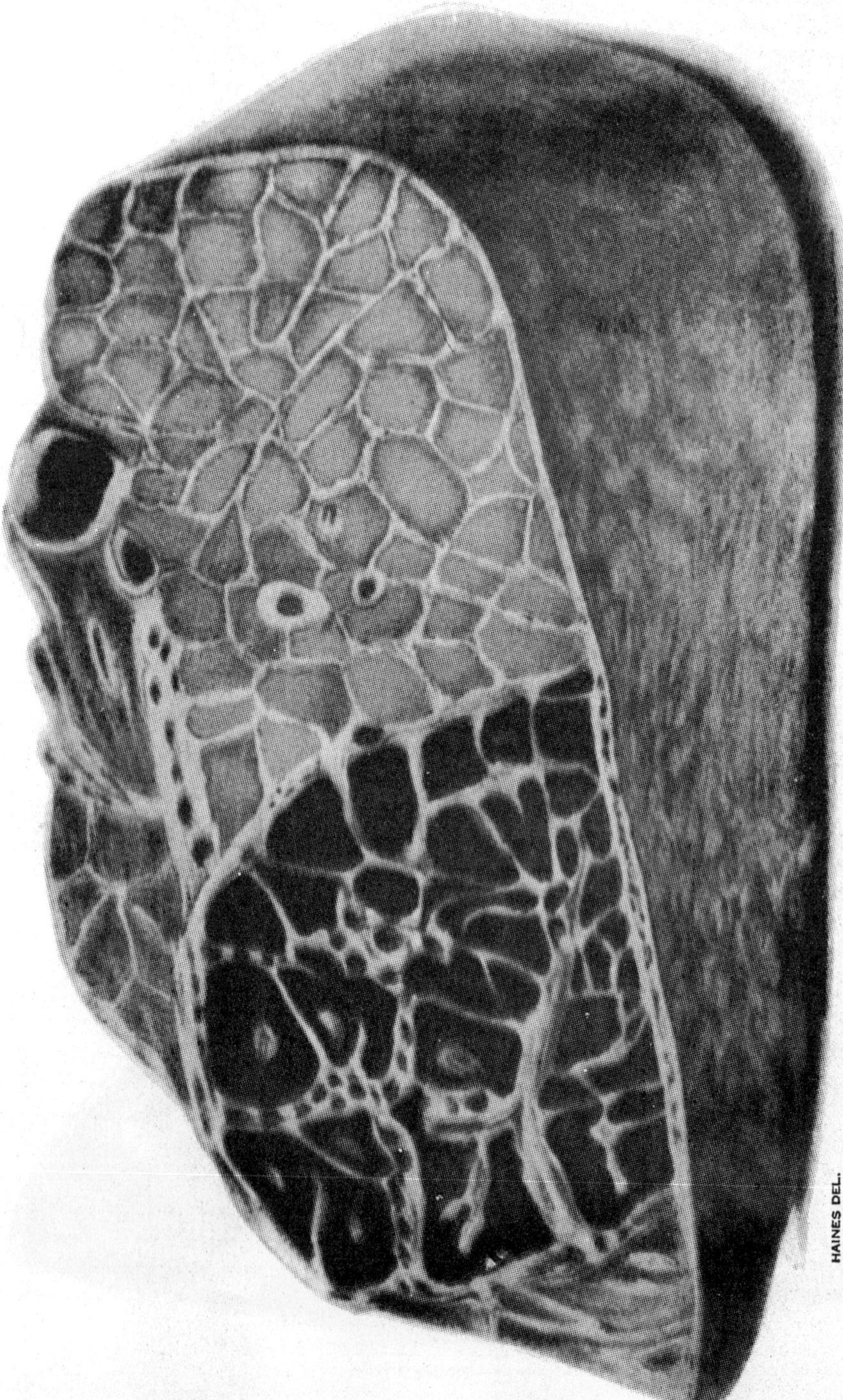

HAINES DEL.

PLATE XXXI. Contagious pleuropneumonia. Appearance of a cow's lung affected with contagious pleuropneumonia when sections or slices are made of it and cut surfaces examined.

Figure 1. Transverse section through the right principal lobe in a case of acute pleuropneumonia. The area drawn includes the air tubes, veins, and arteries, and illustrates the great thickening of the interlobular connective tissue into broad whitish bands and of the walls of the air tubes, veins, and arteries: *a*, Air tube cut obliquely; *a'*, air tube cut directly across; *b*, arteries cut across; *c*, large vein completely occluded by a thrombus or plug formed during life. The great thickening of the walls of the artery and vein is characteristic of this disease. In the healthy lung they are so thin as to be easily overlooked.

Figure 2. Transverse section of the principal lobe in a case of acute pleuropneumonia, illustrating the different kinds of hepatization or consolidation of the lung. These are indicated by the different colors from dark red to reddish yellow. This variation of color is regarded by some as the real marbling characteristic of pleuropneumonia, whereas the whitish bands penetrating the lung tissue in all directions constitute the true marbling according to other observers.

PLATE XXXII. Contagious pleuropneumonia. This illustrates what are called infarctions. The right half of the figure shows nearly normal lung tissue. The left represents a blackish mass, in which the lung tissue is filled with blood and solidified. This is caused by the plugging of the vein carrying away the blood from this portion. The heart forces the blood through the artery into the tissue at considerable pressure, but owing to the fact that its return is prevented, the minute blood vessels rupture and the air vesicles become distended with blood, which coagulates and causes the firmness of the tissue.

Often the attack comes on slowly and the symptoms are much less clear. In the mildest cases there is a cough for a week or two but no appreciable loss of appetite or elevation of temperature. The lungs are but slightly affected and recovery soon follows: Such animals may disseminate the contagion for a long time without being suspected and for that reason are the most dangerous.

A more severe type of the plague is most frequently seen. In these cases the cough is frequent, more or less painful, the back somewhat arched, and the milk secretion diminished. The prominence of these symptoms increases, the appetite is affected, the animal loses flesh, breathing becomes more rapid, the cough more painful, pressure of the fingers between the ribs shows tenderness, the hair loses its gloss and stands erect, the skin becomes adherent, little, if any, milk is secreted, and the temperature rises, varying in different animals from 103° to 107° F. Animals thus affected may continue to grow worse and die in 3 to 8 weeks, or they may after a time begin to improve and make an apparent recovery. The inflammation of the lung does not subside, as a rule, and the organ return to its normal condition, as in ordinary pneumonia, but in pleuropneumonia the life of the affected portion of the lungs is destroyed, the tissue

77431 O—51——24

dies, and a fibrous wall is formed around it to shut it away from the living parts. The tissue, thus encysted, gradually softens, becomes disintegrated, and breaks down into pus. The recovery therefore is not complete; it is only apparent and partial.

To those accustomed to examining the lungs of cattle, other and extremely important symptoms may be apparent during the course of the disease. By applying the ear over the walls of the chest, an area of a certain extent may be found in which the natural breathing sound is diminished or entirely lost. This represents the diseased portion of the lungs. In other cases a loud blowing sound may be heard, quite different from any sound produced when the lung is in a healthy condition. In some cases a crackling sound is heard near the border line of the diseased area and friction sounds produced by the roughened pleura; these can be appreciated, however, only by those whose ears have been trained to distinguish between the different sounds that reach the ear when applied to the chest wall. By percussion—that is by pressing the fingers of the left hand firmly against the wall of the chest and tapping upon the middle finger with the ends of the fingers of the right hand—an area of dullness may be discovered corresponding to the portion from which the respiratory murmur has disappeared. This loss of respiration detected by auscultation and the dullness brought out by percussion are the most important evidences of an inflamed or consolidated lung.

Seriously affected animals remain standing if they have sufficient strength, but those that lie down always lie on the affected side.

The proportion of animals that become affected after being exposed varies according to the virulence of the outbreak, the susceptibility of the animals, and the length of time during which exposure is continued. Sometimes not more than 15, 20, or 30 percent contract the disease when a large herd is exposed; on the other hand, 80 or 90 percent may be affected. The proportion of cases in which the disease proves fatal also varies greatly—it may not exceed 10 and it may reach 50 percent. In general, about 40 percent of the exposed animals contract the disease and about one-half of these cases prove fatal.

Post mortem appearances.—Owing to the complex structure of the lung tissue, its ramifications of bronchial tubes and blood vessels, and its abundant supply of lymphatics, the pathological changes in pleuropneumonia are interpreted with great difficulty. Furthermore, certain kinds of pneumonia have some resemblances to pleuropneumonia and may therefore be confused with it in some of its phases.

If an animal affected with acute pleuropneumonia is killed and the cavity of the chest and lungs examined, the following appearances will be noted:

The thorax may contain more or less serum, which may be clear or clouded. There may be firm adhesions of different parts of the lungs to the chest wall, the extent of which depends on the stage and severity of the disease. The diseased lobes are unusually large and exceedingly firm to the touch. The weight of a single large lobe may reach 40 pounds. Usually only one side is affected and often but a single lobe—most commonly the large or principal lobe. The pleura may be covered with one or more layers of a firm, elastic, grayish membrane, which varies in thickness and sometimes may be pulled away entirely. Sometimes this is absent. The pleura, however, is opaque and apparently much thickened. This is due to the diseased condition of the connective tissue beneath the pleura, as is explained later. When an affected lobe is cut through at right angles to its long diameter, the cut surface shows a variety of interesting changes. In the first place, the spaces between the small subdivisions of the lung (the lobules), which in the healthy lung are barely visible, are distended with a yellowish-white, usually rather firm, substance, which is coagulated fibrin. The cut surface thus appears to be divided into small fields by yellowish-white bands of varying thickness running in different directions through the lung tissue and beneath the pleura (pl. XXXI). These bands may appear honeycombed and the spaces filled with yellowish fluid (serum), or they may be uniformly solid. The space immediately outside of and around the artery, vein, and air tube is similarly broadened by fibrinous deposits. Some authorities look upon these bands as constituting the so-called marbling of pleuropneumonia.

In addition to these changes that have taken place in the connective tissue between the lobules, the lung tissue itself may be markedly altered. Certain areas of the cut surface may be very firm in texture and of a brownish-red color. The cut surface is granular or roughened, not smooth to the eye. Other areas equally firm may be more grayish yellow, and still others may be blackish (pl. XXXII). Besides these areas, which represent solidified (hepatized) lung tissue, there may be others approaching the normal lung tissue in color, are soft, and float in water. From these a milky, purulent fluid may often be expressed. These different shades are represented in plate XXXI, figure 2, within a small compass. Some authorities consider these variations in color on the same cut surface as the so-called marbling of pleuropneumonia. It matters not whether the bands between the lobules or the varying shades of the lobules themselves are regarded as the marbling, provided either or both are peculiar to contagious pleuropneumonia. If the blood vessels appearing on such cut surface are examined, they are usually found to be plugged within the firmly hepatized regions. The artery contains a dark, soft, removable clot, the vein a grayish-pink, granular, fragile plug (thrombus), which adheres firmly to the wall of the vein, and if this is slit open, indications of a diseased condition of the inner coat will be readily detected.

When large regions of the lung tissues are solidified, the main air tube and its branches are usually filled with grayish, cylindrical branched masses of fibrin that are easily removed, as they do not adhere to the mucous membrane.

The views of pathologists differ as to the nature of the earliest changes in pleuropneumonia, and it is not within the scope of this work to present controverted or imperfectly developed theories. In the foregoing description, acute pleuropneumonia in its fully developed phase has been taken as a type and this can scarcely be mistaken for any other disease. It has been shown that there is an inflammatory condition of the connective tissue between the lobules, resulting in the exudation of coagulable lymph. This inflammation is equally marked around the blood vessels and air tubes. It leads to inflammatory changes in the inner wall of the veins, and these cause the deposition of thrombi or plugs in the vessels, which prevent the return of the blood. The blood pumped into the lung tissue through the artery, but unable to get out by way of the vein, leaves the meshwork of capillaries around the air vesicles, enters the latter, and produces the firm, hepatized condition so characteristic of this disease. If one bears in mind that the veins in different parts of the lung tissue are plugged at different times, and that, therefore, the affected regions are in different stages of disease, it will be easily understood how the different shades of color from dark red to grayish or yellowish red are produced.

The complete plugging of the veins may lead to the death of circumscribed masses of lung tissue. A line of separation forms between the living and the dead tissue, and a thick cyst wall of fibrous tissue forms around the latter. The dead tissue for a time preserves the appearance of lung tissue, then undergoes disintegration and liquefaction. The softened mass is finally absorbed, and the walls of the cyst, or capsule around it, gradually collapse and form a cicatrix. This favorable termination takes place only when the dead mass is not too large. It may, however, involve more than half of one of the large lobes. Under such circumstances recovery is improbable. A more favorable termination is the abundant growth of fibrous tissue around and into the hepatized masses. The formation of fibrous tissue may extend to the pleura, or lung covering, and cause firm adhesion of the lungs to the chest wall and to the pericardium, or heart case.

The same peculiar, inflammatory changes that take place between the lobules of the lung and around the bronchi and vessels may invade the pleural cavity, cause extensive membranous and spongy deposits on the pleura, and firm deposits around the heart and large arteries, the gullet, and windpipe.

These are the main features of the lung disease caused by contagious pleuropneumonia. In the typical, acute cases there are a sufficient number of peculiarities to enable one to make a positive diagnosis. There are, however, many cases in which the disease is restricted to small areas or to the interlobular tissue, or in which the changes are still imperfectly developed or so far advanced that doubts may arise as to the true nature of the affection. In such cases all obtainable facts, including the history of the case, the symptoms during life, and the pathological changes observed on post mortem examination must be taken into consideration. Only one who has made a careful study of the disease is fitted to decide in such cases.

Other kinds of lung disease, because of certain features common to most lung diseases of cattle, may be confounded with pleuropneumonia. The inflammation of the connective tissue between the lobules is not infrequently observed in so-called interstitial pneumonia and may lead to the formation of whitish bands intersecting the lung tissues in various directions. On the cut surface these bands may give rise to a decidedly marbled appearance. Again, in traumatic pneumonia, caused, as its name implies, by the entrance of foreign bodies into the lung tissue, generally from the paunch, the connective tissue around the place of disease becomes inflamed and thickened, and the disease itself may simulate pleuropneumonia in its retrogressive stages when it is confined to a small portion of lung tissue. The filling up of the interlobular spaces with fibrin and connective tissue of inflammatory origin is not thus limited to pleuropneumonia but may appear in a marked degree in other lung diseases. It must not be inferred from this statement that these interlobular changes are necessarily the same as those in pleuropneumonia, although to the naked eye they may appear the same. We simply note their presence without discussing their nature.

In general, the distinction between pleuropneumonia and bronchopneumonia it not difficult. In the latter disease the pneumonia generally invades certain lobes. The disease attacks the smaller lobes in their lowest portions first and gradually extends upward, that is, toward the root of the lung or the back of the animal and backward into the large principal lobes. Again, both lungs in advanced cases are often symmetrically affected. In contagious pleuropneumonia, the large principal lobe of one side is most frequently affected, and a symmetrical disease of both lungs is very rare. The lung tissue in bronchopneumonia is not enlarged but rather more contracted than the normal tissue around it. This is well illustrated in plate XXX. Normal, air-containing lobules may be scattered among and around the hepatized portion in an irregular manner. In pleuropneumonia the diseased and healthy portions are either sharply divided off, one from the other, or they shade into each other by intermediate stages.

The hepatized lung tissue in bronchopneumonia, when the cut surface is examined, is usually of a more or less dark flesh color with paler grayish-yellow dots regularly interspersed, giving it a peculiarly mottled appearance. In the more advanced stages it becomes more firm and may contain nodular and firmer masses disseminated through it. The air tubes usually contain more or less soft, creamy, or cheesy pus or a turbid fluid quite different from the loose, fibrinous casts of acute pleuropneumonia. The interlobular tissue may or may not be affected. It sometimes contains loose, fibrinous plugs, or it may be greatly distended with air, especially in the still normal portions of the lung. The pleura is seldom seriously diseased. If these features are contrasted with the firm dark-red hepatizations, the plugging of the veins, the extensive interlobular deposits, and the well-marked pleuritis in pleuropneumonia, there is little chance for confusion between well-developed cases of these two lung diseases.

It should not be forgotten, however, that the lesions of the disease known as contagious pleuropneumonia may be confined to the serous membranes of the thorax or to the parenchyma of the lungs; they may affect a whole lobe or only a small portion of it; they may or may not cause the so-called marbled appearance. In the same way bronchopneumonia may vary as to the parts of the lung affected, the extent of the lesions, the degree and kind of pathological changes in the interlobular tissue, the color of the lung on cross section, and the amount of hepatization. In individual cases, therefore, it is often necessary to take into account the history of the animal, the course of the disease, and the communicability of the affection before a diagnosis can be made between the two diseases.

Prevention and treatment.—The prevention of pleuropneumonia, as of other contagious diseases, consists in handling animals so that they will not be exposed to the contagion. As the disease arises only by contagion, there is no possibility of an animal's becoming affected with it unless it has been exposed. If, therefore, pleuropneumonia exists in a locality, the owner of healthy cattle should make every effort to keep his animals from coming near affected or exposed animals. He should be equally particular not to allow persons who have been on the infected premises to visit his own pastures, stables, or cattle.

If pleuropneumonia breaks out in a herd, every animal in it should be slaughtered, the stables thoroughly cleaned and disinfected, and no other cattle allowed on the premises until 90 days have elapsed.

Medicinal treatment of affected animals is unavailing and should not be attempted. No matter how valuable the diseased animals may have been before they contracted the disease, they should at once be destroyed and the contagion eradicated. This is the best policy for the individual as well as for the community.

The eradication of this disease by local or national governments can be successful only when the same principles are adopted and carried out as here recommended for individual stables. It is, then, a difficult undertaking, simply because the contagion is generally widely disseminated before any measures are adopted, and because most cattle owners will never report the existence of the disease. Regulations must therefore be enforced that will insure the prompt discovery of every herd in which the disease appears, as well as the destruction of all diseased and exposed animals and the thorough disinfection of the premises.

To discover pleuropneumonia sufficiently early for this purpose, the district supposed to be infected should be clearly defined and inspectors should be constantly employed to inspect every herd in it at least once in 2 weeks, or, better, once a week. No bovine animal should be allowed to go out of the defined district alive, and all that enter it should be carefully inspected to insure their freedom from disease. As an assistance to the discovery of diseased herds, every animal that, from any cause, dies in the infected district and every animal that is slaughtered, even if apparently in good health, should be the subject of a careful post mortem examination. Many affected herds may be found in this way.

In addition to these measures, it is also necessary to guard against the removal of animals from one stable to another and the mixing of herds on common pastures or in public highways. The object must be to isolate every herd as completely as possible; otherwise a single affected animal may infect a dozen or more herds. To prevent the sale or trading of cattle without proper authority, each animal must in some way be numbered and recorded in the books kept by the official in charge of the district. In the work of the United States Department of Agriculture, a numbered metal tag was fastened to each animal's ear and index books were so arranged that with a number given the owner could be at once ascertained, or from the owner's name the cattle for which he was responsible could be at once learned. In this way, if an animal was missing from a stable, the fact became apparent at once, or if one too many was found in a stable the number in its ear would indicate its origin.

When pleuropneumonia is discovered by these means, the entire herd should be slaughtered as soon as the formalities of appraisement can be arranged. In country districts the carcasses should be buried, as it is generally impracticable to dispose of them in any other way. In city districts the animals may be taken to a slaughterhouse, with such precautions as are possible to prevent dissemination of the contagion. The animals should be slaughtered under the supervision of an inspector. The healthy carcasses may be utilized for food, but the blood, entrails, and all diseased carcasses should be heated to 212° F. or above and then used for the manufacture of fertilizer.

The disinfection of premises should be thorough and should be carried out by a trained corps of men. The floors of stables should be removed, the accumulations removed from beneath them, the contents of haylofts should be destroyed, and the woodwork and soil beneath the stables should be thoroughly drenched with a solution of bichloride of mercury, 1 part to 2,000 of water. After the flooring is replaced the woodwork should be coated with limewash, containing one-fourth pound of chloride of lime to the gallon of mixture.

Usually in these cases the owners depend on their herds of cows for a living, and consequently it is difficult or impossible to keep the stables vacant for any considerable period. In most instances cattle may be admitted at once to stables so disinfected, without the reappearance of the disease. Occasionally, however, it will reappear without apparent cause. For this reason inspection and other measures must be maintained in the infected district for 6 months or a year after the last case of disease has been disposed of.

Many persons have objected to the slaughter of diseased and exposed animals as an unscientific and expensive method of eradicating the disease. However, it is the only method that has proved to be successful, and in the end it is much more economical than temporizing measures.

RINDERPEST

Rinderpest, also known as cattle plague, is an acute, infectious disease of cattle, in which the digestive organs are mainly involved. Though the disease has never occurred in this country, the importance of having near at hand a few definite facts concerning it, should it ever reach our shores, will be at once appreciated. A knowledge of such facts may aid in an early recognition of the disease. It must not be forgotten, on the other hand, that a superficial knowledge of diseases, such as the layman may gain through reading, not infrequently leads to confounding comparatively harmless, noninfectious maladies with such as are truly dangerous (foot-and-mouth disease and rinderpest, for instance), and causes temporary panics among stock owners.

According to some authorities, rinderpest originated in the territory around the Black Sea and the Volga River; according to others, in central Asia. Thence it has been conveyed at various times by cattle to nearly every country of Europe and Asia, where it has proved to be a veritable bovine scourge. It probably visited Europe as early as the beginning of the Christian era, and since then the migrations of the people from the Far East have from time to time introduced the disease. Especially during the eighteenth century it was more or less prevalent in Europe, owing to the frequent wars, during which herds of cattle were brought from eastern Europe and Asia to supply the demands of the armies. It prevailed in Europe during the Franco-Prussian War. At present it is chiefly confined to portions of Asia and Africa.

The virus is conveyed from one country to another chiefly by means of infected cattle, although infected hides, wool, and feed may play a part in its dissemination. Railroad facilities are particularly likely to aid in the spread of the disease.

In the past, rinderpest was supposed to be identical with various human diseases, among them smallpox and typhoid fever. These suppositions are unfounded, and the view of authorities today is that it is a disease of a peculiar kind, not identical with any other known infectious disease.

Cause.—The cause of rinderpest is a filtrable virus that cannot be seen by the aid of the microscope and that appears to be definitely attached to the white cells of the blood. Experiments indicate that the unseen virus is of such dimensions that it is held by the dense bacterial filters but passes through the more porous ones. Formerly, various authorities supposed that rinderpest virus appeared spontaneously under the influence of deteriorated feed and long and exhausting drives, and also during unusual meteorological conditions. This view, however, is no longer maintained. It is probable that in its home in Asia the disease is perpetuated by continual infection of fresh animals, and some authorities go even so far as to believe that the disease would be entirely stamped out, even in its native haunts, by a destruction of all sick and infected herds. If the virus is found to be strictly parasitic, as the contagion of pleuropneumonia is now believed to be, it might be completely extirpated in this way. If, however, the virus lives and multiplies outside the bovine body, in soil, water, or in some other animal, eradication would be impossible.

The virus may be transmitted in a variety of ways, both direct and indirect, from sick to healthy animals. In the former animals, it is present in the blood, in saliva, and in the various excreta, such as discharges from the nose, the urine, and manure. The virus is believed to retain its vitality for only a short time outside the body but under certain favorable conditions may survive for a considerable time. Fodder and bedding soiled with discharges may convey it. Persons may carry the virus on their shoes, clothing, or implements. Even small animals, such as cats and rats, which frequent barns and stables, have been looked upon as carriers of the virus.

Cattle are very susceptible to the disease, and in its virulent type all those exposed are said to become infected. Buffaloes, sheep, and goats are likewise susceptible, but in a less degree.

It is also claimed that after animals have passed through one attack they are usually successful in resisting future attacks. Inoculation with virus in various forms is said to produce immunity, but in many cases the process of inoculation itself is followed by death. Serum from immunized cattle prevents infection but it must be repeatedly injected to insure continuous protection.

Symptoms.—The symptoms of rinderpest are not very characteristic; hence, the diagnosis of a suspected case in the beginning of an invasion is attended with difficulties. Certain appearances that are characteristic of one epizootic may be absent in another. Different observers do not agree as to the most constant and important.

The period of incubation—the time between exposure to infection and the earliest outward symptoms—varies from 3 to 9 days. The first sign is a very high fever, which may reach 107° F. The heat of the skin varies in different parts of the body and may be felt at the base of the ears and horns. Repeated chills are frequently observed. The pulse reaches 50 to 60 beats a minute and in very severe attacks may rise to 90 or 100.

The animal manifests great debility. The head droops and rests on some object of support. One or both ears may droop. The coat is staring and the muzzle dry. The secretion of milk diminishes rapidly. Within 12 to 20 hours the usual quantity may have become reduced one-half or two-thirds. The back is arched, and the legs are brought together under the body.

As the disease progresses, symptoms with reference to the digestive and respiratory organs become prominent. The mucous membrane of the mouth and the nose, as well as that of the rectum and vagina, becomes reddened, either in patches or diffusely, and assumes a scarlet hue. The discharges, at first firm, become softer, and soon diarrhea sets in. This is said to be one of the most constant symptoms. The rectum may become everted and paralyzed, and the bowels move spontaneously. The discharges become fetid, viscid, and streaked with blood. Coughing is a common symptom and by some is considered characteristic. It is associated with discharges from the nose and vagina and dribbling of saliva from the mouth. The eyes also are affected. There is an increased formation of a viscid secretion that flows down the face.

Another series of changes prominent in some epizootics and mild or absent in others are ulcers, or so-called erosions, in the mouth. These begin as red patches and streaks. The mucous membrane in such localities is converted into a grayish-white slough, which, when shed, leaves a small erosion, or ulcer. At the same time similar changes may go on in the skin of the thighs, the udder, or the scrotum, or about the vagina, which lead to small sloughs.

In severe cases, which are the most common in the susceptible cattle of western Europe, death ensues 4 to 7 days after the first appearance of the disease and is preceded by great emaciation and debility, fetid, purulent discharges from the nose and mouth, and the relaxed rectum and vagina.

If the animal is opened after death and the organs are carefully examined, the chief changes are found in the digestive organs. The lining membrane of the mouth and pharynx is covered with mucus, is reddened in spots, and shows superficial, yellowish-gray, cheesy patches, which represent dead tissue, and when removed expose ulcerated depressions. The same reddening in spots and the yellowish-gray, cheesy deposits or patches are found in the fourth stomach, the small intestines, and more rarely in the cecum, and the third stomach, or manyplies, is more or less impacted with dry, hard feed. Similar changes may be found on the mucous membrane of the nasal cavity, larynx, trachea, the uterus, vagina, and rectum. The lungs may be injected, edematous, or pneumonic. The heart muscle is pale and flabby, and frequently hemorrhages are observed in its internal membrane. The liver may be pale or injected with blood and at times shows hemorrhages beneath its capsule. The bile is thin and watery in consistence. The kidneys may be inflamed or contain small hemorrhages within their substance or under the capsule. The lymphatic glands may be swollen and injected or even hemorrhagic.

Treatment.—On account of the danger of spreading the infection, neither medicinal treatment nor inoculation is permitted in most countries, the exception being those in which the disease is more generally diffused. The most effective method of eradicating rinderpest in those districts in which the disease is not indigenous has been found to be the slaughter of all affected and exposed animals. Where the disease is general, successful efforts adopted for its control have followed the immunization by inoculation of the exposed animals and a strict application of appropriate sanitary measures. This protective inoculation has been practiced with gratifying results in Russia, South Africa, and the Philippine Islands. An active immunity is thus induced in susceptible animals that lasts until the danger from exposure to the disease is over. This immunity may be attained by the (1) inoculation of pure bile from an animal that recently died of rinderpest, (2) inoculation of glycerinated bile, followed by pure bile or virulent blood, (3) simultaneous inoculation of strong standardized serum and virulent blood, or (4) inoculation of virus preparations that have been attentuated by various chemicals.

Some of the latter methods have been used in an endeavor to exterminate the disease in the Philippines and to protect the cattle and carabaos against rinderpest after their importation into those islands. The introduction of cattle into the United States from countries in which rinderpest exists is prohibited by law.

FOOT-AND-MOUTH DISEASE

[Pl. XXXIII]

Foot-and-mouth disease is primarily a foreign livestock malady. This disease has gained entrance to the United States on comparatively few occasions and in each case has been eliminated. The following information is furnished to show the seriousness of this disease and the importance of recognizing it promptly, and of cooperating with veterinary officials in eradicating outbreaks. This highly infectious disease should not be confused with minor diseases and ailments of the mouth and feet; hence the essential facts concerning foot-and-mouth disease are presented even though its presence in the United States has been very infrequent and of short duration.

Foot-and-mouth disease, also known as aphthous fever, epizootic aphtha, and eczema contagiosa, is an acute, highly communicable disease chiefly confined to cloven-footed animals and characterized by an eruption of vesicles or blisters on the mucous membrane of the mouth and on the skin between the toes and above the hoofs. The vesicles rupture and form erosions and ulcerations; there are also salivation, tenderness of the affected parts, loss of appetite, lameness, emaciation, and diminution in the quantity of milk secreted.

The extensive ravages of the disease are seen in the number and variety of the species attacked. Although it may be regarded as essentially a disease of cattle, hogs are also an easy prey. Almost in the same grade of receptivity are sheep and goats. Other susceptible animals are the deer, buffalo, American bison, camel, chamois, llama, giraffe, and antelope. Dogs, cats, and rabbits have been infected artificially but apparently do not contract the disease under natural conditions. Foot-and-mouth disease is transmissible to man, as has been shown definitely by several accidental laboratory infections and several other well-substantiated cases. Investigators have come to believe, however, that man is not readily susceptible.

As in other communicable diseases, the source and origin of foot-and-mouth disease have given rise to much speculation. The disease had been known in Europe for centuries. It is now well established that foot-and-mouth disease is propagated by a specific virus and every outbreak starts from some preexisting outbreak or infection. Experiments have shown that the virus will pass through standard germ-proof filters, thus indicating its minute size and the reason it has not been detected by the staining methods. The contagion may be found in the serum of the vesicles on the mouth, feet, and udder; in the saliva, milk, and various secretions and excretions; also in the blood during the rise of temperature.

A wide distribution of the virus and a rapid infection of a herd are the result. Animals may be infected directly, as by licking, and

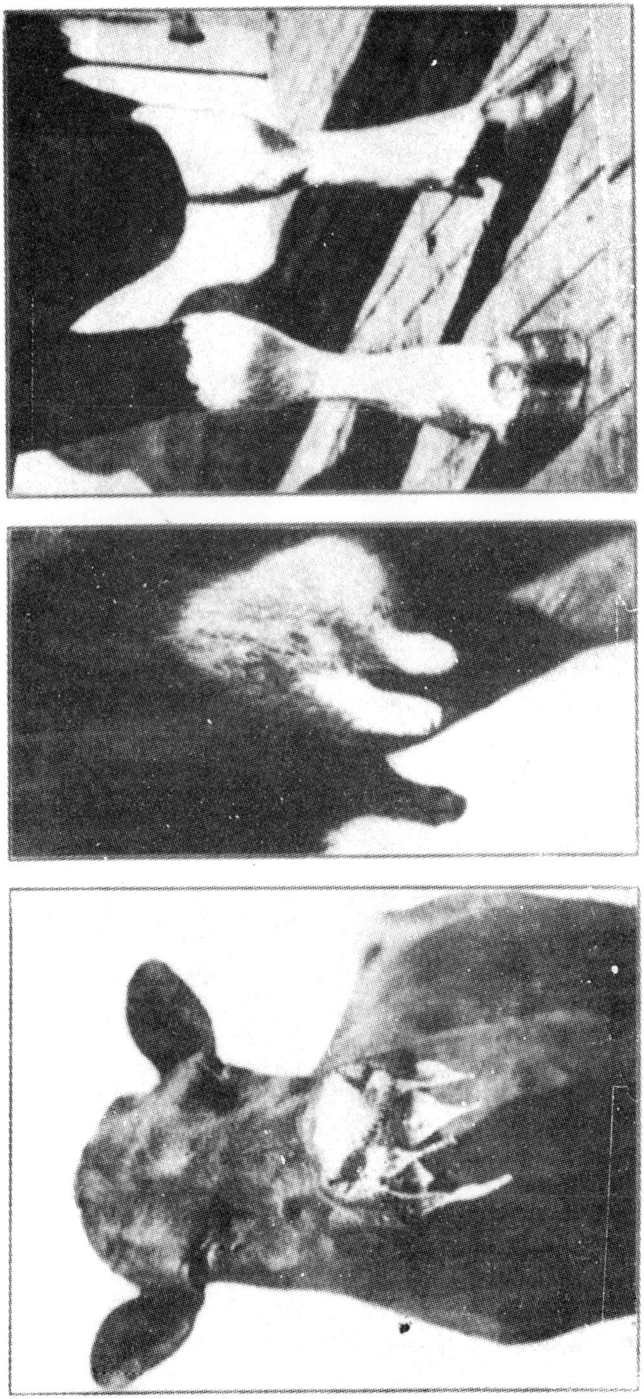

FOOT-AND-MOUTH DISEASE.

calves by sucking, or indirectly by infected manure, feed, utensils, drinking troughs, railway cars, animal markets, barnyards, and pastures. Human beings may carry the virus on their shoes and clothing and transmit it on their hands when milking, since the udder is occasionally the seat of the eruption. It may also be carried by dogs, cats, rats, chickens, pigeons, and other means. Milk in a raw state may also transmit the disease to animals fed with it.

The period of incubation (that is, the time between the exposure of an animal to infection and the development of the disease) is variable, usually from 3 to 6 days. The disease may appear in 24 hours, or, in exceptional cases, it may not appear for 18 days, or even longer.

Losses.—The highly contagious character of foot-and-mouth disease and its rapid spread to practically all exposed susceptible animals lead to heavy losses. Since the mortality is comparatively low, ranging from only 3 percent or less in mild forms to 30 or 40 percent in malignant cases, the havoc caused by the pestilence is sometimes underestimated. But there are other sources of loss that are much more important than the actual mortality. The fever and the difficulty of eating cause a rapid and extreme loss in flesh and a lessening or cessation of milk secretion. The udders often become inflamed and ruined by the formation of abscesses, and cows affected in this way are sometimes rendered permanently valueless for milk production. The inflammation of the feet may cause the horn to drop from the toes, producing great lameness and lasting injury. Abortion is frequent, and typical lesions have been observed in newborn animals. Altogether these losses may amount to 20 or 30 percent of the value of the affected animals.

In addition there are indirect losses of a commercial nature. Dairy farmers are put out of business for a time. Necessary quarantine restrictions greatly interfere with the movement of livestock and such commodities as hay, straw, hides, and farm produce. The business of the stockyards and slaughtering centers is greatly interfered with. Sometimes it is necessary to close stockyards for disinfection. The whole business of marketing, transporting, feeding, and slaughtering is interrupted and deranged. Losses of this character may reach enormous proportions.

That there are great monetary losses to countries in which foot-and-mouth disease has become established is shown by the fact that the estimated direct loss to the livestock industry in Germany during the epizootics of 1920 and 1921 was about $119,000,000. This sum does not include losses caused by disruption of business caused by quarantine restrictions. In Switzerland the losses from this epizootic in 1920–21 were reported to be about $70,000,000. These figures are especially significant in view of the fact that the number of susceptible animals in Switzerland at that time was less than one-fiftieth of the number in the United States and that the area of that country is less than half that of the State of Maine. The figures give some idea of the losses that the disease would cause in this country if it once became established.

The disease in other countries.—As already stated, foot-and-mouth disease has long prevailed in Europe, where it has occasioned great economic losses.

In Italy, France, Germany, the Netherlands, and some other countries of Europe the infection has existed so long and has gained such a foothold that it is economically impossible to fight it with the American methods of slaughter and disinfection, for to do so would kill a large percentage of the livestock of those countries.

The outbreak that appeared in Germany in 1888 increased steadily until 1892, when it diminished gradually for a few years, but the disease again reached great proportions in 1899. Thereafter it continued to exist to a greater or less extent until in 1911 it attained a virulence unequaled before. In that year 3,366,369 cattle, 1,602,927 sheep, 2,555,371 hogs, and 53,674 goats were affected. At that time the total number of cattle, sheep, swine, and goats in Germany was only 51,319,000, whereas there were in the United States 172,572,000, more than 3 times as many. It can readily be imagined, therefore, what it would mean to the United States if the disease were to gain the foothold here that it had in Germany, where, as these figures show, approximately 1 of 7 of the animals susceptible to the disease was affected.

The German Government, of course, has not left the disease to itself. It attempted to control some outbreaks by the method of slaughter, but the pestilence had gained too much headway and was too firmly established in too many portions of the country for this method to succeed, and the slaughter of the infected herds had to be abandoned. It now appears that there is slight hope of getting rid of it. It has been impossible to control it by means of quarantines alone.

Great Britain, Norway, and Sweden, on account of their comparatively isolated positions, have been more successful in keeping out the disease. The outbreaks in those countries have been more sporadic, and by resorting to immediate slaughter the authorities have been able to stamp them out. Great Britain has applied both quarantine and slaughter for many years. The British authorities have succeeded in suppressing each outbreak, but reinfection often occurs from other countries.

In November 1906 the disease reached Belgium from France, where it was prevalent, and by the end of the year every province in Belgium was affected, and the Netherlands as well. Efforts to eradicate it from Belgium were unavailing. The Netherlands apparently succeeded in stamping it out for about 6 months, but it reappeared there. Widespread outbreaks occurred in these three countries and also in Denmark in 1926.

In recent years the disease has been more or less prevalent in Belgium, Czechoslovakia, France, Germany, Netherlands, Italy, Union of Soviet Socialist Republics, Spain, and the Balkan countries. Switzerland, although subject to outbreaks, has been successful in recent years in accomplishing eradication of the disease by the use of the slaughter method. During the 1937–38 outbreak the disease extended to all countries in central Europe except Hungary.

There is less accurate information regarding Asia and Africa, but although Japan and many islands of the South Pacific are apparently free from the infection, it has been reported from India, Algeria, Tunisia, Morocco, Egypt, the Sudan, Nigeria, Rhodesia, Bechuanaland, and other portions of Africa. In 1933 the disease was introduced into the Union of South Africa from the Bechuanaland Protectorate but was successfully eradicated. In 1937 another outbreak occurred in the Union of South Africa. The disease is known to be prevalent in China, the Philippines, and various islands of the East Indies. It is doubtful whether any considerable part of the Orient is free from it.

In South America the disease is reported as common in the principal livestock countries—Argentina, Brazil, Paraguay, and Uruguay—and in all but two or three of the other countries of that continent. It appeared in Jamaica in the summer of 1922 and spread extensively over the island. It was not finally eradicated there until 1927.

In North America, Canada has been free from the disease for many years. In 1926 there was an outbreak in the southeastern part of Mexico, which in December 1927 was officially declared to be eradicated. Since then Mexico and all countries of Central America have remained free from the disease.

Australia and New Zealand have been fortunate in maintaining freedom from the disease for many years.

Outbreaks in the United States.—In 1870, 1880, and 1884 there were outbreaks of the disease in the United States. In each of these the contagion was introduced with imported animals. Since the development of a stringent system of inspection and quarantine of imported livestock, no instance of that kind has occurred.

In November 1902, the disease was discovered in Massachusetts and Rhode Island. The earliest cases were traced to Chelsea, Mass., near the docks, and it was suspected for a time that the infection

77431 O—51——25

was brought in with foreign shipping by some such means as hay, straw, halters, ropes, hides, hair, or wool. Later developments, however, and especially investigations into the cause of an outbreak in 1908, led to the belief that a more probable source of the infection was cowpox-vaccine virus imported from a country where foot-and-mouth disease existed, the vaccine virus being contaminated with the virus of foot-and-mouth disease. The 1902 outbreak involved Massachusetts, New Hampshire, Vermont, and Rhode Island and was eradicated in about 6 months.

The appearance of the 1908 outbreak of foot-and-mouth disease occurred early in November of that year, when it was observed in cattle near Danville, Pa. The infection was traced to the stock-yards at East Buffalo, N. Y., and to Detroit, Mich. The disease appeared in Michigan, New York, Pennsylvania, and Maryland. A careful and thorough investigation made by Mohler, of the Bureau of Animal Industry, and Rosenau, of the Public Health Service, demonstrated that the outbreak started from calves used to propagate vaccine virus at an establishment near Detroit, and that the source of the infection was contaminated Japanese vaccine virus. Vigorous measures of eradication similar to those used in 1902 were at once put into effect and the disease was stamped out in about 5 months.

Another invasion was discovered in the vicinity of Niles, Mich., in October 1914. This became the most serious and extensive outbreak ever known in this country. The disease extended to 22 States and the District of Columbia, ranging from the Atlantic to the Pacific coasts. The work of eradication was not completed for more than a year.

In February 1924, foot-and-mouth disease were discovered in California, the cause being traced to infected garbage from the Orient. Hogs, cattle, sheep, goats, and wild deer were involved in this outbreak, which was apparently eradicated in about 10 months but recurred early in 1925. It was finally eradicated June 10, 1925.

In September 1924, Texas also experienced a separate outbreak of the disease apparently caused by infection entering through a port on the Gulf of Mexico. This outbreak was suppressed in about a month except for a recurrence in one locality, a year later. Eradication was then promptly completed.

The next, which was also the last, outbreak of foot-and-mouth disease occurred in 1929 in southern California in a herd of garbage-fed hogs, the source of infection being meat scraps imported in violation of regulations. This outbreak, which also involved cattle, was of short duration and indicated the effectiveness of the time-tried policy of quarantine, slaughter, and burial of infected and exposed herds.

Details concerning the extent of the various outbreaks are presented in reports of the Bureau of Animal Industry, United States Department of Agriculture.

Symptoms.—Such tissue as the lining membranes of the mouth, tongue, and digestive tract, as well as tissue between the toes and around the top of the hoof, is the first to be affected by the virus. A vesicle or blister forms at the site of entrance of the virus, which is followed in 24 to 48 hours by a rise in temperature and an invasion of the virus into the blood. The virus is carried to distant parts of the body, where it again attacks various tissues and causes blisters to form in the mouth, tongue, lips, and between the toes and around the coronet. The temperature usually drops at this stage of the disease, but the animal shows visible evidence of sickness. There are loss of appetite, a suppression of milk, depression, and evidence of lameness, which increase markedly in a few days. The vesicles or blisters soon rupture and discharge a clear or somewhat cloudy fluid. At the site of the vesicles there remains a raw, eroded surface that may have jagged fragments of loose tissue attached to it. These, however, soon disappear after the rupture of the vesicles. In milk cows vesicles may also appear on the teats and udder (pl. XXXIII).

The various lesions are extremely painful, and in cattle salivation occurs to such an extent that the saliva sometimes hangs in strings from the mouth. Many of the animals make a peculiar smacking sound with the lips. Complications caused by invasion of microorganisms in the lesions follow in most cases.

All four feet may be affected at the same time, but one or more of the feet may entirely escape and remain normal throughout the course of the disease. Ulceration of the tissue between the toes may extend to the ligaments of the fetlock or produce disease of the joint or bone. As the feet become sensitive and sore the animal lies down persistently. Bedsores develop with amazing rapidity in all such cases and wholly baffle all attempts at treatment until after the animal has regained its feet.

The disease may attack some of the internal organs before it appears on any of the external tissues. These cases are likely to be fatal quickly. The animal dies from paralysis of the heart, due to formation of poisonous substances within the system, suffocates by reason of the action of these same poisons on the tissues of the lungs, or chokes to death as a result of paralysis of the throat.

In serious affection of the udder, the erosions are often located within the passages of the teats and result in a "caked" udder. The same toxic poisoning that causes death in the apoplectiform types just mentioned may arise from this source. In any event, the milk from such animals causes fatal diarrhea in suckling calves or young pigs and serious illness in human consumers.

Pregnant animals may abort. In pigs, sheep, and goats the lesions of either the foot or the mouth may be observed, but lesions of the foot are most common.

When the disease has become fully established the duration of the attack varies greatly with different animals. For the recovery of the normal appetite and spirits in mild outbreaks, 10 to 20 days are usually required, whereas the return to a full flow of milk, in the case of milk cows, seldom occurs before the following season.

In the malignant type of the disease it requires 3 months to a year for an animal to recover. The mortality, as already stated, is usually low. The disease is more fatal to young animals that have been fed infected milk and produces death in 60 to 80 percent of these cases as a result of gastroenteritis.

Diagnosis.—The diagnosis of foot-and-mouth disease as a rule is not difficult when the disease is known to exist in the vicinity. However, the far-reaching effect of the pronouncement of foot-and-mouth disease in this country makes the initial diagnosis of great importance. To control the disease effectively its prompt recognition is also of paramount importance. The actual diagnosis of the disease when it first makes its appearance therefore should be left to the judgment of qualified veterinarians skilled in making observations and tests that distinguish this disease from vesicular stomatitis and other somewhat similar maladies (p. 422).

It is the duty of livestock men immediately to call to the attention of the nearest State or Federal veterinary offical animals having symptoms that lead one to suspect foot-and-mouth disease. This is of particular importance when an outbreak exists somewhere in the country.

Eradication.—There are two generally recognized methods of combating foot-and-mouth disease: (1) The slaughter method, which is used in the United States; and (2) the quarantine procedure, which may at times involve some use of the slaughter method.

The slaughter method has for its object the complete eradication of the disease and consists in the slaughter of all infected and exposed animals in the shortest possible time and the cleaning, disinfection, and quarantine of the entire premises. By this method, as amply shown in this country, the disease can be absolutely eradicated.

The quarantine method consists in the main in the isolation and treatment of infected animals. That this method usually will not eradicate the disease is shown by its continued presence in countries where the plan is in use.

The adoption of either of these methods, however logical as a means of dealing with foot-and-mouth disease, depends on certain conditions. In a country free from foot-and-mouth disease and protected from its introduction by geographical situation and quarantine regulations, as for example, the United States, the slaughter method is the logical one to use when the disease makes its appearance. That this method is the most practical one for arresting outbreaks under the above conditions is recognized by all authorities on foot-and-mouth disease.

In countries where foot-and-mouth disease has gained a strong foothold as a result of the long period of activity of the virus, their geographical location, and their consequent inability to prevent the introduction of the disease, the stamping-out method cannot be employed economically and such countries are compelled to adopt the next best means, namely, the quarantine method. Many countries of continental Europe must for these reasons rely on this method in their attempts to control the disease.

The United States has demonstrated that the disease can be entirely eradicated by the stamping-out method and at a much less cost than if the disease once became well established.

Eradication measures in the United States.—The stamping-out or slaughter method is used when foot-and-mouth disease makes its appearance in the United States. This work is actively undertaken by the Bureau of Animal Industry, United States Department of Agriculture, in cooperation with officials of the State in which the outbreak occurs, and the expense of eradication is shared by the Federal Government and the State.

The stamping-out method of eradicating the disease as conducted in the United States includes the following points: Quarantine of premises where outbreak occurs, slaughter of infected and exposed animals followed by burial or burning, cleaning and disinfection of premises and all equipment, and a test of the thoroughness of disinfection by restocking with susceptible animals.

Quarantine.—Because of the highly contagious character of the disease, strict quarantine regulations are put into effect as soon as foot-and-mouth disease is suspected. These restrictions are not removed until the disease has been determined not to be foot-and-mouth disease or until there is reason to believe that the outbreak has been eradicated and that the virus no longer exists on the premises or in the locality.

The necessity of effective quarantine measures is evident from the following: (1) Foot-and-mouth disease is most actively contagious in the early stage; (2) practically all cloven-footed animals are highly susceptible, and the greatest source of danger is removed by slaughter and proper disposal of the involved animals; (3) the virus of the disease may be carried mechanically by persons, dogs, birds, rabbits, or other means, and by any object that may become contaminated with active virus; and (4) conditions may exist in the field under which the virus may remain active for 1 or 2 months or even longer. Cleaning and disinfection after the slaughter of infected animals remove most of the virus, but in spite of these precautions there is danger of further infection. Assurance of complete removal of every vestige of infectious material cannot be given until test animals, introduced on the premises, are found to remain healthy. Further restocking may then take place gradually, but as a safeguard inspections are made at regular intervals.

Importance of prompt reports.—Scientific knowledge concerning foot-and-mouth disease, supplemented by the experience in previous outbreaks, shows the extreme importance of early discovery and diagnosis of this infection as factors in prompt eradication.

Suspicious cases should always be reported *at once* to the nearest Federal, State, or local veterinary official by *telephone* or *telegraph.*

The cooperation of livestock owners and handlers in maintaining established quarantines likewise is essential to early eradication of this disease. They should report at once any unauthorized movement of livestock or mingling of stock with animals on infected or exposed premises.

SEPTICEMIA AND PYEMIA

These two names are applied to diseased conditions that are so nearly alike in their symptoms that it is sometimes difficult to distinguish the one from the other. Indeed, the name "pyosepticemia" or "septicopyemia" is often applied when it is impossible to make a distinction between septicemia and pyemia or when each is equally responsible for the diseased condition. The name septicemia is derived from two Greek words meaning "poison" and "blood" and signifies that the germ lives in the blood; hence the use of the term "blood poisoning" for this disease. Pyemia is likewise derived from two Greek words meaning "pus" and "blood" and is that form of septicemia caused by pus-producing organisms and characterized by secondary abscesses.

Causes.—Except in certain specific infectious diseases, neither of these diseases is brought about, strictly speaking, by any specific organism; hence neither can be looked upon generally as a specific disease. The organisms most frequently found in cases of septicemia are, on the whole, the same as those of pyemia and may be pus cocci, the *Bacillus coli*, or other pus-producing organisms. These organisms are often found as secondary invaders in other diseases, such as advanced cases of tuberculosis, in which cases they are responsible for the formation of pus.

Aside from the causative organism, or, in other words, the active cause, there are many secondary causes. The most important of these in pyemia is a break in continuity of the protective covering, as a wound, which affords an entrance into the tissues for the organisms. Among the different varieties of wounds may be mentioned cuts, bruises, punctures, burns, chemical or frozen wounds, and compound fractures of bones. Injuries received during parturition and infection of the umbilicus in the newly born are also frequent causes of pyemia. Septicemia may follow surgical wounds, local suppuration, metritis, mastitis, pericarditis, enteritis, bronchitis—in fact, wherever there is a local lesion of any kind permitting germs to enter the blood. Septicemia was formerly applied to designate the condition in which the organisms were localized but in which their toxins were diffused in the blood. Pyemia represented that condition when the organisms were localized but in which the pus was transported by the blood. These terms now are applied to conditions in which both the organisms and their toxins, or the pus, are present in the blood. The term "septicemia" is indicated when intoxication is the more pronounced symptom, and "pyemia" if pus formation and metastatic or secondary abscess formation are observed.

Symptoms.—The symptoms of both diseases include primarily a high fever (104° to 107° F.). In addition to this, there is disinclination to move, the animal is depressed and not cognizant of its surroundings. The pulse is rapid, small, and feeble, respiration increased, mucous membrane injected, swollen, and of a yellowish tinge. Appetite is lost and death usually follows in the case of septicemia in from 2 to 4 days. In pyemia the symptoms come on more slowly and are not so intense as in septicemia and the course of the disease is longer, lasting from 6 days to 4 weeks. The mortality is not so great as in septicemia, but the period of convalescence is usually long.

Lesions.—Septicemia is characterized by the destructive changes in the blood, which, after death, is chocolate-colored, noncoagulable, and swarms with bacteria. The lining membranes of the heart are studded with red spots, often running together to form a large hemorrhagic area. The lungs, liver, and kidneys may also contain these hemorrhages. The spleen is enlarged and full of black blood. The carcass decomposes rapidly and in some cases forms great quantities of fetid gas. In pyemia, in addition to these lesions, abscesses are formed in the various organs throughout the body. If the disease develops slowly, a post mortem examination shows the abscesses to be the chief alterations. The pus content is usually stained with blood and contains strings of fibrous tissue and necrosed matter.

Treatment.—Treatment is almost futile in advanced cases of either disease. Septicemia is usually fatal and pyemia frequently so. Prevention and the immediate treatment of local infections are the surest means of combating them. For local treatment of wounds the usual antiseptics are advised, such as a 3-percent compound cresol or carbolic acid or a 2-percent solution of sodium hydroxide. In pyemia, if the abscesses are near the skin and well defined, they should be opened and treated antiseptically by injecting any of the previously mentioned germicides. General and heart stimulants are recommended, such as a drench containing 2 drams of digitalis and 2 ounces of alcohol. Such technical assistance as may be given by the veterinarian is advised.

HEMORRHAGIC SEPTICEMIA (SHIPPING FEVER)

Hemorrhagic septicemia is a name applied to a highly fatal, infectious disease affecting principally cattle and sheep and caused by a micro-organism having definite biological characters and possessing the properties of producing clearly defined and characteristic lesions. As the disease is a septicemia or poisoning of the blood, it often runs a short course and the animal dies quickly. The presence of hemorrhages in the body tissues and organs of animals dead from this disease is usually an outstanding lesion, and because of these characteristics the name "hemorrhagic septicemia" has been applied to this malady. The disease was described by Bollinger in 1878 and named "Wild und Rinderseuche" from its having affected deer, wild boars, cattle, and horses in an epizootic that swept over Germany at that time. Before this, however, several epizootics of what was evidently the same disease had been well described, notably that which occurred in England in 1854. Since then it has occurred in epizootic and enzootic forms in many sections of Europe, Asia, Africa, and North America. Other names given to it are game and cattle disease, buffalo disease, barbone, pasteurellosis bovina, ghotwa, and infectious pneumoenteritis.

Losses appear to be greatest among young animals, especially those that are thin and poorly nourished. A large number of outbreaks of hemorrhagic septicemia in cattle are associated with the shipment of animals from one point to another by rail or truck and their passage through public stockyards. As a result of the rigors of transit, the vitality of the animal is lowered and its resistance to infection is decreased. This disease, therefore, presents a serious problem to stockmen, both from the standpoint of the shipper and receiver. In some years considerable losses may occur as a result of this disease, whereas in other years there are only slight losses.

Cause.—As most of the outbreaks of this disease occur in the fall, winter, and early spring, particularly during inclement weather, it is commonly believed that weather conditions influence its prevalence.

Cattle that appear to be healthy when purchased in the stockyards may arrive on the farm in a run-down condition, owing to prolonged travel and exposure to changeable or severe weather conditions. Overcrowding, irregularity in feeding and watering, hard driving, lack of rest and proper shelter, and the general excitement associated with shipping may reduce the normal vigor and increase the susceptibility to the disease.

The primary cause of hemorrhagic septicemia in cattle has not been definitely determined. Some investigators believe that the principal causative factor is the hemorrhagic septicemia organism, *Pasteurella boviseptica.* Although the organism has been found in the air passages of normal animals and organisms closely resembling it are widely distributed in nature, these investigators believe that the organisms under certain conditions become virulent and that animals whose natural resistance is lowered by severe exposure during shipping and other debilitating influences readily develop the disease.

Others believe that although the hemorrhagic septicemia organism plays a secondary role, such as that of diphtheroids, streptococci and *Bacillus coli* organisms, there is another infective agent, presumably a primary causative factor, concerned in the production of this disease. The nature of this agent, however, is not known but is thought by some to be a virus. It has been observed that, after a hard railroad journey, many cattle manifest symptoms of the disease, and when these affected animals come in contact with local stock the latter often become infected. The extent to which the contamination of yards, buildings, and other equipment, by affected cattle caused the disease in noninfected animals is not known but undoubtedly it is a source of danger. It is worthy of note that the necessary coexistence of two factors (virus and bacteria) as a causative agent in certain infectious diseases has been recognized in recent years, notably in swine influenza.

Symptoms.—Hemorrhagic septicemia usually develops very rapidly in cattle and lasts 2 to 8 days or longer. Affected animals first show an elevation of body temperature, ranging from 104° to 107° F., accompanied with loss of appetite, mucopurulent discharge from the nose, an occasional hacking cough, swollen, watery eyes, general depression, gaunty appearance, stiffened gait, and sometimes diarrhea. Within 3 to 5 days after the first symptoms, affected animals may develop pneumonia and die in 48 to 72 hours, or the disease assumes a chronic course, in which case the sick animals may live for several weeks. In mild attacks of the disease, affected animals may recover in a week or two. During the course of the disease other symptoms sometimes occur. Swelling may appear beneath the skin of the head, throat, or dewlap. These enlargements are somewhat soft and pit on pressure. The tongue is often extensively swollen, and the animal drools and slobbers because of the irritation to its tongue and throat. There may be difficulty in breathing, depending on the degree of involvement of the air passages and of the lungs. Muscular trembling sometimes is evident. There may be a blood-stained discharge from the nostrils, and strings of mucus may hang from the mouth. Examination of the nostrils often reveals the presence of many small hemorrhages, or blood spots, just beneath their lining membranes.

There is an intestinal form of the disease in which the changes are found chiefly in the abdominal cavity, or the intestinal form may develop after the disease has appeared in the lungs. The stomach, intestines, kidneys, and the lymph glands belonging to them become studded with hemorrhages of various sizes, and the intestines become intensely inflamed. As a result, diarrhea sets in, and shreds of mucus and bloody droppings are passed. The intestinal form is rare, as most cases show severe involvement of the lungs and the symptoms of croupous pneumonia. The animals may stand with their forelegs wide apart in order to breathe more freely. They lose flesh very rapidly, their abdomens become "tucked up," and the eyes quickly become sunken. A staggering gait, caused by extreme weakness, sometimes is noticed.

A disease has been described under the name "septic pleuropneumonia" of calves, which apparently is a form of hemorrhagic septicemia caused by the characteristic germ. The symptoms shown by the affected calves are characteristic of hemorrhagic septicemia, and the post mortem findings are also those found in that disease.

Post mortem findings.—The following anatomical changes may be observed in the carcass of an animal dead of hemorrhagic septicemia: Swellings of doughy consistence, containing jellylike material tinged with blood, may be found under the skin. These swellings, if they occur in the region of the shoulder or flank, are sometimes mistaken for blackleg. The lymph glands are enlarged and hemorrhagic. The mucous membranes that line the nose, throat, and air passages of the lungs are inflamed and may contain blood-stained mucus. Hemorrhages may be observed in the fatty tissue around the kidneys and in the serous membranes of the internal organs.

When the disease is chiefly in the chest, the lungs are darkened in color and their fibrous tissues much thickened from the collection of bloody serum in their meshes. There may be solidification of one or more lobes (pneumonia). The diaphragm, heart sac, and heart walls have numerous bloody points and larger collections of blood.

In the intestinal form, hemorrhages into the intestines are present and sloughing of the lining of the intestinal wall is observed, as a result of which the intestinal contents are wrapped in a covering of bloody mucus.

In acute forms of the disease, the animals may die suddenly, and the changes in such cases are not marked. Bacteriological examination of the body fluids may demonstrate the presence of hemorrhagic septicemia organisms.

Diagnosis.—The diagnosis of hemorrhagic septicemia is often difficult because of its similarity to certain other disease conditions in cattle. Owing to its acute course, high fever, and rapid termination, the disease may be mistaken for anthrax, malignant edema, and blackleg. Although certain characteristic features of these diseases may aid in making a tentative diagnosis, a bacteriologic examination, which includes both cultural and laboratory animal-inoculation tests, is sometimes necessary to detect the nature of the disease and especially to differentiate one disease from another.

Other conditions in cattle, such as coccidiosis, cornstalk disease, lead poisoning, sweetclover poisoning, and other forms of vegetable poisoning, may be mistaken for hemorrhagic septicemia. In an outbreak of suspected hemorrhagic septicemia the diagnosis, treatment, and methods of control should be dealt with by an experienced veterinarian.

Prevention and control.—In the consideration of measures for the control and prevention of this disease it is important to remember that hemorrhagic septicemia is the most serious of a group of cattle maladies that commonly result from mishandling, neglect, or exposure of animals in transit or shortly after their arrival at their destination. Therefore, every effort should be made to eliminate predisposing factors to the disease, such as overdriving, overcrowding, overfeeding, and lack of rest, water, feed, and proper shelter during transit.

To maintain the health of livestock in transit and to aid in reducing the heavy losses that hemorrhagic septicemia and kindred ailments have been inflicting on the livestock industry, a committee[1] representing various commercial interests cooperated with the United States Department of Agriculture in studying the situation and in formulating recommendations for improvement. Based on exhaustive studies of both the scientific and practical aspects of the subject, the evidence shows that the losses sustained in the past could have been largely prevented by improved methods of handling and by vaccination with suitable biological products.

Since the infection of hemorrhagic septicemia is commonly harbored in the systems of animals, there is little hope of escaping additional exposure during shipment. It is important to remember, also, that animals of normal vigor usually resist the infection, hence the need of protecting them against devitalizing influences, such as exposure to severe weather, changes in the routine of feeding and watering, excitement, and overexertion. Irregularity in feeding and water-

[1] The committee's membership included: E. C. Brown, representing the National Livestock Exchange; Charles E. Day, the National Traders' Exchange; W. J. Embree, the Western Weighing and Inspection Bureau, and the railroads; L. W. Kube, public stockyards; and F. G. Ketner, the National Livestock Producers' Association.

ing should be avoided to prevent derangement of the digestive processes.

It is especially important to the producer of feeder cattle that his animals reach the market or the feed lot in a thrifty condition. Unthrifty cattle are practically always unprofitable to the owner who feeds them, and this naturally is prejudicial to the interests of producers who have feeder cattle to sell.

For the benefit of shippers, commission men, traders, feeders, and others who handle cattle, the following detailed recommendations are made:

Avoid hard driving and allow ample time for rest before loading. On arrival at the pens the animals should not be allowed to fill up on water but should first have rest and be fed grass or nonlegume hay.

Avoid overcrowding cattle in the cars. In cold weather, bed the car well. In very severe weather, in northern latitudes, it may be well to line the side walls of the car with heavy paper, especially if the cattle are young or unthrifty.

Give feed and water at proper intervals en route. When unloaded for feed, water, and rest, the cattle should have plenty of time to become well rested.

Under the 28-hour law 5 hours' rest is the minimum specified time, and the railroads ordinarily allow that period, exclusive of the time of unloading and reloading. It is better, however, to give stocker and feeder cattle special care, allowing at least 8 hours for feed, water, and rest. Plenty of rest and regular feeding and watering are essential if animals are to arrive at their final destination in the best possible condition. Cows in an advanced stage of pregnancy, commonly termed "springers," should receive particular attention.

The common practice of withholding water from animals until they are very thirsty so that later they will take a heavy fill is harmful. The practice tends to upset the digestive system so seriously that the animals are slow in resuming normal feeding and gain in weight. It is therefore recommended that this damaging process be discontinued through general agreement among livestock owners and handlers.

In stocker and feeder cattle that pass through the public market, the same attention should be given to the shipments back to the country that has been outlined for the shipments to market. After the arrival of cattle at their final destination in the country, they should receive special attention and care to help them over the period of lowered vitality resulting from the hardships of travel.

Feeder cattle on arrival should be given a fill of dry roughage, such as timothy hay, prairie hay, or corn stover. After having access to this roughage a few hours, they should have water but not all that they will drink. By the end of the first day, give free access to dry roughage and water.

Most feeder cattle are raised on grasses different from those found in the fattening areas. Therefore, if they are to be pasture-fed, let them become accustomed to the new grasses gradually, giving them at first only a few hours' grazing each day, especially if the grass is still green.

If feeder cattle are intended for dry-lot feeding with no pasture available, give them access to cornstalk fields or feed them on corn fodder and hay for 10 days to 2 weeks before starting them on the fattening rations.

If the cattle arrive in cold weather, especially if it is wet and stormy, provide adequate dry shelter. Severe exposure to cold and dampness combined, during the period of low vitality, is likely to have serious results. If there is any sign of sickness, segregate diseased animals and keep them quiet.

Biological products and their use in prevention and control.—The use of biological products to prevent hemorrhagic septicemia or to control outbreaks has been successful in many instances, but unsatisfactory results have followed their use in some outbreaks.

Biological products used against hemorrhagic septicemia are either preventive (bacterin and aggressin) or curative (antiserum). Bacterins or aggressins increase the animals' resistance against the infection. They produce an active immunity of long duration, usually several months to a year. For best results feeder and stocker cattle should be treated with bacterin or aggressin at least 10 days before shipment, as the use of these products on animals in transit or a few days after they reach their destination appears to be of little value.

On the other hand, the administration of antihemorrhagic-septicemia immune serum, which contains great numbers of immune bodies, produces an immediate increase in resistance to the disease. This is a passive immunity lasting only a few weeks.

The serum also possesses some curative value. Its use, therefore, is recommended for treatment of cattle in transit or within a few days after they arrive at their destination, particularly if some of the animals in the shipment show symptoms of the disease.

Anaphylaxis (shock or severe reactions) may sometimes follow the administration of the serum or bacterins. To avoid such shock, only homologous serum should be used, and bacterins should preferably be composed of a bacterial suspension in physiological saline free from toxic broth or other foreign protein. The administration of biological products should be left to the discretion of a competent veterinarian.

Treatment.—In most cases medicinal treatment of a fully established case of hemorrhagic septicemia is of little value. In visibly sick animals, especially during the early stages of the disease, the administration of large doses of antihemorrhagic-septicemia serum (one or two injections of 50 cc. or more) frequently assists in bringing about recovery. All apparently well animals should be removed from sick ones by placing them in separate, noninfected quarters. If new cases develop among them in a few days after their removal, the healthy ones remaining should be removed to another locality. In that way the unaffected animals soon will be out of danger of further contamination, especially if they have been given an abundance of good feed and water during the separation.

The administration of sodium bicarbonate has also been reported by some stockmen and veterinarians as being of considerable value, both in the treatment and prevention of this disease.

During 1934, 1935, and 1936, sodium bicarbonate administered in the form of a drench, on the feed, or in drinking water, 1 ounce per hundred pounds of body weight once each day for 14 days, was given by stockmen and stockyard officials to several thousand cattle. Some of the animals were treated in the stockyards and others after arrival on the home premises following shipment. A large number of animals in both groups were untreated and held as controls.

Reports received by the Bureau covering the treatment of these animals showed little difference between the treated and untreated animals in their resistance to hemorrhagic septicemia.

Disinfection of premises.—Inasmuch as hemorrhagic septicemia is an infectious disease, the carcasses of animals dead of the disease should be burned or buried.

Premises usually become infected with hemorrhagic septicemia by stock cattle that have recently passed through some of the larger cattle markets. All stables, sheds, or yards that have contained infected animals should be disinfected. The interior of the stables, especially the mangers and manure trenches, should be washed with a disinfectant, such as liquor cresolis compositus (U. S. P.), 4 ounces to the gallon of water, or carbolic acid, 6 ounces to a gallon of water. The yards may be disinfected by the application of a solution made of 5 ounces of copper sulfate to a gallon of water. The best way to apply disinfectant solutions is by means of a spray pump, such as is used in spraying orchard trees. All refuse and material from the stable and barnyard should be removed to a place not accessible to cattle or sheep. The manure should be spread on fields and plowed under. A plentiful supply of light and air should be provided for the contaminated stables. Open fields or pasture lands are cleansed rapidly by the action of sunlight.

COITAL EXANTHEMA

(VESICULAR ERUPTION OF THE GENITAL ORGANS)

Coital exanthema is more or less prevalent in some foreign countries and has been observed also in parts of the United States. A similar disease of horses and sometimes of other animals occurs, but, so far as is known, the disease is not transmitted naturally from one species to another.

The disease is a highly contagious eruption on the external genital organs of both sexes and accompanied with little or no general disturbance of health. The contagion is transmitted mainly during copulation. The causative agent is considered by most authorities to be a filtrable virus. The bull may have the disease and convey it to all the cows with which he comes in contact, or he may become infected by one cow and, although not showing the disease, he may, during copulation, transmit it for several days to all other cows. Simple contact between two cows may convey the disease, or the sponges used in cleansing the diseased animals may carry the virus to healthy ones. Healthy cows have contracted the disease lying with their hindquarters against infected wooden troughs. Finally, careless examinations of the genital organs may convey the infection from one animal to another.

Symptoms.—The period between the infection and the appearance of symptoms is somewhat variable but is usually 3 to 6 days. It may be briefer or much longer. In cows the mucous membrane of the vagina and the vulva become swollen, inflamed, tender, and covered with dark-red spots. The secretion is abundant and consists at first largely of serum and mucus resembling the white of an egg. Small vesicles then appear, which rapidly burst and are converted into excoriations or deeper ulcerations. The secretion becomes more purulent and is likely to dry in crusts about the root of the tail. The eruption is accompanied with much itching and difficulty in urinating. The walk may be stiff and awkward. In bulls the eruption is situated on the prepuce and the end of the penis and consists of pimples, vesicles, and ulcers, as in cows. It is accompanied with a little purulent discharge from the prepuce, itching, and difficulty in urinating. The discharge frequently mats the hair at the opening of the sheath. In severe cases the inflammation and swelling may extend backward to the scrotum and forward upon the abdomen.

The disease lasts 1 to 4 weeks and always terminates in recovery but sequelae are not uncommon. The acute stage lasts only 4 or 5 days, but complete healing of the inflammation is slow. The eruption is usually accompanied with little general disturbance. If the pain and irritation are severe, there may be a slight loss of appetite and diminished milk secretion in cows. The disease rarely causes abortion. Chronic catarrh of the vagina and permanent sterility frequently follow as sequelae.

Treatment.—No treatment may be necessary except in severe cases. The secretion and exudation may be washed off and a mild antiseptic applied. Care must be taken not to carry the disease from the sick to the well animals by sponges or similar objects that have come in contact with the affected organs. These should be destroyed. In examining and treating animals, cleanliness and antisepsis should be observed by the attendant. To prevent the spread of the disease the infected animals should be isolated until they have recovered, and under no circumstances should infected animals be bred.

RABIES OF CATTLE

Rabies principally affects canines, including dogs, coyotes, and wolves, although all warm-blooded animals, including man, are susceptible to the malady, which is always communicated through bites from a preceding case. It has required many years of patient, scientific research to lead the ablest investigators to a clear comprehension of the cause, nature, and characteristics of this affection. It was known and described several centuries prior to the beginning of the Christian era, and from the earliest dawn of history it has been feared and dreaded. Its terrible manifestations have always been surrounded with an atmosphere of awe and mystery, and it is not surprising that myths, fallacies, and misconceptions in regard to it have been common and widely accepted. Even today fallacies in regard to the disease continue to have a strong hold on the public mind. For instance, it is still a widely prevalent belief that if persons or animals are bitten by a dog they are likely to become rabid if the dog should contract the disease at any future time. There is no foundation for this impression, and it would be a great comfort to many persons who are now and then bitten by animals if the fallacy of this idea were known. All experience, both scientific and practical, shows that rabies is transmitted only by animals that are actually diseased at the time the bite is inflicted, although visible symptoms of the disease are not always evident.

Rabies is an infectious disease involving the nervous system and characterized by extreme excitability and other nervous disorders, and practically always terminating in death. The causative agent belongs to the ever-increasing group of filtrable viruses. Like that of foot-and-mouth disease, it was one of the first members of this class of infective agents to be recognized. It is transmitted naturally from one animal to another solely by bites, and the old idea of spontaneous appearance of the disease is absolutely fallacious. It may be produced artificially by inoculating susceptible animals with an emulsion of the brain or spinal cord, as well as the saliva, and in some cases with the milk, and other secretions of the affected animal. The blood, on the contrary, seems to be free from the infectious principle. The saliva contains the virus, which, under natural conditions, is introduced into or under the skin on the tooth of the rabid animal. The disease is widespread, being found in many countries of Europe, Asia, and Africa, and in many sections of the United States.

Through eradication measures and the rigid quarantine regulations enforced against dogs imported into England, this country has remained free from the disease. Other countries have been protected by import quarantine regulations of dogs. After canines, cattle seem to be the most frequently affected, probably because rabid dogs, next to their morbid desire to attack other dogs, have a better opportunity to bite grazing cattle than any other species of animal. The latter receive bites most frequently on the hind legs and in the hips and about the muzzle. These places are most accessible to dogs, owing to the habit of cattle to drive their tormentors away by lowering their heads and using their horns. Every animal bitten does not necessarily develop the disease, the percentage of fatalities averaging from 25 to 30. Whether or not the disease develops depends on the location and size of the wound, as well as the amount of bleeding produced, and various other conditions. In general, the nearer the bite is located to the central nervous system and the deeper the wound inflicted, the greater the danger of a fatal result. In cases in which the bleeding resulting from the bite is profuse, there is a possibility that the virus will be washed out of the wound and thus obviate the danger of subsequent appearance of the disease.

The virus, after being deposited in the wound, remains latent for an extremely variable period of time, which also depends on the size and depth of the wound, as well as its location and the quantity of the virulent saliva introduced. Experiments have proved that the virus follows the course of the nerves to the spinal cord and along the latter to the brain before the symptoms appear. Gerlach, having collected the statistics from 133 cases, found this time, known as the period of incubation, to vary from 14 to 285 days. Usually, however, the disease is contracted in 1 to 3 months after the bite has been inflicted. It has been clearly demonstrated by the experiments of Roux and Nocard that the bite of a dog is infectious at least 3 days before it manifests symptoms of rabies. At the Athens (Greece) Pasteur Institute infection was noted in the saliva 8 days before the dog showed signs of the disease.

Symptoms.—As in dogs, both furious and dumb rabies occur, the former being more common in cattle. A sharp line of distinction, however, cannot be drawn between these two forms of the disease, as the furious form usually merges into the dumb from the paralysis that appears prior to death. Typical cases of dumb rabies are those in which the paralysis appears at the beginning of the attack and remains until death. The disease first manifests itself by a loss of appetite and

77431 O—51——26

rumination, stopping of the secretion of milk, great restlessness, anxiety, manifestation of fear, and change in the disposition of the animal. This preliminary stage may be followed in a day or two by the stage of excitation, or madness, which is indicated by increasing restlessness, loud bellowing—at times with a peculiar change in the sound of the voice—violent butting with the horns, and pawing the ground with the feet, with an insane tendency to attack other animals and even man, although the desire to bite is not so marked in cattle as in dogs, coyotes, wolves, and other canines. A frequent symptom is the increased secretion of saliva, with a consequent frothing at the mouth, or the secretion may hang from the lips in long strings. These symptoms result from a partial or total paralysis of the throat or other muscles. In some cases of rabies, however, these symptoms may not be present. Constipation is often marked, and there is a continual, although unsuccessful, desire to defecate.

Spasms of the muscles in different parts of the body are also seen at intervals. By or before the fourth day the animal usually becomes quieter and the walk is stiff, unsteady, and swaying, showing that the final paralysis is coming on. This is called the paralytic stage. The loss of flesh is extremely rapid, and even during the short course of the disease the animal becomes exceedingly emaciated. The temperature is never elevated, but usually remains about normal or even subnormal. Finally, there is complete paralysis of the hind quarters, the animal being unable to rise, and but for irregular convulsive movements lies in a comatose condition and dies usually from the fourth to the sixth day after the appearance of the first symptom.

Diagnosis.—It is not easy to decide definitely that an animal has rabies, since the symptoms just given belong in part to a variety of other diseases, among which are the excitement in young animals after close confinement, certain vegetable and mineral poisons, acute enteritis, and alterations of the central nervous system in cattle, such as pseudorabies or other condition.

When rabies is suspected in cattle or when a mad dog has been in the vicinity, a competent veterinarian should be immediately called to examine the sick animals. Since the virus of rabies is found in the saliva of the cattle affected with this disease, human beings may become exposed to infection during attempts to drench the animal or by examination of the mouth and throat of the animal. A definite diagnosis of rabies can be obtained by laboratory examination of the brain of affected animals. The head, packed in ice in warm weather, should be taken to the nearest laboratory equipped for such work. Since the virus of rabies is present in the brain and nerve tissue of animals dead of the disease, rubber gloves should be worn or other protective measures taken during the removal and handling of the head and the carcass. The carcass should be burned or buried deeply.

Transmission of the disease by milk and meat.—Although the virus is most frequently found in the central nervous system and the salivary glands, it may occur also in the other glands and secretions. In a few instances, rabies has been found in the milk or udder tissue.

However, according to available information, such occurrence is exceedingly rare and, therefore, there appears to be little danger in the consumption of milk from even a rabid animal. Milk secretion is usually considerably diminished at the clinical appearance of the disease, with the result that in most cases milk has been consumed only before the animal has shown any evidence of disease. However, the milk from a rabid cow or one suspected of being rabid naturally should be condemned as unfit for consumption.

Likewise, the meat or meat food products of such food animals should not be consumed. The International Rabies Conference held in Paris in 1927 under the auspices of the health committee, League of Nations, made the following recommendation on this point: "Animals bitten by rabid animals, whether treated or not after the bite, should not be butchered between the eighth day at the very least and the end of 3 months following the bite." As this may be a problem of considerable importance in areas where rabies exists, the recommendations just mentioned form a basis for methods of procedure.

Treatment.—This is useless after the first appearance of symptoms. When, however, a wound inflicted by a rabid animal is discovered, it should be immediately cauterized or even completely extirpated, care being taken to cut entirely around the wound in the healthy tissues. For cauterizing the wound, fuming nitric acid, the hot iron, and 10-percent solution of zinc chloride are the most efficacious. To be most effective, this should be done within a few moments after the bite has been inflicted. Since it is often impossible to locate all wounds, it is apparent that even though immediate and thorough cauterization of visible wounds may reduce the chance of infection as far as these wounds are concerned, other unobserved wounds may be present and escape treatment. Animals that have been exposed to infection should be kept in quarantine for at least 3 months.

Pasteur originated and perfected a system of preventive inoculation that has greatly reduced the mortality in human subjects. The Pasteur treatment is rarely administered to animals on account of the expense. Antirabic vaccination, when applied to animals, consists of fewer injections than are administered to persons. From 6 to 14 injection treatments, depending on the severity of the exposure, have been found to produce satisfactory results. The attending veterinarian will be best fitted to recommend the number of injections that should be administered in any specific instance of exposure to rabid-dog bites.

Prevention.—Sanitary regulations to control effectively the disease by exterminating it among dogs are most likely to prove successful. The disposal of farm animals that have been exposed to the bites of rabid dogs or other animals also presents a practical sanitary police problem. The measures adopted to this end cannot be discussed here, but it is a striking fact that where quarantine and other measures have been rigidly enforced, as in England and in certain German districts, the disease has been practically stamped out.

PSEUDORABIES (MAD ITCH, INFECTIOUS BULBAR PARALYSIS)

Pseudorabies is an infectious disease characterized by biting, rubbing, and licking certain parts of the body, symptoms of brain disturbance, and paralysis. The disease was first described by Aujeszky in Hungary in 1902. In Europe and sometimes in the United States it is now referred to as Aujeszky's disease. Although it appears to be less prevalent in North America than in Europe, it is the general opinion of authorities that the disease previously referred to as cutaneous hemorrhagic septicemia in past years in this country was probably pseudorabies, or mad itch. The cause is a filtrable virus. In investigating the disease in Iowa, Shope determined that hogs may carry the virus of the disease without showing marked symptoms, and it seems probable that contact with hogs may be one source of the disease in cattle. In experimental studies made by Shope and others, sheep, goats, dogs, cats, rabbits, rats, mice, guinea pigs, monkeys, and even ducks have also been found to be susceptible to pseudorabies. The disease causes death in many of these species under the conditions in the laboratory but, except for cattle and hogs, other animals are not known to acquire the disease naturally in this country. Horses have been found to react variably to artificial inoculations of pseudorabies virus.

The virus of the disease is present in the blood and secretions of affected animals at certain stages, but the method by which the disease is transmitted naturally has not been determined. Bites by infected rats and blood-sucking insects have been suspected. On the other hand, the disease may possibly be contracted by inhaling virus from another animal.

Symptoms.—A severe itching is usually the first indication of the disease. The affected animal rubs against posts, trees, barbed wire, or other objects and repeatedly licks the skin. It may bite itself or gnaw the skin. The itching seems to be most severe in the hindquarters or on the face, and the constant scratching, licking, and rubbing may remove the hair from spots of the skin, which become leatherlike and smeared with serum. The agonized frenzy of the animal may cause it to lunge and race wildly about as in rabies—hence the name "pseudo (false) rabies." Usually within 24 hours the animal goes down and is unable to rise because of paralysis. Death, preceded by labored breathing, bellowing and, sometimes, by convulsions and a moderate rise in temperature, usually occurs within 2 days after symptoms are first noticed.

Treatment.—No specific treatment is known and cattle rarely or never recover.

Diagnosis.—Diagnosis of the disease is important in order that the spread of the disease may be prevented as much as possible. So far as is known, pseudorabies does not spread from one cow to another through direct contact, and thus it is believed to be not highly contagious. Nevertheless, affected animals like those affected with any disease that may be contagious, should be isolated. A veterinarian should be called, as it is usually desirable to remove the brain for laboratory study. This, when examined microscopically, does not show the presence of Negri bodies as in rabies but does have a more or less characteristic picture in stained sections of the tissue, and the disease is usually inoculable into laboratory animals, such as rabbits, guinea pigs, rates, and mice.

Prevention.—Neither a definite system of prevention nor a preventive vaccine has as yet been developed. For these reasons, the owner of affected animals should cooperate in every way possible with his veterinarian, his State experiment station, and other agencies concerned with the study, diagnosis, and control of diseases in animals, in order that more may be learned of the disease and definite preventive procedures may be developed.

TUBERCULOSIS

[Pls. XXXIV–XXXVIII]

Tuberculosis is an infectious and communicable disease characterized in its early stages by the formation, in various parts of the body, of minute nodules or tubercles, which contain *Mycobacterium tuberculosis bovinus*, the cause of the disease.

The disease, in its various manifestations, has been known for many centuries, and legislative enactments having reference to the destruction of affected animals and forbidding the use of the flesh date far back into the Middle Ages. The opinions regarding the nature and the cause of the malady varied much in different periods and very markedly influenced the laws and regulations in vogue. Thus, in the sixteenth century, the disease was considered identical with syphilis in man. In consequence of this belief very stringent laws were enacted which made the destruction of tuberculous cattle compulsory. In the eighteenth century this erroneous conception of the nature of the disease was abandoned and all restrictions against the use of meat were removed. During the early part of the nineteenth century, the communicable nature of the disease was shown, but it was not until 1882 that the germ causing tuberculosis was first described, and the tide of opinion again turned in favor of repressing the disease and prohibiting the sale of contaminated products.

Occurrence.—The statistics concerning tuberculosis show that it is prevalent in all civilized countries. In some countries, such as the northern part of Norway and Sweden, on the steppes of eastern Europe and Russia, in Sicily and Iceland, and in Algiers, it is said to be quite rare. The returns from testing British cattle with tuberculin frequently show infection of 25 percent or more.

To this fact may be added the evidence of Professor Bang that in the first half of the nineteenth century tuberculosis was brought to Denmark by cattle from Switzerland, Schleswig, and England, and that the same thing occurred in Sweden and Norway, particularly through English cattle. There is also the evidence presented in 1899, by M. Sivori, chief of section at the ministry of agriculture, Argentina, who investigated tuberculosis in that country and who stated that "30 or 40 years ago tuberculosis was unknown in Argentine cattle, and it is still unknown among the native (criollo) cattle. Its appearance dates from the introduction of pure breeding animals."

Moreover, the reports of the royal commission of Victoria, Australia, and of the New Zealand department of agriculture have shown a large proportion of tuberculous cattle in those colonies, where the disease was almost certainly carried by British cattle.

In the same manner that tuberculosis has been carried from Great Britain to Denmark, Sweden, Norway, Argentina, and Australia, it has also been taken to Canada. In one herd of imported cattle slaughtered in the Canadian quarantine station, 13 of the 14 animals were found to be tuberculous. In recent years the bovine-tuberculosis situation has been greatly improved through the adoption and efficient use of tuberculosis-eradication methods.

The slaughterhouse statistics of Prussia have shown 14.6 percent of the cattle and 2.1 percent of the hogs to be tuberculous. In Saxony the percentages were 29 1 for cattle and 3.1 for hogs.

Of 20,850 animals in Belgium tested with tuberculin in 1896, 48 9 percent reacted (Stubbe). Of 25,439 tested in Denmark from 1893 to 1895, 49.3 percent reacted; and of 67,263 tested from 1896 to 1898, 32.8 percent reacted (Bang).

Reports of tuberculin tests made on 400,000 cattle in the United States from 1893 to 1908 by Federal, State, and other officers with tuberculin prepared by the Bureau of Animal Industry show 37,008 reactions, or 9.3 percent. These were mostly dairy cattle.

Later reports of tuberculin tests made in the United States from July 1, 1917, to February 1936 on 171.892,329 cattle by State, county, and Federal officers engaged in cooperative tuberculosis eradication work showed 3,405,447 reactors.

All cattle in the District of Columbia, numbering 1,701, were tested with tuberculin in 1909–10, and 18.9 percent reacted. In 1909–11 herds in Maryland and Virginia supplying milk to the District of Columbia were tested, with 19 and 15.4 percent of reactions, respectively, among 4,501 cattle.

All cattle in the District of Columbia, numbering 1,313, were tuberculin tested in 1920–21, and 5 animals, or about 0.4 percent, reacted, demonstrating that tuberculosis may be eradicated from all the herds in a circumscribed area.

From the statistics just referred to and other data, it appears that, in the more densely populated areas of Europe, 5 to 50 percent of the dairy cattle are affected with tuberculosis, whereas the proportion of beef cattle affected is distinctly less, ranging from 0.14 to 30 percent. This difference is due to a number of causes. Beef cattle, on the average, are younger when slaughtered. They are not so frequently stabled and are for that reason less subject to exposure, and as the males constitute a large proportion of this class of animals the effect of milk secretion in lowering the vital forces is not so apparent.

In the United States it was estimated at one time that approximately 10 percent of the dairy cattle were tuberculous, whereas only about 2 percent of the beef cattle were so infected. By November 1, 1940, all counties in the United States had been designated as modified accredited areas, indicating that the infection had been reduced to less than one-half of 1 percent.

The average extent of bovine tuberculosis, in recent years, has been determined by a series of surveys based on official tuberculin testing. The decreasing percentages in the following tabulation are evidence of the effectiveness of systematic tuberculosis-eradication work:

Year	*Percent of cattle tuberculous*
1922	4.2
1924	3.3
1926	2.8
1928	2.0
1930	1.7
1932	1.4
1934	1.1
1936	0.5

No survey has been made since 1936.

Information concerning the progress and current status of tuberculosis eradication in any part of the United States may be obtained by applying to State livestock officials or to the Bureau of Animal Industry, United States Department of Agriculture, Washington, D. C.

Cause and nature of the disease.—The cause of tuberculosis is the tubercle bacillus, which gains entrance to the body, lodges somewhere in the tissues, and begins to grow and multiply at that point. As this bacillus vegetates and increases in numbers it excretes substances that act as irritants and poisons and lead to the formation of a small nodule, called a tubercle, at the point of localization. As the bacilli are disseminated through the animal body they may affect many parts and cause the formation of an enormous number of tubercles. By the union of such tubercles, masses of tuberculosis material are formed, which in some cases are of great size. The disease is called tuberculosis because it is characterized by the formation of these peculiar nodules, and the bacillus that causes the disease is for the same reason known technically as the *Mycobacterium tuberculosis bovinus.*

There are undoubtedly predisposing conditions that contribute toward the development of the disease; some of these are found in the animal body and others in the environment. An enfeebled condition caused by insufficient feed, exposure to great extremes of atmospheric temperature and insanitary surroundings, or the drain occasioned by heavy production of milk, appears to aid the development of the bacillus, and there is also a special individual susceptibility in some cases that may be otherwise described as an inability of the animal tissues to resist and destroy the bacilli when they have entered the body.

Among the conditions of environment that aid the development of tuberculosis are stabling with lack of ventilation, damp buildings, the keeping of many animals together, drafts of air that cause colds and catarrh, and, in general, everything that prevents the animals from developing and maintaining the highest condition of health. None of these conditions of body or environment are sufficient to cause the disease, however, unless the animals are exposed to the tubercle bacillus.

The principal ways in which the tubercle bacilli find their way into the body area as follows: (1) By inhalation into the lungs; (2) by drinking contaminated water, especially from slow-flowing streams or stagnant pools into which the dung of infected cattle has dropped, or by eating contaminated feed; (3) through the infected milk of a cow to her suckling calf; and (4) through abrasions in the skin. The bacilli can reach the lungs by inhalation only when the bacilli are thoroughly dried and pulverized and in condition to be carried by currents of air. Under suitable conditions bacilli may remain in soil or water for months before they lose their power of producing disease.

They leave the body of diseased animals in several ways. Occasionally a little discharge may be coughed up as a spray from the diseased lungs, or this material may be swallowed and the bacilli carried off with the excrement. There may be a discharge from the vagina when the genital organs are tuberculous. There may also be ulcers of the intestines, from which many bacilli escape with the feces. The bacilli from these sources may become dried and pulverized and carried in the air of the stable and thus be a source of exposure to healthy cattle. The udder often becomes infected in chronic tuberculosis, and tubercle bacilli are given off in large numbers in the milk. Milk may also be contaminated with dung during the process of milking.

The disease of the stomach, intestines, and mesenteric glands is probably the result of feed or water infection, but tubercle bacilli may pass through the intestines without causing a lesion and set up a primary infection in the lungs or adjacent lymph glands.

The source of infection is always some previous case of the disease, for it can never occur spontaneously. It is usually introduced into a clean herd by the addition of an infected animal. No bovine animal should be added to a herd, therefore, until it has been shown by test to be free from the disease. Since the bacilli can be carried by the air, on feed, and by streams, it is not necessary for healthy animals to come in direct contact with cases of disease to become infected.

The bacillus of tuberculosis was discovered by Robert Koch in 1882. It is a slender, rodlike body (pl. XXVIII, fig. 6) from one-third to two-thirds the diameter of a red blood corpuscle in length. As already explained, when the bacillus has become lodged in any organ or tissue it begins to multiply and thereby causes an irritation in the tissue around it, which leads to the formation of the so-called tubercle. The tubercle is composed of several kinds of tissue cells. Soon a change takes place within the tubercle. Disintegration begins, and a soft, cheesy substance is formed in the center, which may contain particles of lime salts. When these tubercles continue to form in large numbers they run together and form masses of various sizes. The disintegration which attacks them leads to the formation of large cheesy masses of a yellowish color, containing more or less lime salts in the form of gritty particles. These large tuberculous masses are surrounded by or embedded in layers of fibrous tissue, which in some cases becomes very dense and thick.

The disease is thus a development of these tubercles in one or more organs or tissues of the body. The distribution and number of the tubercles determine the course of the disease. In a large number of cases the changes are limited to the lungs, lymphatic glands, and the serous membranes[1] of the thorax and abdomen. Other organs, such as the liver, frequently contain tubercles. Though the disease may remain restricted to a single organ, it now and then is generalized, affecting all organs of the body.

In the lungs (pl. XXXIV) the changes observed vary according to the age and intensity of the disease process. They usually begin with the appearance of very minute tubercles. These may appear in large numbers on the surface of the lungs or within the lung tissue. Later the contents become cheesy and partly calcified. When these tubercles are sufficiently numerous to become confluent, large masses may be formed, which undergo the same retrogressive changes of caseation and calcification. In addition to the formation of tubercles in the lung tissue, other changes take place. There is usually bronchitis with abundant catarrhal secretion; this plugs up the smaller air tubes, and the lung tissue supplied with air by the tubes collapses. Subsequently it becomes filled with yellowish, cheesy matter, which greatly distends the small air tubes and air vesicles (bronchopneumonia). The connective tissue between the lung lobules, around the tubercles, and around the air tubes becomes thickened and indurated. In the larynx and the bronchi tubercles may vegetate upon the mucous membrane, and ulcers may result from their breaking down. The inflammatory irritation that the growth of the tubercles on the surface of the lungs arouses gives rise to adhesion of the lungs to the ribs and diaphragm. This adhesion is sometimes so firm and extensive that the lungs appear grown to the chest wall.

When, therefore, the lungs in advanced stages of the disease are cut open there are large yellowish masses, from one-fourth to several inches in diameter, of a cheesy texture, in which calcified, gritty particles may be embedded and which are surrounded by very firm connective tissue. The neighboring lung tissue, when collapsed and involved in bronchopneumonia, has the color and consistency of pale-red flesh. The air tubes, large and small, stand out prominently on the cut surface. They are distended with a pasty, yellowish, cheesy mass, surrounded and enveloped in thick mucus, and their walls greatly thickened. The larger bronchi may be sacculated, owing to the distention produced by the cheesy contents.

The disease usually attacks the bronchial glands, which are situated on the trachea and bronchial tubes at the bifurcation. The changes in the glands are the same as those going on in the lung tissue, and they frequently reach an enormous size.

---

[1] These membranes comprise the smooth, very delicate, glistening lining of the large body cavities. In the thorax the serous membrane (pleura) covers the ribs and diaphragm as well as the whole lung surface. In the abdomen a similar membrane (peritoneum) lines the interior of the cavity and covers the bowels, liver, spleen, etc.

The tubercle formation on the serous membranes covering the lungs and chest wall (pl. XXXVII, fig. 2), which may go on at the same time with the lung disease or independent of it, has been called "pearly disease," on account of the peculiar appearance of the tubercles. These begin as very minute, grayish nodules, which give the originally smooth, lustrous membrane a roughened appearance. These minute tubercles enlarge, become confluent, and project above the surface of the membrane as wartlike masses and attain the size of peas. In this stage their attachment to the membrane is by means of delicate fibers. The attachment is loose, so that the tubercle hangs by a short pedicle or neck and may be moved slightly to and fro. Large masses are frequently formed by a coalescence of many tubercles and the secondary formation of the same. These may be found on the lungs, the ribs, and the diaphragm. These tubercles likewise undergo degenerative changes. The center partly softens and partly calcifies into a grayish mortarlike mass and is gritty. Associated with the formation of tubercles on the pleura, those glands situated back of the center of the lungs between the two main lobes (posterior mediastinal) become greatly enlarged and the center cheesy (pl. XXXVI, fig. 1). They may compress the esophagus and interfere with swallowing. The size attained by these tumors and new growths is well illustrated by the fact that, taken together, they frequently weigh 60 to 80 pounds. The bronchial glands, which in the healthy state are not so large as horse chestnuts, have been found to attain a weight of more than 10 pounds.

In the abdominal cavity tubercles may be found, both in the organs and on the serous membranes covering them. They are situated usually on the omentum, or caul (see pl. XXXVI, fig. 2), the diaphragm, and the walls of the abdomen. In the liver large and small tuberculous masses are occasionally encountered (pl. XXXV). The mesenteric glands, as well as the glands near the liver, may become enlarged and tuberculous. Tubercles may also develop in the spleen, the kidneys, the uterus and ovaries, and the testicles.

Tuberculous affection of the intestines seems to be less common, although ulcers of the large intestines have been observed. Nodules may also form under the serous covering of the intestines.

The brain and spinal cord are occasionally found to be tuberculous. Of 40 cases, Semmer found tuberculosis of the brain in 4. It is probable that, owing to the infrequency of exposing the brain and spinal cord, tuberculosis may have escaped the attention of pathologists, and it may be that it is not so uncommon as is generally supposed. The tubercles occur on the membranes of the brain as well as in the substance of the brain itself. They project into the ventricles as masses, and vary in size from a pinhead to a hen's egg. They finally lead to various inflammatory changes.

Tuberculous lesions have rarely been observed in the bones and muscles of the body. Lesions are more frequently found in the lymphatic glands embedded in the muscular tissue and those that can be felt beneath the skin. These are situated at the joints, under the jaw, and along the neck.

Tuberculosis of the udder in cows (pl. XXXVIII) has received considerable attention from sanitary officials, owing to the infection of the milk with the germs of tuberculosis. The udder becomes swollen uniformly and is rather firm. This swelling, which is painless, frequently attacks but one quarter, more rarely two, these being usually the hind quarters. The larger milk ducts contain yellowish, cheesy particles, in which are many tubercle bacilli. Later larger nodules can be felt within the udder, which undergo the various changes to which tubercles are subject. The udder may become very hard and large, weighing in some cases up to 40 pounds. The milk, at first normal, becomes thin and watery after a month or so and is mixed with flakes and tubercle bacilli.

Symptoms.—The beginning of the disease usually passes unnoticed, inasmuch as it is very slow and insidious and rarely accompanied with fever. When the lungs are involved a dull, short cough is noticed, which may later on become prolonged, convulsive, and very troublesome to the animal. The cough is more frequent in the morning after movement and drinking. The breathing varies. Only when much of the lung tissue is diseased is it labored and accompanied with active movements of the chest and nostrils. Discharge from the nose is rare or absent. At times, however, when the tubercles have broken down and cavities containing cheesy masses have formed in the lung tissue, or when the air tubes have become filled with cheesy and mucous masses, coughing will dislodge them and cause their discharge. In advanced stages the breath may have a disagreeable odor. Pressure on the chest wall may give rise to pain.

The general effect on the body is at first slight. In fact, animals may remain in good flesh for a considerable time. Invariably as the disease progresses loss of flesh and appetite and paleness of the mucous membranes become manifest. These symptoms are accompanied with a gradual diminution of the milk secretion. The debilitated condition of the animal is also manifested by a staring coat and a tough, dry, harsh skin (hidebound). Digestive disturbances are indicated by tympanites, or distention of the rumen by gas, colic, and diarrhea, alternating with constipation. The animal generally dies from exhaustion after a period of sickness that may last months or even years.

Tuberculosis in the generative organs is sometimes signalized by abortion and by abnormal sexual manifestations. When the brain is involved, the disease may cause convulsions, unconsciousness, paralysis, as well as peculiar movements in a circle, oblique position of the head, and other symptoms.

Diagnosis.—A disease so varied in its attack on the different organs of the body and in the extent of the disease processes must necessarily lead to mistakes when diagnosis is attempted by ordinary means of examination. It has been confused with parasitic diseases of the brain, lungs, intestines, and with actinomycosis. A careful examination of the lungs by auscultation and percussion enables the expert to locate large tuberculous masses, owing to dullness, loss of respiratory murmur, and abnormal sounds, such as blowing, whistling, and creaking. In most cases it is exceedingly difficult and impractical to depend on a physical examination alone to detect tuberculosis in cattle, even though the lungs have become seriously involved.

THE TUBERCULIN TEST

The tuberculin test, which is marvelously accurate in its indications, has been universally adopted for the detection of tuberculosis. Tuberculin is a product prepared by sterilizing, filtering, and concentrating the liquids in which the tubercle bacillus has been allowed to vegetate. It contains the cooked products of the growth of these bacilli, but no living bacilli. Consequently, when this substance is injected into or under the skin of an animal or dropped on the eye it is unable to produce the disease, cause abortion, or otherwise injure the animal. In case the injected animal is normal, there is no more effect on the system than would be expected from the injection of sterile water. However, if the animal is tuberculous, a decided rise of temperature follows the use of tuberculin by the subcutaneous method. If the test is made by injecting tuberculin into the skin, or intradermically, usually in the fold under the tail, a swelling develops within 48 to 72 hours. If the tuberculin is dropped on the eye, or ophthalmically, a mucous or milky discharge occurs within a few hours. The value of tuberculin for this purpose was tested in 1890 and 1891 by Guttman, Roeckl and Schütz, Bang and Salomonsen, Lydtin, Jöhne and Siedamgrotzky, Nocard, and many others. It was at once recognized as a remarkable and accurate method of detecting tuberculosis even in the early stages and when the disease had yet made little progress.

In recent years improved methods of producing biological products, by scientists of the Bureau of Animal Industry, have led to the production, from cultures on a new synthetic medium, of a tuberculin that is more efficient as a diagnostic agent than tuberculin produced by other methods. Prior to the development of the new tuberculin, the testing of cattle and other susceptible animals for tuberculosis was conducted with tuberculin made essentially in the same manner as the original product developed by Robert Koch in 1891.

The medium used for the Koch tuberculin consists of a clear broth, made from lean beef or veal, to which 1 percent of peptone, 4 to 7 percent of glycerin, and 0.5 percent of salt are added. This mixture is then inoculated with pure cultures of tubercle bacilli. At the end of the growing period the broth cultures are sterilized, the dead bacteria are removed by filtration, and the clear, sterile filtrate is concentrated to the desired degree. A suitable preservative is then added. The final product, which is used in testing cattle, contains not only the soluble substances derived from the growth of the tubercle bacilli on broth but also any portions of the culture medium that have not been used up during the growth of bacilli. It is generally recognized that the Koch or broth tuberculin is extremely complex. It always contains considerable quantities of unused glycerin. In addition there are unused nitrogenous protein materials derived from the peptone which is added to the broth.

The new synthetic medium contains no protein whatever. The nitrogen required by the bacteria for their growth is supplied by the pure crystals of asparagin, and the other needs of the bacteria are furnished by pure glycerin, dextrose, magnesium sulfate, potassium phosphate, and derivatives of sodium and iron. Tuberculin prepared from such cultures has been found to be much more potent than that derived from cultures on the broth medium.

Another advantage afforded by the use of the synthetic medium lies in the purity of the final product; that is, the tuberculin. As previously stated, the Koch, or broth tuberculin, always contains considerable quantities of unused residues of the culture medium. The newer tuberculin, on the other hand, is essentially a pure solution of the products of the tubercle bacillus. This result was attained by adjusting the constituents of the synthetic culture medium so that the bacteria use practically all of them. The final tuberculin contains only products derived from the tubercle bacillus itself. Since the reaction of tuberculous cattle to tuberculin is caused only by the products of the tubercle bacillus, it is evident that the new tuberculin is much purer than the older product.

The new tuberculin, in comparative tests, has also proved to be more effective when used for diagnosis under practical field conditions. As a result, the tuberculin produced from cultures on the new synthetic medium since April 1934 has been used exclusively by the Bureau of Animal Industry in official tuberculosis-eradication work.

Thus the tuberculin test came into existence and has been developed through careful and thorough scientific experimentation.

The tuberculin should be applied only by a competent veterinarian, capable not only of injecting the tuberculin but also of interpreting the results, and particularly of picking out clinical cases by physical examination.

A great advantage in the use of tuberculin is that it discovers cases in which the lesions are small and obscure. A small lesion today may break down and become widely disseminated in a relatively short period. Therefore any cow affected with tuberculosis, even to a slight degree, must be considered as dangerous not only to the other animals in the herd but also to the consumer of her products.

All animals that give a positive reaction should be separated from the herd, not only in the interest of the public but also in the interest of the owner of the herd. Authorities admit, after studying many thousands of tests, that few mistakes are made in condemning cattle that show a typical tuberculin reaction. Furthermore, in view of the results revealed by numerous tests of vast numbers of animals, tuberculin must be considered as harmless for healthy animals. It has also been clearly demonstrated that tuberculin interferes in no way with the milking function in healthy cattle; neither in the quantity of milk nor in butterfat value has any variation been detected.

Briefly, there is ample evidence to show that tuberculin is the most reliable means of detecting tuberculosis in the living animal and that its use is not attended by any harmful after effects.

Under the plan of eradication herds are tested under State and Federal supervision, and the diseased animals are appraised, removed, and slaughtered under Federal inspection. Retests are then made after suitable periods of time until they show all the animals to be free from the disease.

Details concerning methods of tuberculosis eradication may be obtained by applying to the Chief of the Bureau of Animal Industry, Washington, D. C.

METHODS OF TESTING

The tuberculin test may be applied by three different methods—the intradermic, the subcutaneous, and the ophthalmic.

The intradermic test for detecting tuberculosis has been the method principally used in the tuberculosis-eradication campaign in the United States. When made by those skilled in its application, this test is exceptionally accurate. The double-injection method of applying the test is generally used. This consists in injecting a small quantity of intradermic tuberculin between the layers of the skin in the caudal fold at the base of the tail. A similar injection between the layers of the vulvar tissues at a point along the line of demarcation of the mucous membrane is also made at the same time.

A reaction to the intradermic test consists of a swelling at the point of injection and is observed from 72 to 120 hours after the injection is made. The character of the swelling varies, and a proper diagnosis of tuberculosis by this test can be made only by a competent and experienced person.

The subcutaneous test consists in injecting the proper quantity of tuberculin underneath the skin into the subcutaneous tissue. If an animal is tuberculous, the action of the tuberculin causes a fever, which is indicated by a rise in temperature. This rise, under ordinary conditions, may occur any time between the eighth and twentieth hours after the tuberculin is injected, but in some cases it is desirable to measure the temperature before the eighth hour and continue to the twenty fourth hour or longer.

The temperatures are measured at least three times in advance of the injection, at 2-hour intervals, to learn whether the animal is in proper condition to receive the test. The temperatures after injection are taken every 2 hours until the test is completed. The proper interpretation of the temperatures is made by the person applying the test, and a careful observance of any clinical changes is always important in determining the result. It cannot be set forth too strongly that the test should be attempted only by those who are properly qualified to do the work.

Still another method, the ophthalmic test, has been used to some extent and at one time appeared to possess considerable value. However, at this time it is not generally accepted as an accurate means of diagnosis and is seldom used. In this method a specially prepared ophthalmic tuberculin is placed in one eye and the other eye is used as a control. This procedure is again repeated at the seventy-second hour, and a reaction is indicated by a certain characteristic discharge from the eye receiving the tuberculin, which may occur 3 to 10 hours after the second application or even later. Some swelling and inflammation of the eye and lids are frequently noted.

PREVENTION OF TUBERCULOSIS

Treatment of the disease is not seriously considered at the present time.

The measures to be adopted to prevent the spreading of the disease must take into consideration not only the tubercle bacillus, but likewise all those circumstances that make cattle more susceptible to the disease and that have already been dwelt on. Great care should be bestowed on the breeding, the surroundings, and the feed of the animal, and a tuberculin test should be applied to all cattle before they are introduced into the herd if such animals are not from an area known to be free of the disease.

A rigid exclusion of tuberculous animals and material is necessary to prevent the appearance of the disease in a herd free from infection. The transmission of the human type of the disease to cattle is extremely rare, but cattle may become sensitive to tuberculin by ingesting human tuberculous sputum.

Tuberculosis in cattle must also be considered as bearing on tuberculosis of other domesticated animals, particularly hogs. In Europe and the United States this disease is common among hogs. It usually results from one of the following causes: Allowing hogs to mingle with tuberculous cattle or poultry; feeding pigs skim milk, buttermilk, and whey from creameries, the offal of abattoirs, or garbage.

The carcasses of animals that have died of tuberculosis should be burned or buried deeply so that they cannot be eaten by other animals. This is likewise true of all organs or tissues of slaughtered animals containing tubercles. These should never be fed to other animals, such as hogs, dogs, and cats.

When any of the animals in a herd of cattle show evident symptoms of tuberculosis, or when the tuberculin test proves that they are affected with this disease, the best method of procedure in most cases is to have the affected animals slaughtered and the stables disinfected. A large proportion of the animals that are slightly affected yield carcasses that are perfectly wholesome and fit for human food, but in all such cases there should be an inspection by a veterinarian at the time of slaughter to determine which carcasses or parts of carcasses may be used and which should be destroyed.

Stables may be disinfected by thoroughly cleaning them, scrubbing the floors with hot water, brushing down all loose dust from the walls, and tearing off all woodwork that is partly decayed. Then the whole interior of the stable should be sprayed with a 3 to 4 percent compound solution of cresol or other disinfectants approved by the Bureau of Animal Industry. The choice of a disinfectant, especially for dairy barns, may depend on whether the odor it leaves for a time is objectionable.

Similar precautions should be observed in removing the manure of the infected herd from the barnyard and other places accessible to cattle, since tuberculous cattle frequently eliminate large numbers of tubercle bacilli through the feces. The ground should then be disinfected, either by unslaked lime thickly sprinkled over the soil or other approved disinfectants, and all low, moist places should be drained or filled.

If all the animals that react are destroyed and the stables and yards disinfected in this manner, the herd should remain free from the disease unless other affected animals are added to it.

The disposal of reactors depends on the State laws and livestock regulations of the State in which the herd belongs. The livestock sanitary officials of the State should be consulted and their instructions followed.

RELATION OF BOVINE TUBERCULOSIS TO MAN

Although cattle are extremely resistant to the human type of tuberculosis, human beings can contract the bovine type. They are less

77431 O—51——27

susceptible to the bovine than to the human type, but under continuous or severe exposure the bovine tubercle bacillus can cause every kind of tuberculosis in man that is caused by the human-type germ, such as miliary tuberculosis, lupus, bone and joint, scrofula, kidney infection, and even tuberculosis of the lungs.

Infants are more susceptible than adults to the bovine type of infection, and the disease is usually manifested in miliary tuberculosis, which is a rapidly fatal disease; scrofula (infection of the glands of the neck or throat); lupus (tuberculosis of the skin); and bone or joint tuberculosis. In some European countries, in which 25 to 50 percent of cattle are tuberculous, a large proportion of tuberculous infections, especially in children, is the result of drinking unpasteurized milk from tuberculous cows. The same conditions were observed in this country years ago. In 1917 the bovine tuberculosis eradication campaign was begun in cooperation with the various States, and by November 1, 1940, all States were designated as modified accredited areas, indicating their practical freedom from infection. This campaign, together with the practice of pasteurizing milk, has resulted in such a marked decrease in the bovine type of infection in man that medical experts have stated it is practically impossible to find such cases for the clinical instruction of medical students.

TUBERCULOSIS

DESCRIPTION OF PLATES

PLATE XXXIV. Tuberculosis of the lungs of cattle. The upper figure represents a large cheesy mass, surrounded by a capsule of connective tissue, the whole embedded in healthy lung tissue. The center and lower figures illustrate in section masses of tubercles that have undergone cheesy degeneration, and some of which are surrounded by dense connective tissue.

PLATE XXXV. Tuberculosis of the liver. A large portion of the lobe represented in the plate has undergone tuberculous changes. Numerous nodules are shown in various stages of the disease, the most of which, however, contain the yellowish, partly cheesy, partly gritty areas characteristic of advanced tuberculous degeneration. This large mass involves the surface of the liver and also extends into the liver substance.

PLATE XXXVI. Tuberculosis of lymph gland and of omentum (caul).

Figure 1. A lymph gland from the region of the thorax behind or above the esophagus, or gullet (posterior, or dorsal, mediastinum). The gland is shown cut through and laid open. It is very much enlarged, and the yellowish cheesy masses that represent tissue undergoing tuberculous changes are well shown on the cut surface.

Figure 2. Omentum, or caul, resting on the paunch. The reddish nodules

Pl. XXXVII to be tipped in (pick up cuts)

with which the membrane is beset are tubercles, the product of the disease.

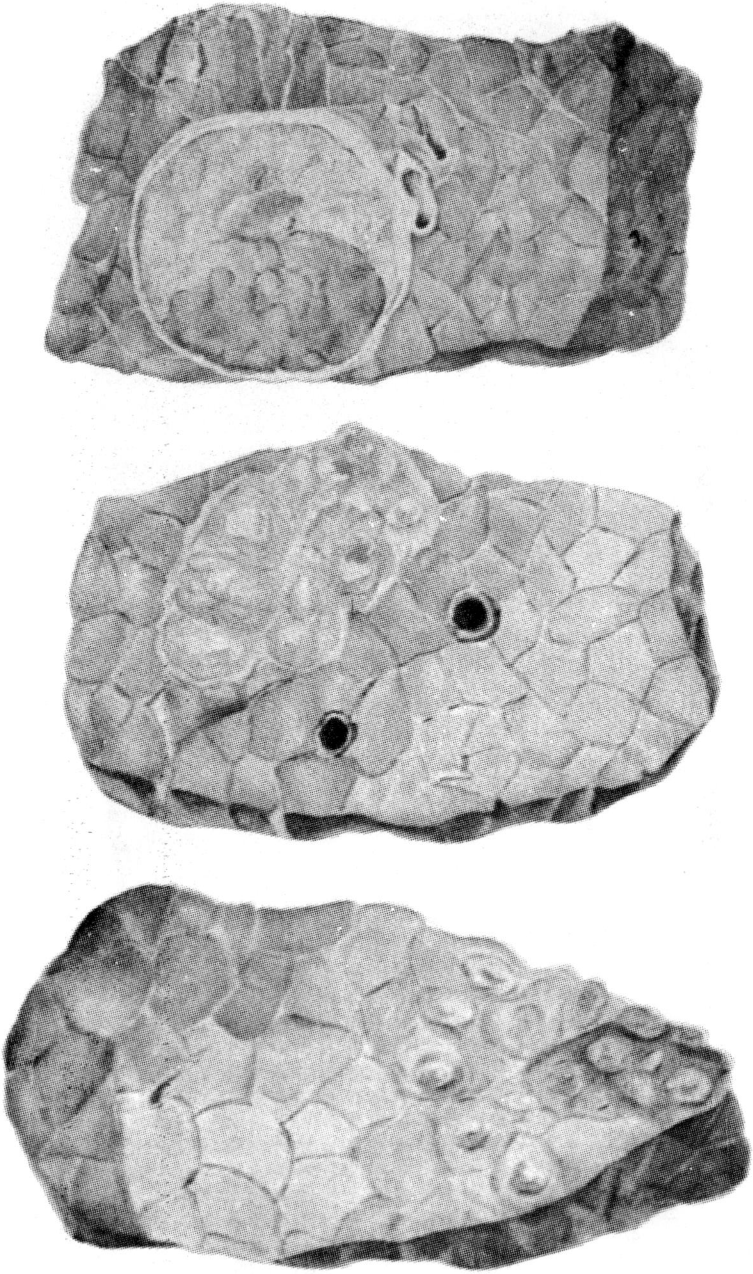

TUBERCULOSIS OF THE LUNGS OF CATTLE.

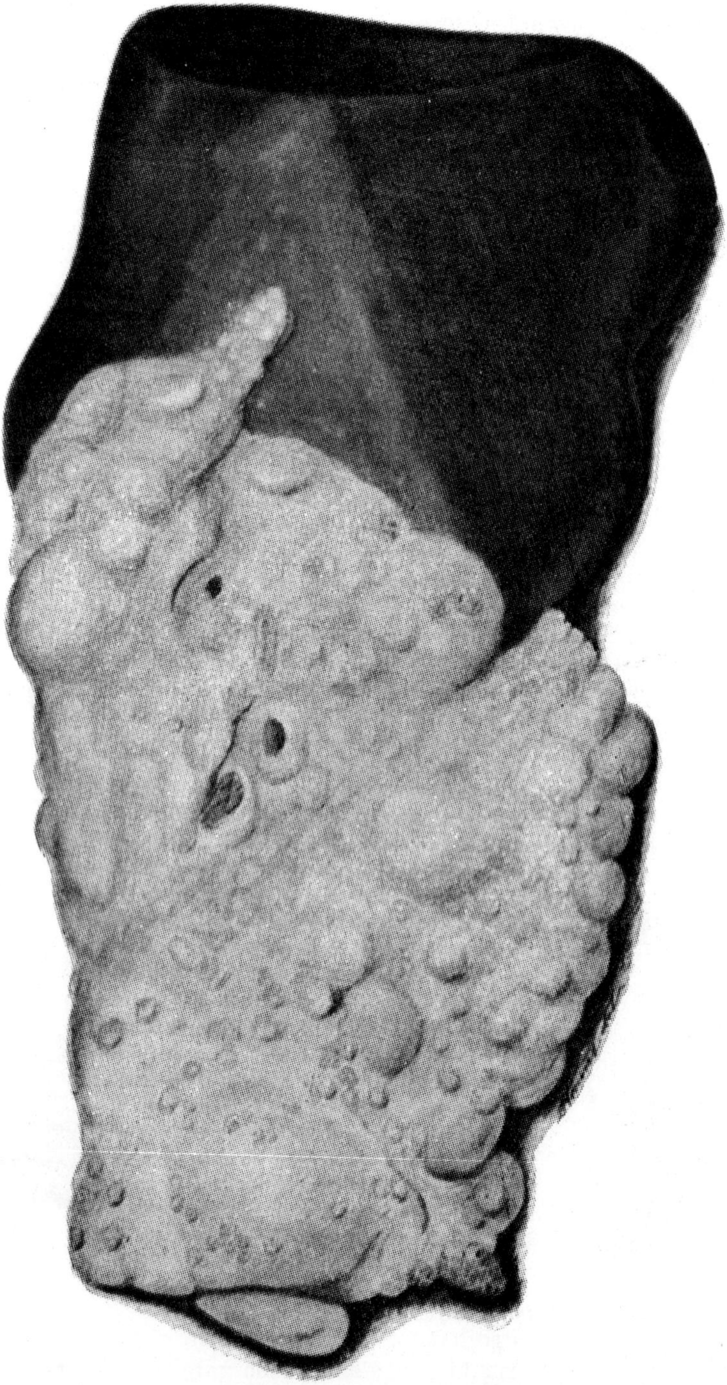

TUBERCULOSIS OF THE LIVER.

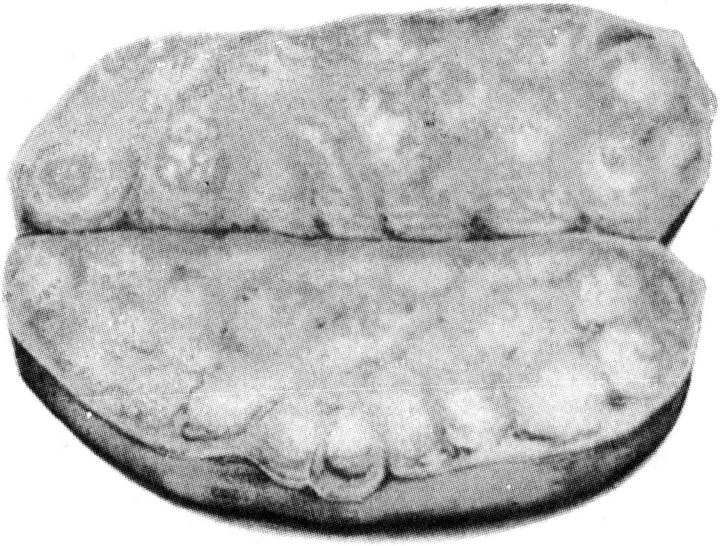

FIGURE 1

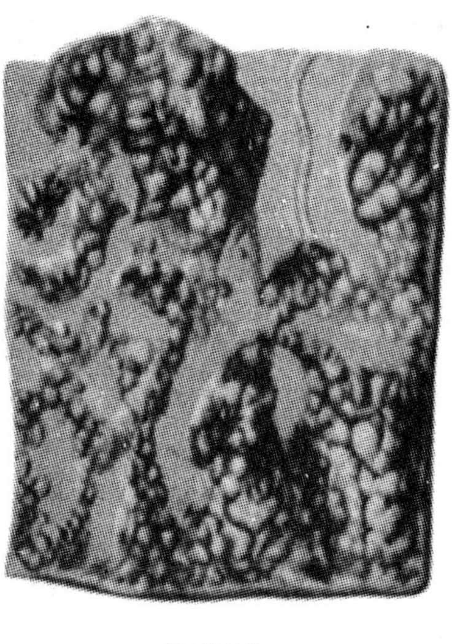

FIGURE 2

HAINES DEL.

TUBERCULOSIS OF LYMPH GLAND AND OF OMENTUM (CAUL).

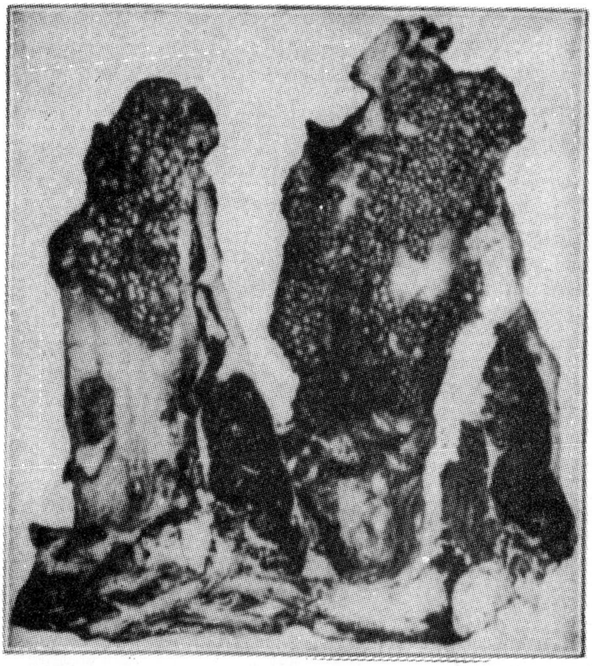

FIGURE 1.—TUBERCULOSIS OF SIRLOIN AND PORTERHOUSE CUTS OF BEEF.

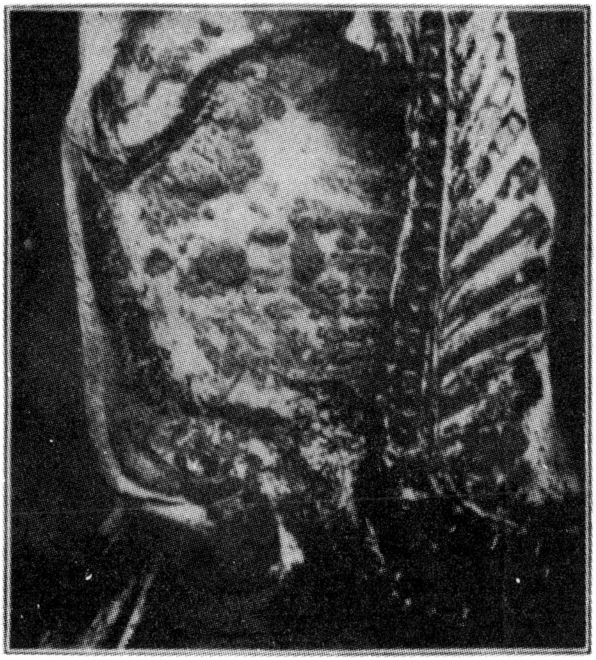

FIGURE 2.—TUBERCULOSIS OF PLEURA OF A COW, SO-CALLED "PEARLY DISEASE."

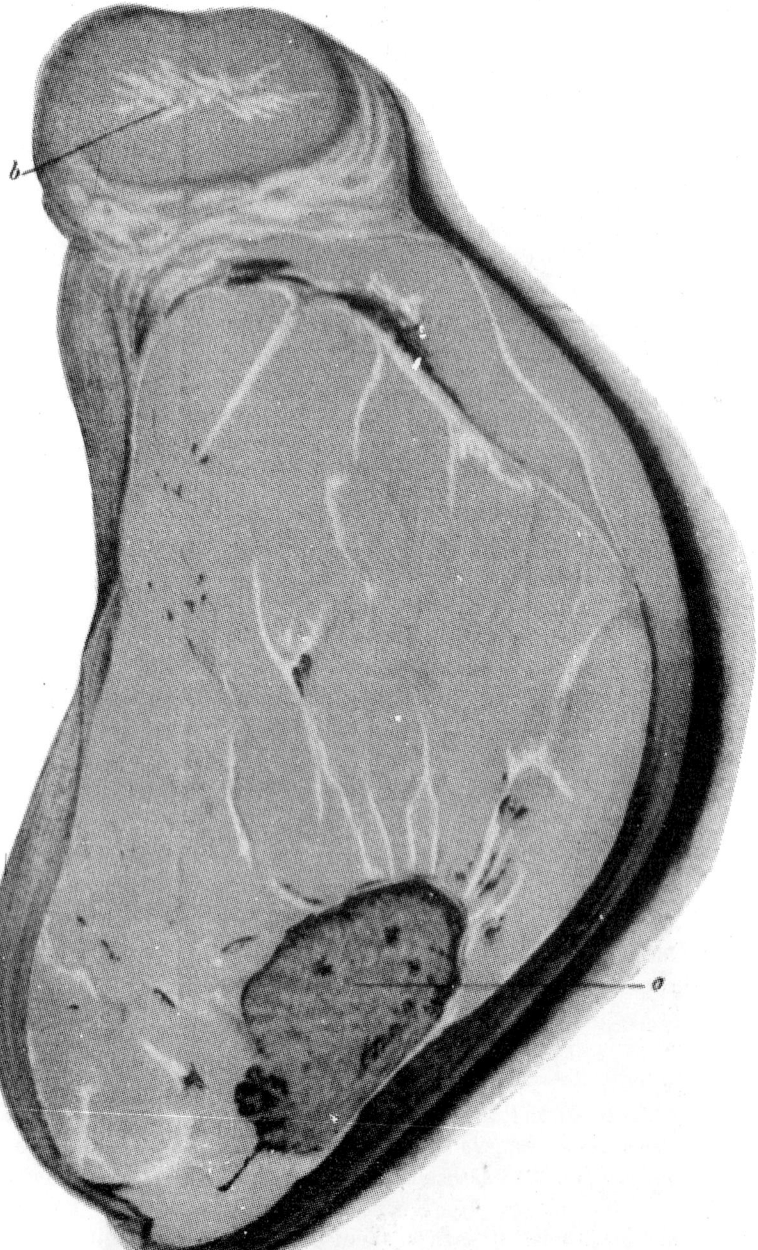

HAINES DEL.

TUBERCULOSIS OF COW'S UDDER.

PLATE XXXVII. Figure 1. Tuberculosis of sirloin and porterhouse cuts of beef. The grapelike tuberculous growths are mainly restricted to the lining membrane of the abdomen.

Figure 2. Tuberculosis of the pleura of a cow, so-called "pearly disease." Notice the grapelike clusters of tuberculous nodules scattered over the lining membrane of the chest (pleura).

PLATE XXXVIII. Tuberculosis of cow's udder. The udder was uniformly swollen and rather firm. Small cheesy foci and yellowish lines of tuberculous material follow the course of the milk ducts. The mucous membrane of the milk cistern (*a*) is ulcerated and covered with yellowish cheesy particles. The supramammary lymphatic gland (*b*) is greatly enlarged and contains many miliary tuberculous foci.

JOHNE'S DISEASE (PARATUBERCULOSIS)

Johne's disease is an incurable, infectious, bacterial dysentery affecting principally cattle, but it may also affect horses, sheep, deer, and goats. It is also called paratuberculosis, bacterial enteritis, chronic hypertrophic enteritis, and chronic pseudotuberculosis enteritis. It was given the name of "pseudotuberculosis enteritis" by some of the early investigators.

Johne's disease was first studied bacteriologically in Dresden, Germany, in 1895 by Johne and Frothingham. It has since been found in India and many countries of Europe, including the Channel Islands. It has also been diagnosed in many sections of the United States, and there is no doubt that the infection has spread to virtually every State. It is not definitely known when the disease first made its appearance in the New World, but it must have been more than a quarter of a century ago; and, like tuberculosis, it was probably brought in with shipments of cattle from Europe. It was first described in this country by Pearson in 1908.

Cause.—The disease is caused by the *Mycobacterium paratuberculosis*, a bacillus, which is usually found in nests and in large clumps in the affected parts of the intestinal mucous membranes and in the lymph nodes of the intestines. In some respects it is like the tubercle bacillus but is different in other ways.

Mode of infection.—The disease is spread from herd to herd by diseased animals being introduced into clean herds, by diseased animals grazing on community pastures with healthy animals, and by drinking contaminated water from pools or slow-running streams. It is spread from animal to animal within a herd by bacilli expelled from the diseased animal's body with the feces, which contaminate the feed and water. From a practical viewpoint, infection of an animal occurs only when the causal agents are taken into the body by the mouth with feed or water, unless the calf is infected in the uterus, which has not been definitely determined.

In planning for the control and eradication of the disease it is necessary to give special attention to such possible sources of infection as ponds, sloughs, slow-running streams, water troughs, and feed boxes. The practice of feeding hay and fodder in field lots on the ground, where it may become contaminated by manure, should be discouraged. Just how long a pasture may remain infected has not yet been definitely determined. The time obviously may be expected to vary under different conditions.

Period of incubation.—Although the period of incubation is not known it is believed that, in some instances, animals become infected when only a few weeks old but do not develop noticeable symptoms until they are 3 or 4 years old.

The evidence at hand indicates that all blood lines and all breeds of cattle are susceptible to infection, but the disease appears to be more prevalent in some breeds than in others.

Symptoms.—The first symptom usually observed in a case of Johne's disease in cows is a severe drop in the milk yield. This symptom is usually followed by intermittent diarrhea or by progressive diarrhea which fails to respond to the usual medicinal agents for the correction of such conditions. The coat becomes rough and the animal looks unthrifty. The appetite may be regained after the first few days and thereafter remain normal. The animal may drink large quantities of water. Although some writers on Johne's disease have not observed any elevation of temperature, others claim that the temperature is sometimes elevated several degrees. In the last stages of the disease the animal becomes greatly emaciated and dies as the result of exhaustion due to the extreme dysentery. Death is often hastened by parturition and has been observed in valuable purebred herds when cows are placed on official test for production. This may be readily explained since in producing large quantities of milk the vitality of the animal is lessened, thereby making it an easy victim to the disease.

Treatment.—No satisfactory treatment for Johne's disease is known. In the earlier stages when the diarrhea is intermittent, temporary relief is sometimes obtained by restricting the feed and placing the animal on a dry diet. Care should be exercised to isolate the suspected cases until such time as a positive diagnosis can be made. Millions of the bacteria which cause the disease are expelled in the feces of the infected animals; therefore, the droppings from suspected and diseased animals should be burned, buried in lime, or disposed of in a cultivated field not accessible to susceptible animals. Treatment should be restricted to preventive measures, as cures cannot be expected, according to present knowledge.

Post mortem appearance.—In advanced cases the carcass will be emaciated and serous fluid may be present in the abdominal cavity. A specific enteritis in both the large and small intestines is sometimes present. The lower part of the small intestine (ileum) and the upper part of the large intestine (cecum and upper colon) are the parts most often affected. In mild cases it may be difficult to detect any abnormal condition in the intestines, but in old, chronic cases the walls of some portion of the small intestines will appear thickened. When this is opened the mucous lining presents an abnormal thickened, wrinkled, or corrugated appearance. This condition should not be confused with the normal furrows found in healthy intestines of cattle. There is little or no general inflammation in any section of the bowels, and in this respect the disease differs from most other conditions which produce diarrhea. The mesenteric lymphatic glands are enlarged, and on their being incised, an increased quantity of milklike fluid escapes.

Diagnosis.—The microscopic examination of feces or pieces of membrane from the intestines will, in some cases, be sufficient to establish a diagnosis.

The post mortem lesions may be characteristic and may suffice to establish the existence of the disease.

At the present time the use of johnin, injected either into the skin (intradermic test) or into a vein, is believed to be the best available means of diagnosing the disease in herds. Johnin, or paratuberculin, is the liquid that is prepared from fluid which has been sterilized, filtered, and concentrated after the growth in it of the organisms that cause Johne's disease. Its nature and method of preparation are much like those of tuberculin, which is widely used in the diagnosis of tuberculosis in animals. Some research workers have reported good results from the use of avian tuberculin intravenously as a diagnostic agent for Johne's disease.

THE JOHNIN TEST

The johnin test is applied to individual animals or herds of cattle in order to ascertain the presence or absence of Johne's disease. The skin or intradermic test is similar to the tuberculin test. Johnin is injected into the skin usually at the base of the tail. An enlargement at the point of injection that persists for 48 hours or longer is considered to be a reaction. The intravenous test is made by injecting the johnin into the jugular vein.

The animals should be arranged as usual in the barn and, throughout the test, water should be withheld from them. Before the application of the test three preinjection temperatures should be taken at 2-hour intervals to be certain that the animals' temperatures are normal. All animals registering a temperature of 103° F. or more should be withdrawn from the test. In very warm weather the test should not be applied, as conflicting results are often obtained from abnormal temperatures. When tests are made under such circumstances they may be given at sundown and continued throughout the night.

The table below shows the record of animals tested with johnin and a comparison of the range in temperature between a healthy cow (No. 62) and two diseased cows (Nos. 44 and 35). Post mortem lesions noted in cows 44 and 35 were typical of Johne's disease and microscopic examinations were positive for acid-fast organisms.

Temperature records and results of testing three cows with johnin; 5 cubic centimeters injected into each cow at 6 a. m.

(Temperatures are degrees Fahrenheit above 100°)

Cow No.	Preinjection temperatures at—			Postinjection temperatures at—													Remarks
	2 a. m.	4 a. m.	6 a. m.	6:30 a. m.	7 a. m.	8 a. m.	9 a. m.	10 a. m.	11 a. m.	12 m.	1 p. m.	2 p. m.	3 p. m.	4 p. m.	5 p. m.	6 p. m.	
44	2.4	2.0	0.8	1.6	1.4	1.4	2.2	2.6	4.1	4.0	4.4	3.8	3.6	2.8	2.8	2.4	Reactor (killed).
35	2.2	2.2	2.6	2.4	2.6	2.8	2.8	3.8	4.3	5.3	4.5	4.4	4.2	4.4	4.5	4.4	Reactor (died).
62	2.0	1.4	1.8	1.8	1.4	1.2	1.5	1.2	.7	1.6	1.9	2.0	2.0	1.7	1.6	1.5	Negative.

Immediately after the third preinjection temperature has been taken, johnin is applied to all the animals intravenously. Postinjection temperatures should be taken, beginning one-half hour later and continued every hour for 12 hours. Reactions may take place in diseased animals 3 to 8 hours after the test has been applied. If there is 1.5° or more rise in temperature above the highest preinjection temperature, the animal should be classed as a reactor. An animal having a rise in temperature, but not sufficiently high to class as a reactor, should be regarded as suspicious and retested at a later date. This test obviously requires technical skill and judgment and therefore is a task for the trained veterinarian.

DIFFERENTIAL DIAGNOSIS

As has already been stated, the principal infection with which Johne's disease may be confused is tuberculosis. However, the latter disease may be readily distinguished from the former through the application of the customary tuberculin test, which will produce a reaction in the tuberculous animal but will have no effect on an animal suffering with Johne's disease.

Various invasions of gastrointestinal parasites may also be mistaken for Johne's disease, but in those instances a microscopic examination of the feces will usually result in the discovery of ova, larvae, or adult parasites from which a diagnosis may be established. However, the presence of such parasites does not necessarily exclude the presence of Johne's disease, as parasitism and Johne's disease may exist simultaneously. On the other hand, it is extremely rare to find both Johne's disease and tuberculosis in the same animal.

INDEMNITY FOR JOHNIN REACTORS

The Bureau of Animal Industry has been granted authority by Congress to pay indemnity to cattle owners for animals that are slaughtered because of reaction to the johnin test. These payments are made on the same basis that indemnity is paid on tuberculous cattle.

Indemnity funds have been available for this purpose since July 1, 1927, from which a number of livestock owners have received benefits. Further details concerning the payment of indemnity on cattle reacting to Johne's disease can be obtained by writing the livestock officials of your State or the Chief of the Bureau of Animal Industry, United States Department of Agriculture, Washington, D. C.

COWPOX OR VACCINIA (VARIOLA)

Cowpox, or vaccinia, is a contagious disease of cattle caused by a filtrable virus that manifests its presence through an elevation of temperature, shrinkage in milk production, and the appearance of characteristic, pustular eruptions, especially on the teats and udders of dairy cows. Although this is a contagious disease, strictly speaking, it is so universally harmless and benign in its course that it is robbed of the terrors that usually accompany all spreading disease and may enter a herd of cattle, run its course, and disappear without exciting any particular notice.

The virus of this disease is believed not to travel through the air from animal to animal, but to be transmitted by actual contact with the skin of some susceptible animal. It may be carried in this manner, not alone from cattle to cattle, but horses, sheep, goats, and man readily contract the disease whenever suitable conditions attend their inoculation.

A similar disease, variola, frequently appears in horses, attacks their heels, and thence extends upward along the leg, producing, as it progresses, inflammation and swelling of the skin, followed later by pustules, which soon rupture and discharge a sticky, disagreeable secretion. Other parts of the body are frequently affected in like manner, especially in the region of the head, where the eruptions may appear on lips and nostrils or on the mucous surfaces of the nasal cavities, mouth, or eyes.

Variola of the horse is readily transmitted to cattle if both are cared for by the same attendant, and, conversely, the disease of cattle may be carried to the horse on the hands of a person who has been milking an affected cow.

The method of vaccination with material derived from the eruptions of cowpox as a safeguard against the ravages of smallpox in members of the human family is well known. The immunity that such vaccination confers on the human subject has led many writers to assert that cowpox is simply a modified form of smallpox, whose harmless attack on the human system is due to a certain attenuation derived during its passages through the system of the cow or horse. The results of numerous experiments to determine the relationship between the disease of the human and bovine families seem to show, however, that, although possessing many similar characteristics, they are, nevertheless, distinct, and that in spite of repeated inoculations from cattle to man, and vice versa, no permanent transformation in the real character of the disease ever takes place.

Symptoms.—The disease appears in 4 to 7 days after natural infection or may appear in 2 or 3 days as the result of artificial inoculation. Young milk cows are most susceptible to an attack, but older cows, bulls, or young cattle are by no means immune. The attack causes a slight rise in temperature, which is soon followed by the appearance of reddened, inflamed areas, principally on the teats and udder, and at times on the abdominal skin or the skin of the inner surface of the thighs. In a few cases the skin of the throat and jaws has been found to be similarly involved. If the affected parts are examined on the second day after the establishment of the inflammation, numerous pale-red nodules will be found, which gradually expand until, within a few days, they reach a diameter of one-half inch or even larger. At this period the tops of the nodules become transformed into vesicles that are depressed in the center and contain a pale, serous fluid. They usually reach their maturity by the tenth day of the course of the disease and are then the size of a bean. From this time the contents of the vesicles become purulent, which requires about 3 days, when the typical pox pustule is present, consisting of a swelling with broad, reddened base, within which is an elevated, conical abscess varying from the size of a pea to that of a hazelnut.

The course of the disease after the full maturity of the pustule is rapid if outside interference has not caused a premature rupture of the small abscess at the apex of the swelling. The pustules gradually become darker colored and drier until nothing remains but a thick scab, which at last falls off, leaving only a slight, whitish scar. The total duration of the disease is about 20 days in each animal, and owing to the slow spread of the infection from animal to animal many weeks may elapse before a stable can be fully freed from it. The fallen scabs and crusts may retain their contagious properties for several days when mixed with litter and bedding on the floor of the stable, and at any time during this period they are capable of producing new outbreaks should other cattle be brought into the stalls and thus come into actual contact with them. Again, the pustules may appear, one after another, on a single animal, in which case the duration of the disease is materially lengthened.

Treatment.—In herds of cattle that regularly receive careful handling no special treatment is usually necessary beyond the application of mild, softening, antiseptic agents to such vesicles on the teats as may have become ruptured by the hands of the milker. Agents containing carbolic acid or cresol compounds are not suited for this purpose, as they are unduly irritant, and, furthermore, milk absorbs their odors. Zinc oxide ointment or boric acid ointment is preferable. In more persistent cases it may be desirable to use a milking tube in order to prevent the repeated opening of the pustules during milking. If this is recommended by the veterinarian, the attendant should obtain and understand instructions pertaining to the cleaning and use of the milking tube. When the udder is hard, swollen, and painful, it may well be supported by a bandage and bathed frequently with hot water. If calves are allowed to suck the cows, the pustules become confluent, and the ulcerations may extend up into the teat, causing garget and ruining the whole quarter of the udder.

As young cows are most susceptible to cowpox, the milker must exercise patience with these affected animals as long as their teats or udders are sore and tender, otherwise the patient may contract vicious habits while resisting painful handling. The flow of milk is usually lessened as soon as the fever becomes established, but is restored with the return of perfect health.

If the affected animals cannot be isolated from the healthy ones and separate attendants cannot be provided, the normal animals should be milked first. Thorough cleanliness in handling or milking affected cattle may prevent, in many instances, the dissemination of the trouble among the healthy animals of the herd, but even the greatest care may be insufficient to check the spread until it has attacked each susceptible animal of the herd.

ACTINOMYCOSIS, ACTINOBACILLOSIS (LUMPY JAW, BIG JAW, WOODEN TONGUE)

The terms "lumpy jaw," "big jaw," and "wooden tongue" have been used for decades to describe chronic infectious diseases characterized by the formation of peculiar tumorlike swellings containing pus of a more or less granular consistence about the head in cattle. These formations are commonly observed in or on the jawbones but may be found in other parts of the body, such as the lungs (pl. XLI, 1 and 2), liver, spleen, lymph nodes, muscles, and even the brain.

Cause.—The cause of actinomycosis is the germ *Actinomyces bovis*, a funguslike organism first observed by Bollinger in 1877 and noted by him to cause the formation in the infected tissues of so-called sulfur granules. Microscopically, these are observed to have the form of peculiar "rosettes" consisting of clublike forms arranged in a rayed formation (pl. XXXIX, fig. 2). The causative organism has thus been commonly referred to as the ray fungus.

In 1902, Lignières found similar rosette formations in the disease now known as actinobacillosis caused by the germ *Actinobacillus lignièresi*. Similar forms have also been observed in staphylococcosis, caused by the common pus-producing *Staphylococcus pyogenes;* coccidioidomycosis, caused by *Coccidioides immitis;* and possibly other diseases. Therefore, what was once believed to be characteristic of actinomycosis and probably one form of growth of Actinomyces, of which there are a large number of various types, is now thought of by some investigators as a product of the reaction of the tissues to one or more of several invading organisms that may vary considerably in nature. At the present time authorities generally agree that *Actinomyces bovis* is the organism usually responsible for actinomycosis that involves the bone, but it may also be found elsewhere. Other organisms that are frequently found in such lesions but are generally considered as secondary invaders include the common pus-producing organisms *Staphylococcus pyogenes* and *Corynebacterium pyogenes*. On the other hand, *Actinobacillus lignièresi* is known to attack the soft tissues especially, notably the lymph nodes, muscles, skin, and so forth.

Actinomycosis and actinobacillosis somewhat resemble each other not only in the common presence of rosette formations but also in the character of the pus. Also, both tend to cause the formation of considerable excess connective tissue in the lesions of the two respective diseases. Without the aid of laboratory procedures, usually including a culture of the causative organisms, it is impossible exactly to classify the two diseases. In fact, without identifying procedures, even tuberculosis may be confused with actinomycosis and actinobacillosis.

Methods of infection.—*Actinomyces bovis* and other disease-producing actinomyces, together with *Actinobacillus lignièresi*, are believed to gain entrance to the body tissues through abrasions or lacerations usually in the mouth. Particularly dry, harsh, rough feeds frequently injure the mucous membranes of the mouth. The sharp, barbed awns of barley and other grains and of foxtail and other grasses, which are sometimes found in feeds, commonly penetrate the membranes of the mouth and throat and become buried in the deeper tissues. The infection may travel into the tissues with these feeds, or, if present from other sources, find ready access to the body through the wounds caused by such substances.

When cattle are teething, the gums are always more or less tender and lacerated and thus afford another avenue for the ingress of the infection. Finally, the organisms in these tissues may also invade other parts of the body; for example, the spermatic cord and the udder, usually through wounds.

Description of lesions.—The commonest lesion of actinomycosis is in the bones of the jaws—the mandible, or lower jaw, or the maxilla, or upper jaw. The spongy tissue of the bone is replaced by tumorlike formations consisting largely of connective tissue. The pus formed in the pockets of the diseased tissue is granular and often viscous in consistence and of a yellow, greyish-yellow, or yellow-green color. The framework of the bone is partially softened, and the growth of inflammatory tissue causes more or less swelling of the bony substance accompanied with actual thickening of the outer dense osseous tissue.

In the early stages the swelling is scarcely perceptible, but with the progress of the disease huge disfiguring swellings may develop with masses of fungoid tissue appearing through the skin or along the gums. Meanwhile adjacent tissues, such as the submaxillary or the parotid salivary glands or the tissues of the throat, may be involved. The lungs (pl. XLI), the brain and its membranes, or the liver or other abdominal organs may be invaded.

In the early stages only the local swelling with little disturbance of health is noticeable. Later, however, the teeth may be so dislocated as to make mastication difficult or even impossible. In these cases and those in which serious lesions develop in the internal organs, there may be marked loss of condition and an increasing weakness followed by death.

The commonest lesions of actinobacillosis, on the other hand, are in the tongue or elsewhere in the mouth or throat. When the tongue is affected, the earliest evidence of the disease is usually found on the top of the organ just in front of the ridge and groove across its face. Here penetrating substances from the feed are likely to become lodged and offer entrance to the causative germ of actinobacillosis or ordinary pus-forming bacteria. In the former, greyish-yellow ulcers or deep-seated abscesses occur.

The mucous membrane of the mouth, also the lips, may develop fungoid growths. With the progress of the disease in the tongue the organ may become increasingly stiff and sore, the entire musculature being diffusely infiltrated with fibrous tissue and small abscesses from the size of millet seeds to that of small walnuts. Eating becomes increasingly difficult, and the tongue protrudes helplessly from the mouth. Such cases are commonly referred to as wooden tongue or woody tongue. Lesions of variable extent thus sometimes appear in large numbers of calves and yearlings on one farm or ranch.

As a part of the above-described process or through infection by other avenues, lesions may appear in the lymph glands or other soft tissues anywhere in the body. These are commonest about the head, especially the throat, where they may be confused with actinomycosis, but any of the internal organs may also be invaded.

Prevention.—The question as to how and where animals contract these diseases is one largely still in the stage of conjecture, because there is actually little information concerning the life history of the organisms concerned. Most observers believe that animals become infected from the feed, although some believe that the organisms may normally exist in the mouth, awaiting the opportunity to invade the body. In either case it is generally believed that the contagion is, as it were, inoculated into the affected part. This inoculation is performed by the sharp and pointed parts of plants that penetrate the mucous membrane and carry the germs with them. Actinomycosis is considered to be inoculable rather than contagious. However, there is some evidence that actinobacillosis may be contracted from contaminated premises. The mere presence of the diseased animal will not give rise to disease in healthy animals unless pus or infected tissue passes directly from the diseased animal into some wound or abrasion of the healthy one or drops on the feed that is consumed by the latter. When the disease appears on any premises, the affected animals should be isolated as soon as discovered and kept separate from the rest of the herd until these affected animals are either cured or slaughtered. This procedure is required by most milk ordinances.

The most certain method of treatment is surgical removal of the affected tissue. However, if this is to be undertaken it must be done before extreme involvement or spread to several organs has occurred, in which case surgical treatment is rarely practicable.

Many cases, particularly of actinobacillosis, respond miraculously to the administration of various compounds of iodine, a treatment first reported by Nocard in 1892. According to the nature of the case, variable doses of one or several such compounds may be given by the mouth or by injection into the affected tissue or into the blood stream. Such treatment should be administered or at least supervised by the veterinarian in order to insure the greatest possible efficacy and to avoid iodine poisoning. Repeated doses for a considerable period of time are usually required when the iodine is given by mouth. When it is injected into the vein, much less extended

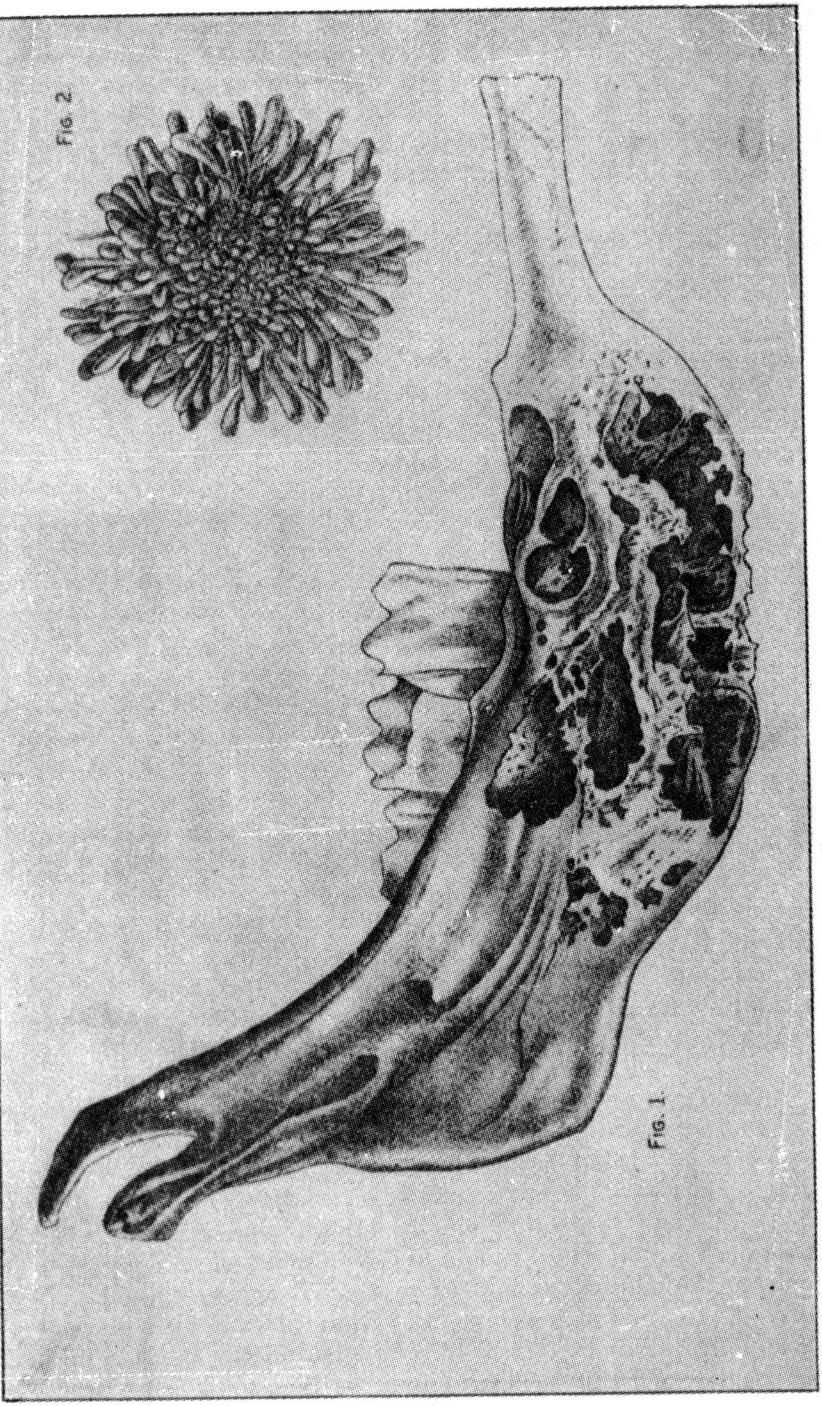

ACTINOMYCOSIS

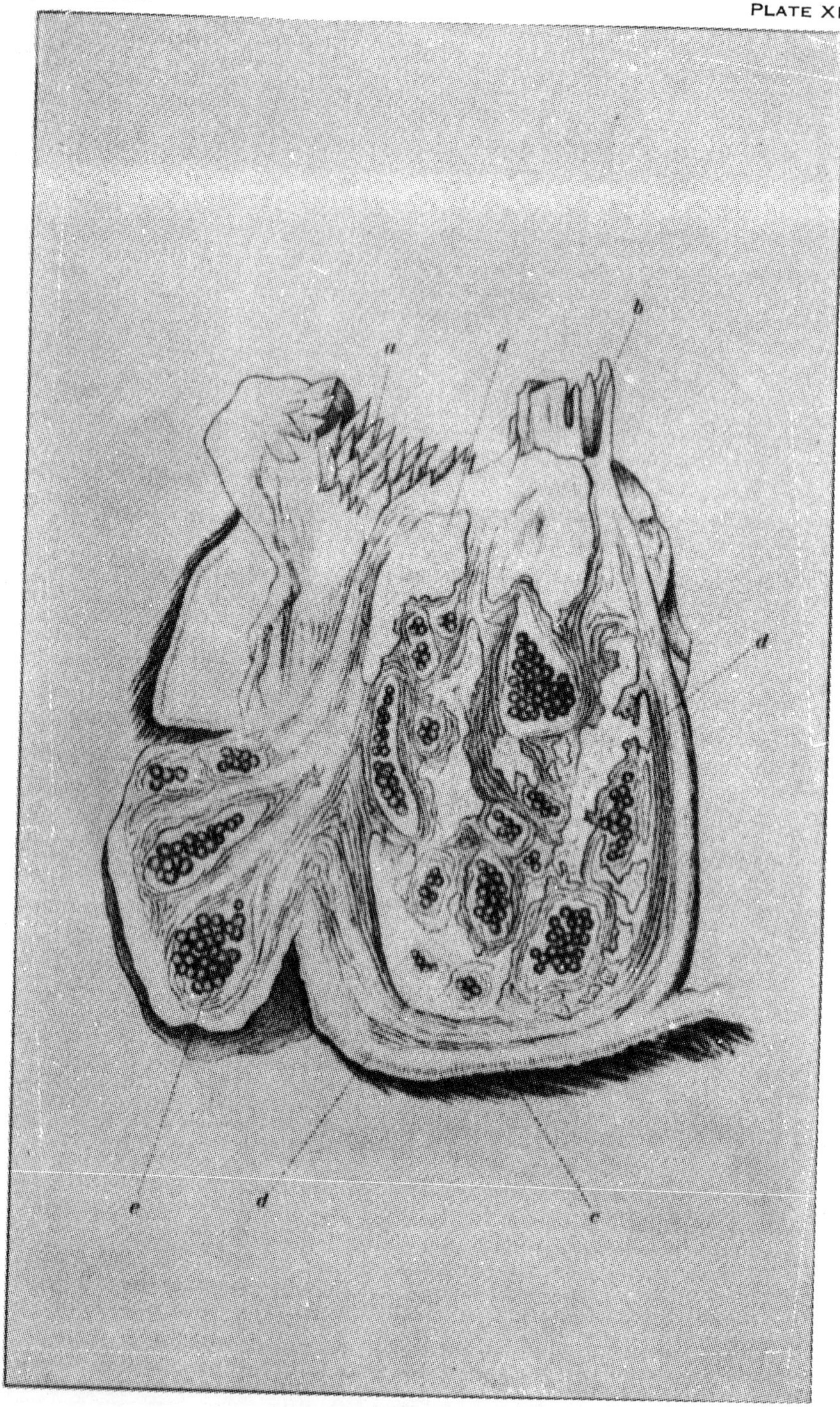

ACTINOMYCOSIS OF THE JAW

treatment is usually required but the dangers are increased; also, the dosage must be more closely graded according to the size and condition of the animal being treated.

Some animals are believed to be rendered sterile by long-continued administration of iodine. Such treatment may also result in abortion and frequently causes a marked reduction of milk flow. A portion of the drug is secreted in the milk, which is thus rendered undesirable for human consumption.

Some cases do not respond to iodine therapy. Some are so extensively and severely affected, particularly by actinomycosis, that they cannot be economically treated. In such instances it may be preferable to fatten the animals, if possible, and send them to slaughter. Since both actinobacillosis and actinomycosis may affect man, it is advised that the carcass of any animal affected with these diseases be inspected as to suitability for food. So far as is known, man does not contract the affections directly either from infected cattle or from carcasses. That he may become diseased through some unknown intermediate agency, however, can scarcely be denied, and under no conditions should diseased parts be used as food.

The Federal meat-inspection regulations require condemnation of carcasses showing generalized actinomycosis or actinobacillosis. If carcasses are in a well-nourished condition and show only uncomplicated localized lesions of these diseases, they may be passed for food after the infected organs or parts have been removed and condemned. When the disease of the jaw is slight, strictly localized, and without pus formation, fistulous tracts, or lymph-gland involvement, the tongue, if free from disease, may be passed. Affected heads, including the tongue, must be condemned, except that when the lesions in the jaw are strictly localized and slight in extent the tongue may be passed if uninvolved.

ACTINOMYCOSIS, ACTINOBACILLOSIS (LUMPY JAW, BIG JAW, WOODEN TONGUE)

DESCRIPTION OF PLATES

PLATE XXXIX. Actinomycosis. (From Jöhne's Encyklopädie d. gesammt. Thierheilkunde.)

Figure 1. Actinomycosis of the jaw. The lower jawbone has been extensively eaten away by the disease.

Figure 2. Microscopic appearance of the rosette formation in an actinomycotic tumor of the jawbone in cattle, magnified 550 times.

PLATE XL. Actinomycosis of the jaw. (Reduced one-half. From Jöhne's Encyklopädie d. gesammt. Thierheilkunde.) The lower jaw is sawed through transversely (from right to left), and shows the disease within the jawbone itself; *a*, within the mouth, showing the papillae on the mucous membrane of the cheek; *b*, front view of a molar tooth; *c*, the skin covering the lower surface of the jawbone; *d*, the jawbone hollowed out and

77431 O—51——28

enlarged by the formation of cavities within it, which are filled with the soft growth of the actinomycotic tumor. The section makes it appear as if the bone were broken into fragments and these forced apart; *e*, a portion of the tumor that has broken through the bone and the skin and appears as a tumor on the cheek. The little roundish masses represent the granulomata (minute tumors) in which the fungus vegetates.

PLATE XLI. Actinomycosis of the lungs.

Figure 1. Transverse section of the ventral lobe of the right lung, from a case studied in the laboratory. The yellowish dots represent the places where the actinomyces fungus is lodged. The larger yellowish patches are produced by the confluence of a number of centers. The entire lobe is of a dark flesh-red color, due to collapse and bronchopneumonia.

Figure 2. The cut surface of a portion of the principal lobe of the same lung, showing the recent invasion of antinomycosis from the other lobe; *a*, large air tube; *b*, artery; *c*, a pneumatic lobule; *d*, lobule containing minute yellowish dots. In these the actinomyces fungus is lodged.

Figure 3. Cut surface of a small portion of another lung, showing a few lobules; *a*, the fungus is sprinkled throughout the lung tissue in the form of yellowish grains, as shown in the illustration. The pleural covering of the lung tissues is shown in profile above.

ANTHRAX

Anthrax is an infectious disease of livestock caused by a specific micro-organism or germ, known as the anthrax bacillus (*Bacillus anthracis*) and characterized in its most common form by rapidly fatal course or by sudden death. The disease causes annual losses of many millions of dollars to the livestock industry. As it is also infectious to man, anthrax is a menace to public health.

Practically all animals are susceptible in some degree to anthrax, but the herbivorous animals are most susceptible. Cattle, horses, sheep, goats, and wild herbivorous animals are most commonly affected, and in these animals the disease usually appears in the acute forms which rapidly terminates in death. Dogs and other carnivorous animals may become infected by eating the carcass of an animal dead of anthrax. Poultry, however, are not susceptible to the disease under ordinary conditions. Mice, guinea pigs, and rabbits, which are commonly used in laboratory diagnosis, are very susceptible, whereas rats are less so.

Man acquires the infection through the handling of anthrax-infected carcasses, hides, wool, or hair. The disease manifests itself as a local infection of the skin or as an infection of the respiratory or digestive tracts. In the latter forms, the disease spreads rapidly throughout the body and terminates in death.

The germ that causes anthrax is indigenous to the soil in certain areas, wherein it survives for long periods, especially in areas that are subject to periodic inundations or in low-lying marshy land. These organisms in their active state (vegetative forms) are cylindrical in shape and grow in the presence of air. When they gain access to the

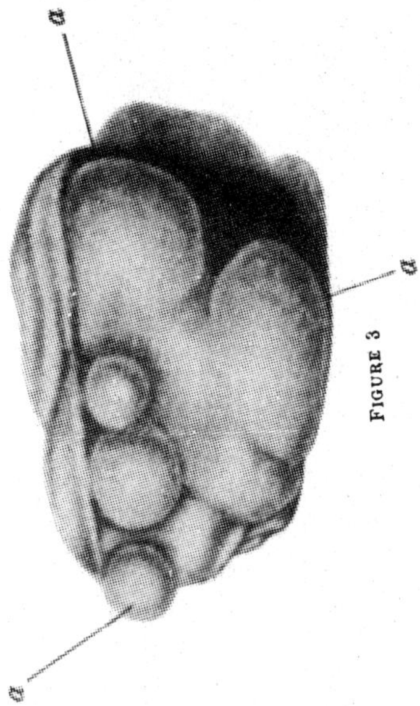

FIGURE 3

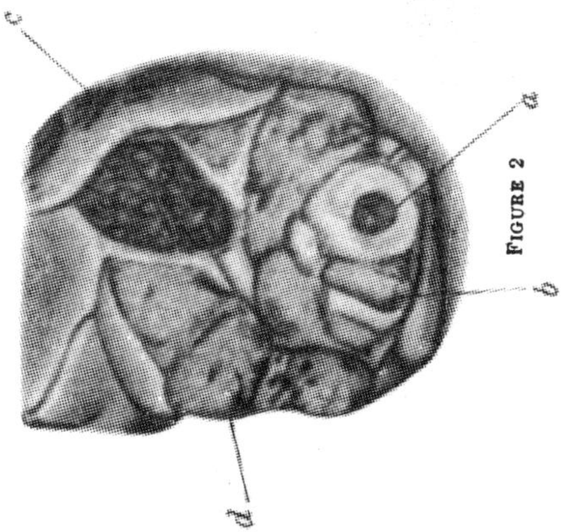

FIGURE 2

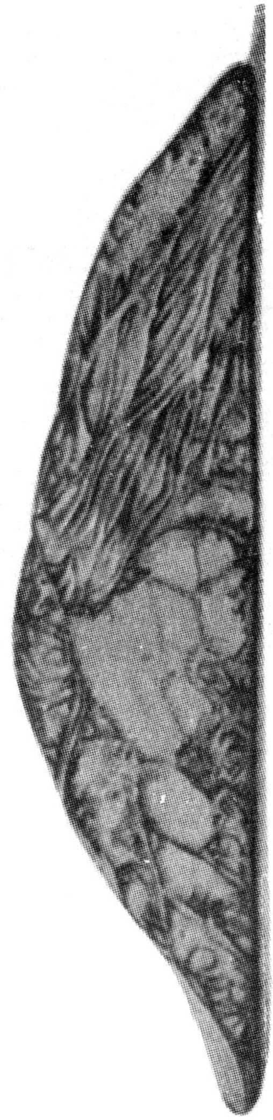

FIGURE 1

ACTINOMYCOSIS OF THE LUNGS.

HAINES DEL.

animal body they multiply rapidly and invade the blood stream, producing a rapidly fatal blood infection or septicemia. When these cylindrical rods are released from the animal body they produce, on access to the air, elliptical bodies known as spores, similar in nature to seeds, which are remarkable for their viability and very resistant to heat, cold, drying, and exposure to disinfectants. In the soil these spores may live for years, ready to reproduce the disease in susceptible animals that may come in contact with them.

Anthrax is recognized as one of the oldest and most destructive diseases recorded in history. Although it existed in very early times and acquired its name through the dark color of the blood of its victims, its nature was unknown until 1836, when its infectiousness was established through the transfer of the disease from one animal to another by inoculation and the ingestion of diseased blood.

The specific rod-shaped microscopic germs were first observed in the blood in 1849 by the German investigator, Pollender. The microorganisms were also observed in 1850 by the French investigator, Davaine, who later (1865) showed their causal relationship to anthrax. In 1876 the German investigator, Robert Koch, cultivated the anthrax bacillus outside the animal body on an artificial culture medium and definitely demonstrated it to be the specific causative agent of anthrax.

Anthrax is widely distributed, as it has appeared on every continent. Before the disease was known to be infectious and before systematic measures were taken to suppress it, heavy losses were sustained in many countries.

Being indigenous to the soil, anthrax is more or less confined to certain districts, where it occurs almost every year; these are commonly designated as anthrax districts. In these the disease constitutes a perennial problem. It makes its appearance during a more or less definite period of the year, the anthrax season, usually the late summer and early fall. In such districts, where widespread outbreaks may occur, the disease can be kept in check by appropriate preventive measures. Isolated cases, however, may occur at any time, including the winter months, when stock are not on pasture.

Since anthrax-contaminated soil is the source of the disease in livestock, most outbreaks occur when the animals are on pasture. It has been observed that hot, dry summers with scant growths of pasture, necessitating grazing close to the soil, are frequently followed by unusually large numbers of cases of anthrax. Likewise, a period of rainy weather followed by warm days appears to favor the occurrence of the disease. Heavy losses from anthrax often follow in the wake of floods and periodic inundations of low-lying land. In certain years the disease assumes a very virulent form and appears simultaneously at a number of places. New centers of infection occur in rapid succession, and soon it covers large areas and occasions heavy losses of livestock. The cause of these cyclic waves is as yet unknown.

Modes of infection and dissemination.—Anthrax infection, for the most part, occurs by way of the digestive tract. Spore-laden soil is taken in with the feed principally while the animal is on pasture, although hay made on anthrax-contaminated lands may harbor virulent spores and cause the disease in stable-fed animals.

Contaminated drinking water is also a potent source of infection. Water may become contaminated through the surface drainage of anthrax lands or from the carcasses of animals that died of anthrax, especially when they lie close to or in an upper branch of a stream or in a pond.

Infection may also occur by way of the skin through anthrax spores from the soil lodging in wounds and abrasions or through punctures made by biting insects that had previously fed on a diseased animal. Antrax organisms may penetrate the unbroken skin, reach the deeper structures, and set up infection. Such evidence has already been obtained in human cases at least. Infection may also take place through the respiratory tract, the inhaled spores setting up a rapidly fatal form of pneumonia. This form of anthrax is recognized in man more often than in the lower animals.

As previously stated, soils contaminated with anthrax frequently remain dangerous for long periods and require only favorable climatic and moisture conditions to cause repeated outbreaks of the disease and the consequent reinfection of the land. Additional territory may in turn become contaminated through the wandering of diseased animals, which spread the germs with their excreta as they go and finally contaminate new land heavily with the countless numbers of micro-organisms that escape from the natural openings of their dead bodies.

Dogs and other carnivores, as well as the carrion-eating animals and birds, are potential spreaders of anthrax from one area to another. After feeding on an anthrax-infected carcass, their bodies doubtlessly are heavily contaminated with anthrax spores and these may be carried to distant fields. Virulent anthrax spores were found, in an experiment, in the droppings of buzzards that previously had fed on an anthrax-infected carcass.

Some of the flying insects must be considered as potential spreaders of anthrax, feeding as they do on the blood of living animals or on the materials that escape from the natural openings. Animals sick of anthrax become easy prey to myriads of flies and other insects, both biting and nonbiting. Virulent anthrax organisms have repeatedly been found in or on the bodies of several species of flies including blowflies taken from the carcasses of animals dead from anthrax. Some of these flies and other insects travel great distances.

Streams contaminated with surface drainage from anthrax-infected land or by carcasses of animals dead of anthrax may convey the germs many miles downstream and infect the territory through which they pass.

Anthrax may spread from one country to another through the interchange of infected hides, hair, wool, bonemeal, fertilizer, forage, and other items closely related to animal life. The Government endeavors to prevent introduction of this disease into the United States through the administration, by the Bureau of Animal Industry, of regulations governing the sanitary handling and control of animal products, animal byproducts, and hay and straw of foreign origin.

Form and symptoms.—According to the course of the disease, anthrax is recognized in three forms: A peracute form, in which the interval between the first outward manifestation of symptoms and death is but a few hours or even minutes; an acute form, in which the disease lasts for a day or two; and a subacute form, in which the period between first symptoms and death or recovery extends beyond several days.

In the peracute or apoplectic form of the disease, death occurs so quickly that clinical symptoms are seldom observed. In most instances, animals that when last seen were apparently in perfect health are found dead. Less often a seemingly healthy animal is seen to fall to the ground, go through a few convulsive movements, and die. Closer examination frequently shows blood-stained discharges from the nose, mouth, and anus. Peracute anthrax occurs most often in the beginning of an outbreak among cattle and is the most common form of the disease in sheep. Sudden death in cattle, sheep, and horses in areas where anthrax previously existed should always be viewed with suspicion, and the owner should be on the lookout for anthrax.

In cattle, in addition to the peracute form of the disease in which few symptoms are seen, acute and subacute infections develop. In these forms there is first a stage of excitement, which is soon followed by depression. In this stage the animal lags behind, with the head hanging low, refuses to eat, and prefers to stand still or to lie down. Respiration is more rapid than normal and appears to be labored. Rumination ceases, and in milking cows the milk secretion is materially lessened. Pregnant animals may abort. At this stage of the disease the body temperature is elevated and may reach 108° F. Bloody discharges usually come from the natural body openings. When diarrhea sets in, the feces are usually blood tinged. Small hemorrhages may be noted on the visible mucous membranes. Soft swellings that pit on pressure may develop over the body, but the more common sites are about the external genitalia and on the lower wall of the abdomen. The tongue also may show extensive swelling and dark discoloration.

Shortly before death respiration becomes extremely labored, the mucous membranes take on a bluish cast, and the temperature falls below normal.

In man, anthrax usually occurs as a primary localized infection of the skin in the form of a carbuncle or as an infection of the lungs known as "woolsorter's disease." In countries where the flesh of animals dead of disease is eaten, an abdominal form of anthrax has been reported.

Skin infections result from the handling of carcasses of animals dead of anthrax or the hides, hair, or wool from such carcasses. Originating as localized infections in the form of small pimples, the lesions develop rapidly and may terminate in a fatal septicemia or blood poisoning. Prompt medical attention is most important whenever anthrax infection is suspected.

The pulmonary form of the disease results from the inhalation of anthrax spores in factories where hair and wool are processed. The course of this form of anthrax is very rapid and terminates fatally.

Anatomical changes.—If anthrax is suspected, the stockman should consult a competent veterinarian at once rather than open up a carcass for the purpose of making a definite diagnosis. The seriousness of such a mistake can hardly be overestimated owing to the greatly increased danger of spreading the disease when the body is opened and discharges from it escape. Post mortem examination in suspected cases of anthrax should be made only by a competent veterinarian who is prepared to take all necessary precautions against infecting himself and the premises.

Carcasses of animals dead of anthrax decompose rapidly and soon become greatly bloated. The natural post mortem stiffening of the muscles is incomplete. Dark blood escapes as a rule from the natural openings, and the visible mucous membranes are dark blue in color and frequently show hemorrhages. The blood is considerably darker than normal, does not clot readily, and is frequently spoken of as being tarry. Hemorrhages beneath the skin are common. Clear or somewhat blood-tinged gelatinous exudates are found between the muscles and beneath the skin, especially in the areas where the swellings were seen before death.

With rare exceptions the spleen shows characteristic changes, which are of considerable assistance in making a diagnosis of anthrax. This organ is greatly enlarged, and the splenic pulp is dark red to blackish in color and soft or even semifluid in consistence. The liver and kidneys are congested and enlarged and frequently have areas of hemorrhage on their surfaces. The heart muscle is grayish red and flabby. The lungs are congested and contain serum. The mucous membranes of the trachea and bronchi are red and dotted with hemorrhages of varying sizes. The mucous membrane of the intestines is greatly swollen and hemorrhagic.

Diagnosis.—When an animal dies within an anthrax district or on or near premises where the disease has appeared previously, it is very important to know definitely whether the death was due to anthrax. Lack of such information has often been responsible for heavy losses of livestock and, at times, the loss of human lives. Whenever there is a possibility of anthrax, it is advisable to have the cause of death determined by a competent veterinarian. If local veterinary service is not available the State livestock sanitary officials should be consulted.

The diagnosis of anthrax from clinical symptoms, because of its similarity to other disease conditions, may at times be difficult, especially when the disease occurs at a time when it is not prevalent and on premises that have formerly been free from the infection. A definite diagnosis of anthrax in such instances can be made only by laboratory examination. In peracute anthrax, for example, death is so sudden and the clinical symptoms are so meager that a definite diagnosis is impossible without the aid of laboratory examination. Cerebral hemorrhage, sunstroke, lead poisoning, or some acutely fatal digestive disturbance may be confused with peracute anthrax especially if it occurs in the so-called anthrax districts.

In the less acute cases of anthrax, there may be an escape of bloody exudate from the natural openings, together with swellings beneath the skin. However, somewhat similar swellings are observed in malignant edema, hemorrhagic septicemia, tick fever, and sweetclover poisoning of cattle and purpura hemorrhagica in horses. Although swellings are found in blackleg of cattle, such swellings crackle under pressure because of their air content and are readily distinguishable from the gasless swellings of anthrax that have a doughy consistence and pit on pressure. In all the above diseases, with the possible exception of malignant edema, blood-stained discharges may at times be seen.

Any previous occurrence of anthrax on the premises is sufficient reason for considering anthrax as a possible cause of any deaths among livestock that cannot be clearly attributed to other causes. In a large number of such instances a tentative diagnosis of anthrax can be substantiated by laboratory examination. When a laboratory examination is desired, suitable specimens should be collected by a competent veterinarian. In case professional services are not available and the samples are to be collected by others, the greatest care should be taken by the operator to prevent infecting himself. Heavy rubber gloves should be used to prevent the infectious material from coming in contact with the hands.

A few drops of blood deposited in a small wide-mouthed bottle or jar and the container rolled around so as to spread the blood in a thin film that will dry quickly on the bottom or side walls makes a very satisfactory specimen for bacteriological examination. Larger quantities of blood are unsatisfactory in that putrefaction may set in and destroy any anthrax organisms that may be present. Furthermore, the forwarding of larger quantities of such blood by common carrier is a dangerous procedure that should not be undertaken. The few drops of blood that are required may be collected from a small cut made over the jugular vein or at the base of the ear immediately before the carcass is buried or cremated. The blood may be absorbed by small pieces of blotting paper, chalk, or preferably sterile cotton swabs, which should be allowed to dry and then placed in a sealed container. The container should be enclosed in an unbreakable outside receptacle, such as a metal mailing tube, for shipment to the laboratory for examination.

Another method of obtaining a specimen, but a less satisfactory one, is as follows: Remove an ear, place it in a tight container, and pack it in a strong box for shipment to the laboratory. As in the case of large quantities of blood, however, there is danger of putrefaction setting in.

After the samples are collected, it is advisable to destroy the operating knife with the carcass and thoroughly disinfect the hands and arms with a solution of 1 part bichloride of mercury to 1,000 parts of water. This solution should be mixed in and used from a wooden bucket or stoneware crock. As this disinfectant, if swallowed, is very poisonous to man and animals, precautions should be taken accordingly.

No attempts should be made by the layman to collect specimens of the internal organs. The body cavities should be opened only by an experienced veterinarian who is able to protect himself and the premises should the animal's death be due to anthrax.

Control measures.—Anthrax is a menace to the livestock industry and requires the concerted defensive action of livestock sanitary officials, local veterinarians, and owners. When the disease threatens or invades one's herd, it is advisable to obtain the assistance of a competent veterinarian or State official, who is in a position to advise intelligently on the most effective means of control.

When a diagnosis of anthrax has been made, the following measures are the most effective means of control:

(1) Prompt and proper disposal, either by complete burning or deep burial, of animals dead of the disease, together with all the manure, bedding, blood-stained soil, and similar material that has been contaminated by these animals.

(2) Careful examination of the herd for animals showing early symptoms of the disease, prompt isolation of sick animals, and immediate treatment with large doses of antianthrax serum.

(3) Vaccination of the apparently well animals in the herd as soon as possible for prevention, in accordance with methods recommended by the State livestock sanitary officials and other experienced veterinarians.

(4) Immediate change of pastures if practicable. This precaution alone in many instances has helped to reduce losses. If the outbreak occurs during the fly season, it is best to move the herd at night so that most of the infection-carrying flies will be left behind.

(5) Strict quarantine of premises, rigidly enforced, to prohibit positively the movement of livestock or other commodities of a contraband nature within or into the infected area.

In the control of anthrax prompt and effective disposal of carcasses is of greatest importance. It is good practice to dispose of all animal carcasses properly, especially in an anthrax district, even though the possibility of anthrax may at the time seem remote. This can be accomplished either by complete cremation or deep burial under a layer of quicklime covered with at least 6 feet of earth. Carcasses should not be buried in low swampy land or adjacent to streams where overflow might inundate the grave, or on a hillside where there is a possibility of subsurface drainage reaching the surface at lower places nearby. The area above and around the grave should be saturated with oil and burned over. The method to be employed will be governed by the prevailing weather conditions and the relative promptness and ease with which each procedure can be carried out at the place where disposal becomes an issue.

In disposing of a dead animal the following method is recommended: Immediately after finding the animal, cover it with kerosene or crude oil to keep flies, dogs, buzzards, crows, and vermin from the carcass until it is disposed of. If conditions permit, cremate or bury the carcass where it is found. If moving to a more suitable site is necessary, take the greatest care to prevent any discharges or hair from contaminating the soil over which the carcass is moved. Consequently, never permit a carcass to be dragged. A stone boat or sled may be used as a means of conveyance. Thoroughly disinfect or burn any equipment used in moving anthrax-infected carcasses. Avoid actual contact with the germ-laden body; this can be done through the use of properly applied ropes and poles, which may then be burned. Prepare a solution of bichloride of mercury to disinfect the hands and boots or shoes of the operator after the disposal of the carcasses has been completed. It is advisable, if possible, to have the disposal of anthrax-infected carcasses conducted under the supervision of a competent veterinarian who from experience can advise on the most effective and economical means of destroying the carcass and disinfecting whatever materials may have become contaminated by the animal or carcass.

The cremation of the carcass of a sheep or hog is not difficult, but the complete destruction of that of a horse or cow is more of a problem. Several methods give satisfactory results in the cremation of large carcasses. One of these is to dig two trenches approximately 2 feet wide and 18 inches deep, crossing each other at right angles, over which a grating of green posts is laid, followed by several layers of dry rails or split logs. After the carcass is placed on this pyre, straw and either kerosene or oil are used to start a good fire. Additional fuel is added as needed. A covering of sheet iron or green logs tends to conserve the heat and hasten the destruction of the carcass.

Another method requires no trenches. Oil is applied freely to the carcass, which is then covered with a liberal quantity of straw, and this in turn is covered with a thick layer of heavy, moderately dry manure. Burning the straw generates sufficient heat to start the manure burning, which continues slowly until the carcass is reduced to ashes. This method is slower than the one that involves the use of a rail pyre. There should be plenty of oil, straw, and manure, and the carcass should be fully covered.

When anthrax is prevalent, it is advisable for the owner to keep his dogs tied up and in every possible way to discourage stray dogs from coming on the premises. There is always a possibility that such dogs will eat the carcass of an animal dead from anthrax and so become spreaders of the infection. For the same reason action should be taken to protect livestock from the dangers of buzzard and crow roosts. Protection from flies and biting insects so far as practicable is advisable also.

When anthrax occurs in stabled animals, prompt and thorough disinfection of the quarters should follow the removal of the dead animals. When sick animals are being treated, every precaution should be taken to prevent spread of the infection through contaminated excreta. There is always a possibility that rats or mice will transfer contamination to the hayloft or feed storerooms. Therefore, special effort should be made in anthrax districts to get rid of these pests.

When an outbreak of anthrax occurs in a dairy herd, the dairy should be placed under strict quarantine and all milk withheld from distribution until the public-health officials and State livestock sanitary officials consider circumstances satisfactory for issuing a clean bill of health. Precautions should be taken to prevent the contamination of milk cans, mechanical milkers, buckets, and other dairy equipment from direct or indirect contact with diseased animals and their excreta.

Of the disinfectants, lye is one of the most effective. For disinfection of premises against anthrax, a 5-percent solution is recommended. To prepare such a solution 2½ pounds of commercial lye containing 94 percent of sodium hydroxide is dissolved in 5½ gallons of water. When a whitewash is not objectionable, water-slaked (not air-slaked) lime may be added to the lye solution in the proportion of 2½ pounds of lime to each 5½ gallons of lye solution to prevent the transformation of the active principle, sodium hydroxide, into sodium carbonate, which is considerably less effective as a germicide. It is advisable to use the lye or lye-and-lime solution as soon as it is prepared. All places to be disinfected should be thoroughly soaked with the disinfectant, which should be allowed to remain on for at least a day and then thoroughly washed off with clean water before the livestock are returned.

Manure from a stable where deaths from anthrax have occurred should be burned or deeply buried or, if this is impracticable, disinfected with very liberal applications of a 5-percent solution of lye. However, it is questionable whether any reasonable heavy applications of lye solution would disinfect completely large quantities of manure. It is impossible, therefore, to make general recommendations on the disposal or disinfection of manure that would be efficient and practicable under all conditions. Methods of procedure, therefore, should be left to the judgment of a competent veterinarian.

Preventive vaccination.—Where anthrax appears more or less regularly each year, vaccination affords the best means of keeping the losses low. Proper immunization against anthrax is a highly technical problem that involves an understanding of the principles of immunity, as well as expert knowledge of the available immunizing agents, the nature of each product, the immunizing value of each, and its limitations. Anthrax vaccination, therefore, should be under the immediate supervision of a competent veterinarian.

Where vaccination is necessarily an annual procedure, it should be performed in advance of the anthrax season or at least before anthrax makes its appearance. There is a possibility that vaccination may be followed by an initial state of lowered resistance preceding the establishment of immunity, and exposure to anthrax during this period of increased susceptibility may prove costly. In fact, field observers have frequently witnessed the rapid development of cases of anthrax within several days after vaccination when it was performed after the disease had begun. This, it was believed, could have been avoided had the vaccination been performed before the outbreak occurred.

It should be borne in mind, however, that vaccination is not 100-percent effective regardless of the method or of the vaccine used. It is not uncommon for anthrax to develop in an occasional animal even when it is vaccinated with an anthrax biologic that apparently affords protection to the rest of the herd. Whether this is due to the failure of the individual to respond properly to vaccination or whether that particular animal picked up a sufficient number of anthrax spores to break down any degree of immunity cannot be determined. In experimental work in which a number of similarly vaccinated animals are given identical exposures to anthrax, the occasional loss of a properly vaccinated animal seems to point to the failure of the particular individual to respond properly to the vaccination that was given rather than to a fault in the vaccine. With the knowledge that anthrax vaccination is not 100-percent effective an occasional loss from anthrax in a vaccinated herd does not constitute grounds for questioning the value of the biologic that was used; neither does it justify hasty revaccination of the herd.

Immunizing agents and their use.—The following varieties of anthrax-immunizing agents are now available in the United States: Antianthrax serum, anthrax bacterin, antianthrax serum and anthrax-spore vaccine, single-injection anthrax-spore vaccine (in liquid or pill form), double- or triple-injection anthrax-spore vaccine (in liquid or pill form), anthrax-spore vaccine (intradermic), anthrax-spore vaccine in saponin solution or in alum solution. The first two of these comprise the sterile anthrax products and the remainder the living-spore anthrax products. The selection of the anthrax biologic to be used on a given lot of animals should be left to the local veterinarian or State livestock sanitary officials who, because of their experience and knowledge of the local conditions, are in a position to know which products are best suited to the needs of the herd.

Antianthrax serum is made from the fluid part of the blood of horses, mules, or cattle that have undergone a process of hyperimmunization to anthrax. This process consists in beginning with injections of small quantities of weakened anthrax cultures, followed by a number of injections both larger in quantity and of increased virulence, until the animal can withstand enormous doses of virulent anthrax culture. By this means the blood serum of the hyperimmunized animal becomes heavily charged with anthrax-immune bodies. When such serum is collected, properly preserved, and stored it will retain its potency for several years. The serum contains no living micro-organisms or spores. Antianthrax serum injected into animals produces increased resistance to anthrax as soon as it is absorbed, and the resistance is in direct proportion to the quantity of serum that is given. It is of value both as a preventive and as a curative agent. The immunity that it confers, however, is relatively short. Under experimental conditions the serum afforded complete protection at 4 days after its administration, but 16 days after vaccination the protection was reduced by one-half. As a preventive, therefore, the use of antianthrax serum is advisable when immediate protection is the principal object even though the immunity is but temporary. When serum alone has been given to the apparently healthy animals in an infected herd, it should be followed 10 days later by vaccination with a biologic that will produce a more enduring immunity.

Anthrax bacterin differs from antianthrax serum in that it stimulates the treated animal to produce immune bodies (active immunity), whereas the serum treatment is merely a mechanical transference of already produced immune bodies to the treated animal (passive immunity). Naturally the protection afforded by bacterin would not become established so early as that by serum, but it would be of longer duration. This product, being sterile, is, in itself, incapable of producing disease in the treated animal and is therefore safer than the living-spore anthrax vaccines.

All anthrax-spore vaccines are composed of living anthrax spores and are prepared in either liquid or solid form (pellets). These products may be used alone or in combination with antianthrax serum. The spores in these vaccines are so weakened that under ordinary conditions they will not produce the disease in livestock, if the vaccines are administered according to directions. However, a few individual animals are unusually susceptible and may react severely to vaccination with these spore vaccines, and occasionally an animal may die as a direct result of the vaccination (vaccination anthrax). For this reason, it is ordinarily inadvisable to use living-spore anthrax vaccines on premises where the disease has not existed previously or where there is reason to believe that previous infections have died out.

When these living-spore vaccines are used to control anthrax, the greatest care should be taken to prevent contamination of the soil with the vaccine. Although the spores have been weakened, there is no definite assurance that they may not, under favorable soil conditions, again return to a virulent state and establish a new center of infection. Thorough disinfection of the restraining chute and the floor or ground where the vaccination was performed and prompt disposal of the empty vaccine containers by burning are recommended.

Experience has shown that the living-spore vaccines produce a higher degree of immunity than do the sterile anthrax products and as a rule vaccination with any of the living-spore vaccines, used either alone or in combination with serum, is followed by an active immunity that lasts sufficiently long to carry the animal through the usual anthrax season. However, in some years anthrax makes its appearance in a highly virulent form, and in these years the artificial immunity that can be produced by vaccination does not always protect against infection. To overcome or prevent these post-vaccination outbreaks after the use of anthrax-immunizing agents of ordinary strength, stronger spore vaccines known as Nos. 3 and 4 have been prepared. The use of these stronger vaccines is not without danger and requires considerable discretion.

Favorable results following the use of the intradermic method of vaccination with anthrax spore vaccine have been reported by investigators and veterinary practitioners, both in Europe and the United States. Reports from the field indicate that in recent years this vaccine is gradually growing in favor, particularly in badly infected anthrax districts, and that the results obtained from its use have been highly satisfactory. During 1939 and 1940, more than 6,000 head of cattle on five Indian reservations located in known anthrax districts were vaccinated by the intradermic method under direct supervision of Bureau of Animal Industry veterinarians, with excellent results.

In this method of vaccination the spore vaccine is injected directly into the skin (intracutaneous) and not under the skin (subcutaneous), the usual method in other forms of vaccination. This method also has the advantage of requiring but one injection.

Other control measures.—An additional line of defense against anthrax consists in appropriate measures to prevent the introduction of the infection on anthrax-free premises and keeping livestock off the most dangerous parts of infected premises.

The principal concern of owners of anthrax-free premises is to prevent the introduction of the infection. Although the disease can be introduced through means that are beyond man's control, every effort should be made to guard against possible introduction by needless or faulty vaccination with living-spore anthrax vaccines, roaming dogs, especially when anthrax is prevalent in the vicinity, and the use of hay, straw, or other forage originating on premises where anthrax infection is known to exist. Livestock should also be protected from the potential dangers of buzzard and crow roosts. This can to a certain extent be accomplished by fencing off a small area about each tree containing a buzzard or crow roost.

Thorough inspection of premises where outbreaks of anthrax have occurred may disclose pools or marshlands that are potential sources of infection. Such places, as well as parts of pasture lands known to be heavily infected, should be fenced off as far as is practicable, since vaccination may fail to produce an immunity strong enough to protect against the heavy exposure that might be acquired in such heavily infected places.

Treatment.—When the progress of the disease is not too rapid, treatment with large doses of antianthrax serum administered by a competent veterinarian is frequently successful. When the serum is used either as a preventive or as a curative there is no danger of giving an overdose, but there is a possibility of giving quantities which are insufficient to accomplish their purpose. No other known product, drug, or combination of drugs can be depended on to cure an established case of anthrax in animals.

INDIVIDUAL RESPONSIBILITY AND COOPERATION

From both an economic and public-health standpoint, anthrax is a dreaded disease against which every means of suppression needs to be exerted. The suddenness with which anthrax strikes, the heavy toll that it takes, the long life of the infection in the soil, and the many ways in which the disease may be spread, make the problem of control a common cause to which every livestock owner should be a contributor. To this end, all persons concerned are in duty bound to put into effect every known measure of combating the disease and to cooperate to the fullest extent with the local veterinarian and livestock sanitary officials who are charged with the responsibility of controlling diseases of livestock.

BLACKLEG

Blackleg (also known as black quarter, quarter ill, symptomatic anthrax, and emphysematous anthrax) is an acute infectious disease that attacks principally young cattle. It is characterized by swellings or tumors beneath the skin, due to gas formation in the tissues, usually accompanied with high fever. It follows a rapid course and nearly always results in death. The disease is more or less restricted to definite localities, such as pastures, where the soil is infected with the blackleg organism and where outbreaks may occur year after year unless prevented by vaccination.

Blackleg was formerly regarded as identical with anthrax, but there is little doubt that it has existed for many centuries and that a large number of outbreaks of destructive disease among cattle, referred to by early historians as anthrax, were really blackleg. This supposition is based on the fact that their description of the symptoms and post mortem appearances in many cases corresponds more exactly to our present knowledge of blackleg than of anthrax. Investigations by various scientists in recent times have definitely proved the entire dissimilarity of the two affections from the standpoint of both cause and clinical appearance.

Following the work of Pasteur on anthrax, three other French investigators—Arloing, Cornevin, and Thomas—in 1879 proved that blackleg is caused by an entirely different organism and consequently is a distinct disease. The following year the same authors published a description of the blackleg organism and demonstrated that the disease could be produced in susceptible animals by inoculation and that immunity might be produced by introducing the organism into the circulation of such animals under certain favorable circumstances. This discovery was the beginning of a series of experiments that finally led to the introduction of preventive vaccination.

Blackleg occurs in nearly all parts of the world from which definite information regarding animal diseases is obtainable. The ravages of the disease are not confined to certain zones or altitudes, but occur as frequently in the extreme north as in tropical regions, and as often on mountain pastures as in the lowlands. It is therefore evident that the infection possesses great power of resistance to the destructive influences of varying climatic conditions.

In Europe blackleg occurs in Norway as far north as cattle are kept, also in Sweden, Denmark, Germany, the Netherlands, Belgium, France, Switzerland, Austria, Hungary, Italy, and Great Britain. On the summer pastures in the Alps in Switzerland, where for 5 months of the year the ground is covered with snow and ice, it has appeared regularly in summer when the cattle were brought from the lowlands and has been known to carry off as high as 25 percent of the young stock. In France blackleg has been regarded as the most destructive disease among the cattle, and the greatest losses have occurred in the dairy districts and on the mountain pastures.

In Africa blackleg occurs both in the northern and southern colonies, especially in the French possessions in Algeria, where it frequently takes 10 percent of the young stock. Also in the southern British provinces, especially Natal and the Transvaal, it has been reported to be very prevalent. The same seems to be the case with the English colonies in Asia, although no definite statistics are available. In South America the disease prevails extensively throughout Argentina and has been observed in Chile. Cattle in Cuba and Australia also suffer from it.

Investigations made and reports received by the Bureau of Animal Industry have shown that blackleg occurs in nearly all parts of the United States with the possible exception of some of the Southern Atlantic and Eastern Gulf States. The greatest losses have taken place in the great cattle-raising and cattle-feeding regions of the West, bounded on the north and east by the Missouri and Mississippi Rivers and on the west by the Rocky Mountains, and including Texas, New Mexico, Oklahoma, Kansas, Nebraska, Colorado, North Dakota, and South Dakota. In the Far West the disease prevails to a considerable extent also in Montana, Idaho, Washington, Oregon, California, Utah, and Arizona. In the East a number of outbreaks have been reported from Virginia, West Virginia, and Pennsylvania, and scattering outbreaks have occurred in Vermont, New York, Ohio, Kentucky, Tennessee, and North Carolina. In the Central States outbreaks have been reported from Michigan, Indiana, Illinois, Wisconsin, Minnesota, Iowa, and Missouri.

Cause.—The cause of blackleg is a micro-organism known as *Clostridium chauvoei.* This organism, which is in the form of a short rod, produces spores or seeds in one end (pl. XXVIII, fig. 4). The relation of the rodlike organism to the spore is somewhat like that of a plant to its seed. The spores, like grains of wheat or corn, are very resistant to destruction by heat, cold, drying, or chemical disinfectants, whereas the form of the organism that corresponds to the plant is easily killed by these agencies. The spores may lie dormant for several years, in a pasture for instance, retain their vitality, and still germinate and cause the disease when favorable conditions are present. The blackleg germ belongs to the class of bacteria known as anaerobes, which develop only in the absence of oxygen.

The germs gain entrance into the body of the animal through abrasions or punctures of the skin, and perhaps in rare cases through the mucous membrane of the mouth, tongue, throat, or gastrointestinal tract. As it is necessary that air be excluded in order that the spores may develop, the introduction of the disease is favored by minute punctures carrying the organisms through the skin and into the underlying tissues, whereas cuts or open wounds are not favorable to its development even though the infection is present in abundance. Slight puncture wounds of the skin, such as those received from barbed-wire fences or from stubble, thorns, spines, briers, grass burs, or sharp or pointed parts of feed, seem to be the most likely method of infection, since they correspond most closely to the only manner in which the disease may be produced artificially, namely, by injection of the virus under the skin or into the muscle. Several observers have found the organisms in the mud of swamps. By placing a little of the mud under the skin the disease has been produced.

Susceptibility.—Every stock owner who lives in a district where blackleg occurs knows that the young cattle, especially those between the ages of 6 and 18 months, are most likely to become affected. From a number of infected districts, however, it has been reported that calves frequently die at the age of 4 to 5 months, and cases of blackleg in even younger animals are not exceedingly rare, although not numerous enough to be of practical importance. Increase in number of cases with increase in age is very characteristic and suggests that natural or inherited immunity from blackleg, which is so pronounced in young animals, gradually wears off with the approach to the fateful half-year mark. It is unusual for cattle in the United States to contract the disease when past 2 years old. According to Swiss statistics (Hess) cows, when past 3 years old, are almost immune to blackleg.

As to the class of cattle most frequently affected by blackleg, the majority of reports agree that purebred or high-grade stock are more subject to the disease than low-grade cattle. In this country it was noticeable that blackleg began to increase when stock owners began to improve their cattle. A large number of ranchmen have stated that their losses from blackleg were insignificant before they im-

77431 O—51——29

proved the breeding of their stock. On large ranches where both low- and high-grade stock are kept it has been observed that most of the deaths from blackleg occur among the better stock. The common range cattle of Texas and the Western States are very hardy, and it is probable that in regions where blackleg has prevailed for a number of years the native stock have acquired or inherited a partial or complete immunity from the disease. In view of the nature of the disease and the manner in which the infection takes place, it seems that the more thin-skinned the animal the more likely it is to become infected, and that the thicker and tougher the skin the less likely is infection to occur.

Whether one sex is any more predisposed to blackleg than the other is very doubtful. A number of reports state that steer calves are more frequently affected than heifers, but the great majority of stock owners are of the opinion that both sexes are equally susceptible. In older animals there seems to be a greater susceptibility to blackleg among the males.

As to the condition of the animals, there seems to be a greater susceptibility in young cattle that are rapidly improving in flesh, as is the case when they are turned on fresh grass in the spring. On the other hand, the change from grass to hay in the fall in many localities seems to have an equally fatal effect on the stock. Some stock owners attribute the appearance of blackleg to a lack of exercise and state that driving the herd for a considerable distance temporarily checks the disease. There is reason to believe that lack of exercise while the grass is fresh and abundant is a predisposing factor in the appearance of blackleg.

Sheep and goats are subject to blackleg, and a few cases have been reported in swine, but man, horses, dogs, cats, and fowls appear to be immune.

Seasonal occurrence.—The spring and the fall are the seasons when blackleg is principally observed. The disease is not confined to the seasons, however, but appears at all times of the year with more or less frequency. In the North, for instance in the Dakotas, the real blackleg season lasts from April to September or October, but outbreaks are reported in every month of the year. In Nebraska, Colorado, and Kansas the outbreaks are more evenly distributed over the whole year, with a slight increase in the spring and the fall. In Oklahoma and the Panhandle of Texas it is difficult to single out any season as being more favorable to blackleg than others; but in central and western Texas the greatest number of outbreaks occur during the fall, winter, and spring, with but few cases during June, July, and August.

The occurrence of the disease in various parts of the world and under all sorts of climatic and weather conditions indicates that location, geological formation, climate, and weather have no influence either favorable or unfavorable to the development of blackleg.

Symptoms.—The symptoms of blackleg are so characteristic that the disease is usually easily recognized, especially by the veterinarian. The first symptoms may be either general or local, though more frequently the latter. The general symptoms are high fever, loss of appetite, and suspension of rumination, followed by great depression. Breathing becomes more rapid. The animal moves about with difficulty, frequently lies down, and, when water is near at hand, drinks at short intervals and but a little at a time. The visible mucous membranes are at first red and congested, but they change in the course of 12 hours to a dirty leaden or purplish color.

The most important characteristic of the disease is the development of a tumor or swelling under the skin. The swelling may appear on any part of the body and legs except below the knee or hock joint and on the tail. It is frequently seen on the thigh or shoulder, and, owing to the extensive discoloration of the swollen parts, as observed after the animal has been skinned, the disease has been popularly named "blackleg" or "black quarter." Tumors may also appear on the neck, chest, flank, or rump. At first they are small and very painful. They increase rapidly in size and in a few hours may cover a large portion of the body. One or more of these tumors may form simultaneously and when in close proximity to one another may unite. The neighboring lymph glands become considerably swollen. When slight pressure is made on a tumor, as in stroking or handling it, a peculiar crackling sound under the skin is heard. This is due to a collection of gas formed by the organisms as they multiply. At this stage the tumor is cool to the touch and painless in the center, and the skin over it is dry and parchmentlike. If the swelling is cut into, a frothy, dark-red fluid is discharged.

The swellings usually appear before the general symptoms, and they may even reach such an extent as to cause complete paralysis of the affected parts while the animal still looks bright and has a good appetite. This condition is, however, of short duration. As the swelling increases in size the general symptoms become more intense. The temperature may reach 107° F., and the respirations may exceed 140 a minute. The animal is unable to rise; the extremities become cold, and some time before death the temperature falls and may become subnormal. There is trembling of the muscles, which, as death approaches, may develop into violent convulsions.

With few exceptions the disease terminates fatally in 12 to 36 hours after the first appearance of the symptoms. A few cases linger for 3 to 4 days, and the disease may occasionally terminate in recovery.

Appearance after death.—The carcass of an animal that has died from blackleg soon becomes very much distended by gas, partly through fermentation in the intestines and partly through the formation of gas in the tissue under the skin. This distention, which is especially pronounced in the region of the blackleg tumors, extends for a considerable distance from the tumors and in the directions where it meets the least resistance—that is, where there is plenty of loose tissue. This is especially the case on the back and sides of the chest, on the shoulder, between the shoulder and the chest, and on the outer surface of the hind quarter. This inflated condition frequently causes the two legs on the upper side of the carcass to stand out straight without touching the ground.

A dark, blood-colored, frothy discharge flows from the nostrils and the anus. Decomposition takes place soon after death, except in the affected muscles, which retain a sweetish-sour odor without developing any putrid odor, even when the rest of the carcass has decomposed.

On the surface of the body may be seen one or more of the characteristic blackleg tumors. The skin covering these swellings is affected with dry gangrene. The connective tissue beneath the skin is infiltrated with blood and bloody serum and is distended with gas. The distended muscles are dark brown or black, are easily torn, and the spaces surrounding them are filled with bloody liquid and gas. The muscle tissue is distended with numerous smaller or larger gas-filled cavities, often to such an extent as to produce a resemblance to lung tissue (pl. XLII). On incision it does not collapse perceptibly, as the gas cavities are not connected with one another. The discoloration is deepest at the center, shades off toward the edges, and becomes brighter by contact with the air. On compression thick blood escapes, which is charged with gas and has a disagreeable odor, somewhat like that of rancid butter. The blood in the remaining parts of the carcass is normal, coagulates easily after death, and forms a solid clot. The abdominal cavity sometimes contains a considerable quantity of bloody effusion. The mucous membrane of the intestine may be congested or inflamed, and the contents of the bowels may be covered with blood. Blood spots are found also on the heart and lungs. The liver is congested, but the spleen is always normal.

For the same reasons outlined under anthrax, a blackleg carcass should never be unnecessarily opened, and the operation is always preferably done by a veterinarian. If it must be done by a layman, every effort should be made to limit spreading of the infective blood, exudates, and other possible sources of infection.

Differential diagnosis.—Among the features of blackleg that distinguish it from anthrax are the unchanged spleen and the ready

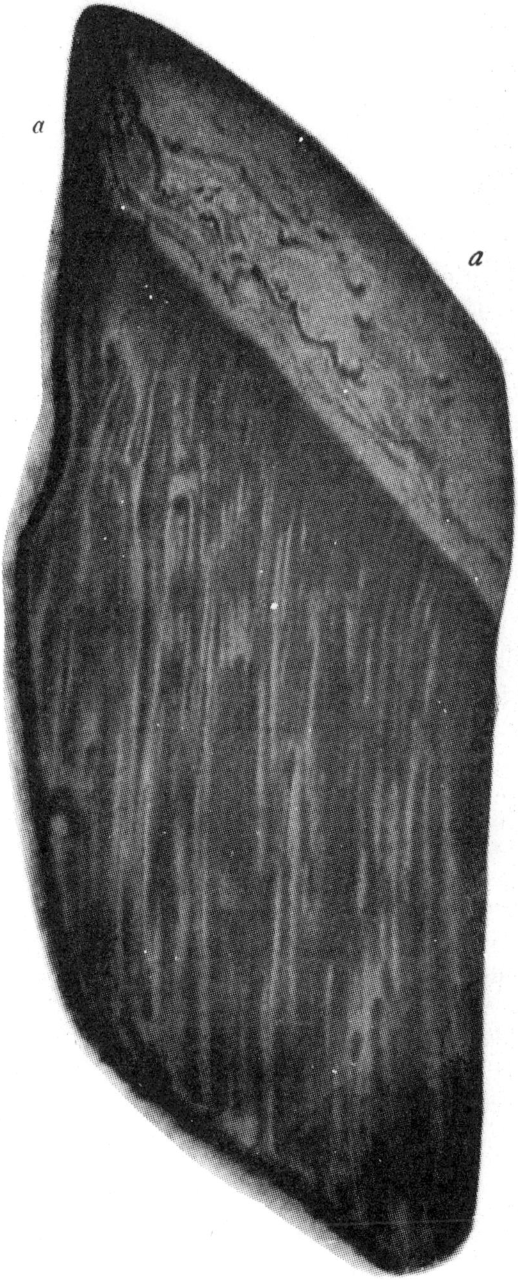

HAINES DEL.

SECTION OF MUSCLE FROM A BLACKLEG SWELLING.

a. Gas bubbles.
b. Cavities due to gas formation.

clotting of the blood. In anthrax the spleen is very much enlarged and the blood is tarry, and coagulates feebly. The anthrax carbuncles and swellings differ from the blackleg swellings in not containing gas, in being hard and solid, and in causing death less rapidly.

It is difficult to distinguish between the swellings of blackleg and those of malignant edema, as they resemble each other very closely, and both are distended with gas. Malignant edema, however, generally begins from a wound of considerable size. It often follows surgical operations and does not result from the small abrasions and pricks to which animals are subjected in pastures.

Hemorrhagic septicemia may be differentiated from blackleg by its affecting cattle of all ages, by the locations of the swelling usually about the region of the throat, neck, and dewlap, by the soft, doughy character of these swellings without the presence of gas bubbles, and finally by the characteristic hemorrhages widely distributed throughout the body.

Bacteriological tests, including microscopic examination of diseased tissues, which are best selected for character and suitability by the veterinarian, together with inoculation of test animals, afford the most reliable means of distinguishing between infectious diseases and identifying infection. Inoculation experiments on guinea pigs, rabbits, and chickens will disclose the differences between blackleg, anthrax, and malignant edema, as all these species are killed by the germ of malignant edema, but only the first two by the anthrax germ and only the first one by the blackleg infection.

Treatment.—Medicinal treatment has thus far proved unavailing in the treatment of blackleg. Some writers have recommended the use of certain drugs, which have seemed to be beneficial in a few cases, but a thorough trial has shown them to be valueless. Others have advised that the swelling be opened by deep and long incisions and that a strong disinfectant, such as a 5-percent solution of carbolic acid, be applied to the wounds. Such a procedure cannot be too strongly condemned. As nearly all the animals attacked die in spite of every kind of treatment, and as the opening of the tumors scatters the germs over the stables or pastures and causes danger to other animals, such measures do more harm than good and should be discarded as dangerous.

Other methods formerly practiced but now generally condemned are bleeding, "nerving," setoning or roweling, and violent exercise. "Nerving" is a term sometimes applied by laymen to severing the artery between the hoofs. Setoning or roweling consists in producing a large running sore in the dewlap or on the shoulder by the insertion of a piece of tape or other suitable substance, thus draining the animal's vitality. This method has been used extensively in

England, where public opinion was opposed to vaccination, but leading English veterinary authorities consider it useless. The evidence indicates, in fact, that none of these measures have either curative or preventive value, whereas they are open to objection on the ground of cruelty. In particularly valuable animals, the use of antiblackleg serum may be resorted to, but the expense involved and the uncertainty of results make this practice impractical.

Vaccination.—The only effective and reliable means known for protecting animals against blackleg is vaccination, which has been thoroughly tried and proved to be efficacious.

The three French veterinarians already mentioned (Arloing, Cornevin, and Thomas) devised a method of inoculation with attenuated (weakened) blackleg spores that produce immunity from natural or artificial inoculation of virulent blackleg germs. Their method of vaccination, which became popularly known as the French method, the Arloing method, or the Lyons method (their laboratories are located at Lyons, France), was introduced in 1883 and was generally adopted during the following 2 years. According to this method the material used for vaccine is obtained from a fresh blackleg tumor, and after being dried and ground into a powder it is mixed with water to make a dough, spread on thin plates, and attenuated by heating in an oven to a temperature of 100° to 104° C. for 7 hours. The material is then pulverized, mixed with sterile water, and injected under the skin of calves, producing a partial immunity. This immunity is later reinforced after 8 or 10 days by a second injection of a vaccine that has been heated for the same length of time but at a temperature of 90° to 94° C.

Later Kitt, a German scientist, modified the French method so that but one injection of vaccine was required instead of two. The Kitt method was further modified by Nörgaard, of the Bureau of Animal Industry, in 1896, by heating the virus to 94° or 95° C. for 6 hours, and this modification was used for many years by the Bureau of Animal Industry in the preparation of Government powdered vaccine. Vaccines prepared after the above-mentioned methods are put out in the usual pellet or powdered form.

Other improved methods of protecting cattle against blackleg include the use of forms of vaccine known as aggressins and filtrates. The principal advantage of these new immunizing agents is the impossibility of producing the disease itself in the treated animals, but, as a rule, they are somewhat more expensive than the powder vaccine.

Antiblackleg serum is also being produced for treating calves already affected with blackleg, as well as for producing a passive immunity in exposed animals of an infected herd. This serum is prepared by inoculating horses with repeated injections of washed cultures of the blackleg organism into the veins and later under the skin, and afterwards drawing the blood to obtain the serum. This product, however, is rarely used at the present time in the United States.

Although directions for the use of blackleg vaccine accompany the packages, it should be realized that vaccination against any disease is not simply a mechanical procedure but one which, if improperly done, may not only fail to protect the animal injected but may actually spread other unrecognized diseases from one animal to another. Therefore, whenever possible a competent veterinarian should perform this service.

In order to avoid danger from complicating disorders, it is well to refrain from castrating, spaying, and dehorning at the time of vaccination. When animals to be vaccinated are gentle and accustomed to being handled, vaccination may be performed on the standing animal. Range cattle or other half-wild animals must be thrown or otherwise secured, as, for example, in a chute such as is used for branding and dehorning. The immunizing properties of vaccine are not usually imparted until 10 or 12 days after vaccination. As vaccine is thus a preventive and not a curative agent, it is not advisable to vaccinate an animal after the symptoms of blackleg have developed, though the serum mentioned previously, if available at the onset of the disease, might be efficacious in such cases.

Vaccination is generally followed by insignificant symptoms. In some cases there is a slight rise in temperature, and sometimes a slight swelling may be noted at the point of injection. The immunity conferred by vaccination varies according to the character of vaccine used; aggressin and filtrate apparently confer the longest immunity, which may last for 18 months or longer. Animals vaccinated with powder vaccine before they are 6 months old and those in badly infected districts should be revaccinated before the next blackleg season.

In 1897 the United States Department of Agriculture began the preparation and free distribution of blackleg vaccine to stock raisers. Up to that time the "single vaccine" could not be obtained in this country. The effect of vaccine in preventing losses and in reducing the prevalence of blackleg was highly satisfactory. In the 25 years of Government distribution about 47,000,000 doses were supplied. Reports indicated that as a result of the use of the vaccine the losses from blackleg were reduced from about 10 percent to less than one-half of 1 percent of the number of calves produced annually in the infected districts. The distribution of the Government blackleg vaccine was discontinued July 1, 1922, in compliance with the provision of an act of Congress. Although public notice was given of the discontinuance at the time, numerous requests for vaccine have continued to reach the Bureau of Animal Industry. Stock owners can avoid delay by applying directly to their veterinarian, commercial concerns, or other sources for one of the immunizing agents previously mentioned.

PREVENTING AND DESTROYING INFECTION

When blackleg occurs with more or less regularity in a pasture, feed lot, or stable, it is due to the presence of the blackleg germ either in the ground of these places or in materials—coarse feed, for instance—brought there regularly. Whenever an animal becomes affected the germs multiply by the million in its system, and their liberation, through natural or artificial means, tends to preserve, increase, or spread the infection. When attempts are made to "doctor" affected animals by opening the swellings, the infection is scattered with the bloody discharge. Infection may be spread over wide areas by dogs, wolves, coyotes, and buzzards which attack and devour the carcasses of animals that have died of blackleg.

It is, therefore, of the utmost importance that cattle owners in infected districts realize that an animal affected with blackleg may be the cause of great subsequent losses from the same disease, perhaps not immediately, but within a period of years to follow; and it cannot be too urgently recommended that they make every effort to reduce the danger by taking adequate measures to destroy as completely as possible this source of renewed infection.

Proper disposal of carcasses.—Where wood is plentiful the best method of destroying an infected carcass is to burn it. In order to insure its complete destruction, the dead animal should be placed on two logs and plenty of dry wood heaped around it. About 2 quarts of kerosene should then be poured on and fire set to it. It is necessary that the carcass be entirely destroyed; if any part of it remains, another fire should be built around it.

In a pasture where wood is scarce the carcass may be buried. This method is less satisfactory as the infection is not destroyed but merely removed to a few feet below the surface, whence it may return through various means—for instance, as demonstrated by Pasteur, through the agency of earthworms. Therefore the hole in the ground should be made at least 6 feet deep and the carcass well covered with quicklime before the earth is filled in. A place should be selected that is free from danger of contaminating the water supply. The place where the animal was lying before being buried, as well as the top of the grave, should be freely sprinkled with a strong disinfecting solution, such as compound cresol solution (at least 4 ounces to the gallon of water) or one of the recognized commercial coal-tar dips or disinfectants.

Because of the difficulty of destroying the infection, it is well to kill an affected animal as soon as the disease has been definitely determined to be blackleg and to burn the carcass immediately without removal. The fresh virus is much more easily destroyed than the dried, and by quick action a better result is always assured. If an animal dies from blackleg in a stable, it becomes necessary to remove the carcass to a proper place for burning or burial. For the purpose, a low sled or wagon, should be used instead of the carcass being dragged over the ground. Care should be taken to scatter straw or hay wherever there is a possibility of infecting the stable floor or the ground with the discharges from the carcass while it is being removed. All litter should be removed from the stable and burned, together with that used in removing the carcass. The woodwork and floors of the stable should be thoroughly and repeatedly soaked with a disinfectant of the kind already mentioned.

Freeing pastures of infection.—Eradication of blackleg infection from pastures is difficult. The method of preventing the renewal of infection by keeping susceptible animals away from a pasture until the infection has died out, which is effective against some diseases, is impracticable in the case of blackleg because of the long time that the spores retain their vitality. Outbreaks of blackleg have been reported as appearing in pastures where no previous case had occurred for 11 years. Even if the actual time necessary to insure freedom of premises from infection were known, few persons could afford to keep a pasture unstocked for a sufficient length of time for the infection to die out. A change of stock from one pasture to another nearby is likely to be ineffective because as a rule the conditions are very much alike in all pastures on the same farm or ranch.

It has been asserted that complete drainage and cultivation of the soil for several years will prevent further outbreaks, but where the question concerns large pastures that are unsuitable for anything but cattle raising this measure is, of course, out of consideration.

Probably one of the most effective methods for freeing a pasture from blackleg infection is to allow the grass to grow high and when it is sufficiently dry to burn it off. One burning is not sufficient to destroy all infection; hence the process should be repeated several years in succession. This method, however, is often impracticable, as but few cattle owners can afford to carry it out.

After all it appears that immunization by means of vaccination is the only known practicable and effective means, not only of protecting individual animals against blackleg, but, by repeated application year after year, of eventually ridding pastures of infection by preventing the development of new cases during the long period necessary for the old infection to disappear.

NECROTIC STOMATITIS (CALF DIPHTHERIA)

(Pl. XLIII)

Necrotic stomatitis is an acute, specific, infectious inflammation of the mouth, occurs mostly in young cattle, and is characterized locally by the formation of ulcers and caseonecrotic patches and by constitutional symptoms, chiefly toxic. This disease has also been termed "calf diphtheria," gangrenous stomatitis," "necrobacillosis," "ulcerative stomatitis," "malignant stomatitis," and "diphtheritic patches of the oral mucous membrane."

During the last several years farmers and cattlemen in the United States, especially in the West and Southwest, have noted an increasing occurrence of enzootics of "sore mouth" among the young animals of their herds. These cases usually occur during the winter months when cattle are often corralled under insanitary conditions. Instead of healing of themselves as do the usual forms of sore mouth, those caused by necrotis stomatitis, if untreated, result in death. Careful study of some of them has resulted in their identification with cases reported in 1877 by Dammann, from the shore of the Baltic; in 1878 by Blazekowic, in Slavonia; in 1879 by Vollers, in Holstein; in 1880 by Lenglen, in France; in 1881 by Macgillivray, in England; and in 1884 by Löffler, who isolated and described the micro-organism that produces the disease. Bang obtained this organism from the diphtheritic lesions of calves in 1890, and Kitt likewise recovered the bacillus from similar lesions of the larynx and pharynx of calves and pigs in 1893.

Cause.—The cause of necrotic stomatitis, as demonstrated by Löffler and since confirmed by other investigators, is *Actinomyces necrophorus*, often spoken of as the bacillus of necrosis. This organism varies in form from a coccoid rod to long, wavy filaments, which may attain a length of 100μ; the width varies from 0.75μ to 1μ. Hence it is described as polymorphic. It does not stain by the Gram method but takes the ordinary aniline dyes and often presents especially the longer forms, a beaded appearance. A characteristic of the organism, of great moment in the treatment of the disease, is that it grows only in the absence of oxygen, from which fact it is described as an obligate anaerobe.

Few organisms have a wider range of pathogenesis. According to clinical observation, *Actinomyces necrophorus* is pathogenic for cattle, horses, hogs, sheep, reindeer, deer, kangaroos, antelope, and rabbits. Experimentally it has been proved to be pathogenic for rabbits and white mice. Dogs, cats, guinea pigs, pigeons, and chickens

PLATE XLIII

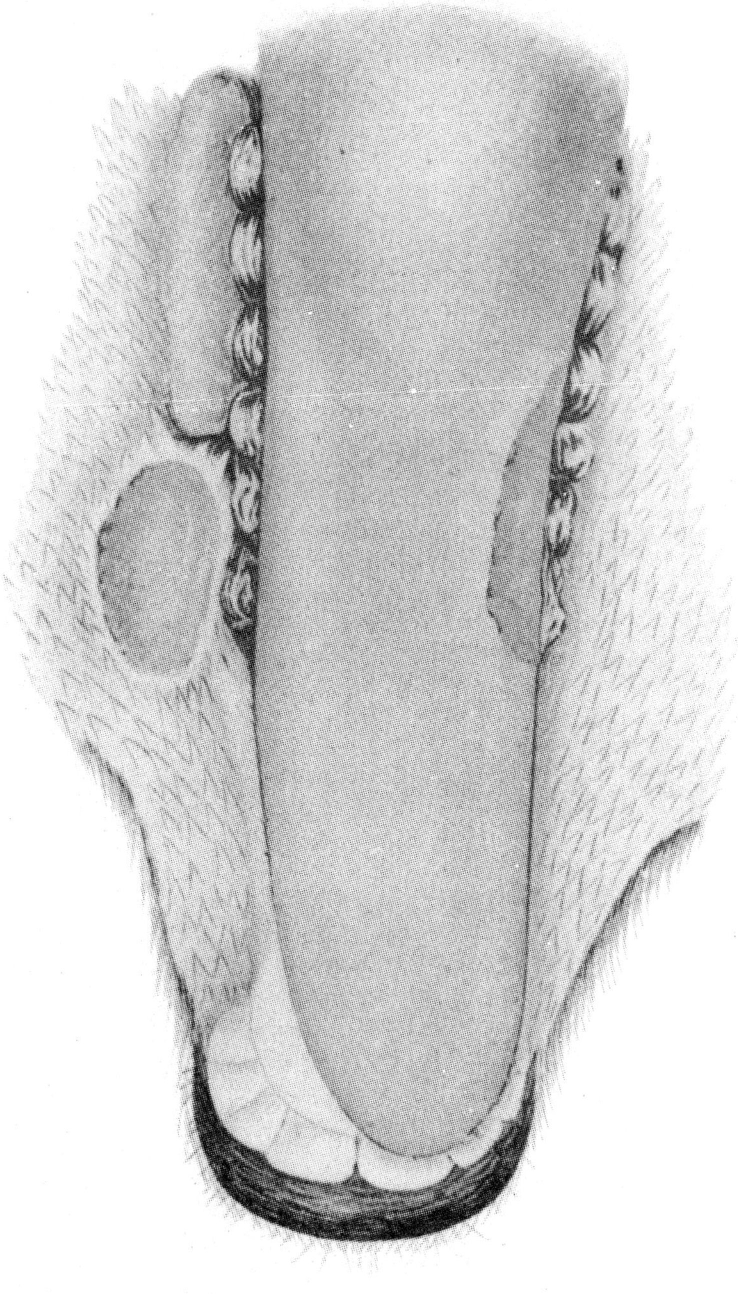

HAINES DEL.

NECROTIC STOMATITIS (CALF DIPHTHERIA).

appear to be immune. A few cases of infection attributed to this organism have been described in man.

The importance of this bacillus is far beyond even its relation to necrotic stomatitis. Besides this disease it has been incriminated as the causative factor in foot rot, multiple liver abscesses, disseminated liver necrosis, embolic necrosis of the lungs, and necrosis of the heart, in cattle; gangrenous pox of the teats and diphtheria of the uterus and vagina, in cows; diphtheritic inflammation of the small intestines of calves. Among horses it is often involved in the production of necrotic malanders, quittor, and diphtheritic inflammation of the large intestine. In hogs it has been found in necrotic or diphtheritic processes in the mucous membrane of the mouth, necrosis of the anterior wall of the nasal septum, and pulmonary and intestinal necrosis, accompanying hog cholera. Abcesses of the liver, gangrenous processes of the lips and nose, and gangrenous affections of the hoof in sheep, have been attributed to this organism.

Pathology.—The principal lesions in necrotic stomatitis occur in the mucous membrane of the mouth and pharynx. The alterations may extend to the nasal cavities, larynx, trachea, lungs, esophagus, stomach, intestines, and hoofs. The oral surfaces affected are, in the order of frequency, tongue, cheeks, hard palate, gums, lips, and pharynx. In most cases the primary infection seems to occur in the tongue (pl. XLIII).

According to present information, infection takes place by inoculation. Some abrasion or break in the continuity of the mucous membrane of the mouth occurs. The origin may be connected with the eruption of the first teeth after birth, or, in animals somewhat older, the entrance of sharp-pointed particles of feed, such as barley beards or foxtail awns. Gaining an entrance at this point, the bacilli begin to multiply. During their development they elaborate a toxin, or poisonous substance, that causes the death, or necrosis, of the epithelial, or superficial, layer of the mucous membrane and also of the white blood cells that have passed through the vessel walls to the defense of the tissues against the bacillary attack. This destruction of the surface epithelium seems to be the essential factor in the production of the caseous patch, often called the false membrane. From the connective-tissue framework below is poured forth an inflammatory exudate highly albuminous or rich in fibrin-forming elements. When this exudate and the necrosed cellular elements come into contact, the latter furnish a fibrin ferment that transforms the exudate into a fibrinous mass. This process is known as coagulation necrosis, and the resulting fibroid mass, containing in its meshes the necrosed and degenerated epithelium and leucocytes, constitutes the diphtheritic or false membrane. In this connection, the disease has no relation to diphtheria of man. If the process ceased at this point, it would be properly called a diphtheritic inflammation, but it does not. A caseating ferment is supplied by the bacilli, and this, acting on the fibroid patch, transforms it into a dry, finely granular, yellowish mass of tissue detritus resembling cheese, and therefore described as caseous.

Frequently this caseous inflammation results in the formation of one or more ulcers with thickened, slightly reddened borders, surmounted by several layers of this necrosed tissue. The floor of the ulcer is formed by a grayish yellow, corroded surface, under which the tissue is transformed into a dry, friable, or firm cheesy mass. In the tongue this may progress to two fingers' thickness into the muscular portion; in the cheek it may form an external opening, permitting fluids to escape from the mouth; on the palate it frequently reaches and includes the bone in its destructive course; on the gums it has produced necrosis of the tooth sockets, causing loss of the teeth. In the advanced forms, caseous foci may be seen in the lungs and in the liver and necrotic patches observed on the mucous membrane of the gastrointestinal tract.

Symptoms.—Necrotic stomatitis ordinarily does not affect a large number of animals at one time. It is both a local and a systemic affection but is primarily the former. The local lesion is the caseo-necrotic patch or ulcer developed as a result of the multiplication of the bacilli at the point of inoculation. The general affection is an intoxication, or poisoning, of the whole system produced by a soluble toxin elaborated by the bacilli.

The stage of incubation is 3 to 5 days. The first symptoms are a disinclination to take nourishment, some drooling from the mouth, and an examination of the mouth will show on some portion of its mucous membrane a circumscribed area of infiltration and redness, possibly an erosion. The latter gradually extends in size and depth and forms a sharply circumscribed area of necrotic inflammation. Its size varies from that of a 5-cent piece to that of a silver dollar or even larger. It has the appearance of a corroded surface, under which the mucous membrane or muscular tissue seems transformed into a dry, friable, or firm cheesy mass. It is grayish yellow in color and is bordered by a zone of thickened tissue slightly reddened and somewhat granulated. The necrotic tissue is very adherent and can be only partially peeled off. It is homogeneous, cheesy, and may extend two fingers' depth into the tissues beneath. The general symptoms are languor, weakness, and slight fever. In spite of plenty of good feed the calf is seen to be failing. It stops sucking, or, if older, altogether refuses to eat. The temperature at this time may be 104° to 107° F. The slobber becomes profuse, swallowing very difficult, opening of the mouth painful, and a most offensive odor is exhaled. The tongue is swollen and its motion greatly impaired. Sometimes the mouth is kept open, permitting the tumefied tongue to protrude. One or more of the above symptoms direct the attention to the mouth as the seat of disease; or, the debility and disinclination to eat having been noticed, an examination of the animal may show a lump under the neck or swelling of the throat or head.

The general affection at this time manifests itself by dejectedness, extreme weakness, and emaciation, constant lying down, with stiffness and difficulty in standing.

The disease frequently extends to the nasal cavities from which there is a thin, yellowish, or greenish yellow, sticky discharge that adheres closely to the borders of the nostrils. Their edges also have caseous patches similar to those in the mouth. Sometimes the nasal passage is obstructed by great masses of the necrosed exudate, thus causing extreme difficulty in breathing. When the caseous process involves the larynx and trachea there result coughing, wheezing, and dyspnea, together with a yellowish mucopurulent expectoration.

When life is prolonged 3 or 4 weeks, caseous foci may be established in the lung, giving rise to all the signs of a bronchopneumonia. Many of these cases are associated with a fibrinous pleurisy. The invasion of the gastrointestinal tract is announced by diarrheal symptoms. This disease principally attacks sucklings not more than 6 weeks of age, but calves 8 and 10 months old are frequently affected, and several cases in adult cattle have been reported.

In its very acute form many cases run their course in 5 to 8 days. In these the local lesions are not strongly marked, and death seems due to acute intoxication. In other enzootics most of the affected animals live 3 to 5 weeks. In these, pulmonary and intestinal symptoms are occasionally present and caseonecrotic lesions sometimes develop in the liver. Ordinarily affected animals show no tendency to spontaneous cure. Left to themselves they usually die. On the contrary, if taken in hand early, the disease is often readily amenable to treatment. In the latter event the prospects of recovery are usually good.

Differential diagnosis.—Necrotic stomatitis may be differentiated from foot-and-mouth disease by the fact that in the latter there is a rapid infection of the entire herd, including the adult cattle, as well as the infection of hogs and sheep. The characteristic lesion of foot-and-mouth disease is the appearance of vesicles containing a serous fluid on the mucous membrane of the mouth and on the udder, teats, and feet of the affected animals. In necrotic stomatitis vesicles are never formed; necrosis occurs from the beginning and is followed by the formation of yellowish, cheesy patches, principally in the mouth. Mycotic stomatitis occurs in only a few animals of the herd. chiefly the adult cattle, and the lesions produced consist of an inflammation of the mouth and lips and of the skin between the toes, followed in a few days by small irregular ulcers in the mouth. This disease appears sporadically, usually in the early fall after a dry summer, does not run a regular course, and cannot be produced by inoculation.

Prevention.—As the disease is seldom seen in animals on pasture, pasturing is preferable to confinement whenever weather and other conditions permit.

As soon as the disease appears, the healthy animals should be separated from the sick animals and placed in clean quarters. A daily inspection of the exposed animals serves to disclose cases of the disease in an early stage and therefore facilitates treatment and prevents spread of the infection.

All barns, sheds, corral fences, floors, and troughs should be thoroughly cleaned and disinfected with some such disinfectant as 3-percent solution of compound cresol solution. The litter, discharges, and material scraped from the mouth should be burned or buried.

In going from sick to healthy animals, one should pay particular attention to cleanliness, especially of the hands and clothing.

It is conceivable that exposure to cold might so disturb the normal circulation of the oral tissues as to make the mucous membrane an excellent location for the causative factor of the disease. There is another possibility, however, that relates to the disinfection of barns, sheds, and other places mentioned. The so-called diphtheritic inflammations of the vagina and uterus in cows are caused by the same organism that induces necrotic stomatitis. A European writer has pointed out the almost constant relation of such attacks to previous occurrences of foot rot in the same or other cattle on the place. In all likelihood, in such cases the stalls and sheds are the harborers of this germ. It is possible that many of these outbreaks have some relation to preceding cases of the above-mentioned diseases and the greater use in winter of the stalls and sheds, thus harboring the *Actinomyces necrophorus.*

Treatment.—The varying results of treating the condition seem to depend on whether the lesion is advanced or in an early stage and on whether the deepest part of the diseased tissue is exposed to the antiseptic to be used. If the lesion is in an easily accessible part of the mouth or throat it is first to be curetted—that is, the dead tissue is removed by means of a curette—or a small spoon may be employed. Incidentally, all accumulated fibers of feed are to be removed, and the mouth may be thoroughly washed twice daily with an antiseptic solution, such as 4-percent boric acid or 5- to 10-percent potassium permanganate solution. The base of the ulcer may be painted with tincture of iodine every day until healing begins. If the lesions are inaccessible, the calf often dies, as other than diligent treatment of the site of the infection seldom suffices.

MYCOTIC STOMATITIS OF CATTLE

Numerous letters have been received by this Bureau relative to the existence of a disease affecting the mouths and feet of cattle in certain Eastern and Central Western States. Later reports indicate that the malady has made its appearance in the Southwest where it has caused much alarm among stockmen owing to its similarity to the foot-and-mouth disease of Europe. The disease which is discussed under the name "mycotic stomatitis," has been carefully investigated on various occasions, and it is with the view to giving the results of these clinical investigations as well as to assert its noninfectiousness and to differentiate it from the virulent foot-and-mouth disease, which it so closely simulates, that this article is prepared.

The name "stomatitis" signifies that there is present in the affected animals an inflammation of the mucous membrane of the mouth. This inflammation, which quickly develops into ulcers, is one of the principal and most frequently observed lesions. Mycotic stomatitis refers to that form of stomatitis that presumedly results from eating feed containing irritant fungi. Thus the name not only suggests the cause of the disease, but also indicates the location of the earliest and most prominent symptoms. Other names that have been applied to this disease by different writers are sporadic aphthae; aphthous stomatitis; sore mouth of cattle; sore tongue, benign, simple, or noninfectious foot-and-mouth disease; mycotic aphthous stomatitis; and sporadic stomatitis aphthosa.

Mycotic stomatitis is a sporadic, apparently noninfectious disease which affects cattle of all ages that are on pasture, especially milk cows. It is characterized by inflammation and ulceration of the mucous membrane of the mouth, producing salivation and inappetence, and secondarily affecting the feet, which become sore and swollen. Superficial erosions of the skin, particularly of the muzzle and of the teats and udders of cows, may also be present, with some elevation of temparture and emaciation.

Cause.—This disease, as its name indicates, is believed to be caused by the eating of forage containing fungi or molds. It is probable that more than one fungus is involved in the production of this disease, but no particular species has been definitely proved to be the causative factor. Several attempts have been made by the writer to determine the exact cause and also to transmit the disease to other animals by direct inoculation, but with negative results. Suspicion, however, has been directed by various observers to the *Uromyces* and the red and black rusts that occur on clovers. These fungi cause severe irritation of the lining membrane of the mouth, producing sometimes a catarrhal, at other times an aphthous, and occasionally an ulcerous stomatitis. The fungus of rape and similar feeds (*Polydesmus excitiosus*) is very irritating to the mouths and feet of cattle, and causes severe inflammation and in some instances symptoms that have been mistaken for foot-and-mouth disease. The fungi (Penicillium and Puccinia) found on grasses have also been credited with the production of stomatitis. The fact that this disease disappears from a locality at a certain time and reappears at irregular intervals suggests the probability that certain climatic conditions are essential for the propagation of the causative fungi, since the malady becomes prevalent after a hot, dry period has been followed by rain, thus furnishing the requirements necessary for the luxuriant development of molds and fungi. Owing to this fact, the disease is observed in one locality during one season and in an entirely different section another year, but reappears in the former center when favorable conditions prevail. In this way the affection has occurred at irregular intervals in certain sections of both the United States and Canada. Attempts to transmit the disease by transferring diseased tissue from an affected animal to a normal one have generally failed, tending to support the belief that the condition is non-infectious.

Symptoms and lesions.—Among the first symptoms observed in mycotic stomatitis are inability to eat, suspension of rumination, frequent movements of the lips with the formation of froth on their margins, and in some cases a dribbling of saliva from the mouth. There is a desire to eat, and frequent attempts to take food are made, but this is very difficult. If, however, food is placed on the back of the tongue, it is readily masticated and swallowed. If the mouth is examined at this time, it will be found red and hot, and exceptionally small blisters will be seen, which, however, quickly become eroded and developed into active ulcers varying in size from ⅛ to 1 inch in diameter. Where several ulcers have coalesced a large and irregularly indented patch is formed. These erosions are most frequently found on the gums around the incisor teeth, on the dental pad, inside the lips, and on the tip of the tongue, but they also occur on the cheeks, interdental space, and dorsum of the tongue. The ulcers have a hemorrhagic border, a depressed suppurating surface, and contain a brownish or yellowish colored debris, which is soon replaced by granulation tissue. As a result of this sloughing of the tissues and the retention of food in the mouth, a very offensive odor is exhaled. The muzzle becomes dry and parched in appearance, which condition is shortly followed by erosions and exfoliations of the superficial layer of the skin. Adherent brownish crusts and scabs form over the parts, and similar lesions are seen around the nostrils and external surface of the lips.

In some cases there are associated with these alterations a slight swelling and painfulness in the region of the pasterns, at times affecting the forefeet, at other times the hind feet, and occasionally all four feet. In a few cases the swelling may extend above the fetlock, but it has never been observed above the knee or hock. The skin around the coronet may occasionally become fissured and the thin skin in the cleft of the foot eroded and suppurated, but without the formation of vesicles. As a result of these foot lesions, the affected animal may assume a position with its back arched and the limbs propped under the body as in a case of founder, and will manifest much pain and lameness in walking. If the animal lies down, it shows reluctance in getting up, and although manifesting no inclination to move about, when forced to do so there is more or less stiffness and a tendency to kick or shake the foot as if to dislodge a foreign body from between the claws.

In some outbreaks the milk cows have slight superficial erosions on the teats that at times extend to the udder. The cracks in the skin are filled with serum and form brownish-colored scabs. The teats become tender and the milk secretion diminishes; in some cases it disappears. A similar tendency toward the formation of fissures and scabs on the skin of the neck and shoulders manifested itself in an outbreak in Texas, and this feature was likewise noticeable in the disease when it occurred in Maryland and Virginia in 1889.

In mild cases only the mouth lesions may be observed, or these alterations may be associated with one or more of the other above-described symptoms, but in severe cases, where there is a generalized mycotic intoxication one animal may show all these alterations. When the disease is well developed the general appearance of the animal is one of great lassitude, and it either stands off by itself with hind feet drawn under the body and its forefeet extended, or it assumes a recumbent position. Owing to the inability to eat and to the general systemic disturbance present, the animal loses flesh rapidly and becomes greatly emaciated in the latter stages of the disease. The temperature and pulse are somewhat increased, the former 2 or 3 degrees, the latter to from 75 to 90 beats a minute. The fever is not lasting, and these symptoms are soon modified. The animal has an anxious look, and in a few cases there is a gastrointestinal

77431 O—51——30

irritation, the feces being thin, of a dark color, and of an offensive odor.

Prognosis and mortality.—Mycotic stomatitis is not a serious disease, and in uncomplicated cases recoveries soon follow the removal of the cause and the application of the indicated remedies. In such cases complete restoration may take place within 1 week. In mild outbreaks a large percentage of the animals recover without treatment, but that the disease is fatal is shown by the fact that animals which develop an aggravated form of the affection succumb if not treated. In such animals death occurs in 6 to 8 days, but the mortality in the serious outbreaks thus far investigated has been less than 0.5 percent. The course of this disease is irregular and runs from 7 to 15 days, the average case covering a period of about 10 days.

Differential diagnosis.—In examining a case of mycotic stomatitis it is important not to mistake it for foot-and-mouth disease, which has appeared in this country on 9 occasions up to 1941. This may be accomplished by taking into consideration the fact that in the contagious foot-and-mouth disease there is a rapid infection of the entire herd, as well as of any hogs and sheep that may be on the premises. It is also readily transmitted to neighboring herds by the spread of the infection from diseased animals, but it never occurs spontaneously. The characteristic lesion of foot-and-mouth disease is the appearance of vesicles containing serous fluid in the mouth and on the udder, teats, heels, and coronary bands of the affected animals. Drooling is profuse, and there is a peculiar smacking sound made by sucking the affected lips.

Mycotic stomatitis occurs sporadically on widely separated farms and affects only a few animals in each herd. The lesions produced consist of erosions without the typical vesicular formations of foot-and-mouth disease. The failure of the vesicles, if any appear, to spread extensively in the mouth, the absence of these blisters on other portions of the body—notably the teats and udder, and characteristically the feet—together with the absence of infection in the herd, and the inability to transmit the disease to calves by inoculation, distinguishes between this affection and foot-and-mouth-disease. The erosions of the mouth are not so extensive and they heal more rapidly in mycotic stomatitis. The swelling of the feet and stiffness of the animal are also more marked in mycotic stomatitis. The difference between mycotic and vesicular stomatitis is shown in the chapter on Vesicular Stomatistis (p. 422).

The lesions resulting from ergotism may be differentiated from those of mycotic stomatitis by the lack of ulcerative eruptions in the mouth and by the location of the lesions at the tips of the ears, end of the tail, or on the lower part of the legs, usually below the knees or hocks. The lesions of ergotism do not take the form of ulcers or festers, but the end of the leg affected is entirely diseased and the eruption extends entirely around the legs followed soon afterwards by a distinct line of demarcation between the healthy skin above and the diseased skin below. The absence of suppurating sores between the claws and on the mucous membrane of the mouth, the knowledge that the lesion on the leg in question extends uninterruptedly around it, and the presence of ergotized seeds in the hay or grain fed the animals should point conclusively to a diagnosis of ergotism.

In foot rot, or foul foot, of cattle, the inflammation of the skin and toes usually affects but one foot. It begins as a superficial inflammation followed by sloughing, ulceration, and the formation of fistulous tracts that may involve the tendons, bones, and joints. The mouth remains unaffected, and the presence of the disease may be traced to filth and poor drainage.

In necrotic stomatitis (calf diphtheria) there is a formation of yellowish, cheesy patches in the mouth without any lesions of the feet or udder. It affects suckling calves chiefly and is caused by the *Actinomyces necrophorus*.

Treatment.—The treatment of mycotic stomatitis should consist in first removing the herd of cattle from the pasture in which they have been running. If possible, the affected animals should be brought to the barn or corral and given soft, nutritious feed, such as bran mashes, ground feed, and gruels. A bucket of clear, cool water should be kept constantly in the manger, so that the animals may drink or rinse their mouths whenever they wish. It will be found beneficial to dissolve 2 heaping tablespoonfuls of borax or 1 tablespoonful of potassium chlorate in each of the first two buckets of water taken during the day. If the animals are gentle enough to be handled, the mouth should be swabbed out daily with antiseptic washes, such as a 2-percent solution of carbolic acid or a 1-percent solution of compound solution of cresol or of potassium permanganate, or 1 part of hydrogen peroxide to 2 parts of water. This should be followed by astringents, such as one-half tablespoonful of alum, borax, or potassium chlorate placed on the tongue. Probably a more satisfactory method of administering the antiseptic treatment to a large number of animals would be to mix thoroughly 2 teaspoonfuls of pure carbolic acid every morning in a quart of bran mash and give to each affected animal for a period of 5 days. Range cattle may be more readily treated by the use of medicated salt placed in troughs accessible to the animals. This salt may be prepared by pouring 4 ounces of crude carbolic acid upon 12 quarts of ordinary barrel salt, after which they are thoroughly mixed. The lesions of the feet should be treated with 2-percent solution of carbolic acid, whereas the fissures and other lesions of the skin will be benefited by the application of carbolized petrolatum, or zinc ointment. If the animals are treated in this manner and carefully fed, the disease usually disappears rapidly.

VESICULAR STOMATITIS OF CATTLE

Vesicular stomatitis is known in Europe and South Africa and has been observed occasionally in sporadic form in the United States. Early in the fall of 1916 it became very extensive in certain sections of this country, especially in Nebraska, South Dakota, Colorado, and Wyoming. Other extensive outbreaks of the disease have been encountered in later years.

Notwithstanding the fact that the disease affects horses and mules primarily, it may spread to cattle under certain conditions, but thus far it has not been observed under natural conditions among hogs and sheep. Evidently the necessary conditions for its spread from horses to cattle were present in Nebraska, as a shipment of cattle from that locality to the Kansas City stockyards in the fall of 1916 was found to be infected. Much excitement resulted, since the disease was suggestive of foot-and-mouth disease. However, a series of careful experiments was at once begun from which the true nature of the disease was ascertained and the diagnosis of vesicular stomatitis made.

The name "vesicular stomatitis" not only indicates the location of the lesions in the mouth but also suggests that the vesicles or blisters are characteristic features, being observed at the beginning of the disease. Other names that have been applied to this affection are: Sporadic aphthae, stomatitis vesiculosa, stomatitis aphthosa, erosive stomatitis, sore mouth, blue tongue, and pseudo foot-and-mouth disease.

Cause.—Vesicular stomatitis is caused by a virus that has been shown to pass through bacteria-retaining filters. The virus is contained in the contents of vesicles that develop in the course of the disease, in the epithelium covering them, and also in the blood during the febrile stage and for a short period afterward. It has not thus far been demonstrated to occur in the milk of cows except as a contaminant from vesicles, which sometimes form on the teats. The virus disappears from the mouth of the affected animals within a few days after the rupture of the vesicles.

Though little work has been done to determine the resistance of the virus to sunlight, drying, and disinfectants, indications are that it is rapidly destroyed by these means. However, fragments of the epithelial coverings of vesicles kept in a moist state either in 50-percent glycerin or without it, placed in test tubes, sealed with paraffin, and kept in the dark in the ice box, have been found in some instances to contain active virus at the end of a month.

Virus kept alive for several years, by successive passages through guinea pigs, still appeared to have lost little of its virulence. On the other hand, the disease often appears to die out in naturally infected herds without infecting more than a small proportion of the animals.

Plurality of types of virus.—In 1925 the Bureau of Animal Industry proved the existence in the United States of at least two types of vesicular stomatitis that appear to be indistinguishable clinically, just as three types of foot-and-mouth-disease virus have been found in Europe. The general characteristics of the two viruses of vesicular stomatitis seem to be the same, but one type of virus does not immunize against the other, although it does against itself. An animal recovering from one type might suffer from a fresh attack of the disease caused by the second type within a few weeks, whereas it would be immune to the first type for months and possibly years. Animals immune to either type of vesicular stomatitis have not been found to be immune to foot-and-mouth disease.

One of the two types of virus was found to be responsible for an outbreak of vesicular stomatitis in the Middle West early in 1925, another in New Jersey late in 1925, and a third outbreak in Alabama in 1929.

Symptoms and lesions.—The first phenomenon of vesicular stomatitis is an acute rise in temperature that is immediately followed by formation of reddened patches on the buccal mucosa, especially of the tongue. These are quickly succeeded by vesicles or blisters of grayish-red color only slightly elevated, from the size of a dime to that of a silver dollar, and filled with clear or yellowish serous fluid. These blisters may be isolated but frequently they coalesce to form a large vesicle. They usually rupture in a short time, which accounts for their not being recognized at times even in the early stages of the disease. With the rupture of the vesicles the temperature drops to normal within a few hours. The rupture of the vesicles also results in exposing the raw underlying surfaces, which appear as reddened erosions with the grayish-white fragments of the torn mucous membrane of the preexisting vesicles still attached to the irregular borders like a fringe. These erosions may become confluent, and vary from the size of a dime to that of the palm of the hand. Healing usually occurs rapidly in 8 to 15 days in uncomplicated cases.

In horses these lesions are principally confined to the upper surface of the tongue, but they may involve the inner surface of the lips, the angles of the mouth, and the gums. The susceptibility of horses to vesicular stomatitis is of importance to cattle owners, since the horse, as shown later, is one of the best test animals for differentiating vesicular stomatitis from foot-and-mouth disease.

In cattle, lesions may occur on the tongue, hard palate, lips, and gums, and sometimes extend to the muzzle and around the nostrils. In a few cases fresh cows have shown similar lesions on the teats when their infected calves have been sucking them. In one outbreak in which the disease seemed to be of unusual virulence and infected more than 30 herds, a large proportion of the cows in 3 dairy herds developed large vesicles on the teats, the virus evidently being carried on the hands of the milker from cow to cow. In none of the affected cows were vesicles observed on the udder proper.

A few cases in which foot lesions developed in cattle have been observed in the field. In nearly all these cases the lesions were confined to a single foot of the affected animal. The lesions consisted of a very large vesicle in the interdigital space, and extended over its entire area. Other vesicles appeared around the coronet. In some of the affected feet observed there was considerable separation of the horny from the deeper structures at the heels. The lesions of the feet were practically identical in appearance with those of foot-and-mouth disease, but, unlike them in the cases observed, were confined to one foot. Furthermore, only a small proportion of affected animals had lesions of the feet, whereas in foot-and-mouth disease the feet, as well as the mouth, usually become affected.

Immediately before or simultaneously with the appearance of the vesicles, the animal is usually depressed. After the vesicles rupture, a more or less profuse flow of saliva follows, which dribbles from the mouth and consists of a thin, stringy, or frothy fluid. Frequently salivation is the first indication that the animal is sick. Owing to the painful condition of the mouth at this stage, there is loss of appetite or at least inability to eat, and smacking noises are heard as in foot-and-mouth disease. This sensitiveness, as a rule, remains for several days, after which healing commences. The sick animals begin to eat very soon, even while their tongues are still eroded. Although eating well, they do not regain their original thrifty appearance for some time. In dairy cows, in addition to shrinkage in flesh there is a noticeable reduction in the normal flow of milk for a few days.

So far as observations of the writer are concerned, the period of incubation of vesicular stomatitis, after natural exposure, varied from 36 hours to 9 days, but the greatest number of cases occurred in 2 to 5 days after exposure. After inoculations, vesicles are seldom more than 48 hours in appearing, are usually present after 38 to 44 hours, and occasionally appear in 24 hours. The temperature begins to rise between the eighteenth and twenty-fourth hours and may reach 105° or even 107° F. in cattle. No losses have been reported from uncomplicated cases of this disease.

Contagiousness.—That the malady is contagious has been definitely shown by the transmission of the disease from sick to healthy animals by inoculation. The degree of contagiousness, however, varies between wide limits. Experiments have proved that the virus is most virulent at the time the blisters rupture or shortly thereafter, but when the lesions are 5 or 6 days old the virus of the disease has practically disappeared.

The virus is evidently of short life and is transmitted only by close contact. Probably the infected environment remains dangerous longer than the affected animals. Several instances have been reported in which a line fence or a board fence in a double corral has been sufficient to prevent transmission of the disease from the infected animals on one side to the healthy animals on the other.

Investigations indicate that the disease is seldom communicated by owners or caretakers of affected animals visiting other farms. As a rule the disease appears to spread by direct contact with recently affected animals or by recently infected feed troughs, water troughs, bridles, or pails. However, in one outbreak in which the virus seemed unusually virulent, the disease appeared to spread in some other way in addition to these, possibly by a person who visited infected herds and then handled susceptible cattle. In this outbreak, which lasted about a month, 33 herds, containing in all approximately 700 animals, became infected.

Differential diagnosis.—Although the disease has not the great economic importance of foot-and-mouth disease, it nevertheless is contagious and causes considerable alarm owing to its close resemblance to the dreaded European disease. As this infection in cattle may be readily confounded with foot-and-mouth disease, a prompt and exact differentiation is accompanied with numerous difficulties. These difficulties are best appreciated by those who have faced them with the consciousness that their pronouncements if mistaken would lead on one hand to unnecessary and serious economic disturbances and on the other hand to the spread of one of the most dreaded and easily communicated among animal plagues. Vesicular stomatitis, therefore, is a menace whenever and wherever it appears. For these reasons it is strongly urged that local quarantines to prevent its spread be imposed by State livestock officials in whose territory the disease may be found. All owners and handlers of horses, mules, and cattle, particularly liverymen, managers of stockyards, and stockmen, should be directed to separate sick from well animals, clean and disinfect contaminated premises, and have all infected animals appropriately treated.

The opinion that the malady is not foot-and-mouth disease is based on the fact that persistent observation of sick animals has failed to reveal certain typical symptoms that would be expected in an outbreak of foot-and-mouth disease. The drooling, vesicles, and erosions are similar in appearance to those produced by foot-and-mouth disease, but in only a small number of the animals examined in the field has there been found any soreness of the feet, which is a common symptom of foot-and-mouth disease. Moreover, many horses have this particular ailment, but horses have not been observed to contract foot-and-mouth disease in any of the foot-and-mouth outbreaks in the United States. Hundreds of hogs exposed to the disease and in association with the sick animals in pastures have shown no signs of the malady, which is regarded as significant, because in the 1914 outbreak of foot-and-mouth disease hogs were as susceptible to that disease as were cattle. Exposed sheep also failed to show vesicular stomatitis, yet these cloven-footed animals are susceptible to foot-and-mouth infection. In a number of cases of vesicular stomatitis the lesions appeared to be continuous or progressive, and not explosive, as in foot-and-mouth disease. In these instances, secondary lesions were apparent, on a number of consecutive days, in the mouths of both horses and cattle, and vesicles were observed on the bases of tongues, the free portions of which were almost denuded of mucous membrane as a result of the rupture of similar vesicles 6 or 7 days before.

Complications are extremely rare in vesicular stomatitis, and neither mammitis nor chronic diseases of the hoof have been observed following it. Suckling calves are seldom affected with the disease, and rarely in other than a mild form, whereas an attack of foot-and-mouth diseases in calves is always serious and frequently fatal. The vesicles in foot-and-mouth disease, as a rule are larger than in vesicular stomatitis and are more tightly filled with serious fluid.

The percentage of animals infected in herds of cattle and the history of exposure without transmission of the disease except by immediate contact, indicate that this ailment is not the highly contagious foot-and-mouth disease that, once it is introduced into a herd, quickly affects practically 100 percent of the cattle and hogs on all the farms to which the virus may be carried.

The result of this study of vesicular stomatitis suggests the necessity of inoculating horses with suspected material in any future outbreak of disease bearing a resemblance to foot-and-mouth disease.

Finally, it must be apparent that vesicular stomatitis more closely resembles foot-and-mouth disease than either mycotic or necrotic stomatitis, and that a reliable differential diagnosis can be made only after inoculation experiments and careful observation lasting a number of days.

In mycotic stomatitis portions of the lining membrane of the mouth become inflamed, and in a few days it changes to a croupous membrane that peels off and leaves a raw surface, while the thin skin between the toes may also be inflamed. Swelling of the feet and stiffness of the animal are frequently evident in mycotic stomatitis. The previous history of the case, the absence of its spread to horses exposed to the infection, and the complete negative results obtained by the inoculation of calves, distinguish this disease from vesicular stomatitis. Lastly, mycotic stomatitis occurs in only 10 to 15 percent of the cattle in a herd, usually late in the summer or early in the fall after a dry spell, and it does not run a regular course.

Necrotic stomatitis may be distinguished from vesicular stomatitis by the fact that although it affects cattle, especially calves, it may also involve pigs and sheep, but its spread among the animals of a herd shows a much lower degree of infectiousness than vesicular stomatitis. In necrotic stomatitis blisters are never formed, destruction of the tissues occurring from the beginning and being followed by the formation of yellowish, cheesy patches principally involving the lining membrane of the mouth, especially the tongue and cheeks, or in other cases the lining of the larnyx. The cause is *Actinomyces necrophorus* (*Bacillus necrophorus*).

Another vesicular disease called vesicular exanthema of swine, which has occurred in California in garbage-fed hogs since 1932, is very similar in its manifestations to vesicular stomatitis and foot-and-mouth disease. The disease cannot be transmitted to cattle or guinea pigs by inoculation or natural exposure but some strains of the virus can produce symptoms and lesions in horses by inoculation although they are but slightly similar to those of vesicular stomatitis.

Treatment.—The treatment of vesicular stomatitis consists in first removing affected animals from healthy ones and isolating the former until fully recovered. Such isolation, together with the adoption of rigid sanitary precautions, greatly reduces the prevalence of the disease. Medicinal treatment or undue handling of the affected parts should not be attempted until after the true nature of the disease has been determined, as the lesions may be so mutilated as to make diagnosis difficult. Animals affected with vesicular stomatitis should not be fed hay for the first few days, but instead bran or other soft feed should be given. If the animals are treated in this manner, the disease should rapidly disappear.

MALIGNANT CATARRH

Malignant catarrh, or infectious catarrhal fever, is an acute, infectious disease of cattle involving mainly the respiratory and digestive tracts, although the sinuses of the head, eyes, and the urinary and sexual organs are frequently affected. Through researches originating in Germany, the cause of the disease has been proved to be a filtrable virus. It is relative rare in the United States, being more common on the continent of Europe. Outbreaks occur, however, from time to time in this country. The disease appears to be most common in stables with damp floors, low ceilings, poor ventilation, and insanitary conditions in general. Usually only a few animals on a given farm develop the disease at one time, but once the disease has made its appearance it is likely to reappear every year or so, over long periods. One European veterinarian reports an instance in which the disease remained for 25 years on the same farm and attacked 225 animals, the mortality being about 98 percent.

The disease is most common in late winter and early spring, at all altitudes, and has a special preference for young, well-nourished cattle, although older animals are not immune. In natural cases, the incubation period—the time between the entrance of the infective agent into the body of the animal and the appearance of the first symptoms—is probably about 20 to 30 days. Fortunately, it does not spread to any great extent or cause severe losses; hence, legislative enactments for its restriction have not been adopted.

Symptoms.—These are extremely variable, according to the point of localization of the lesions. The disease is usually ushered in with a chill, followed by a marked rise of temperature (104° to 107° F.) The head droops, the skin is hot and dry, and the coat staring. Quivering of the muscles in various parts of the body is frequently observed. Marked dullness of the animal, passing, according to some observers, into an almost stupefied condition later on, is common. The secretion of milk stops in the beginning of the disease, and loss of flesh, invariably associated with the disease, is extremely marked and rapid. The lesions of the eyes may best be likened to moon blindness (periodic ophthalmia) in horses.

There is first an abundant secretion of tears, which run down the face. The lids are swollen and inflamed, and this condition may be so marked as to cause involuntary eversion, exposing the reddened conjunctiva to view. Sunlight causes pain, as is shown by the fact that the animal keeps its eyes continuously closed. This inflammation may extend to the cornea, causing it to assume a slightly clouded appearance in mild cases or a chalky whiteness in more severe affections. Cases of ulceration of the cornea followed by perforation and subsequent escape of the aqueous humor, leading to shrinking of the eyeball and permanent loss of sight, have been recorded, but these are relatively rare, although slight inflammation of the deeper structures of the eye (iris) are more frequent. In mild cases this inflammation may undergo complete resolution, but more frequently permanent cloudiness of the cornea, either diffuse or in spots (leucoma), is the result. The mucous membranes of the mouth, nose, sinuses of the head, throat, and lower respiratory passages are also involved. It is first catarrhal in character, but soon a false or diphtheritic membrane is formed, with the production of shallow ulcers. There is dribbling of saliva from the mouth and discharge from the nose, at first watery, then becoming thicker and mixed with blood and small masses of cast-off croupous membrane, emitting a very fetid odor. These croupous areas when they form in the throat, larynx, or windpipe may lead to narrowing of the passages, with consequent difficult breathing and even suffocation. Various respiratory murmurs may also be heard, caused by the movement of mucus and inflammatory deposits to and fro along the air passages. There is also inflammation of the sinuses and horn core with consequent loosening of the horn shell, and the horns are thus readily knocked off by the uneasy, blind sufferer.

The animal may refuse all feed from the time of the initial rise of temperature. In less severe cases, especially when the lesions of the digestive tract are not so marked, the appetite may remain until the disease is well advanced. Constipation is common at the commencement of the attack, followed by diarrhea and severe straining, the evacuations becoming very soft, fetid, and sometimes streaked with blood. Cases of the evacuation of desquamated patches of diphtheritic membrane from the intestinal mucosa 6 to 9 feet in length have been reported. The kidneys and bladder are usually inflamed, the urine being voided with difficulty and the animal evincing signs of pain. Inflammatory elements, as albumin and casts, may be found on examination of the urine. In cows the mucous membrane of the vagina or vestibule is congested, swollen, and may contain ulcers and an excessive quantity of mucus. Abortion during advanced pregnancy is not infrequent, following a severe attack. In connection with these various symptoms there may be much uneasiness on the part of the animal, leading in some cases to madness and furious delirium; in others, to spasms and convulsions or paralysis, thus simulating encephalitis, rabies, pseudorabies, and similar diseases. A vesicular eruption of the skin may occur, seen principally between the toes and on the inside of the flank and in the armpits, with subsequent loss of hair and epidermis.

Like other infectious diseases, malignant catarrh pursues a longer or shorter course in accordance with the severity of the attack. In acute cases death may take place 3 to 7 days after the appearance of symptoms. Recovery, if it occurs, may take 3 or 4 weeks. According to statistics, from 50 to 90 percent of the affected animals die.

If animals that have died of this disease are examined, in addition to the changes in the mucous membrane of the mouth and nasal cavities referred to previously, shallow ulcers in these situations will be found occasionally. These necrotic processes may pass beneath the mucous membrane and even involve the underlying bony structure. In severe cases membranous (croupous) deposits are found in the throat. Similar deposits have been found on the mucous membrane of the fourth stomach and intestine. There is more or less inflammation of the membranes of the brain, kidneys, and liver, and some degeneration of the muscles. In countries where rinderpest appears, it may be difficult to distinguish between it and malignant catarrh, owing to a general similarity of the symptoms. The principal points to be observed in differentiating between the two are the irregular transmissibility of the latter as compared with the intense contagiousness of the former, and the tendency of malignant catarrh to run a more chronic course than rinderpest, which usually results fatally in a few days. As a result of quarantine and the vigilance of veterinarians, rinderpest does not exist in the United States.

Treatment.—There is no specific treatment for this affection. Therefore, all that can be done is to attempt to improve the animal's condition by treating each symptom according to its nature. Antiseptic washes applied to the eyes, nose, and mouth, with ice poultices over the crest of the head and frontal region, may be helpful symptomatic treatments. Intestinal and respiratory symptoms are handled according to the necessity in each case. General stimulants may be beneficial. There is much greater success in preventive measures than in attempted treatment. The former consists in the removal of the healthy from the infected animals (not vice versa) and thorough cleaning and disinfection of the contaminated stables. If these measures are thoroughly and carefully carried out, the contagion should be destroyed and the danger of the reappearance of the disease in a great measure lessened. Severely affected animals might best be killed, according to the discretion of the attending veterinarian. The carcasses should be destroyed by burning or burial in quicklime.

MALIGNANT EDEMA

Malignant edema, also termed "gangrenous septicemia," is an acute, inflammatory disease of domestic and wild animals and man, resulting from the introduction of a specific organism, *Clostridium septicum*, into the deep connective tissues of a susceptible animal and proving fatal in many instances within 24 to 48 hours. The disease may be inoculated from one animal to another but only by inserting the virus deeply below the skin. It is seldom met with in cattle as an uncomplicated disease but may develop following contamination of accidental or surgical wounds. Malignant edema sometimes follows the use of hypodermic syringes and needles by careless or untrained persons.

Clostridium septicum, like other clostridia (spore-bearing organisms that grow in the absence of air), are sometimes present in the lesions of blackleg, and some cases diagnosed clinically as blackleg have been found, on laboratory examination, to be malignant edema. Blackleg bacterin, according to the regulations of the United States Department of Agriculture, must be prepared from pure cultures of *Cl. chauvoei*, the cause of uncomplicated blackleg, but biologics prepared from mixtures of cultures of *Cl. chauvoei*, *Cl. septicum*, and other clostridia are sometimes prepared for use in connection with infections due to the several organisms.

Unlike the germs that cause anthrax and blackleg, which are confined to certain districts, the germ of malignant edema is widely distributed and is generally present in soil and in the intestinal tract of Herbivora. The introduction of the germ into minor superficial wounds rarely does any harm, but if the organism reaches the deeper tissues excluded from the air, it develops quickly, forming a soluble toxin, or poison, which is the fatal agent.

Symptoms.—Usually the first symptoms are overlooked. In the early stages the animal appears listless, disinclined to move about, and lies down in shady and quiet places. If the animal is forced to move about, the hind legs are drawn forward with a peculiar, stiff, dragging movement, and there may be slight muscular trembling over all the body, which becomes more intense as the disease progresses. When driven, the animal shows signs of fatigue, ultimately dropping to the ground completely exhausted. Breathing becomes fast and painful, with frequent spasmodic jerks.

The pulse is quick and weak and the temperature is 106° to 107° F. An edematous, doughy, and painful swelling appears at the point of infection. This tumefaction spreads more and more and crackles on pressure. In case of an open wound, a fetid liquid and frothy discharge is observed. The center of the swelling may appear soft and jellylike, and the margin is tense, hot, and painful. The symptoms increase rapidly, resulting in coma and death.

Lesions.—After death, the fat and subcutaneous tissues surrounding the infected area are infiltrated with a gelatinous material containing foam, due to the presence of gas bubbles. The muscles at this point are darkly discolored, friable, spongy, dissociated by gas, and with a blood-tinged exudate. A peculiar characteristic odor is present. The intestines are generally normal, but, together with the peritoneum, they may be inflamed, and the lungs are often the seat of edema. The spleen, liver, and kidneys usually retain their normal appearance, in marked contrast with anthrax.

Differential diagnosis.—Unlike blackleg, this disease rarely appears as an epizootic but in isolated cases. It may also be differentiated from the former by the history of a recent parturition or surgical operation, by the presence of an external injury at the site of the swelling accompanied with a fetid liquid discharge, and the gangrenous appearance of the tumefaction. Man is susceptible to malignant edema but not to blackleg. Malignant edema may also be differentiated from anthrax in that the blood and spleen are generally normal in appearance, whereas in the latter disease the blood is usually dark and tarlike, and the spleen appears swollen, injected, and softened. The local tumor in malignant edema contains gas bubbles, which are absent in anthrax swellings. Inoculation experiments with guinea pigs, rabbits, and chickens also disclose the differences among the above-mentioned three diseases, since all these species are killed by the germ of malignant edema, only the first two species by the anthrax bacillus, and the guinea pig alone by the blackleg infection. Finally, bacteriological cultures also serve to differentiate the three diseases.

Treatment.—Treatment of this disease is rarely successful in animals. Free incision and drainage of the swellings and treatment with antiseptic solutions may be tried. In some cases a specific serum, prepared chiefly for use against the disease in man, may be a practical treatment. Usually the disease, when observed, has advanced to such an extent that medicinal aid is without avail. Preventive treatment is by far the most desirable and consists, essentially, in a thorough disinfection of all accidental wounds, the cleansing of the skin, sterilization of all instruments, and the exclusion of soil, filth, and bacteria during surgical operations of any nature. Sheds, barns, and stables should receive a thorough cleaning and disinfection after all litter and rubbish have been removed and burned. All dead animals should be burned or deeply buried after covering well with quicklime.

TICK FEVER (CATTLE TICK FEVER, SPLENETIC FEVER, PIROPLASMOSIS)

(Pls. XLIV–L)

Tick fever, or piroplasmosis (commonly known in the United States as Texas fever) is an infectious, febrile disease caused by various species of a genus of one-celled (protozoan) organisms called *Babesia* by Starcovici (1893) in honor of Babes, who in 1888 described the organisms, which he discovered in the blood of cattle dying of hemoglobinuric fever. In the United States and other parts of the Western Hemisphere two species of the genus, namely, *Babesia bigemina* (*Piroplasma bigeminum*) and *Babesia argentina* (*Piroplasma argentinum*) are responsible for this disease. These organisms were described and figured by Smith and Kilborne in their epoch-making publication on tick fever in 1893, but the parasites were not then recognized as separate species.

History.—The minute animal parasites that are the cause of the disease were first seen in the red blood cells as early as 1869. The general idea was entertained by farmers and stockmen for many years that southern cattle, even though apparently in good health, were able to (bring about) transmit disease to northern cattle with which they came in contact or which occupied premises previously occupied by southern cattle. There was also a widespread belief that the ticks harbored by the southern cattle were responsible in some way for the disease in the northern cattle.

The earliest account of this disease in the United States dates back to 1814, when it was stated by James Pease, before the Philadelphia Society for Promoting Agriculture, that the cattle from a certain district in South Carolina so certainly produced disease in all others with which they came in contact in their progress to the North that they were prohibited by the people of Virginia from passing through the State; that these cattle infected others while they themselves remained in perfect health; and that cattle from Europe or the interior taken to the vicinity of the coast area of the Southern States were attacked by a disease that generally proved fatal. Similar observations had also been made in regard to other districts in the southern part of the United States.

The facts that supported the supposition that cattle ticks were in some way concerned with the spread of tick fever finally became so numerous and convincing that the Bureau of Animal Industry inaugurated a series of experiments to determine the cause of the disease and the exact role of the tick in its transmission. According to Cooper Curtice (1889), the experiment of allowing native cattle to live on the trail of Texas cattle had been repeated a number of times and always with the same result—namely, the native, or nonimmune, animals invariably became sick and a large percentage of them died. However, these experiments, although strongly suggesting that the ticks infesting the southern cattle were in some way connected with the illness later developing in the native animals, did not prove the point. Curtice, however, appears to have been so strongly convinced that the ticks were responsible for causing the disease that he suggested a series of experiments to determine the truth or falsity of his ideas. The experiment, which was made by Kilborne in 1889, consisted in placing a group of northern cattle with a group of cattle from North Carolina after all ticks had been removed from the latter and in placing a second group of northern cattle with a group of

North Carolina cattle on which the ticks were left. The first group of northern cattle remained healthy but the second group died of what was then called Texas or southern-cattle fever. The result of this experiment indicated that ticks were an essential factor in producing the disease. About this time Cooper Curtice made a careful study of the life history of the cattle tick which greatly contributed to settling the question of the part that this tick played as the transmitter of tick fever and also laid the foundation for the tick-eradication project that was to follow.

In 1889, the report of the Chief of the Bureau of Animal Industry records the finding by Theobald Smith of peculiar bodies in the red corpuscles of cattle suffering from southern-cattle fever. These bodies, identified by Smith as Protozoa, were associated with the destruction of the blood corpuscles and were named by Smith and Kilborne *Pyrosoma bigeminum.*

Symptoms and post mortem appearance.—Animals suffering from tick fever have high fever, increased respiration, rapid pulse, anemia manifested by paleness of the visible mucous membranes, dullness. loss of appetite, atony of the rumen, constipation, decrease and sometimes cessation of milk flow, and hemoglobinuria or bloody urine. The last symptom manifests itself in severe cases near the termination of the disease.

Post mortem examination shows enlargement of the spleen. On incision of this organ, its contents have the appearance of a dark blackberry jam. In some cases they may even be fluid and appear as a dark red, almost black, fluid mass. The liver is swollen and icteric or yellowish in appearance. When it is incised this yellow color, which is due to the large quantity of bile present, is even more noticeable. The gall bladder is distended with bile, which holds in suspension a large quantity of yellow flakes. When the gall bladder is opened the contents have what is commonly called a coffee-grounds appearance. The carcass is usually emaciated and the blood thin and watery. The kidneys are congested, and the urine in the bladder varies in color from a light claret to a deep port wine. The heart usually shows a number of ecchymotic hemorrhages (patches of blood extravasation).

Diagnosis.—The diagnosis of tick fever is based on clinical symptoms in the presence of cattle-fever ticks and the demonstration of the causative organism in the red blood cells.

Clinically and on post mortem examination tick fever caused by *Babesia bigemina* and that caused by *B. argentina* can hardly be differentiated, and examination of the organisms found in the red blood cells will be necessary in making a definite diagnosis. The disease must also be differentiated from anaplasmosis, which resembles tick fever in its clinical symptoms and post mortem lesions. In cattle tick-infested areas the period of incubation, the temperature, the yellow discoloration of the visible mucous membranes and unpigmented parts of the skin, also referred to as icterus and jaundice, will aid in differentiating these diseases. In tick fever, or piroplasmosis, the period of incubation, that is, the time elapsing between the exposure of the animal to tick infestation and the appearance of symptoms of disease, is usually 7 to 12 days, whereas in anaplasmosis it is usually 30 to 40 days. As a rule, the temperature in cases of piroplasmosis exceeds that in anaplasmosis. Jaundice is more common in anaplasmosis than in piroplasmosis. In areas that have been freed from the cattle-fever tick, any animal showing the above-mentioned symptoms does not have piroplasmosis since this disease does not occur in the absence of the cattle-fever tick. In cattle tick-infested areas, severe and rapidly fatal cases of tick fever may be confused with cases of anthrax at necropsy because in both diseases the spleen is enlarged. An examination of the blood for piroplasms and of the blood and tissues for *Bacillus anthracis* should aid in the differentiation of these two diseases.

Life history of ticks.—In the United States tick fever, or piroplasmosis, is transmitted only through the cattle-fever ticks, *Boophilus annulatus* and *B. annulatus* var. *microplus* (-*Boophilus annulatus* var. *australis*). The males of these two ticks can be differentiated by the presence of a small spine on the posterior margin of the body of *B. annulatus* var. *microplus*. The ticks are blood suckers, and when they engorge on cattle suffering from tick fever they ingest the piroplasms. These organisms enter the eggs of the tick and are passed through the eggs to the larvae or seed ticks of the next generation. The tick-fever organisms become lodged in the salivary glands of the larval ticks, which attach themselves to susceptible cattle and thereby transmit the disease organisms. The organisms multiply in the blood of susceptible cattle and after a suitable period, a case of tick fever develops.

The cattle tick has four stages in its life history—namely, the egg, larva, nymph, and adult. The adult female tick, when fully engorged, releases its hold on the host, drops to the ground and immediately begins to search for a hiding place that may serve as a protection from unfavorable conditions and enemies. Egg laying may begin in 2 to 3 days or may be delayed for several weeks, depending on external conditions. In warm weather the preoviposition period (period elapsing before egg laying begins) is usually short, whereas in the fall and winter this period is usually prolonged. The eggs are small, about one-fiftieth of an inch long, elliptical, and at first of a light amber color, which later changes to a dark brown. They are

77431 O—51——31

coated with a sticky secretion, which causes them to adhere in clusters and keeps them from drying out. The eggs must undergo a period of incubation before they are ready to hatch. This period varies with the temperature, being as short as 19 days in summer and as long as 200 days in fall or winter. The six-legged larvae or seed ticks, hatching from the eggs, remain more or less quiet for a few days, after which they become very active if the weather is warm and ascend the nearest vegetation. The seed ticks take no food, do not increase in size, and unless they reach hosts on which to live as parasites they die of starvation. They are, however, able to live without food for several months.

After reaching a favorable host, such as a cow, the seed ticks attach themselves to those parts of the body where the skin is soft and pliable, and the hair scanty, namely, the escutcheon, inside of thighs, and dewlap. They begin to suck blood, and in 5 to 12 days after attachment they undergo their first molt. The ticks emerging from this molt are known as nymphs. They have eight legs but are still sexually undifferentiated. The nymphs again begin to suck blood and in from 5 to 11 days undergo the second molt, from which they emerge as males and females. The males are active, moving about on the skin of the host. The females never show much activity, seldom moving far from their original point of attachment. After mating, the females increase rapidly in size, about 10 to 25 days being required for their complete engorgement. After engorgement, the females drop from the host and begin the cycle over again. It is clear from the life history of the cattle ticks that the engorged female tick, the egg, and the seed tick occur on the pasture and that the seed tick, nymph, and unengorged adult occur on cattle. Measures for the eradication of the ticks and, therefore, for the control of tick fever, may be directed either to the pasture or the cattle or both.

Dr. Cooper Curtice (1892) appears to have been the first person to suggest that in order to combat tick fever the cattle should be freed from ticks as far as possible and to express the belief that this would so free the pastures that what at first would seem a formidable task would grow easier and easier. In 1896 he urged tick eradication over the State of Virginia and other infested States. In 1899, he inaugurated a tick-eradication campaign in North Carolina, which was continued by Tait Butler, and in 1906 when the Federal Government began its tick-eradication campaign, 20 counties in North Carolina had been freed from cattle ticks.

Prevention.—If southern cattle are entirely free from the species of tick known as *Boophilus annulatus* and *B. annulatus* var. *microplus* they may be allowed to mingle with the most susceptible animals without danger. Furthermore, these ticks infest pastures only transiently, never permanently, and usually mature on cattle or equines. Their extermination is possible, and the disease they cause may thus be prevented. Therefore, the various methods of prevention and elimination should be directed toward the destruction of ticks on cattle as well as their eradication from the pastures.[1] In freezing pastures of ticks, the method followed may be either a direct or an indirect one. The former consists in excluding all cattle, horses, and mules from pastures until all the ticks have died from starvation. The latter consists in permitting the cattle and other animals to continue on the infested pasture and treating them at regular intervals with agents destructive to ticks and thus preventing engorged females from dropping and reinfesting the pasture. The larvae on the pasture, or those that hatch from eggs laid by females already there, will eventually die. Such of these as get on the cattle from time to time will be destroyed by the treatment, and those that fail to find a host will starve in the pasture.

Animals may be freed of ticks in two ways. They may be treated with an agent that will destroy all the ticks present, or they may be rotated at proper intervals on tick-free fields until all the ticks have dropped. The method most generally used is dipping the cattle in a solution of arsenic. The pasture-rotation method is not only more complicated, but the necessary tick-free fields are seldom available.

Value of dipping.—The dipping vat is the best and cheapest means of applying the tick-destroying solution. The great advantage of dipping over spraying and applying remedies by hand lies in the fact that thoroughness of the treatment is practically assured.

When eradication is undertaken, all the cattle, and also the horses and mules if they harbor ticks, are treated regularly every 2 weeks until the ticks have disappeared. The purpose of the treatment is to destroy all ticks that get on the animals before they have had a chance to mature and drop, thus preventing them from reinfesting the pasture, farm, or range. If the treatment used were absolutely effective in destroying every tick on the animals treated there would be no renewal of the infestation after the treatment is begun. The cattle would act simply as collectors of ticks, which would be destroyed regularly by the treatment applied every 2 weeks. However, in most instances, either because of the lack of efficiency of the dip or imperfect application, or because of failure to dip all cattle systematically, some ticks escape treatment and reproduce, thus prolonging the time that otherwise would be required for eradication.

[1] Only a general outline of methods of eradication are given here. For detailed information, including directions for the construction of dipping vats and for the preparation of dips, the reader is referred to Farmers' Bulletin 1057, which may be obtained free on application to the Department of Agriculture, Washington, D. C.

If ticks apparently disappear from the cattle after they have been under treatment for some time, the dipping should not be discontinued until a number of careful inspections show that the cattle are free of ticks. If ticks continue on cattle until cold weather and then finally disappear, in all probability eradication has not been accomplished and there may be engorged females, unhatched eggs, and inactive seed ticks on the farm or range. Even if the cattle should remain free of ticks during the winter they may become reinfested the following spring. In any case in which ticks disappear from the cattle and treatment is discontinued, the cattle should be watched carefully for ticks until ample time has elapsed to leave no doubt that eradication has been accomplished.

As a general rule, if dipping is begun in March and systematically and thoroughly done, all cattle being dipped every 14 days until November, complete eradication will be obtained. In dipping, each animal should be completely covered by the dip. To prevent any animals from going through the vat without becoming wet all over, a man provided with a forked stick should be stationed at the middle of the vat to shove under those that had not been completely submerged.

Dipping is the most satisfactory method of treating animals for ticks. In cases of emergency, however, or where there are not cattle enough within a radius of several miles to warrant the construction of a vat in which all the cattle of the community may be dipped, spraying may be advisable. In spraying animals the work should be done with great thoroughness and every portion of the body treated. An animal cannot be sprayed properly unless it is tied or otherwise held, nor can good results be obtained unless the hair and skin are thoroughly wet.

Arsenical dips.—Many substances and preparations have been experimented with in an effort to find a practical and satisfactory application that will destroy the tick and not injure the cattle. The arsenical cattle dip best meets these requirements and is now the dipping bath generally used in the treatment of cattle for the removal of ticks. Proprietary brands of arsenical dips are readily available, or the arsenical cattle dip may be prepared as a home-made product from the raw materials, as explained in Farmers' Bulletin 1057.

Treatment.—When tick fever has broken out, all animals, the sick as well as the healthy, should be freed from ticks immediately and removed to a noninfested pasture. Although this may not check the disease, it may save the lives of some animals by removing them from the possibility of attack by more young ticks. Removal from infested pastures likewise prevents a second attack, which is caused by another generation of ticks. It is important to remove all ticks from sick animals, since they abstract a considerable quantity of blood and thereby retard final recovery.

In the United States the medicinal treatment of tick fever has received little attention. The efforts of the Bureau of Animal Industry and State livestock sanitary officials have been directed toward the elimination of tick fever by the eradication of the ticks, which serve as definitive hosts and transmitters of the tick-fever organisms.

As tick fever is caused by protozoan organisms within the red blood cells and as in that respect it closely resembles malaria, formerly there was a tendency to regard the disease as animal malaria. It was, therefore, natural that quinine should have been recommended for its treatment. It was not until Nuttall and Hadwen (1909) demonstrated that tick fever of dogs caused by *Babesia canis* was favorably influenced by treatment with trypan blue, that a specific drug treatment for tick fever caused by one species of *Babesia* became available. In the tick-quarantine area, as well as in other parts of the world in which tick fever occurred, the treatment with trypan blue met with indifferent success. In many cases the results were all that could be expected; in many other cases the treatment had no influence whatever on the course of the disease. These contradictory results were disappointing and mystifying. The mystery was cleared up when it was discovered that tick fever as originally described by Smith and Kilborne was in reality a mixture of piroplasmosis and anaplasmosis, and that in some instances more than one type of *Babesia* was involved, only one of which, *B. bigemina*, was affected by the trypan blue treatment. The other disadvantages of trypan blue are that it must be injected intravenously, it stains the tissues, and the flesh of animals treated with this drug retains the stain for a long time after the treatment has been compleed. Another drug that has been reported to have been used apparently with considerable success is trypaflavin. According to Hörlein this drug has a larger field of action than trypan blue and a more intensive action on the individual types of causal organisms. It is as effective as trypan blue and causes only a slight staining of the flesh. It must, however, be injected intravenously. Other preparations have been used in various countries and the reports of their efficacy vary; none of them are completely satisfactory.

About 1935 Schönhöfer and Heneaka introduced a new synthetic drug for the treatment of piroplasmosis. This drug has the trade name of acaprin and chemically is a urea compound of the quinoline series known as N–N[1] (Bismethylchinolylium-methylsulfate-6-urea). According to reports from various parts of the world, this drug is effective in the treatment of tick fever or piroplasmosis regardless of the species of *Babesia* responsible for the disease. The drug is dispensed in both solid and liquid forms. The solid form known by the trade name of aciron consists of tablets containing 0.25 gram of the drug and the dose is one or two tablets dissolved in 5 to 10 cc. of water. The liquid form, called acaprin is prepared and dispensed in sterile ampoules each containing 6 cc. of a 5-percent solution of the drug. The dose is 1 ampoule. The drug can be administered subcutaneously or intramuscularly. It is colorless and does not stain the flesh. Treatment should be instituted as soon as the disease is suspected. If the first dose does not reduce the fever sufficiently, a second dose may be given 24 hours later. Muscular tremors, salivation, and other evidence of toxic effects of the drug may occur occasionally and have been described, but these do not appear to be serious.

QUARANTINE REGULATIONS

The sanitary regulations issued by the United States Department of Agriculture and the States containing ticky areas for the control of cattle shipments from the infested districts have for their initial purpose the prevention of the transportation of ticks from such districts to those that are not infested, either on cattle or in stock cars or other conveyor. They are based on the fact that tick fever is carried only by the cattle tick, and the exclusion of this parasite from the noninfested territory has in every instance been found to be a certain method of excluding the fever. The regulations governing the movement of cattle from the quarantined area are made by the Secretary of Agriculture. These regulations define the boundary of infested districts, which are shown in maps issued periodically.

In consequence of the enforcement of these quarantine regulations, tick fever has been practically prevented in the noninfested districts for several years, and little hardship has been caused to stockmen handling cattle from infested districts. Prior to the adoption of these regulations the tick-infested area was rapidly extending northward, but since the quarantine line was established and systematic eradication methods enforced, the quarantined area has been gradually reduced and now embraces less than 1 percent of the area infested in 1906.

BENEFITS OBTAINED FROM TICK ERADICATION

Systematic cooperative work by the Federal Government and the affected States for the eradication of cattle ticks that transmit tick fever was begun in the summer of 1906 under authority given by Congress in the act making appropriations for the Department of Agriculture for the fiscal year ended June 30, 1907. Funds have been provided for this project in succeeding Department appropriation acts. Liberal appropriations have also been made for this work by the States and counties concerned.

The eradication work thus provided for has resulted in the freeing from ticks and release from quarantine of a large part of the territory originally infested and has paved the way for a profitable cattle industry in those areas.

Great improvement has resulted from this work in the released territory. More cattle are being raised, and a better grade of breeding stock is being introduced; calves grow faster, and cattle put on flesh more rapidly during the grazing season and go into the winter in better condition because of the absence of the ticks; they can be marketed without quarantine restrictions, and higher prices are being obtained; dairy cows give a larger yield of milk; and values of farm lands are enhanced.

The difference between the prices realized for cattle from the tick-infested region and the prices of cattle of similar grades from outside the quarantine area has ranged from $2.25 to $5 a head at the principal northern livestock markets, without taking into account the improvement in quality and weight of cattle because of the eradication of the ticks. The extermination of the ticks means a large total annual increase in the prices obtained for southern cattle sold in northern markets. In addition to this, the increase in prices of cattle sold locally in the South represents a large sum. This local increase has amounted to $3 to $15 a head in territory freed from ticks. An agricultural official of one of the southern States has reported that calves in the tick-free area bring double the prices that can be obtained for similar calves in the tick-infested region.

Heretofore it has been impracticable to improve the quality of southern cattle by introducing fine breeding animals from other sections, because such animals were likely to contract tick fever and die unless protected by inoculation. Furthermore, it is impossible for animals to attain good growth and to thrive when they are heavily infested with ticks. With the eradication of the ticks, however, the southern farmers are enabled to introduce good breeding animals and to improve the grade of their stock.

TICK FEVER (CATTLE TICK FEVER, SPLENETIC FEVER, PIROPLASMOSIS)

DESCRIPTION OF PLATES

PLATE XLIV. Normal spleen and spleen affected by tick fever.

Figure 1. Spleen of an acute, fatal case of tick fever. The narrow end of the spleen is here represented.

Figure 2. Spleen of healthy steer. Though the latter animal weighed one-half more than the former, the weight of the diseased spleen (6⅞ pounds) was nearly three times that of the healthy spleen (2⅜ pounds).

PLATE XLV. Tick fever.

Figure 1. The cut surface of a healthy liver taken from a steer slaughtered for beef.

Figure 2. The cut surface of the liver in tick fever.

Figure 3. Appearance of the urine in an acute, fatal case of tick fever.

Figure 4. Red corpuscles, magnified 1,000 diameters, containing the parasite of anaplasmosis; compare with figure 5. This parasite appears as a blue point *a* near the edge of the corpuscle. The blood was taken from a skin incision. The case was nonfatal and occurred late in the fall.

Figure 5. Red corpuscles from the blood of an acute, fatal case of tick fever, 20 hours before death. The tick fever organisms *a* are shown as pear-shaped bodies, stained with methylene blue, within the red corpuscles. The larger body on the right, *b*, is a white blood corpuscle, also stained with methylene blue. (Magnified 1,000 diameters.)

PLATE XLVI. The cattle tick (*Boophilus annulatus*), the carrier of tick fever.

Figure 1. A series of ticks, natural size, from the smallest, just hatched from the egg, to the mature female, ready to drop off and lay eggs.

Figure 2. Eggs, magnified 5 times.

Figure 3. The young tick just hatched (magnified 40 times).

Figure 4. The male after the last molt (magnified 10 times).

Figure 5. The female after the last molt (magnified 10 times).

Figure 6. A portion of the skin of the udder, showing the small ticks. From a fatal case of tick fever produced by placing young ticks on the animal. (Natural size.)

Figure 7. A portion of the ear of the same animal, showing same full-grown ticks ready to drop off. (Natural size.)

PLATE XLVII. The cattle tick (*Boophilus annulatus*).

Figure 1. Dorsal view of male. (Greatly enlarged. Original.)

Figure 2. Ventral view of male. (Greatly enlarged. Original.)

Figure 3. Dorsal view of replete female. (Greatly enlarged. Original.)

Figure 4. Ventral view of female.

PLATE XLVIII. Portion of a steer's hide, showing the fever tick (*Boophilus annulatus*). (Natural size. Original.)

PLATE XLIX. Figure 1. Tick-infested steer.

Figure 2. Dipping cattle to kill ticks.

PLATE L. Facsimile of poster used to show the difference between cattle of similar breeding raised on a tick-free farm in one case and on a ticky farm in the other.

ANAPLASMOSIS

Anaplasmosis is a serious infectious, protozoan disease of cattle. When properly prepared and stained, a varying number of the red blood cells of cattle suffering from this disease show on the margin or in the center of the cells small, deeply stained bodies. These bodies, generally considered the causative agent, are called *Anaplasma marginale* if they are predominantly located on the margins of the red blood cells and *A. centrale* if they are predominantly located in the centers of these cells.

Transmission.—The cattle fever tick, *Boophilus annulatus*, or *B. annulatus* var. *microplus*, is known to serve as a carrier and transmit-

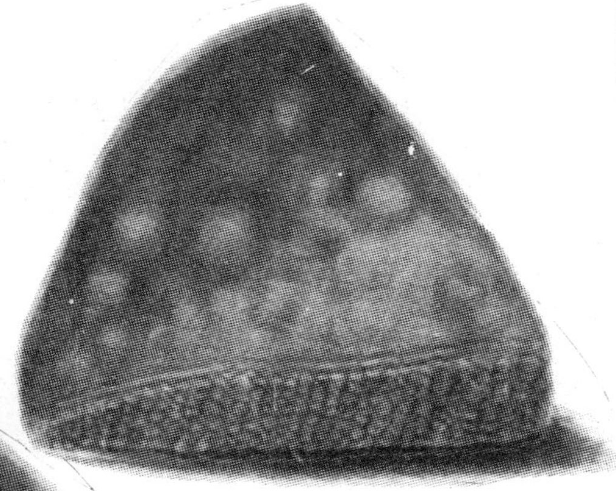

FIGURE 2

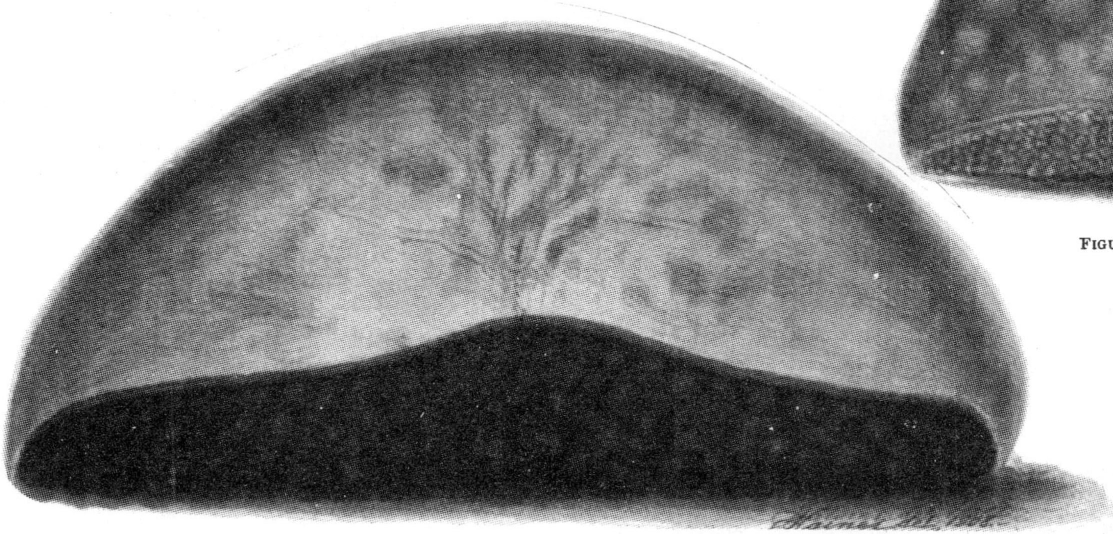

FIGURE 1

NORMAL SPLEEN AND SPLEEN AFFECTED BY TICK FEVER.

FIGURE 1.—Spleen of an acute, fatal case of tick fever.
FIGURE 2.—Spleen of healthy steer.

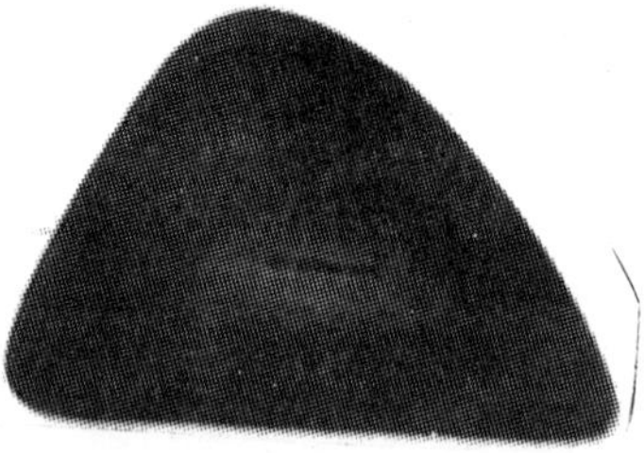

FIGURE 1

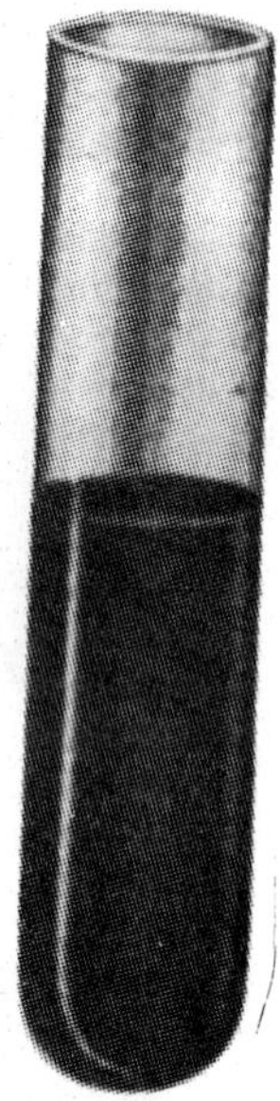

FIGURE 3

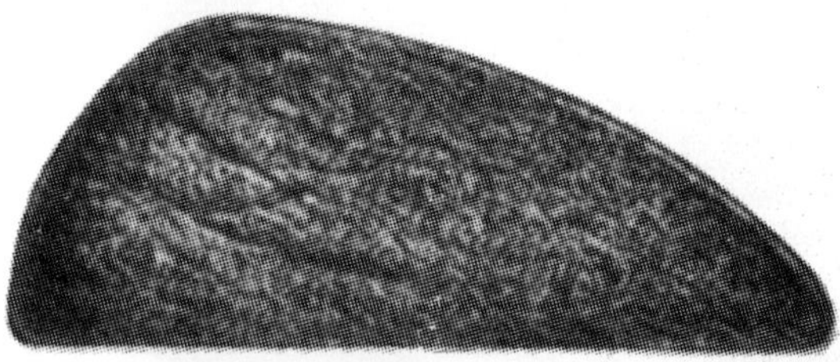

FIGURE 2

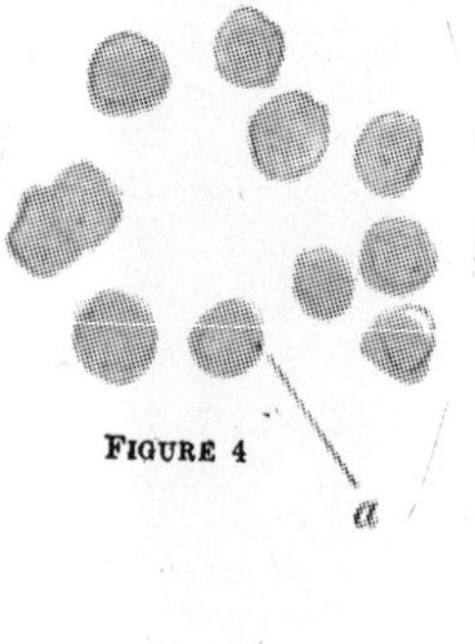

FIGURE 4

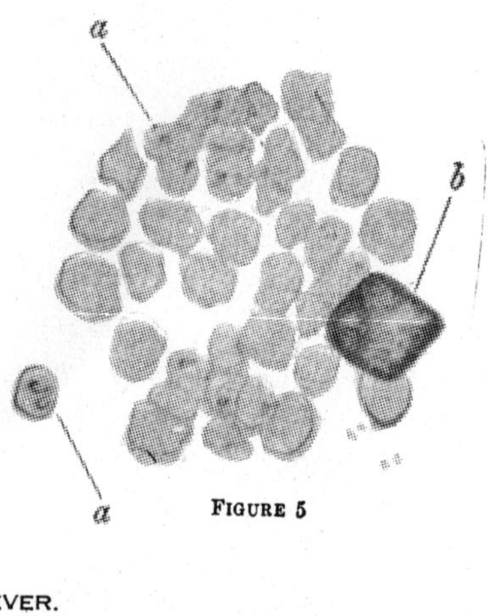

FIGURE 5

TICK FEVER.

PLATE XLVI

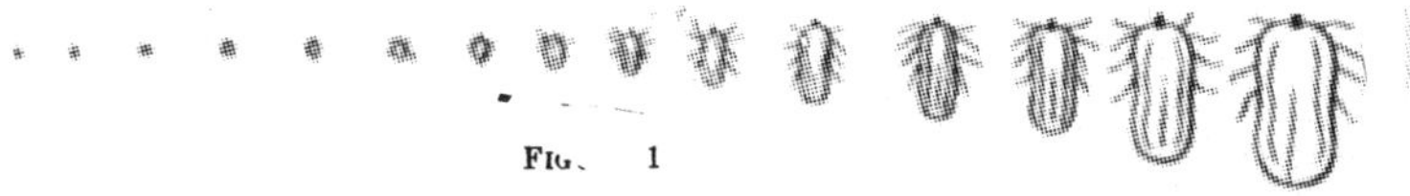

FIG. 1

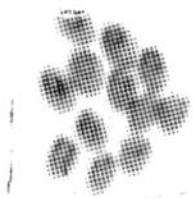

FIGURE 2

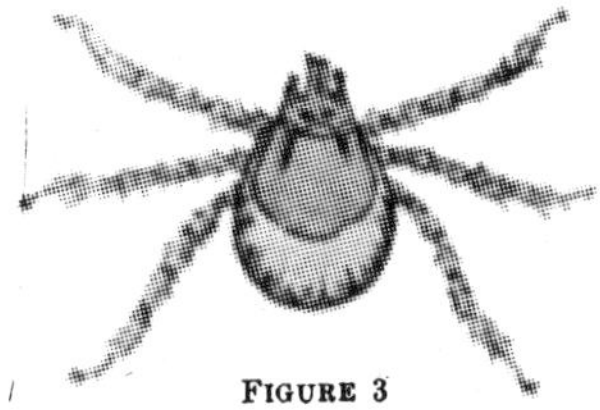

FIGURE 3

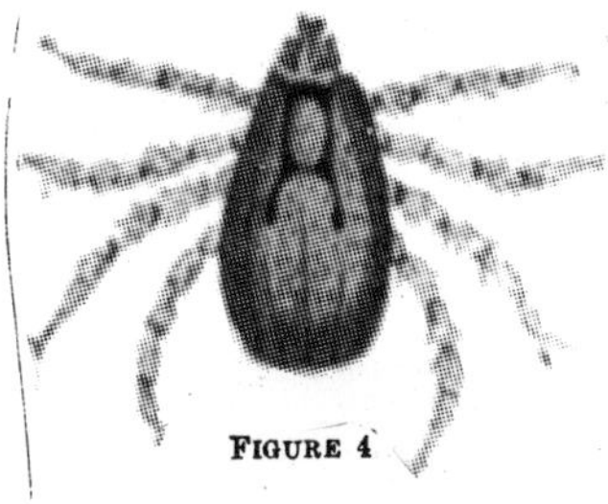

FIGURE 4

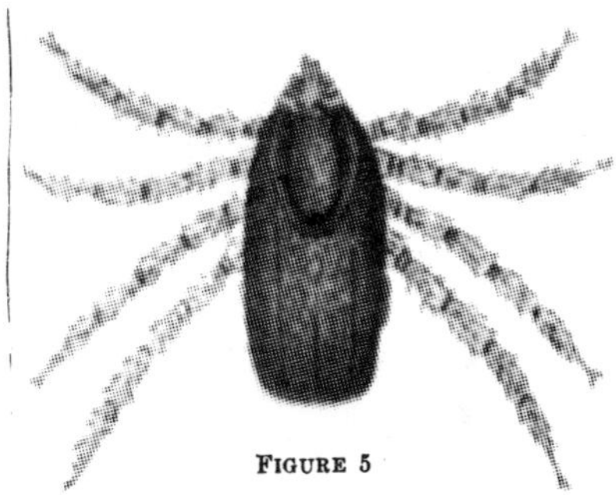

FIGURE 5

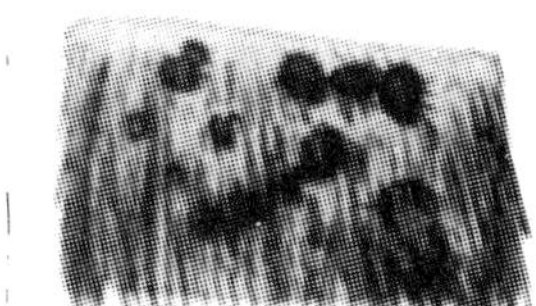

FIGURE 6

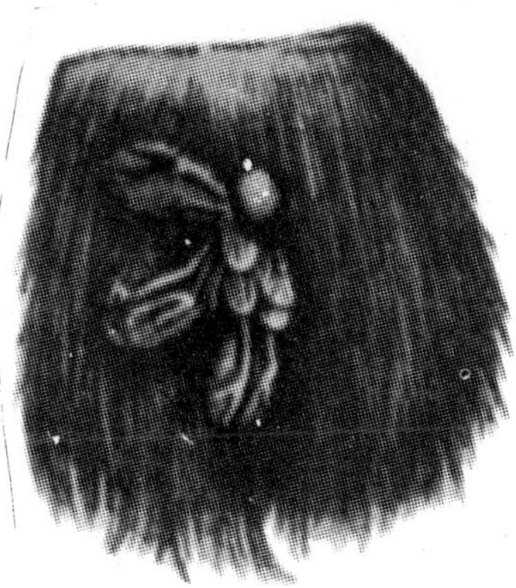

HAINES DEL.

FIGURE 7

THE CATTLE TICK (BOOPHILUS ANNULATUS), THE CARRIER OF TICK FEVER.

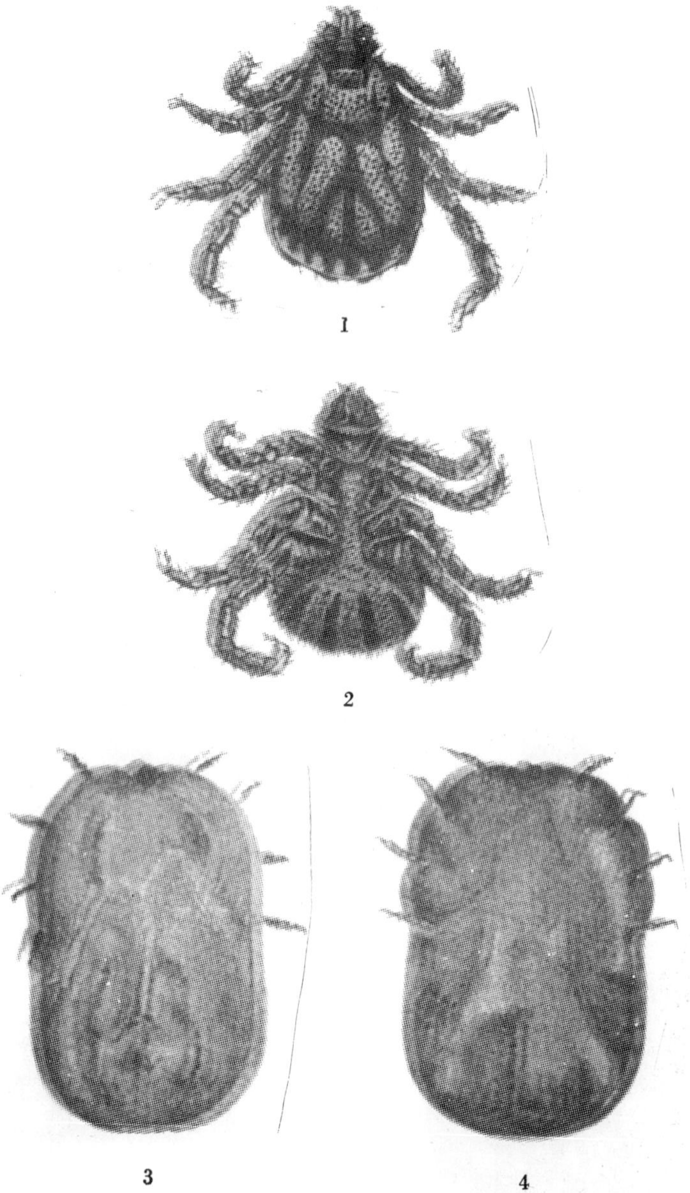

HAINES DEL.

THE CATTLE TICK (BOOPHILUS ANNULATUS).

FIGURES 1 and 2.—Dorsal and ventral views of male.
FIGURES 3 and 4.—Dorsal and ventral views of replete female.
(Greatly enlarged.)

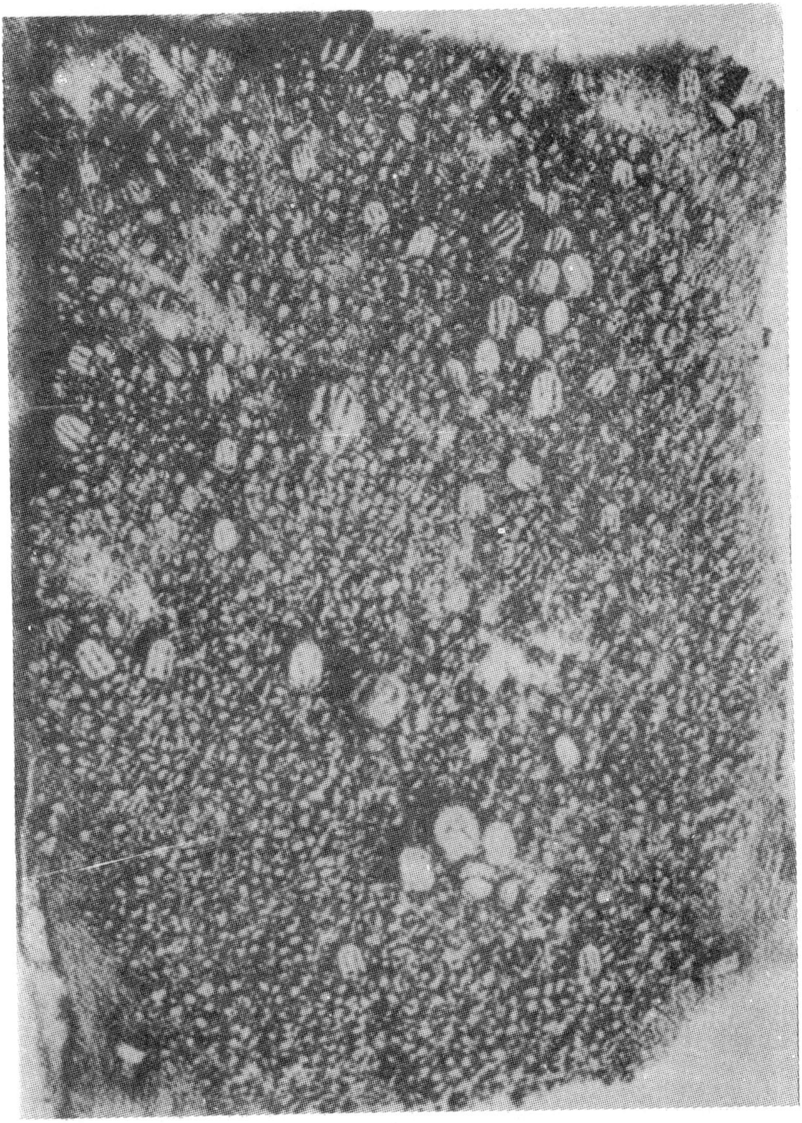

PORTION OF A STEER'S HIDE, SHOWING THE FEVER TICK (BOOPHILUS ANNULATUS) OF THE UNITED STATES. NATURAL SIZE. ORIGINAL.

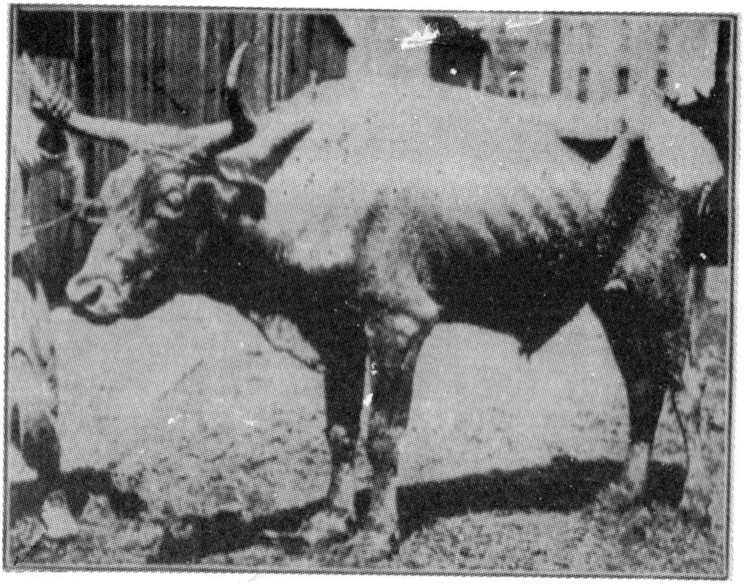

FIGURE 1.—TICK-INFESTED STEER.

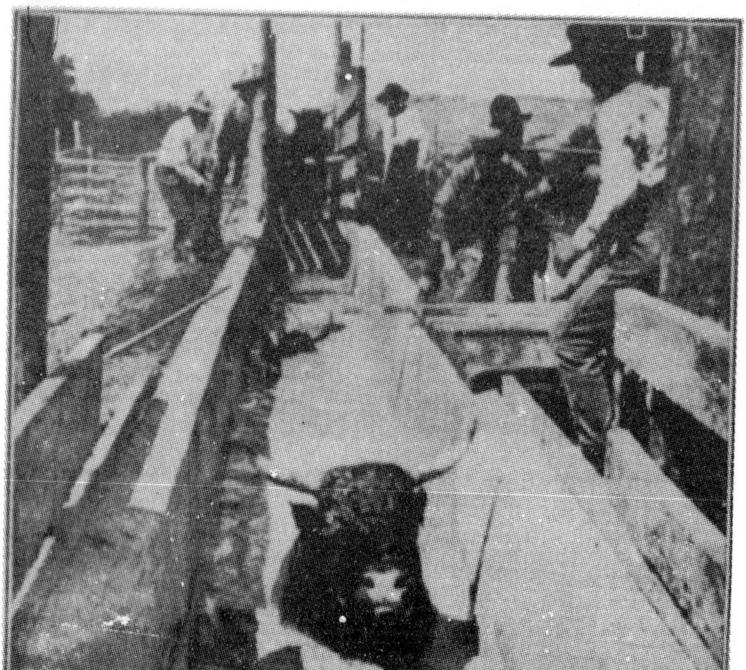

FIGURE 2.—DIPPING CATTLE TO KILL TICKS.

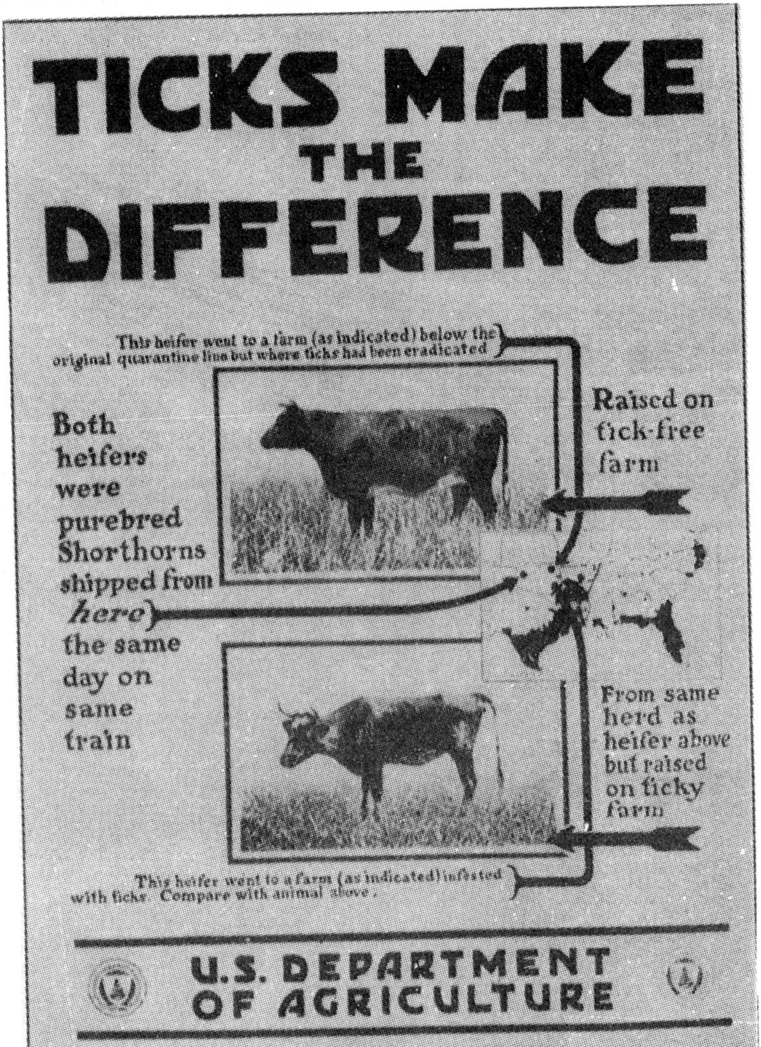
TICKS MAKE THE DIFFERENCE
This heifer went to a farm (as indicated) below the original quarantine line but where ticks had been eradicated
Raised on tick-free farm
Both heifers were purebred Shorthorns shipped from here the same day on same train
From same herd as heifer above but raised on ticky farm
This heifer went to a farm (as indicated) infested with ticks. Compare with animal above.
U.S. DEPARTMENT OF AGRICULTURE

FACSIMILE OF POSTER USED IN TICK-ERADICATION WORK.

ter of tick fever and anaplasmosis, and both these diseases may occur in the same animal at the same time. Scientists have also demonstrated that a number of other ticks are capable of spreading anaplasmosis under experimental conditions but just how important they are in the transmission of the disease under natural conditions in the field is not known. Certain species of horse flies and deer flies have also been shown to be capable of transmitting this disease. It has been reported that anaplasmosis may also be transmitted by the mosquitoes, *Psorophora columbiae* and *P. ciliata.*

Mechanical transmission by hypodermic needles, dehorning apparatus, and other surgical instruments has been responsible for many outbreaks of anaplasmosis.

Symptoms.—In the early stages of anaplasmosis there is a marked rise of temperature, ranging from 103° to 105° F. When the disease has fully developed, the temperature may become normal and later subnormal before the animal dies. Many affected animals have a rapid, tumultuous heart action with a pulse rate of 80 to 140 a minute. The breathing is accelerated and labored, the respiration ranging from 50 to 60 a minute. Other symptoms are exhaustion, great debility, and suspended rumination. The skin, udder, teats, mouth, vagina, sclera of the eyes, and all visible membranes become yellow and anemic. Pica, or depraved appetite, manifested by eating dirt or chewing bones, is sometimes observed. The animal may lie down frequently, and when walking, a stiff, weavy, unsteady gait is occasionally noted.

The urine is rarely bloody, as in tick fever. Cerebral symptoms are rather common, and afflicted animals are disposed to fight. Muscular tremors of the neck, shoulders, or flanak are often observed. The bowels are usually constipated, and the feces are dark in color, often blood tinged and partly covered with mucus. Glandular swellings, a puffiness of the eyes, and a roughened coat may be noted. Abortion in advanced cases of pregnancy is common. Death may occur within 24 hours after the appearance of the first symptoms, but usually follows an illness of 2 or 3 days' duration. In cases that recover improvement takes place slowly, many days or weeks being required for restoration to be complete. Clinically recovered animals may remain carriers of the disease for many years.

Losses.—There is a wide range of mortality in outbreaks of anaplasmosis. Occasionally only a single death may be recorded in small herds of afflicted animals. At other times a high percentage of sick cattle succumb to the malady. The mortality ranges from 30 to 50 percent of the animals affected. There may be considerable immunity where the disease has existed for some time. The death rate is highest in sick animals in which a high proportion of the red cells (25 to 50 percent) are affected with the parasites. When the number of cells involved is not more than 5 to 10 percent, the mortality is much less.

In addition to the direct loss of cattle by death from this disease, there is a loss from the poor condition of the flesh and the low weight of those animals that seem to recover, particularly range cattle and younger animals. In dairy herds, milk production not only may be greatly reduced but sometimes fails completely until the following period of freshening. As already noted, anaplasmosis may also cause abortion, the fetus usually being expelled near the end of the gestation period during the acute onset of the disease.

Post mortem findings.—Death occurs usually without violent struggling. Externally, there is no evidence of hemorrhage or injury. All visible mucous membranes and the skin show anemia and jaundice. Internally, the lymph glands are slightly enlarged, edematous, and watery in appearance without marked swelling or hemorrhagic appearance. The heart is usually enlarged and flabby, and its surface well sprinkled with petechiae (pinpoint blood spots). The blood is thin, watery, and light colored. The lungs are colorless and anemic and appear to be filled with air bubbles.

The liver is usually enlarged with hemorrhagic areas on its surface. When incised, this organ appears to be saturated with bile. The gall bladder is greatly distended and contains a viscid, thick, and flocculent, dark-green fluid. Externally, the kidneys may appear normal, aside from a tinge of yellow discoloration, but internally a slight congestion may be noted.

In most cases the spleen is enlarged, the pulp is softened, dark colored, resembles blackberry jam, and is disintegrated. An occasional case may fail to show the splenic enlargement.

The urinary bladder usually contains a considerable quantity of dark, straw-colored fluid, which often contains traces of bile and sugar. An occasional pin-point hemorrhage is noted on the inner walls of the bladder, but bloody urine is seldom found. The gastrointestinal tract shows nothing characteristic; however, the third stomach is usually somewhat drier than normal. Dry hard masses of feces are often seen in the large bowel; they may be streaked with a bloody mucus, indicating a catarrhal enteritis. The entire internal structure, including muscle, fat, connective tissues, brain, and other organs, usually show a lemon-yellow discoloration.

Diagnosis.—The disease may be accurately diagnosed, either during life or after death, by the microscopic examination of properly prepared and stained smears made with the blood of the affected or dead animal. The inoculation of blood from suspicious cases or carriers into a suitable susceptible animal will likewise conclusively prove whether the disease is present.

Within quarantined areas anaplasmosis may be confused with tick fever. In the latter disease, bloody urine is usually present, whereas in the former it is rarely so. Microscopic examination of the blood should disclose parasites characteristic of either disease. The presence of the fever tick, together with bloody urine, indicates tick fever.

Anaplasmosis may be erroneously diagnosed as anthrax at necropsy because the spleen is abnormal in appearance in both diseases. Cultures, microscopic examinations, and animal inoculation will aid in arriving at the correct diagnosis.

Anaplasmosis has also been confused with hemorrhagic septicemia. In the latter disease, however, there are no marked changes in the blood, the lymphatic glands are engorged and enlarged, and the lungs are deeply congested. A positive diagnosis may be made by growing the *Pasteurella* organism, followed by serological tests and animal inoculations.

In simple gastrointestinal disorders the illness would probably be of short duration and not fatal. In encephalitis there would be subnormal temperature, paralysis of the throat, and other symptoms of that illness.

Treatment.—There is no specific medicinal treatment. Animals suffering from anaplasmosis should be kept in the shade, given plenty of clean water and a little green feed, and protected against fly annoyance. Good care is essential in helping animals to resist the disease. Unnecessary driving or rough handling of sick cattle may hasten their death.

As most cattle sick with anaplasmosis are constipated, the use of saline purges or other cathartics to flush the bowels is ordinarily beneficial, but the dose must be moderate in order to prevent too drastic an effect. Mineral oil or mild cathartics may be of value and without danger to the animal.

Arsenical preparations have been used in the treatment of this disease, and good results have been reported from the intravenous injection of 1 quart of 5-percent dextrose solution to which sodium cacodylate has been added. The sodium cacodylate is dissolved in water in such proportions that each cubic centimeter contains about 5 grains of the drug. The dose of sodium cacodylate is 25 to 30 grains per 100 pounds of live weight, that is, 5 to 6 cc. of the sodium cacodylate solution. The value of such drugs, however, has not been demonstrated by well-controlled experiments with untreated sick animals as controls. In some herds the mortality has been high even when this drug was used in large doses.

Stimulative treatment with injections of camphorated oil or strychnine may be advisable to assist the heart action.

Prevention.—As it is not known with any degree of certainty how anaplasmosis is spread under field conditions, no preventive measures can be recommended. However, proper precautions should be taken against spreading the disease by dehorning, castrating, drawing blood, and similar means. Thorough disinfection of all instruments used in these operations is essential.

NAGANA

Nagana, also called tsetse-fly disease, is an infectious fever occurring chiefly in horses and cattle, characterized by alternating paroxysms and intermissions and produced by specific flagellate protozoan (*Trypanosoma brucei*) in the blood. It is probably transmitted from animal to animal solely by the bites of flies, particularly the tsetse fly. This insect is something like a large house fly, and when it settles on a diseased animal, sucks the blood and infects its proboscis. On biting a second animal, it infects the latter by direct inoculation. This disease is found throughout a large portion of central and southern Africa, along the low-lying and swampy valleys. It has never occurred in the United States, nor it is known to be present in the Philippines, but its relation to surra and the possibility of its appearance in one of our island dependencies are the reasons for including a few remarks at this time.

Symptoms.—The chief symptoms in addition to the fever, which is usually about 104° or 105° F., are the muscular wasting, progressive anemia, and loss of power, together with the edema most marked about the head, legs, abdomen, and genital organs. The urine is yellow and turbid and occasionally contains albumin and blood. There is paralysis of one or both of the hind legs, difficult urination and defecation, labored breathing, discharge from the eyes and nose, extreme thirst, and gradual extension of paralysis to other parts of the body. The disease runs a chronic course, lasting from 3 to 6 weeks in horses, and from 1 to 6 months in cattle. Besides these animals, the mule, ass, sheep, goat, hog, buffalo, antelope, hyena, camel, and dog contract the disease naturally, and the sheep, goat, cat, and small laboratory animals succumb to artificial inoculation.

Lesions.—The spleen and lymphatic glands are enlarged. There are serofibrinous exudates in the body cavities, the liver is enlarged and engorged, heart flabby, and a catarrhal condition is present in the respiratory passages. Pathological changes occur in the spinal cord. The finding of the *Trypanosoma* by microscopic examination of the blood is conclusive evidence for diagnosis.

Treatment.—Treatment has not proved satisfactory. Quinine, arsenic, various dyes, and other drugs have been used but without consistent success. Endeavors thus far made to produce immunity from this disease have likewise been unavailing.

CATTLE FARCY

This is a chronic disease of cattle formerly observed frequently in France, and is now common in the island of Guadeloupe, West Indies, and certain other tropical and subtropical countries. It is characterized by caseating, nodular swellings, first of the skin and afterwards of the superficial lymphatic vessels and glands, finally proving fatal within a year by extension to the viscera. The swellings rupture and discharge a purulent yellowish fluid, which contains the causative organism. This affection, called farcin du boeuf by the French, resembles cutaneous glanders or farcy of horses, but is caused by an entirely different organism, *Actinomyces farcinicus*. Moreover, cattle are immune from glanders, and for this reason the name, unfortunately applied to this disease, should not lead to any confusion with the cutaneous glanders or farcy of horses.

Treatment.—Treatment consists in making incisions into the swellings and syringing them out with an antiseptic solution such as 2-percent compound cresol solution. The cavities may then be packed with cotton soaked in 5-percent zinc-chloride solution. The swollen lymphatics may also be bathed or covered with cloths wrung out in this solution.

OTHER INFECTIOUS DISEASES

The following are also infectious diseases of cattle, discussions of which are found in other chapters:

	Page
Brucellosis (Bang's disease)	142
White scours of calves	219
Infectious catarrhal conjunctivitis (pink eye)	302

77431 O—51——32

Parasites of Cattle[1]

By B. H. RANSOM, Ph. D.

[Revised by GERARD DIKMANS, D. V. M., Ph. D.]

EXTERNAL PARASITES

Parasites of cattle comprise more than a hundred different species. Fortunately not all these parasites occur in the United States, and of those present many are uncommon. There is a wide range from highly pathogenic forms to forms not known to be injurious and rated as apparently harmless. Some of the common forms are of distinct importance to the American stockman on account of the known damage for which they are responsible. These definitely injurious parasites are the ones considered here, for the most part.

FLIES

Of the various species of flies that infest and injure cattle, some are blood suckers and cause annoyance and pain due to their bites. Some transmit diseases or parasites from the blood of diseased animals to that of healthy cattle. Others, which in the winged adult state do not bite, live as parasites in cattle during their larval stages.

THE STABLEFLY (STOMOXYS CALCITRANS)

The stablefly closely resembles the housefly, but unlike the latter it is a biting fly. It is common about stables and often enters dwellings, especially in cloudy weather. According to Noé, it is the agent of transmission of a parasitic roundworm of cattle (*Setaria cervi*, p. 484). This fly is capable of transmitting anthrax from diseased to healthy animals, and under some conditions it may transmit surra, a disease (not present in the United States) caused by a blood parasite that affects horses, cattle, and other livestock.

The stablefly is widely distributed throughout the world. It is found in every part of the United States but its abundance in different localities varies greatly. Annoyance to livestock by the fly is most common in the Central States from Texas to Canada, and it is a more or less persistent pest in all irrigated regions. It seldom becomes

[1] For more complete information regarding any of the parasites that affect cattle, write to the U. S. Department of Agriculture, Washington, D. C.

abundant before early summer and causes most of its injury during August and September.

Although stableflies transmit some important cattle diseases, according to the Bureau of Entomology and Plant Quarantine, these insects are important principally because of the annoyance and worry produced by their attacks and the loss of blood caused by their repeated engorgements. During warm weather, animals must keep up a constant fight against the flies. The loss of blood during severe attacks is of considerable importance. Each fly ingests several drops of blood while feeding. This blood is soon digested and the feeding is then repeated. Animals serving as the source of supply for several thousand flies therefore lose a large quantity of blood.

In fly-infested zones milk production in dairy cattle is reported to be reduced as much as 60 percent during severe outbreaks, and beef cattle lose flesh rapidly.

The stablefly breeds in moist accumulations of straw, chaff, cow or horse manure, and various fermenting vegetable substances. The debris collecting in and under outdoor feed troughs and the remains of straw stacks are favorable breeding places for the stablefly. Under the most favorable conditions about 3 weeks is required for development from the egg to the adult stage.

The proper care of straw and the proper disposal of stable manure are necessary in the control of stableflies. Straw stacks should be carefully built to shed rain, and loose straw or chaff should be scattered or burned. Straw not required for winter feed should be promptly disposed of by scattering and plowing it under or by burning. Stable manure should be hauled out and scattered at regular intervals, preferably every 3 days, and the vicinity of stables should be kept free from accumulations of straw and hay that become wet and serve as breeding places for the flies.

The annoyance to cattle and horses from stableflies is much lessened if the stables are darkened. The screening of doors and windows, however, if preferable, as ventilation is not interfered with as it is in darkened stables. For milk cows, coverings made from burlap (double thickness), including trouserlike coverings for the legs, may be used when the flies are very numerous and troublesome. Fly traps fitted to the windows of dairy barns are useful in destroying stableflies. The United States Bureau of Entomology and Plant Quarantine has found that a mixture of fish oil 1 gallon, oil of pine tar 2 ounces, oil of pennyroyal 2 ounces, and kerosene 1 pint is fairly effective for a short time when applied lightly, but thoroughly, to the portions of animals not covered with blankets.

THE HORN FLY (HAEMATOBIA IRRITANS)

The horn fly (fig. 1), now found nearly everywhere in the United States, was introduced into this country from Europe about 1885.

Horn flies, when present in large numbers, have the habit of clustering about the base of the horn (fig. 2), whence the name by which they are popularly known. They do not damage the horn and congregate there only to rest. In view of the general practice of dehorning cattle, the name "horn fly" is less distinctive than it once was. Moreover, horn flies rest on other parts of the body more than on the horns, and the classical picture of horn flies illustrated in figure 2 is rarely seen now in the country although it was common when the fly was first introduced.

When flies are resting, the wings are held down close to the body (fig. 1); when feeding, their wings are held out nearly at right angles, ready for flight. Characteristically, horn flies rest with their heads downward on cattle.

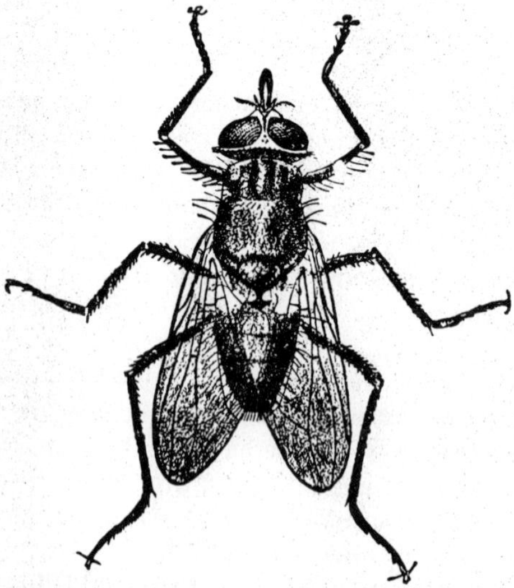

FIGURE 1.—The horn fly (*Haematobia irritans*) in resting position. Greatly enlarged.

The fly lays its eggs in freshly dropped cow manure, where they hatch in about 24 hours. The larvae, or maggots, develop in 4 to 5 days to the pupal stage, which lasts from a week to 10 days. In warm weather the pupal stage may last only 4 to 5 days, according to the Bureau of Entomology and Plant Quarantine. The flies emerging from the pupae may begin feeding on cattle in 2 to 3 hours. Mating has been observed as early as 2 days after emergence and egg laying 1 day later. The entire life cycle from egg to egg may, therefore, be completed in 12 to 14 days during the summer The adult lives approximately 3 weeks.

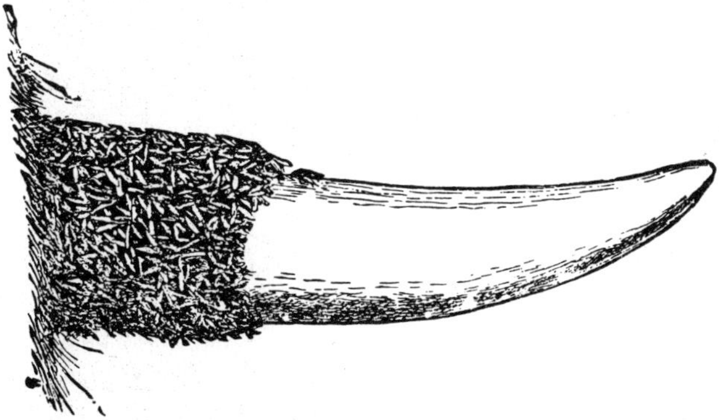

FIGURE 2.—Horn flies (*Haematobia irritans*) on cow horn.

Horn flies appear with the first warm days of spring and are present on cattle until fall, when cool weather halts their activities. Warm, damp weather is ideal for their propagation; hot, dry weather and low temperatures are unsuitable for their development.

The flies puncture the skin and suck blood and usually attack the upper parts of the body, which are out of reach of the animal's head or tail. Unlike most flies, they remain on the animal more or less constantly, day and night.

The annoyance and irritation caused by horn flies are responsible for a considerable loss of flesh in all classes of cattle during the season when the flies are abundant. Cattle often refuse to graze during the day and seek protection by hiding in brush or tall grass until nightfall, when the flies are less active. In areas where screwworms are present, the wounds caused directly by the flies and indirectly by the attempts of the animals to escape the flies or to rid themselves of the flies by licking, kicking, running through brush or rubbing against trees, are potential places of screwworm infestation.

Horn flies are easily killed by most of the livestock fly sprays now in common use and they can be controlled effectively by systematic spraying. Obviously this method of control is most suited to the control of the flies in dairy establishments, the sprays being designed to kill the flies rather than to prevent infestation. The Bureau of Entomology and Plant Quarantine has developed a cattle fly trap,[2] which is stated to have been found effective for the control of horn flies on many farms, dairies, and ranches. In order to be effective

[2] For detailed information concerning the construction and operation of this trap, consult the Bureau of Entomology and Plant Quarantine.

as a control measure, this trap should be so located that animals are compelled to pass through it on their way to water, salt, or to enter a barn.

Dipping cattle in a vat provided with splashboards set at the proper angle destroys most of the horn flies present on the animals. Unless the splashboards are used, all but a few of the flies succeed in escaping as the cattle plunge into the bath and later the flies return to the animals. Scattering the droppings of cattle, either with a shovel or with brush dragged over pastures in order to insure the rapid drying of the manure and consequent destruction of the larvae, is an efficient means of reducing the number of these flies.

BUFFALO GNAT

These small flies, also known as black flies, are about one-eighth inch long and have a characteristic "humped" back (fig. 3). They breed in running water and appear in swarms during spring and summer, often in enormous numbers, causing great annoyance to stock and human beings on account of their bites and their entrance

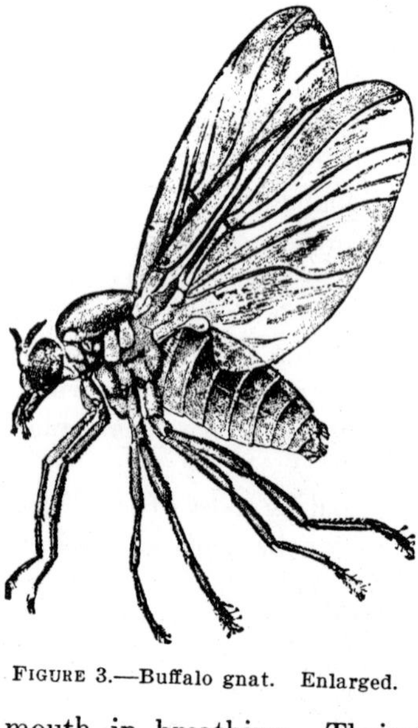

FIGURE 3.—Buffalo gnat. Enlarged.

into the nose and mouth in breathing. Their bites appear to be poisonous, and in seasons especially favorable to the gnats heavy losses of horses and cattle often occur.

Buffalo gnats are more troublesome during bright sunny weather than during cloudy weather, and animals that have not shed their winter coats suffer more from their attacks than those with smooth coats. Cattle kept in darkened stables are not molested.

The use of smudges that produce a dense smoke is a remedy much used in the South for the temporary protection of livestock. The animals soon learn the value of the smoke as a gnat repellent and will stand in it for hours at a time when the pests are present in great numbers. During the season when gnats are likely to appear, animals should never be kept under fence in river-bottom pastures where they have no chance of seeking shelter from buffalo gnats when they suddenly appear.

The most commonly used repellents consists of mineral oils, such as crankcase or "burnt" oil, in which a little pine tar is dissolved. Commercial "gnat oils" also are widely used by those able to afford them. These oils are usually mopped on the animals, and the hair and hide gradually becomes so oil soaked that in the case of work animals they may become overheated while working, and considerable injury undoubtedly results therefrom. Preliminary tests to develop a nonoily repellent for use against buffalo gnats indicate that a 5-percent pine-tar-oil emulsion is very promising for this purpose. It is made by boiling ½ pound of soap in 1 gallon of water, and then adding 0.6 ounce of refined pine-tar oil slowly while stirring vigorously. By mopping this material on an animal in the morning and giving light sprayings during the day as needed, comparative freedom from the gnats is obtained.

SCREWWORM

Screwworms are the maggots of the fly *Cochliomyia americana*, as shown in figures 4 and 5. Adult screwworm flies are bluish-green blowflies with three dark stripes along the back between the wings and with a yellowish-red face. This insect is a true parasite of warm-blooded animals and attacks wounds of all types. The screw-

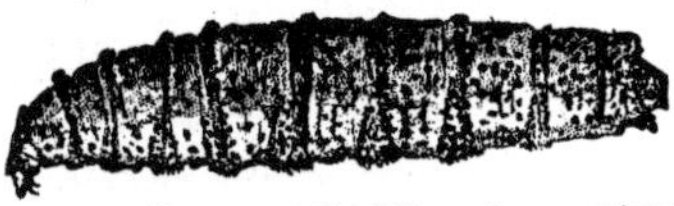

FIGURE 4.—Screwworm (larva of *Cochliomyia americana*). Enlarged.

worm flies lay their eggs in regular, oval, shinglelike masses and cement them to the edges of wounds or blood spots. The eggs hatch in about 12 hours and the larvae or maggots, or so-called screwworms, begin to burrow into the flesh and continue burrowing and feeding for 4 to 10 days, after which they leave the wound, drop to the ground and crawl into the earth, there transforming into the quiescent pupal stage. This stage is usually completed in about 7 days but may last much longer. The mature flies then emerge from the pupal envelope and are soon ready for egg laying. From 18 to 24 days, therefore, is required for the entire life cycle, although under certain conditions a month or longer is often required.

The fly is exterminated each winter by low temperatures in all areas except the extreme southern portions of the United States. In this area the fly persists mainly because of wintertime surgical operations, the birth of young livestock, the wounding of game animals, and lack of treatment. More than 90 percent of the December and January screwworm cases in southern Texas have been found to be in wounds caused by birth of young domestic animals and by surgical

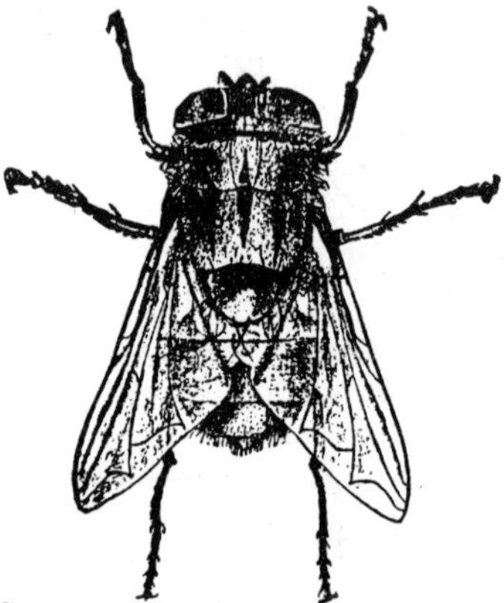

FIGURE 5.—Screwworm fly (*Cochliomyia americana*). Enlarged.

operations. The screwworm fly is migratory and spreads from its overwintering area with the onset of spring and warm weather.

The shipping of screwworm-infested animals from infested to noninfested areas has been known to cause destructive outbreaks in the latter areas.

Screwworm fly attacks and the resultant loss are proportional to the number of flies present. If the flies are limited in number, the wounds are not all infested, and infested animals usually survive the initial attack and a few subsequent reinfestations without treatments. As the number of flies increases, all open unprotected wounds may become infested. Even slight scratches and fly and tick bites may become infested, and the larger wounds may be so grossly attacked that animals, unless treated, may die in 2 or 3 days. Even under favorable weather conditions, and in the presence of many untreated wounds, 2 to 3 months is required for large numbers of flies to be present.

According to the Bureau of Entomology and Plant Quarantine, screwworms attack any warm-blooded animal, and cattle, sheep, hogs, horses, mules, and dogs are infested in about the order named. Deer and other wild animals are frequently infested and man also may be attacked. The place of attack depends on the location of the injury and any abrasion, cut, or wound in any part of an animal may become the site of screwworm infestation.

Treatment.—Since every case of screwworm infestation must be treated individually, infested animals should be placed where they can be examined thoroughly and treated with a minimum expenditure of time and labor and with a maximum protection from injury that may result from handling. The Bureau of Entomology and Plant Quarantine has found that benzol is the best general killer of screwworms, and it recommends the commercial grade (90 percent) for the killing of screwworms in infested wounds. It is best applied with a syringe or an oil can but may be poured into the wound from a narrow-necked bottle. Wounds should be cleansed with absorbent cotton before the benzol is applied because this product will not mix with blood; hence the screwworms may escape its destructive action in uncleansed wounds. In a wound with a small external opening, it is well to plug the opening with a piece of cotton after the benzol is applied. The worms are usually killed in 2 to 3 minutes, but care should be taken that the worms in all the pockets and crevices are actually dead. To insure this, it is best to apply a little more benzol 2 to 3 minutes after the first application. The wound and the area around it should then be lightly coated with commercial pine-tar oil (specific gravity 1.065, dehydrated).

In areas where screwworms are present every year the Bureau of Entomology and Plant Quarantine strongly recommends the use of the following mixture known as Smear No. 62:[3]

	Parts by weight
Diphenylamine (technical grade)	3½
Benzol (commercial)	3½
Turkey red oil (pH-10 or neutral)	1
Lamp black	2

After the use of this preparation it is not necessary to remove the dead worms, as large numbers of them soon drop out of the wound. As they carry with them a considerable portion of the preparation used, it is therefore necessary to repeat the treatment in 24 to 48 hours. It is recommended that regular treatment be given twice each week until the wound is healed.

Prevention of infestation.—It is best not to castrate, dehorn, mark, brand, or perform any surgical operation on cattle during the screwworm season. If such operations must be performed during that time, pine-tar oil or the preparation mentioned above should be applied to and around the wounds and the animals kept where they can be closely observed and treated when necessary. Avoid anything that may injure animals. Handle livestock carefully. Re-

[3] For details concerning the preparation and use of this mixture consult the Bureau of Entomology and Plant Quarantine.

move all projecting boards and nails from around stables and corrals, and separate animals that are likely to fight. Treat all wounds, cuts, and abrasions promptly.

The Gulf coast tick, *Amblyomma maculatum*, which attaches itself to the ears of cattle and other animals, produces a condition that is favorable to screwworm attack. It occurs from June to November in the coastal areas of the Southern States and is seldom found as far as 100 miles from the Gulf of Mexico or the South Atlantic seaboard. The ears of infested animals should be treated with a mixture of 3 quarts of pine-tar oil, 1 quart of linseed oil, and 1 pint of benzol applied by hand both to the inside and outside of the ear. This preparation causes the death of the female ticks before they lay eggs and prevents other ticks from attaching for a period of about 2 weeks. It also protects against screwworm attacks for a few days.

Infestation with the spinose ear tick, *Ornithodorus megnini*, may also favor screwworm infection. This tick attaches itself deep in the ear. To control this species the mass of debris and ticks found in the ears of infested cattle should be loosened with a wire loop and the ear swabbed with a mixture of 3 parts of pine-tar oil and 1 part of linseed oil or crude cottonseed oil. This treatment should be repeated at intervals of about 30 days.

The use of dogs to catch animals may lead to trouble with screwworms. Animals caught by dogs suffer a number of minor injuries, each of which may become the site of screwworm infestation.

In areas where screwworm flies are present throughout the year, the birth of young should be timed to coincide with the season of least activity of the flies.[4] In dairies where it is considered necessary to distribute calving throughout the year, special care should be given during the fly season to both the cow and the calf at the time of parturition. A few days before the date of calving the cow should be treated with a light application of pine-tar oil (dehydrated, specific gravity 1.065) about the vulva. After calving the cow should be examined and given an additional treatment with pine-tar oil. The navel of the calf should be treated with iodine, and pine-tar oil should be applied to the belly around the navel to repel the flies.

Provide small pastures for wounded and screwworm-infested animals where they can be examined carefully every day and treated promptly when necessary.

Watch all animals closely during the fly season for indications of screwworm infestation.

Several kinds of blowflies that normally breed in carrion may also attack wounds of various kinds. This is especially true of the black

[4] For suggestions concerning ranch practices dealing with such factors as times of parturition in screwworm infested areas, consult the Bureau of Entomology and Plant Quarantine.

blowfly, *Phormia regina*, which has been found to attack wounds resulting from dehorning.

GRUBS, WARBLES, BOTS

Warbles are whitish or, when full grown, dark-colored grubs or maggots that develop from the eggs deposited on the hairs of cattle by certain flies known as warble flies. In the United States there are two species of warble flies, sometimes called ox warbles or grubs, tech-

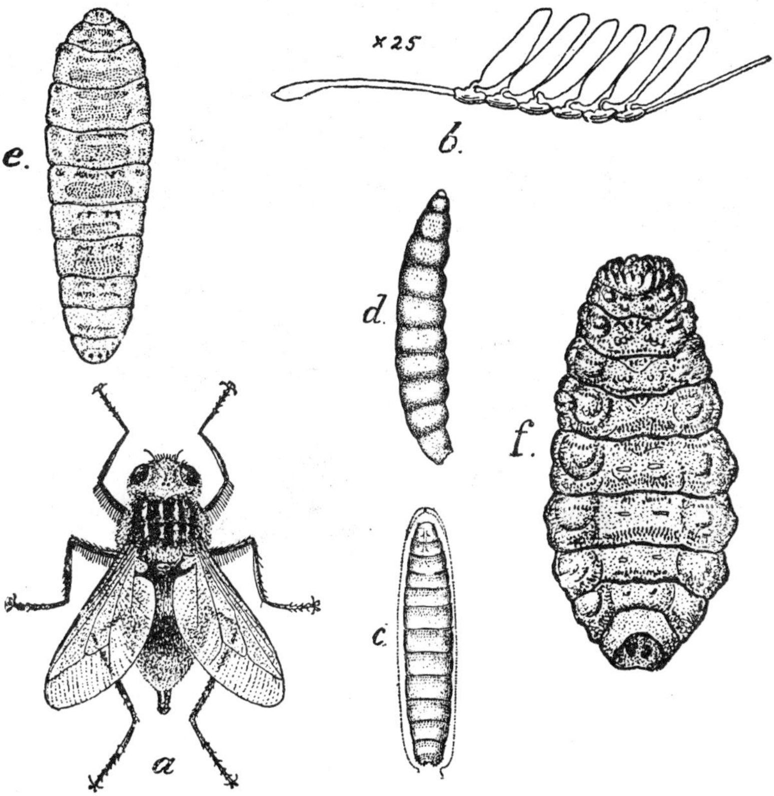

FIGURE 6.—The warble fly (*Hypoderma lineatum*) : *a*, Adult female ; *b*, eggs attached to a hair, × 25 ; *c*, larva as seen in eggs ; *d*, larva from esophagus of a cow ; *e*, later stage of larva from beneath the skin of the back ; *f*, larva or warble, at the stage when it leaves the back of cattle and falls to the ground—all enlarged (after Riley).

nically known as *Hypoderma lineatum* and *H. bovis* (fig. 6). These flies somewhat resemble bees in their general appearance but, like all flies, have only two wings.

The first named, *H. lineatum*, is commonly called the heel fly and is more generally distributed over the United States than the other species. The tail has a distinctive reddish-orange color and the legs are rough and hairy. This fly commonly deposits its eggs about the coronet, whence the name of heel fly, and on the fetlocks, knees, and hocks. When cattle are resting, eggs are deposited along the line of contact of the body with the soil. Cattle are often indifferent to the activity of this fly in depositing its eggs but not infrequently may be stampeded by it. Commonly 8 to 10 eggs, sometimes as many as 14, are attached to a single hair.

In the United States, the distribution of the other warble fly, *H. bovis*, is limited, at least as far as is known at present, to the Northern and Central States. The tail is orange yellow, lighter in color than that of the other species, and the legs have but few hairs. This fly commonly deposits its eggs on the outside of the hindquarters and above the fetlocks when the animals are moving, or lower down if they are quiet. Cattle are usually much disturbed by the activity of this fly and frequently appear terror stricken. The eggs are attached singly, one egg to a hair near its base.

The eggs of the warble flies hatch, as a rule, in 3 to 6 days, the time varying with local conditions. The young maggot is about 1 mm. (one twenty-fifth of an inch) long. It crawls to the base of the hair and burrows into the skin. This burrowing produces much irritation, causing the animal to kick and stamp and to lick the affected parts. The penetration of the larvae into the skin usually causes a considerable flow of serum with pus formation, which results in the matting of the hair on affected areas of the skin and in scab formation. The larvae, after penetrating the skin, migrate through the body and ultimately reach the backs of the cattle. In latitudes north of Kansas, *H. lineatum* usually appears near the surface of the skin about the middle of January, and *H. bovis* about a month later. During their migrations, before they reach the back, the young larvae of *H. lineatum* spend a considerable period in the wall of the esophagus, or gullet, and may be found in this location as early as August 15. During the fall and winter a large proportion of the gullets of cattle that are slaughtered are found to be infested with warbles and, in the packing houses, are known as grubby gullets or weasands.

When the warbles first appear in the back they are about three-fifths of an inch long. They cause swellings about the size of pigeon's eggs, each swelling having a small hole in the center, which has been punctured in the skin by the warble to enable it to breathe. Through this hole the warble leaves the back of the cow when it has completed its parasitic stage of development, at which time it is nearly an inch in length. The minimum period of development in subcutaneous tissue of the back is about 35 days.

The full-grown larvae, or warbles, begin to leave the backs of the cattle early in the year, and in northern latitudes the last ones leave before the middle of July. After leaving the backs of cattle they burrow into the ground, lie quiescent for about a month, and became transformed into mature flies. In northern latitudes the mature flies of the species *H. lineatum* may be observed during April and May, and those of the other species during June and July.

The damage caused by warbles includes injury to stampeding cattle frightened by the flies, decreased milk flow, diminished growth of infested animals, and injury to hides, the last item being especially serious. The total loss to this country on account of the warble fly is extensive and has been estimated to be as much as $50,000,000 to $100,000,000 a year.

Treatment.—During the winter and spring, examine the cattle for the presence of warbles. By passing the hand over the backs of the animals the swellings marking the location of the grubs may be readily found. Pressure properly applied to the swellings will cause the grubs to "pop out" if they have reached a late stage of development. They may be more easily removed by means of slender forceps inserted into the opening made by the warbles. In order that none may escape, it is advisable to examine the cattle every 2 weeks late in the winter and spring and remove the grubs that have developed sufficiently to cause perceptible swellings.

Other methods of treatment are the application of salves to the grub holes and the injection of insecticides into these holes. The Bureau of Entomology and Plant Quarantine reports that an ointment consisting of petrolatum, 10 parts, and powdered derris root, 1 part, has given excellent results. As insecticides injected into the grub holes with an oil can, both benzol (commercial 90 percent) and carbon tetrachloride killed more than 90 percent of the grubs treated. Derris has also been used in the form of powder and as a wash. When used as a powder it should be applied to the entire back of the animal after first ruffling the hair with the hand or with a stiff brush. The powder should be rubbed in thoroughly with the fingers. A wash made of 1 gallon of water, 4 ounces of soap, and 12 ounces of derris powder containing 4 percent of rotenone, briskly rubbed in with a stiff fiber brush, has given excellent results.

This wash may be applied to cattle with a sponge, cloth, or brush, but a more convenient and sanitary way is to use an ordinary glass pint jar equipped with a metal cover. Remove the porcelain lining from the metal cover and punch a number of small holes in the top of the metal cap. Fill the jar with the well-stirred mixture and apply the liquid from the jar along the middle line of the back of the animal. As the liquid flows from the jar it should be spread with the brush into the hair coat and onto the skin of the back and upper part of the sides of the animal. The liquid should be applied slowly to the part of the back and the side that is being scrubbed. One pint of wash usually is sufficient for an average-size animal. More liquid is required for large cattle having long hair than for small, short-haired cattle. In preparing washes for mixed herds it is customary to allow an average of 1 pint of wash for each animal to be treated.

If the wash is properly used and applied at the right time, one treatment with derris or cube wash can be depended on to kill practically all grubs that have reached their location in the backs of cattle at the time treatment is applied. Derris and cube powders remain in the hair coats and on the skins of treated cattle for several weeks or longer and kill the new grubs that reach their location and form holes in the skin after the washes are applied. The exact time that the powders continue to be effective on treated cattle is not definitely known. Probably this varies considerably, depending on rainfall and other factors.

The proper time to apply washes for the destruction of cattle grubs must be determined in each locality by examining cattle and noting the appearance of the first grub openings or holes in the skins of the cattle. About 25 days, and not more than 30 days, after the first grub holes appear in the skin the wash should be applied. If the work is delayed longer than 30 days, some of the grubs may emerge, pupate, and form a new crop of flies.

One treatment with the washes, in localities where the common species of cattle grub is the only one present, usually kills 90 to 95 percent of the grubs. One treatment during the grub season, therefore, cannot be depended on to eradicate the common species of cattle grub but it will, if generally applied, afford a considerable measure of control. Two treatments, given about 30 days apart, probably will kill all grubs that appear in the treated cattle during the grub season.

In localities where both species of grubs are present, or where *Hypoderma bovis* is prevalent, one treatment a season is of little value, since the grub season in such localities is so much longer than the period of effectiveness of one treatment. Three to four treatments, applied 30 to 40 days apart, probably could be depended on to kill most of the grubs in the treated cattle in such areas.

Prevention.—In localities where it is practicable to examine cattle systematically and remove the grubs, it is possible to reduce the number of grubs greatly in two or three seasons. To do this, the herds must be comparatively small and subjected to the close supervision of their owners, who will be able to remove enough grubs so that only a very small percentage will survive to be transformed into flies.

LICE

Cattle in the United States are commonly infested with three species of lice, two of them sucking lice, commonly known as blue lice—*Haematopinus eurysternus*, the short-nosed cattle louse, and *Linognathus vituli*, the long-nosed cattle louse—and one biting louse, *Bovicola bovis*, commonly known as the red louse.

Blue lice (figs. 7 and 8) suck the blood of cattle and are more injurious than red lice (fig. 9). Unless very abundant, the latter cause

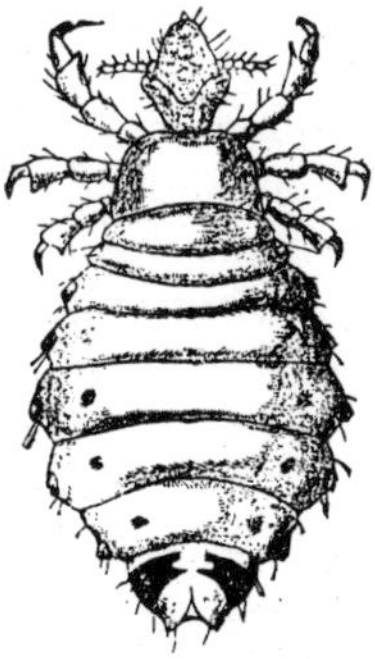

FIGURE 7.—Short-nosed blue louse (*Haematopinus eurysternus*) of cattle. Enlarged.

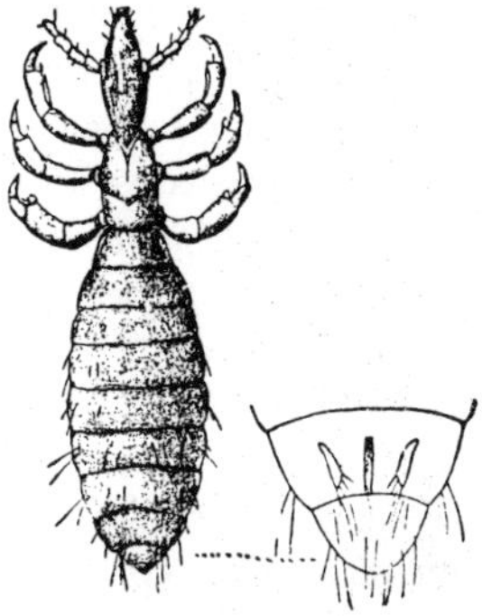

FIGURE 8.—Long-nosed blue louse (*Linognathus vituli*) of cattle. Enlarged.

little injury. If numerous they irritate and worry their host probably more by their sharp claws than by their bites, as their food seems to consist entirely of particles of hair and dead skin. They produce hairless patches on the skin.

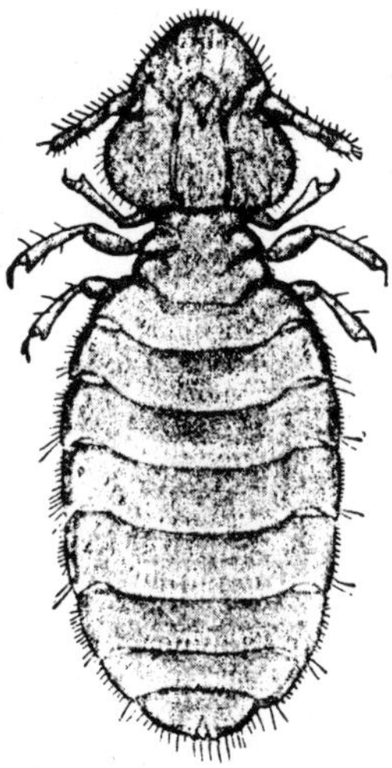

FIGURE 9.—Red louse (*Bovicola bovis*) of cattle. Enlarged.

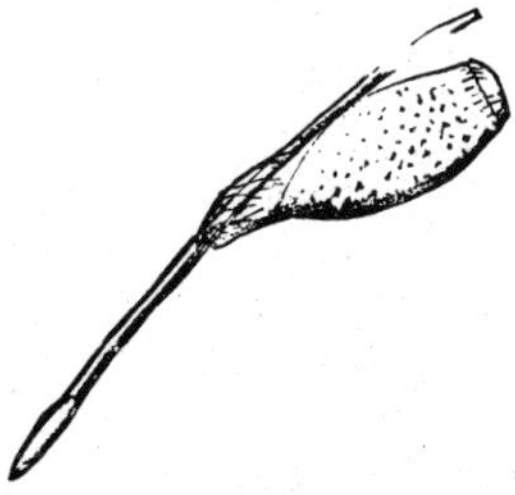

FIGURE 10.—Egg of short-nosed blue louse (*Haematopinus eurysternus*) attached to a hair. Enlarged.

Cattle lice reproduce by means of eggs or nits (fig. 10), which they fasten to the hair. Blue lice infest chiefly the neck and shoulders; red lice, when present, may be found almost anywhere on the body but are usually most numerous on the neck and shoulders and at the root of the tail.

On account of the itching caused by the lice, infested cattle rub against posts, trees, and other objects and lick themselves, the hair sometimes coming out and the skin becoming thickened so that mange may be suspected.

Treatment.—Cattle may be treated for lice by means of hand applications, spraying, or dipping. Dusting powders and fresh, finely ground derris or pyrethrum are of value in helping to hold lice in check when the weather is too cold for dipping or spraying. The application of greases and insecticidal liquids by hand is fairly effective and practicable when only a few animals are to be treated. The following remedies have proved effective when applied by hand, the treatment being repeated if necessary, in about 16 days: (1) Cottonseed oil and kerosene, equal parts; (2) kerosene, one-half pint, mixed with lard, 1 pound; (3) crude petroleum; (4) any of the dips recommended for use in dipping cattle, as coal-tar-creosote and nicotine dips (p. 465), diluted in the same proportions as for dipping. Oils or greases should not be used in very warm or very cold weather. The remedies mentioned may be applied with brush or a cloth. They should be distributed in a thin, even coating over the surface of the body, care being taken that there is no excess quantity at any point.

Any of the dips recommended for lice may be applied as a spray when properly diluted. It should be spread over the entire body by means of a spray pump. Thorough wetting of the skin and hair is important, and a second treatment should be given 15 to 16 days later.

When a considerable number of animals are to be treated, the most satisfactory method is by the use of a dipping vat. Two dippings should be given 15 or 16 days apart. Dipping in the fall is good insurance against risk of loss from lice during the winter. All animals in the herd should be treated regardless of the number showing infestation. Either coal-tar creosote or nicotine dip may be used. Both are sold under various trade names. The directions for dilution given by the manufacturer should be carefully followed. As coal-tar creosote dips do not mix well with all kinds of water, they should be tested by mixing some of the dip in the proper proportion with the water in a clean and clear glass bottle or jar. If an oily layer or mass of globules collects either at the top or the bottom of the mixture after standing an hour, the dip is not suitable for use with that kind of water. Imperfectly mixed coal-tar creosote dips are likely to poison animals even when not used in stronger solutions than that recommended by the manufacturers and also are likely to be ineffective.

The lime-sulfur dip, which is highly efficacious as a mange remedy, is of little value for destroying lice, especially blue lice. The arsenical dip used in tick eradication is a good louse remedy, but its use is not advisable on account of its poisonous nature, except under the supervision of persons who know how to use it and what precautions should be taken.

The long-nosed sucking lice and the biting lice are much more easily eradicated than the short-nosed sucking lice. One treatment with arsenical dip or coal-tar creosote dip is usually sufficient to eradicate the first two species, but, as a rule, one treatment does not eradicate the short-nosed sucking lice. In fact, two treatments sometimes fail to eradicate it, especially in the case of infested bulls. When a herd is infested with all three species the animals should be given two treatments 15 to 16 days apart. After the second treatment the animals should be examined at frequent intervals, and if live lice are found a third treatment should be given about 16 days after the second treatment.

MANGE, ITCH, SCAB

Cattle are subject to four kinds of mange, of which common mange, or psoroptic mange, is the most important.

PSOROPTIC MANGE

Psoroptic mange of cattle is caused by small mites (fig. 11) that multiply rapidly and are spread from diseased to healthy cattle by contact or by pens, stables, or railroad cars recently occupied by mangy cattle. The mites attack the skin and cause it to become thickened and covered with crusts and scabs, with a consequent loss of hair. Intense itching accompanies the disease, and affected cattle are more or less constantly rubbing and licking themselves. Psoroptic mange commences at the root of the tail or on the neck or withers, gradually extends over the back up to the head and over the sides, and may finally affect nearly the entire body except the legs. In serious cases the skin may become ulcerated; the animals are greatly weakened and emaciated and finally die. By taking scrapings from the edges of scabby patches and placing them on a piece of black paper in a warm place, the mites may be seen as tiny white objects over the paper. They may be seen more distinctly if a magnifying glass is used. Mange may be confused with lousiness, ringworm, or any condition in which there is itching or loss of hair, but if mites are found there is no question of the diagnosis. The disease is worse during cold, wet weather. Mangy cattle, when on good pasture during the summer, often seem to recover, but in the fall the disease may appear again in a severe form.

Treatment.—The most generally used and most satisfactory method of treating cattle mange consists in dipping the animals in a vat

774310—51——33

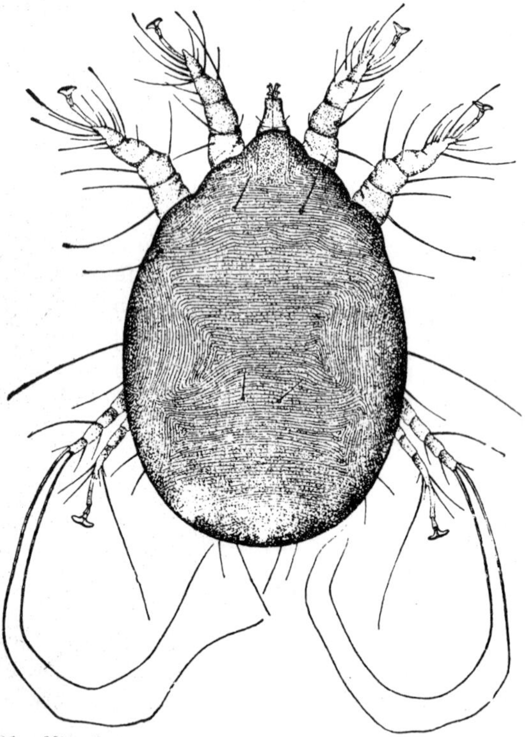

FIGURE 11.—Mite that causes psoroptic mange. Enlarged about 100 times.

filled with a liquid of such a nature that it will kill the parasites without injuring the cattle. Vats for dipping cattle are built of wood, stone, or concrete and vary in length from 30 to 100 feet or more. They vary in width from 3 to 7 feet at the top and 1½ to 3 feet at the bottom, and the depth may be 7 to 10 feet. A narrow chute through which the cattle are driven leads to one end of the vat, where a steep slide pitches the cattle into the dipping fluid, through which they swim. The cattle climb out of the vat at the other end, where a slope, provided with cross cleats, gives the animals a foothold. A draining pen with a floor sloping back toward the vat is generally provided. The dip should be used warm, 100° to 105° F., and the cattle held in the vat for 2 minutes to insure thorough action of the dip. The head of each animal should be ducked at least once. Care should be taken that the vat contains a sufficient depth of fluid to swim the animals to be dipped. The dipping fluid may be heated from a steam boiler by pipes or hose, or water heated in large iron cauldrons or tanks may be used for charging the vat. Hot water with a proper quantity of dip should be added from time to time as the dipping fluid becomes cool.

If crude-petroleum dips are used, one dipping is usually sufficient, and the dip is used cold. Crude-petroleum dips are rarely used for common, or psoroptic, mange but are of special value for another kind of mange, known as sarcoptic mange, which is cured with difficulty by the ordinary dips. In the treatment of common mange with lime-sulphur or nicotine dips, two dippings are necessary, the second being given 10 to 14 days after the first. The second treatment kills the few parasites that sometimes escape at the first treatment.

LIME-SULFUR DIP

The lime-sulfur dip is made in the proportion of 12 pounds of unslaked lime (or 16 pounds of commercial hydrated lime—not air slaked lime), 24 pounds of flowers of sulfur, and 100 gallons of water.

Directions for preparing 100 gallons of dip.—Weigh out the lime, 12 pounds (or hydrated lime, 16 pounds), and sulfur, 24 pounds. Place the unslaked lime in a shallow, water-tight box similar to a mortar box, or some other suitable vessel, and add water enough to slake the lime and form a lime paste or lime putty. Sift into this paste the flowers of sulfur and stir well. Then place the lime-sulfur paste in a kettle, boiler, or tank containing 30 gallons of water, the water first being heated nearly to the boiling point. Boil the mixture for 2 hours at least, stirring frequently; add water occasionally to maintain the original quantity. Allow the mixture to settle in the tank, or draw the entire contents of the kettle or boiling tank into a large tub or barrel placed near the dipping vat and provided with a bunghole about 4 inches from the bottom, and then allow ample time to settle—2 to 3 hours, or more if necessary. When the mixture is fully settled, draw off the clear liquid into the dipping vat, and take care not to allow any of the sediment to accompany it, as this is likely to render the dip caustic. The clear liquid thus obtained requires only the addition of sufficient clear warm water to bring the total to 100 gallons. Flowers of sulfur must be used and the lime must be of good quality.

The dipping bath should be used at a temperature of 100° to 105° F. and for official dippings must be maintained at all times at a strength of not less than 2 percent of "sulphide sulphur" as indicated by the Bureau of Animal Industry field test for lime-sulfur baths.

NICOTINE DIP

The nicotine dip is made with sufficient extract of tobacco, or nicotine solution to give a mixture containing not less than 5 one-hundredths (0.05) of 1 percent of nicotine and 2 percent of flowers of sulfur. Sufficient nicotine is therefore furnished for 96 gallons (about 800 pounds) of dip by 1 pound of a 40-percent solution of nicotine. The formula for this dip is as follows: Nicotine, 0.4 pound; flowers of sulfur, 16 pounds; water, 96 gallons.

To calculate how much nicotine solution or extract of tobacco should be used for 96 gallons of water, divide the quantity of nicotine required in the dip by the proportion of nicotine in the extract. For example, if the nicotine solution contains 25 percent of nicotine, we have $0.40 \div 0.25 = 1.6$. Therefore, in this case it would require 1.6 pounds of nicotine solution for the 96 gallons of dip. Or if a tobacco extract is used, having, for example, 2.4 percent of nicotine, the formula would be as follows: $0.40 \div 0.024 = 16.66$; and, therefore, 16.66 pounds would be required for 96 gallons of dip. Do not use any preparation the strength of which is not given on the outside of the package.

In preparing these dips the nicotine solution and flowers of sulfur should be mixed with water before being added to the water in the dipping vat. On no account should the dip be heated above 110° F. after the nicotine solution is added, as heat is likely to evaporate the nicotine and weaken the dip.

For official dippings, the bath should be used at a temperature of 100° to 105° F. and at all times must be maintained at a strength of not less than 0.05 percent of nicotine as indicated by a field test approved by the Bureau of Animal Industry.

CRUDE PETROLEUM DIPS

Crude-petroleum dips, which are valuable for the treatment of sarcoptic mange, are not often used for the treatment of psoroptic mange or of chorioptic mange. Besides unprocessed crude petroleum, processed petroleum from which the gasoline and other light hydrocarbons have been removed may be utilized in the treatment of cattle for mange, particularly sarcoptic mange. There are a number of proprietary brands of crude-petroleum dips on the market, consisting of processed crude petroleum with other substances added, mainly lighter oils to give the dip a suitable consistence. In dipping cattle in crude-petroleum dip, fill the vat with water to within 1 foot or 18 inches of the dip line and then add the oil until the surface is flush with the dip line. The oil floats on the water, and as the animals pass through the vat their bodies become coated with oil. When cattle are dipped in any of the crude-petroleum dips, a cool, shady place should be provided near the dipping vat where they may be quiet and protected from the sun for several days. If this is impossible the oil dips should not be used, as serious injury is likely to result from exercise or exposure to bright sunshine soon after dipping in oil. These dips should not be used in cold weather.

CHORIOPTIC MANGE

Chorioptic mange, due to a species of mite different from that causing common mange, is confined almost entirely to the region at the root of the tail and if not treated may persist for years. The treatment is the same as for psoroptic mange.

SARCOPTIC MANGE

Sarcoptic mange, frequently called barn itch, is caused by a mite very similar to that which causes itch in human beings. It commonly affects the head and neck but may occur also on various other parts of the body. Bulls are particularly likely to be affected with this form of mange. Cattle may become infested not only from other cattle but also from horses, goats, dogs, sheep, and hogs. As a rule sarcoptic mange in any species of animal, if acquired from an animal of another species, is likely to run a short course and to terminate in spontaneous recovery.

The treatment likely to be most efficacious is that of dipping in a crude-petroleum dip, one treatment as a rule being sufficient. (See Crude-Petroleum Dips, page 466.) If lime-sulfur dip is used, four or five successive treatments, or even more, at weekly intervals, may be necessary before a cure is effected.

DEMODECTIC MANGE

Demodectic mange, which is caused by a small parasite that lives in the hair follicles, causing pustules, especially on the neck and shoulders, occurs in cattle in this country and is of importance on account of the injury to the hide. When tanned, hides infested by this parasite are pitted, the pits, in some cases, being so deep that they form holes. No practicable treatment is known for this disease.

TICKS

About 10 species of ticks have been reported as parasites of cattle in the United States. The most common and most important is the species known as *Boophilus annulatus*, which transmits tick fever. Information concerning this tick and tick fever has been given elsewhere in this volume (p. 432).

The spinose ear tick (*Ornithodorus megnini*) is frequently found in the ears of cattle in the western part of the United States and commonly occurs also in the ears of horses, dogs, cats, and other animals. When its parasitic stage of development is completed, the ear tick leaves its host. Mating of ticks occurs after they have cast their skins following the abandonment of their host. They usually crawl up some distance from the ground and secrete themselves in cracks and crevices of trees, walls of buildings, or similar places, where the females deposit their eggs. After the eggs hatch, the larval ticks that emerge from them seek a host, enter the ears, and gradually develop to the stage at which they are ready to leave the host animal. The females may live several months, or even years, if they do not find mates. After mating they may deposit their eggs intermittently. Hatching of the eggs may occur as early as 10 days after deposition. The larvae may live for 80 days without a host. The parasitic period has been observed to vary from about 2 to 7 months.

Treatment.—On account of their habits and great vitality and their occurrence in various kinds of animals besides cattle, complete eradication of these ticks is difficult. The only effective treatment known is to introduce directly into the ear passages a remedy that will kill the ticks. Cattle may become reinfested from exposure to infested ranges or enclosures. The following mixture, however, in addition to killing the ticks in the ears, will protect against reinfestation for about 30 days: Ordinary commercial pine tar, 2 parts by volume, and cottonseed oil, 1 part—animals to be treated are confined in a chute, and the mixture is injected into the ears with a syringe, after the wax and other debris in the ears have been cleaned out with the loop end of a wire probe as illustrated in Farmers' Bulletin 980.

PARASITES OF THE STOMACH

The stomach of cattle consists of four compartments, of which the first and fourth are most likely to be the seats of parasitic infestation. The first stomach, or paunch, contains large numbers of minute organisms known as protozoa, which are too small to be seen with the naked eye. These organisms are not known to be injurious.

FLUKES

In the States bordering on the Gulf of Mexico and also in some other sections of the United States cattle commonly harbor, in the rumen or paunch, small numbers of parasites known as rumen flukes. These flukes are from one-fifth to one-half of an inch in length, pinkish in color when alive, and generally conical in shape; hence the name "conical flukes," by which they are also known (figure 12). They are usually found attached to the leaflike papillae near the opening of the paunch into the reticulum, or honeycomb stomach.

Their life history is similar to that of the common liver fluke, and the snails that serve as intermediate hosts of the liver fluke may serve in a similar capacity for the rumen fluke. After being swallowed in grazing, the young flukes pass through the stomachs and into the duodenum, or anterior portion of the small intestine. According to Mönnig (1934), they remain in the small intestine for about 6 weeks and then migrate to the rumen. When present in small numbers,

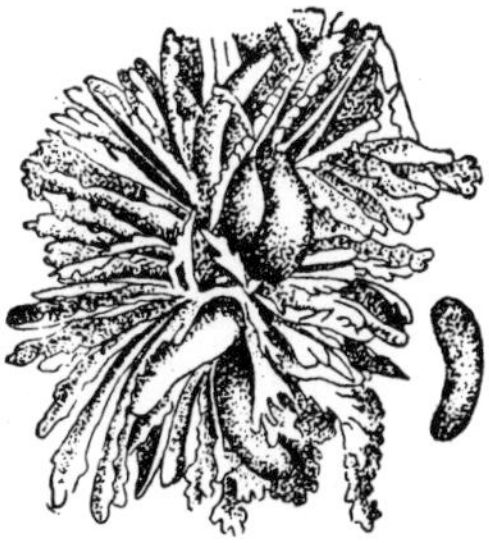

FIGURE 12.—Portion of the wall of the first stomach of a cow with conical flukes attached. Slightly enlarged.

these parasites are generally considered to be harmless. However, in heavy infestations they have been reported by South African, Australian, and Indian workers as causing severe, persistent diarrhea, marked retardation of growth, weakness, progressive emaciation, and death, the severity of the symptoms depending on the degree of infestation. In fatal cases death may occur in 10 to 14 days after the onset of symptoms.

The flukes responsible for the symptoms manifested by infected animals are immature; consequently, a diagnosis cannot be made by fecal examination. A tentative diagnosis based on circumstantial evidence and the elimination of other causes of diarrhea may be made, but a definitely positive diagnosis is possible only by finding the immature flukes in sufficient numbers in the duodenum at necropsy. No treatment for this trouble has been described.

ROUNDWORMS

Several species of roundworms may occur in the fourth stomach. The most important of these are the twisted stomach worm, *Haemonchus contortus*, and the lesser stomach worm, *Ostertagia ostertagi.*

THE TWISTED STOMACH WORM (HAEMONCHUS CONTORTUS)

The twisted stomach worm (*Haemonchus contortus*, figs. 13, 14, and 15) is sometimes found in enormous numbers in the fourth stomach of cattle. Sheep, goats, and other ruminants also may be infested with it. Among the symptoms caused by this parasite are anemia, loss of flesh, general weakness, dullness, capricious appetite, and excessive thirst. The anemic condition is seen in the paleness of the skin and mucous membranes of the mouth and eye and in the

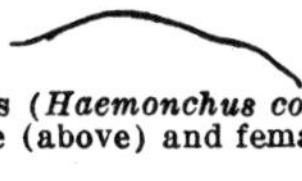

FIGURE 13.—Twisted stomach worms (*Haemonchus contortus*). Outlines showing natural size of male (above) and female (below).

watery swellings that often develop under the lower jaw, a condition known as bottle jaw or poverty jaw. If the fourth stomach of a dead animal is cut open and the contents examined carefully, the parasites, which are from ½ to 1¼ inches in length anad about as

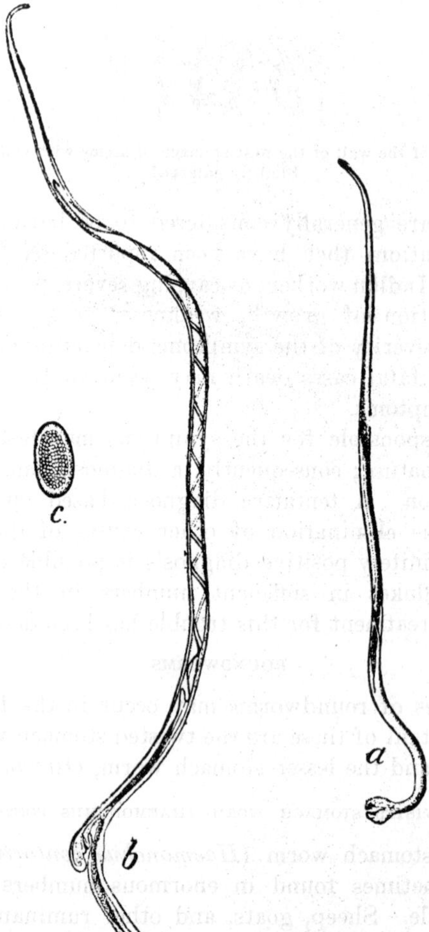

FIGURE 14.—Twisted stomach worms (*Haemonchus contortus*). (Male (*a*), female (*b*), and egg (*c*). Enlarged.

thick as an ordinary pin, may be seen, if present in any considerable numbers, wriggling about actively like little snakes.

Cattle become infected with these parasites by grazing on pastures on which infested cattle, sheep, or goats have grazed and scattered their droppings. The worms in the stomach produce a multitude of eggs (fig. 14, *c*) of microscopic size, which pass out of the body in the feces. In warm weather these eggs hatch in a few hours, provided sufficient moisture is present. At temperatures below 60° F. the eggs do not develop. Freezing temperatures and drying kill them. The larvae that hatch from the eggs are microscopic in size and, like the eggs, are very susceptible to freezing and drying until they have developed to a certain stage. In very warm weather the larvae complete their development to the infective stage in 2 or 3 days. In cooler weather the time required for this development is

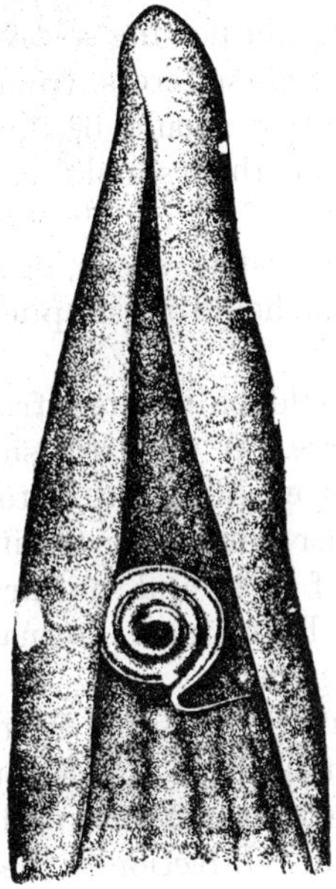

FIGURE 15.—Larva of twisted stomach worm (*Haemonchus contortus*) coiled on tip of grass blade. Enlarged.

longer, and at temperatures below 70° F. 10 days to several weeks may be necessary. The larvae are then ready to be taken into the body. The eggs and early stages of the larvae do not develop if swallowed. In the infective stage the larvae migrate up grass stalks (fig. 15) or other objects and show activity whenever the air is saturated with moisture, that is, during rains, fogs, and dews. When the air becomes dry and the moisture evaporates from the grass, the young worms cease their activity and resume their migrations when the air again becomes overladen with moisture. Larvae that have developed to the infective stage, unlike the eggs and early larval stages, are able to survive long periods of freezing and dryness. In 2 weeks to a month after the embryos are swallowed the worms reach maturity and begin producing eggs.

Prevention.—Preventive measures are important. As moisture favors the development of the embryos, high sloping ground is preferable for pastures. If low ground is used, it should be drained properly. The pasture should not be overstocked. Burning over the pasture will destroy most of the young worms on the grass and on the ground, and this means of disinfection under certain circumstances is very advantageous. The herd should be changed to fresh pasture as often as possible. Cattle should be watered preferably from tanks or troughs raised above the ground and supplied with clean, pure water from wells, springs, or flowing streams.

As calves are the chief sufferers from parasitic infestation, the major efforts at prevention should be directed toward their protection. Whenever possible they should be pastured separately from older infested animals. They should not be put on pastures recently occupied by older cattle, sheep, or goats. When the pastures become short the calves should be supplied with sufficient quantities of other feeds.

Affected animals should be isolated from the rest of the herd in hospital pens or pastures. A plentiful supply of nourishing feed is an important factor in enabling cattle to withstand the attacks of stomach worms and other intestinal parasites. The stabling of cattle, with the maintenance of clean and sanitary surroundings and liberal feeding, will often stop losses from internal parasites, even though no medicinal treatment is given.

Treatment.—In dosing animals for stomach worms it is advisable to treat not only animals that are seriously affected but also the rest of the herd, since the parasites with which they are infested will remain as a source of reinfection to the others. The cattle should be removed to fresh pasture after treatment, if possible.

The animals to be treated should be deprived of feed for 12 to 16, or even 24 hours before they are dosed, and if the bluestone treatment is used the cattle should receive no water on the day they are dosed until several hours after dosing. In drenching, a long-necked bottle or a drenching tube may be used. If the former is employed, the dose to be given may be first measured off, poured into the bottle, and the point marked on the outside with a file, so that subsequent doses may be measured in the bottle itself.

A simple form of drenching tube (fig. 16) consists of a piece of rubber tubing about 3 feet long and ½ inch in diameter, with an ordinary tin funnel inserted in one end and a piece of brass or iron tubing 4 to 6 inches long, of suitable diameter, inserted in the other end. The metal tube is placed in the animal's mouth between the back teeth, and the dose is poured into the funnel, which is either held by an assistant or fastened to a post. The flow of liquid through the tube is controlled by pinching the rubber tubing near the point of union with the metal tube. It is important not to raise the animal's head too high on account of the danger of the dose entering the lungs. The nose should not be raised higher than the level of the eyes. The animal may be dosed either when standing or when lying on its side.

The standing position is preferred by some authorities, who believe that more of the remedy is likely to reach the fourth stomach when the animal is dosed standing than when in other positions.

Great care should be used in dosing to prevent the entrance of the

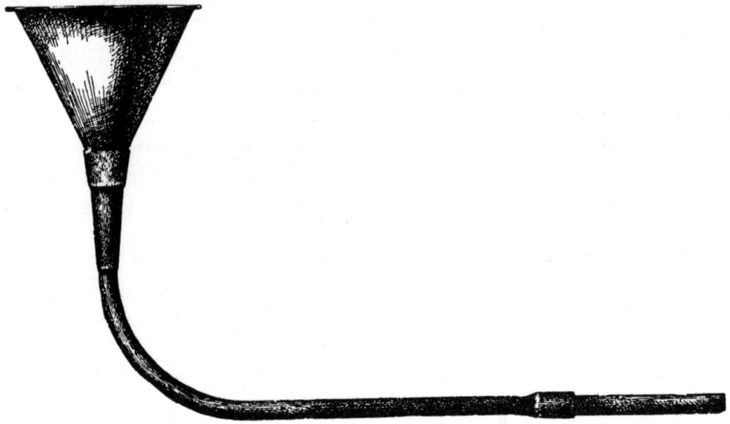

FIGURE 16.—A drenching tube made from an ordinary tin funnel, a piece of rubber hose, and a piece of brass pipe.

liquid into the lungs, and in the preparation and administration of the remedy to avoid getting the solution too strong or the dose too large. Bluestone, or copper sulfate, has been used extensively throughout the world in the treatment of sheep and cattle for stomach worms. To prepare the solution, take 1 pound (avoirdupois) of pure bluestone, powder it, and dissolve in 9½ gallons of warm water. It is better first to dissolve the bluestone in 2 or 3 quarts of boiling water, then add the remaining quantity of cold water, and mix thoroughly. This solution may be given to cattle in the following doses:

	Fluid Ounces
Calves	3½ to 4
Yearlings	6
Two-year-olds and over	12 to 16

In making up the solution only clear blue crystals of bluestone should be used. Bluestone with white patches or crusts should be rejected. It is especially important that the bluestone and water be accurately weighed and measured, and the size of the dose graduated according to the age of the animal.

Phenothiazine administered in gelatin capsules at a dose rate of 30 grams (approximately 1 to 1.5 ounces) for calves and 50 to 60 grams (2 ounces) for yearlings and older animals may be used also in the treatment of cattle for stomach worms. In a limited number of experiments this drug has been found to be effective in the treatment of cattle for stomach worms, hookworms, and nodular worms. Phenothiazine has also been used successfully at a dose rate of 0.1 gram per pound or 10 grams (2.5 drams) per 100 pounds of body weight for stomach worms and nodular worms. The capsules should be lubricated with mineral oil to facilitate swallowing. Dry capsules are difficult to administer. It is advisable to use the ½-ounce capsules for small calves to prevent choking. The drug may also be administered in the feed, with or without preliminary fasting.

The value of medicated salts advertised under various trade names as preventatives against worms is problematical. Often they contain little besides common salt, the other substances being in such small quantities that their therapeutic effect is practically negligible. There is no definite evidence that they are more efficacious than common salt and their use is not recommended.

THE LESSER STOMACH WORM (OSTERTAGIA OSTERTAGI)

This parasite is as thick as a fine hair and less than one-half of an inch in length. The developing larvae of this worm are found in small nodules in the mucous layer of the wall of the stomach (fig. 17), and the adults occur free in the stomach, generally in the pyloric end, that is, the end nearest the small intestine. They are usually covered by a layer of mucus. The symptoms caused by this parasite are very similar to those produced by the twisted stomach worm. The life histories of the two worms also are similar. Consequently, measures recommended for the prevention of infection with the twisted stomach worm may be used also for the lesser stomach worm.

Treatment.—Tetrachlorethylene administered in hard gelatin capsules at a dose rate of 5 cubic centimeters for each 100 pounds of weight, after the animal has been fasted for 24 hours, is of some value in the treatment of animals infested with this parasite. The treatment must be repeated every few weeks in warm weather to control the infestation. Tetrachlorethylene may be followed immediately by sodium sulfate (Glauber's salt) given in capsules or in solution in water at a dose rate of 2 ounces for calves and 1 pound for full-grown animals. Tetrachlorethylene should not be given to animals with febrile diseases, and the dose rate should be diminished for those suffering from emaciation and debility. The drug should be given only by a competent veterinarian. Phenothiazine administered at a dose rate of 30 grams for calves and 50 to 60 grams for yearlings and older animals is reported to be an effective treatment for the removal of these worms.

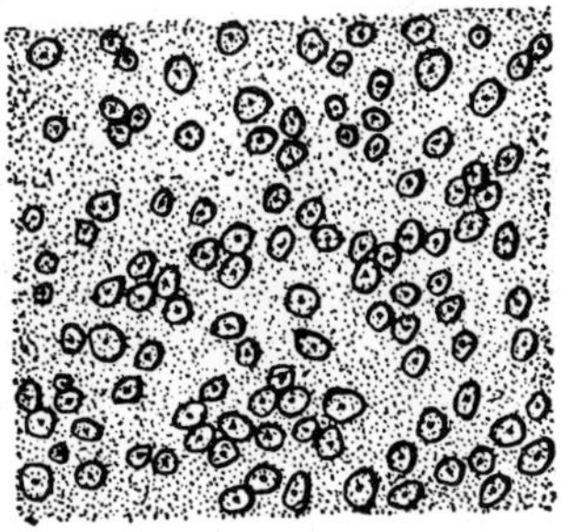

FIGURE 17.—Piece of lining of fourth stomach showing lesions caused by the lesser stomach worm (*Ostertagia ostertagi*). Natural size.

INTESTINAL PARASITES

TAPEWORMS

Two species of tapeworms (fig. 18) are known to occur in the small intestine of American cattle. They sometimes grow to a length of several yards and to a breadth of three-fourths of an inch. Small portions of tapeworms, consisting of one or more segments, are occasionally seen in the droppings of infested cattle.

As the segments dry they burst and liberate large numbers of eggs. These and other eggs passed in the manure may be ingested by certain free-living mites, *Galumna* sp., known as beetle mites. In the mites the eggs develop into cysticercoids or larval tapeworms. Cattle become infested with tapeworms by swallowing infected mites in grazing. The mites occur on open pastures and are present on the grass during the cooler parts of the day and on warm, cloudy days. During periods of intense sunlight and when high, drying winds prevail, the mites leave the grass and are found on the grass roots and in the soil. Saturation of the soil due to heavy or continued rains causes the mites to migrate to the grass blades.

Calves infested with tapeworms, as shown by the passage of segments in the manure, often have diarrhea and are unthrifty, and these evidences of injury are commonly attributed to the tapeworms. However, calves infested with tapeworms usually harbor various species of roundworms and the symptoms shown by tapeworm-infested animals may be due to the roundworms rather than to the tapeworms. Sheep experimentally infested with tapeworms only, did not show any marked evidence of infestation. The feces became somewhat softened and there was a slight retardation of growth. The severity of the symptoms depends on the age of the animal and the degree of infestation.

Treatment.—Medicinal treatment for tapeworms in cattle is usually unsatisfactory, but the bluestone treatment recommended for stomach worms (p. 472) sometimes expels tapeworms. Arsenic in doses of 1½ to 3 grains has been claimed to give good results in the treat-

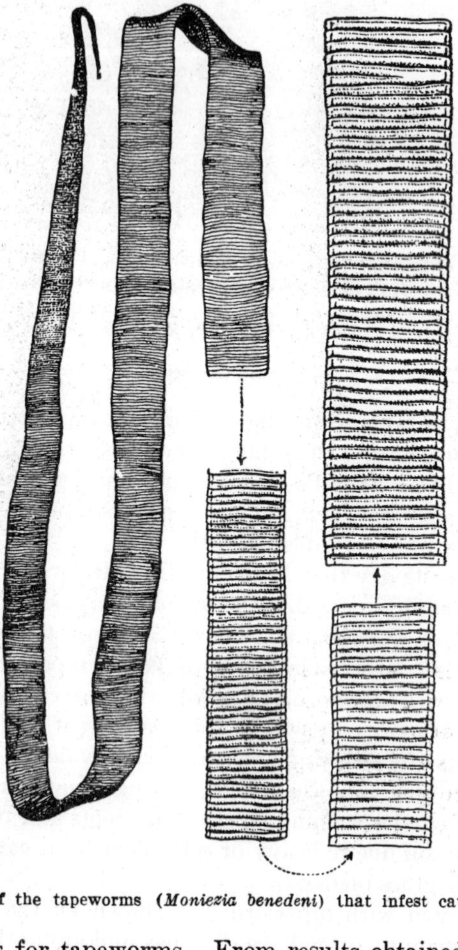

FIGURE 18.—One of the tapeworms (*Moniezia benedeni*) that infest cattle. Natural size.

ment of calves for tapeworms. From results obtained at the Oklahoma Agricultural Experiment Station in the treatment of sheep for tapeworms, it appears that the efficacy of the bluestone treatment against these parasites may be increased by the addition of nicotine. For use in cattle, the bluestone-nicotine mixture may be prepared by adding 1 ounce of 40-percent nicotine solution to 1 gallon of 1-percent copper sulfate, or bluestone, solution. The doses of this solution are the same as for the simple copper sulfate solution, namely:

	Fluid ounces
Calves	3½ to 4
Yearlings	6
Two-year-olds and over	12 to 16

ROUNDWORMS

A large roundworm (*Neoascaris vitulorum*), 6 to 12 inches in length, is sometimes found in the intestines of cattle, especially calves. Infection occurs through the swallowing of the eggs of the parasite in feed or water that has been contaminated with the feces of infested cattle.

In the course of their migration through the lungs, the larvae of these worms, provided they are present in sufficient numbers, may cause a verminous pneumonia similar to that produced in pigs by the larvae of *Ascaris lumbricoides*. The adult worms may cause unthriftiness and general digestive disturbances.

A number of other species of roundworms, ¼ to 1 inch or more in length, occur in the intestines. The most important of these are the hookworm, *Bunostomum phlebotomum;* the cooperids, *Cooperia punctata*, *C. oncophora*, and *C. pectinata;* and the nodular worm, *Oesophagostomum radiatum*.

Hookworms are relatively large white worms. When present they are usually attached to the wall of the anterior portion of the small intestine. When numerous they cause anemia and other symptoms similar to those caused by stomach worms.

The species of *Cooperia* frequently found in the small intestine of cattle are all relatively small, hairlike worms about one-fourth to one-half of an inch long and of a brownish-red color when freshly collected. *C. pectinata* appears to be confined to the Southern States, *C. oncophora* has a more northerly distribution, and *C. punctata* has been found in cattle in both northern and southern parts of the United States. *C. punctata* is definitely known to be pathogenic. Profuse, watery diarrhea, anemia, rapid loss of flesh, and death have been observed in calves heavily infested with this nematode. Deaths of calves due, at least in part, to infestation with *C. punctata*, have been reported from several States. Cases of enteritis due to *C. oncophora* have been reported from New York and Vermont.

The adult nodular worm, *Oesophagostomum radiatum*, is found in the cecum and colon of cattle. The larvae or immature worms are found in nodules in the walls of the posterior part of the small intestine, cecum, and large intestine. The free-living phase of the life history of this parasite is similar to that of the stomach worm, that is, the eggs pass out with the manure and develop on pasture to infective larvae. The larvae are ingested in grazing and after being swallowed migrate to the posterior part of the digestive tract. They penetrate the wall of the intestine and encyst there, causing hemorrhagic nodules. After a few days the larvae, which have grown considerably in the meantime, leave these nodules and develop into adults in the large intestine. The symptoms shown by animals infested with nodular worms are diarrhea, capricious appetite, and loss of weight. These symptoms are manifested principally during the time that the larvae invade the wall of the intestine. The severity of the symptoms depends on the degree of infection.

Treatment.—According to reports of the Oklahoma Agricultural Experiment Station, the combined copper sulfate and nicotine solution, as used for the treatment of cattle for stomach worms, has proved effective for the removal of hookworms, the dose being the same as that given for the treatment of stomach worms. Tetrachlorethylene is also fairly effective against cattle hookworms. Although it will not remove all the worms, it removes enough to stop death losses and restore emaciated animals to a condition of relative thriftiness. Phenothiazine has been found to be very effective in the treatment of animals for both hookworms and nodular worms, but is only partially effective for the removal of the cooperids. The doses are the same as those recommended for the treatment of cattle for stomach worms.

Oil of chenopodium may be used for the removal of the large roundworm from calves. The animals should be fasted for 24 hours before treatment. The oil of chenopodium is administered at a dose rate of 0.1 cubic centimeter for each kilogram (2.2 pounds) of body weight and is immediately preceded or followed by castor oil, at least 4 ounces for young calves and more for older ones. Oil of chenopodium should not be given to calves suffering from severe diarrhea, inflammation of the stomach or intestinal tract, chronic constipation or febrile diseases, or to very weak and emaciated animals. Treatments should be given by a competent veterinarian.

PROTOZOA

A number of different kinds of protozoa have been reported as parasites of the intestines of cattle. Of these minute parasites, one genus, *Eimeria*, comprising several species, causes a condition known as coccidiosis, or red dysentery, which appears to be widespread throughout the United States. The resting or spore forms of these parasites, which are the forms usually found on microscopical examination of fecal specimens, are oval or ovoid in shape and range in size from slightly larger to about four to five times as large as a red blood cell, averaging about 0.001 inch in length.

The life history of this parasite is very complicated. The resting, or spore forms, known as oöcysts, pass out of the body with the manure. Under favorable conditions there develop within the oöcyst four bodies known as sporocysts. Within each sporocyst there develop two sporozoites, so that at maturity the oöcyst contains eight sporozoites. This is the infective stage of the parasite. When taken up by a susceptible animal in feed or water, these sporozoites are liberated in the intestine and invade the wall of this organ. The preferred site in which the parasite undergoes its development is the large intestine; to a much lesser extent it develops in the small intestine. Here the parasites reproduce and multiply asexually. After awhile male and female forms develop, fertilization takes place, and oöcysts are formed.

Symptoms and lesions.—The first symptom is diarrhea. In the early stages blood is on the outside of the fecal mass, but as the disease progresses and the feces become more diarrheic it may be mixed throughout the fecal mass. The animals are dull, lie down a great deal, eat little or nothing, and become emaciated rapidly. The skin becomes tight, the hair coat rough, the abdomen assumes a tucked-up appearance, and the tail and buttocks become stained with feces. Peristalsis is diminished, and the feces are passed with a great deal of straining. The pulse and temperature may be slightly increased. Depending on the severity of the attack, the post mortem lesions are: A catarrhal condition of the small intestine with congestion and thickening of the wall of the cecum and colon; or, in severe cases, the mucous membrane lining the walls of the cecum, colon, and rectum is red and contains numerous small hemorrhages. The colon and rectum may contain considerable quantities of blood.

In young animals the acute manifestations usually last 10 to 12 days. In severe cases death may occur in a few days. In animals that recover the period of convalescence lasts several weeks, depending on the severity of the initial infection. Recovered animals usually become carriers, that is, they continue to discharge oöcysts for a long time.

Treatment.—Calves affected with coccidiosis should be segregated in separate pens, which should be cleaned and supplied with fresh bedding daily. The sick animals should be disturbed as little as possible, as movement tends to increase the straining and hemorrhage. Soft nutritious feeds should be given in small quantities several times a day. Milk and barley water especially are advised. There is no satisfactory medicinal treatment for coccidiosis. Attention should be directed toward keeping up the strength of the animal and in controlling symptoms as they appear. Intestinal astringents are used to

77431 O—51——34

control the diarrhea and prevent severe hemorrhage. Rectal injections of such drugs appear to be most useful. For this purpose, ichthargan, a silver preparation, may be used in the proportion of 1 gram (15 grains) dissolved in 1 quart of boiled water, or tannic acid in the proportion of 1 gram in 100 cubic centimeters of boiled water, injected far into the rectum. A mixture of creolin (20 minims), aromatic spirits of ammonia (1 dram), and mineral oil (2 ounces), is sometimes given by mouth, although the value of drugs administered in this manner is questionable.

Prevention.—As calves are the most severely affected and as the disease is spread by means of oöcysts, which are very resistant to unfavorable external conditions, efforts at prevention should be directed toward keeping calves away from sources of infection in areas where the disease is prevalent. Soiled bedding should be burned or disposed of in such a manner as to be no longer a source of infection for susceptible animals. After the affected animals have either recovered or died, the stalls or pens should be thoroughly cleaned and disinfected.

MISCELLANEOUS PARASITES

FLUKES IN LIVER

Two species of flukes occurring usually in the liver and sometimes in the lungs are known to affect cattle in the United States. These parasites are flat, leaflike worms, one of which, the common liver fluke (*Fasciola hepatica*, fig. 19), is less than an inch in length, and the other, the large American fluke (*Fascioloides magna*, fig. 20), is considerably larger when full grown. These flukes depend on snails as intermediate hosts. At a certain stage of development the young flukes leave the snails, become encysted on stalks of grass (fig. 21) or on the surface of drinking water, and are swallowed by cattle in drinking or grazing.

The large American fluke, *Fascioloides magna*, occurs in cysts in the parenchyma of the liver. The cysts are dark in color, about the size of a walnut, and when superficial are usually somewhat elevated above the surface of the liver. There is a black discoloration of the mesentery, peritoneum, and lymph glands. Apart from rendering the liver unfit for food it appears to cause little injury to cattle. These animals appear to be abnormal hosts of this parasite, and the eggs found in the cysts remain there and are not found in the feces of the infested animal. Cattle, therefore, do not aid in the spread of this parasite.

The common liver fluke occurs in the bile ducts and is never found in the liver tissue except when very young. This fluke never causes cyst formation as in the case of the large American fluke.

Symptoms.—The symptoms of fluke disease in cattle, caused by the common liver fluke, are similar to those produced by other worms, namely, unthriftiness, anemia, and related conditions. These symptoms are less pronounced, however, in cattle than in sheep. In cattle the bile ducts are greatly thickened and often calcified, and they remain in this condition even after the flukes have been eliminated. These permanently thickened bile ducts cause the condemnation of the

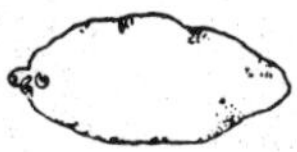

FIGURE 19.—The common liver fluke (*Fasciola hepatica*). Natural size.

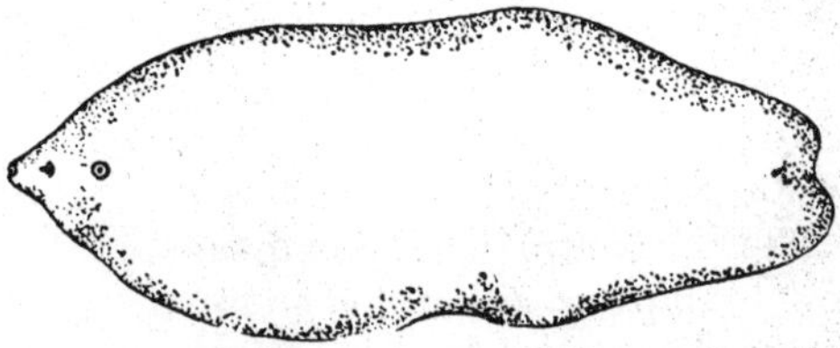

FIGURE 20.—The large American fluke (*Fascioloides magna*). Natural size.

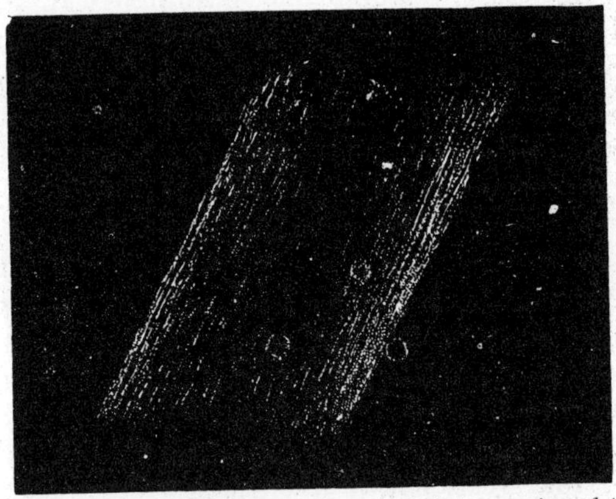

FIGURE 21.—Portion of grass stalk bearing three encysted cercariae of the common liver fluke (*Fasciola hepatica*). Enlarged.

liver in meat inspection. In severe infestations the flukes may invade the lungs and cause fairly large abscesses.

Treatment.—Extract of male fern has been recommended for the treatment of cattle suffering from fluke disease due to the common liver fluke, *Fasciola hepatica.* The average dose for cattle is 1 gram (15 grains) of the extract for each 10 kilograms (22 pounds) of body weight, that is, 10 grams (2.5 drams) for a young animal weighing 100 kilograms (220 pounds) and 50 grams (about 1.5 ounces) as a maximum for large animals weighing 500 kilograms (1,100 pounds) or more. The extract is mixed with about five times as much non-purgative oil. After the animal has been fasted overnight, the dose is administered each morning for 5 consecutive days 2 hours before the animal is allowed to feed. The extract of male fern used should contain at least 15 percent, and preferably 24 to 25 percent, of filicin and 3.5 percent of filicic acid.

Kamala powder also has been used for the treatment of liver fluke disease due to *Fasciola hepatica.* The dose for cattle is 0.139 to 0.26 gram (approximately 2 to 4 grains) per kilogram (2.2 pounds) of body weight. Alicata (1941) reports having obtained good results from the administration of a mixture of hexachloroethane (10 grams), and kamala extract (1.75 grams) for each 70 pounds of body weight. The drugs are administered in capsules over a 2-day period. There is no effective treatment for fluke disease due to the large American fluke.

Prevention of fluke disease.—The destruction of the snails, the intermediate hosts of the flukes that infest cattle, is the most important control measure. This may be accompanied by draining or filling infected wet or swampy areas or by eliminating such areas from pastures by fencing or other means. Where conditions make the above-mentioned measures impossible or impractical, snails may be destroyed by the application of copper sulfate, or bluestone. For the destruction of snails on swampy areas copper sulfate mixed with a suitable carrier, such as fine sand or land plaster in the proportion of 1 part of copper sulfate to 4 to 8 parts of the carrier, may be scattered by hand, power duster, or, in large marshy areas inaccessible by ordinary methods, by airplane. For the destruction of snails in small streams or streams confined within definite banks, gunny sacks containing crystals of copper sufate may be placed in the head waters. To reach snails on the banks or in low wet areas adjoining them, dams may be thrown across the stream at various places, depending on the fall of the stream, to raise the treated water to cover the snails. Usually one treatment of a stream or pasture is enough for that year, but if live snails are subsequently found, a second treatment should be given. The concentration of copper sulfate needed to kill snails is not injurious to livestock drinking the treated water and it will not kill the grasses. Copper sulfate will kill algae and moss and when used in sufficiently high concentrations it will kill certain fish; therefore, in treating waters stocked with fish, the water should be treated only along the banks, or other precautions taken to protect the fish.

TAPEWORMS CAUSING CYSTS OF VISCERA AND BRAIN

Cysts from three kinds of tapeworms—hydatids (*Echinococcus granulosus*), thin-necked bladder worms (*Taenia hydatigena*, or *Cysticercus tenuicollis*), and bladder worms (*Multiceps multiceps*, or

Coenurus cerebralis)—are found in the viscera of cattle. All of them are the intermediate stages of tapeworms that live when mature in the intestines of dogs, wolves, and other carnivores. The eggs of the tapeworms are scattered over the fields in the droppings of infested dogs or wolves and, when swallowed in feed or water by cattle, hatch and the embryos migrate to the liver, mesentery, lungs, brain, or other organs, where they develop into cysts, variously known as hydatids, bladder worms, and water balls. When organs of cattle thus infested are eaten by dogs or wolves, the cystic worms also are likely to be swallowed, and these then develop into mature tapeworms. To prevent cattle being infected with these parasites, they should be protected from stray dogs, wolves, and coyotes. Dogs allowed on the premises should be kept free from tapeworms. As a precaution against infection with tapeworms, the viscera of cattle, sheep, or hogs should not be fed to dogs unless cooked.

Hydatids (*Echinococcus granulosus*) form tumors (fig. 22), some-

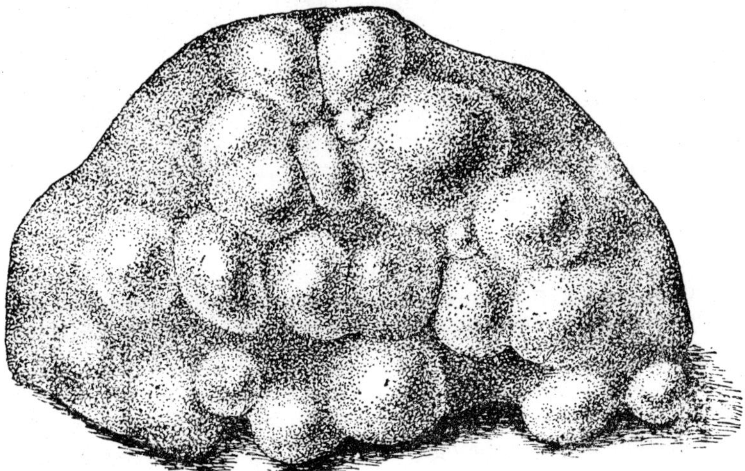

FIGURE 22.—Hydatids (*Echinococcus granulosus*) in portion of liver.

times as large as 6 inches in diameter, in the liver, lungs, and other organs. Their contents are liquid, resembling water. The presence of these parasites cannot be detected in the living animal and there is no medicinal treatment for them. It is especially important that organs containing hydatids should be destroyed by burning in order to prevent their being eaten by dogs as these animals, when infested with the tapeworm stage of this parasite, may infect human beings. Hydatids develop in man if the eggs of this parasite are swallowed.

Thin-necked bladder worms (*Taenia hydatigena*, or *Cysticercus tenuicollis*, fig. 23) are most commonly found attached to the mesentery and omentum. There is no medicinal treatment.

Bladder worms (*Multiceps multiceps*, or *Coenurus cerebralis*), which are occasionally found in the brain of cattle and which cause gid, "turnsick," or "staggers," deserve mention. These worms are the intermediate stage of a tapeworm found in dogs. Cattle harboring this parasite show symptoms indicating an affection of the brain, walking or turning in circles, dizziness, uneven gait, and impaired vision. Treatment consists in trephining the skull and removing the parasite, an operation that requires a skillful operator and is frequently unsuccessful. Unless the parasite is removed affected cattle almost invariably die.

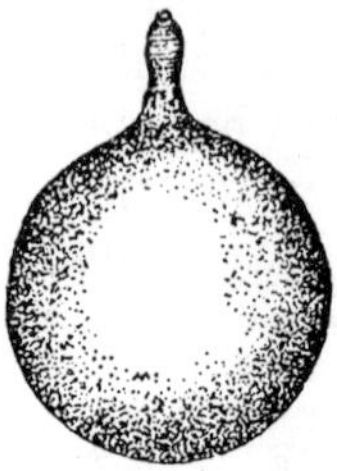

FIGURE 23.—Thin-necked bladder worm from abdominal cavity of a steer. Natural size.

TAPEWORM CAUSING CYSTS IN THE MUSCLES, BEEF MEASLES

Small tapeworm cysts (*Cysticercus bovis*), about the size of a pea, and found in the muscles of cattle, are the larvae of the common tapeworm (*Taenia saginata*) of man. Cattle become infected from feed or water that has been contaminated by the feces of persons harboring the adult tapeworms, and human beings in turn become infected by eating raw or rare beef infected with the larval stage (measly beef). To prevent cattle from becoming infested with this parasite, care should be taken that human feces are not placed where they will contaminate the feed or drinking water.

This parasite is very common in cattle in the United States, at least 1 percent of cattle being infested. As a result, a considerable loss is entailed through condemnations of beef carcasses by meat inspectors because of the presence of tapeworm cysts. All this loss could be avoided and the danger of tapeworm infestation in human beings from this source could be removed by the observance of proper precautions in disposing of human excreta.

THREADWORMS

Threadworms (*Setaria cervi*), 2 to 4 inches long, are frequently found in the abdominal cavity. They seem to cause little trouble. The larvae produced by these worms enter the blood vessels. According to Noé, they are spread from one animal to another by stableflies (p. 448), but this has not been proved definitely. Some of the roundworms found occasionally in the anterior chamber of the eye (p. 486) are immature forms of this species that have reached this location during their migration.

LUNGWORMS

Lungworms (*Dictyocaulus viviparus*, fig. 24) in cattle are thread-like worms 2 to 4 inches long, found in the bronchial tubes and producing a condition known as verminous bronchitis. The life history of this lungworm is similar to that of the twisted stomach worm, and infection is acquired on the pasture on which the animals graze. In the later stages of the disease the cattle cough, especially at night. Young cattle are more seriously affected than older animals.

Treatment.—Various treatments have been advocated for lungworms, including fumigating with different substances and injections of remedies into the trachea by means of a large hypodermic syringe or by a special spraying apparatus, but none have been very successful from a practical standpoint. About all that can be done is to feed affected animals well and protect them from exposure by removing them from the pasture and keeping them in dry yards or stables maintained in a sanitary condition. The methods of prevention in general are similar to those described under the discussion of the twisted stomach worm (p. 469).

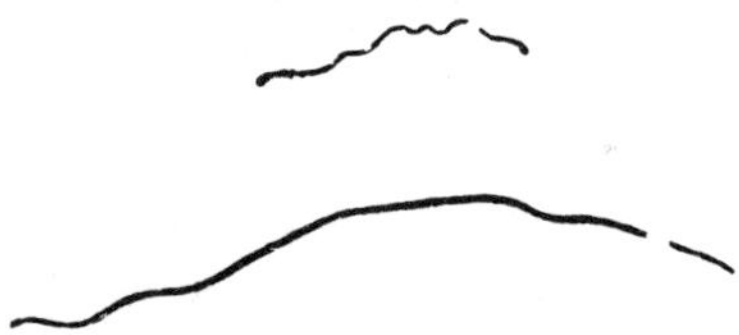

FIGURE 24.—Lungworm (*Dictyocaulus viviparus*) of cattle. Outlines showing natural size of male (above) and female (below).

ROUNDWORM PARASITES OF THE EYE

Small roundworms, about one-third to four-fifths of an inch in length, may occur in the ducts of the tear glands between the eye and the lids or under the nictitating membrane. Of the several species, all belonging to the genus *Thelazia*, one species, *T. rhodesi*, has been reported as occurring in the eyes of cattle in California; other species have been found in the eyes of sheep and deer in the United States.

T. rhodesi normally occurs in the ducts of the tear glands, but they may escape from their usual location and be found on the surface of the eyeball beneath the lids, under the nictitating membrane, or even in the eyeball. These worms are white, slender, and attenuated at both ends. The males are one-third to one-half inch long, and the females one-half to 1 inch long. Their life history is unknown, but they probably have an intermediate stage in some arthropod. This worm has been reported only from cattle in California.

According to Griffiths, the first symptoms shown by infested animals are profuse lachrymation (secreting of tears), photophobia (sensitiveness to light), and cloudiness of the cornea, to be followed later by definite opacity of the cornea. As a result of the invasion by pus-producing organisms, the cornea may become ulcerated and this, in turn, may lead to an inflammation of the iris and other structures of the eye. If the worms are not removed, the eyelids and the nictitating membrane may become swollen and owing to the drying of the purulent discharge exuding between the eyelids, the lids may adhere to each other. The globe of the eye becomes more and more affected and is finally destroyed. Mechanical injuries due to loss of sight and the fixation of the nictitating membrane, which is unable to function because of its swollen condition, may aggravate the primary condition.

The presence of these eyeworms may be suspected when one or more animals in a herd show signs of photophobia with profuse lachrymation. The parasites are most easily found in animals showing the earliest stages of the clinical manifestations, namely, lachrymation with slight opacity of the cornea and little, if any, purulent discharge. The septic processes due to secondary infection appear to kill off the nematodes or, at least, to confine them to the depths of the lachrymal ducts. The worms are not always seen in a hasty examination of the eye because of their unusual habitat. It is necessary, therefore, to examine the parts thoroughly by exposing the under surface of the nictitating membrane and the eyelids, where the worms can be detected by their active wriggling movements in the lachrymal secretion. They appear to be washed up with the tears from the lachrymal duct, as any manipulations or applications of dressing that tend to increase the secretion of tears facilitates the recovery of specimens from infected animals.

Until the life history of these worms is known, no preventive or control measures can be recommended.

Treatment consists in the mechanical removal of the worms from the eye. After these have been removed, the eyes should be treated as in cases of inflammation due to other causes.

TRICHOMONADS OF THE GENITAL TRACT

A species of *Trichomonas*, called *T. foetus*, may be found in the genital tract of cattle and, when present, is responsible for the genital disease called bovine trichomoniasis.

Trichomonas foetus is a one-celled, microscopic organism varying in length from 10 to 25 microns and in width from about 8 to 10 microns. (A micron is 1/25000 inch.) It has three anterior flagella (whiplike appendages), each about as long as the body, and a posterior flagellum constituting the marginal filament of the undulating membrane and projecting postericrly beyond the membrane as a free flagellum. The posterior flagellum is about as long as the anterior ones. There is a dorsally placed undulating membrane extending almost the entire length of the body; this membrane has four or five undulations. In general, *T. foetus* is somewhat larger than the polymorphonuclear leucocytes and somewhat smaller than the epithelial cells commonly found in vaginal smears.

When examined alive the organism is actively motile. It moves across the field of vision of the microscope with an undulating motion; at times it turns and twists and assumes varying shapes. It may appear pear-shaped, oval, or rounded. The rapidity of its movements depends to some extent on the medium in which it is examined. When studied in a drop of physiologic saline, the movements of *T. foetus* are rather rapid, but in a collection of somewhat tenacious vaginal mucus the movements are considerably restricted.

The organism reproduces by division, each organism splitting and dividing into two. It is usually transmitted from one animal to another by coitus. The disease is most common in bred heifers and older bulls but *Trichomonas foetus* has been reported as occurring in the vagina of virgin heifers and in the prepuce of a young bull that, as far as is known, had never been used for breeding purposes.

As a result of infection in females one of several things may happen: (1) The animal fails to conceive; (2) conception takes place, but due to uterine infection there is abortion; (3) following conception the fetus dies, but instead of being expelled it becomes macerated, and the uterus is filled with a characteristic thin, grayish-white, almost odorless fluid; or (4) a normal gestation and parturition occurs in spite of infection.

Animals that fail to conceive may develop a uterine infection manifested by a vaginal discharge that is continuous or intermittent. Estrual periods may become irregular owing to infection with *Trichomonas foetus* and the discharge may be most marked at this time.

Abortion due to trichomoniasis may occur at any time during the period of gestation, but it usually takes place in 8 to 16 weeks after conception. There are usually no signs of estrum during this period. A few days before abortion there is often a vaginal discharge indicating the approaching abortion. At times only a small quantity of whitish mucoid fluid is expelled instead of the fetus. The abortion may pass unobserved, especially if it occurs at night, in a dark stable, or on pasture. A few days after such an abortion the animal usually comes in heat, and this is often the first indication of infection.

When the fetus becomes macerated and is not expelled, the animals generally behave like those normally pregnant. They show no signs of illness, but the usual outward signs normally indicating approaching parturition fail to appear. At the end of the period of gestation there is no calf, and on examination the uterus is found to be filled with fluid.

Inflammation of the prepuce accompanied with pus formation and discharge has been reported in recently infected bulls. In such cases, the preputial mucosa and penis are found to be inflamed and to contain many small nodules similar to those occurring in bulls affected with nodular venereal disease. Trichomonads have been reported as occurring in the epididymis and in the ampullae of the vas deferens where these enter the urethra. They have been found also in the anterior portion of the urethra, but in most cases they appear to be confined to the glans penis and the area of prepuce surrounding the glans. The infection usually becomes chronic in bulls.

The diagnosis of trichomoniasis is based, in part, on the breeding history of the herd and of affected animals within the herd. However, the demonstration of the organism in vaginal or uterine discharges is necessary to make the diagnosis complete. The immediate microscopic examination of material taken from the vagina is the most direct method of making a diagnosis. For this purpose a cotton swab, moistened with physiologic saline, is introduced into the vagina and the material adhering to the swab is placed on a slide and immediately examined under the low power of the microscope. If the organisms are present there is no difficulty in recognizing them. In case no microscope is available the contents of the swab may be washed into a tube of physiologic saline, a few drops of Lugol's solution of iodine or 10-percent formalin solution added, the tube tightly closed, and then sent to a laboratory for examination. Where facilities are available and direct microscopic examination fails to reveal the organisms, culturing the material removed from the vagina may prove to be of great assistance. This will often show the presence of the organisms when they are too few in number to be detected by direct examination.

A similar procedure may be followed in bulls. The cotton swab moistened in physiologic saline is introduced into the sheath and then examined in the same manner as the vaginal swab. However, a negative examination is by no means conclusive, and it may be necessary to make several examinations extending over a considerable period. With cows and heifers, the best time for an examination appears to be during the estrual periods. Vaginal examination of a cow or heifer in 14 to 21 days after service has been suggested as a means of determining whether the bull used is transmitting trichomoniasis. If so, the infection in the cow will be vaginal and can be demonstrated at that time. The diagnosis, therefore, is made on the basis of the breeding history of the individual animal and of the herd and the demonstration of the presence of the organism.

There is no specific treatment. The disease should be handled in the same way as any other form of genital infection in cattle.

Cows that abort early in the period of gestation usually recover spontaneously provided the abortion is complete and the animals are given a period of sexual rest for about 3 months. If the abortion is incomplete and there is a persistent discharge, the animals should be handled in the same manner as cases of uterine infection due to other causes. This also applies to cases of pyometra. In some cases of pyometra the cervix relaxes when the end of the normal gestation period approaches and there is discharge of uterine contents. In other cases the cervix remains tightly closed and the only way to make a diagnosis is by manual examination per rectum. In these cases the uterus should be emptied and douched in the usual manner. Whether such animals will return to breeding efficiency depends on the extent of the damage to the uterine mucosa.

Cows that fail to conceive after repeated services, as a result of trichomonad infection, should be given sexual rest until the estrual cycle returns to normal. Treatment should consist of uterine and vaginal douches, ovarian massage, and removal of yellow bodies when present. This treatment should be administered by a competent veterinarian.

Infected bulls are generally considered as incurable and their destruction as a means of eliminating sources of infection has been advocated. This advice, while theoretically sound, is not always practical. A treatment that has been used in a few cases with apparent success consists in casting the animal, unsheathing the penis under epidural anesthesia, and injecting 50 to 100 cubic centimeters of a 0.1-percent solution of trypaflavine into the urethra and rubbing a 0.5-percent trypaflavine ointment into the inner surface of the prepuce. The treatment should be repeated in a week. Douching the sheath of the bull before and after service has also been recommended.

As the disease is spread principally by coitus, the utmost caution should be exercised in the introduction of mature animals as permarent additions to the herd. The breeding histories of all such animals, whether male or female, and the breeding histories of the herds from which they come, should be carefully examined. Cows known as hard or difficult breeders should not be brought to the premises for breeding purposes unless it can be definitely determined that they are not infected with trichomoniasis. Cows known to be free from trichomoniasis should not be bred away from home. They may acquire the disease in the process and later serve as sources of infection to animals in the herd to which they are returned. In herds in which the infection has become established, the use of infected bulls should be restricted to cows that have either passed through an attack of the disease or that have at least been previously exposed. Cases of trichomonad infection in heifers have been attributed to contact with infected animals. There is no experimental evidence that such infection can occur, but until the question is definitely settled it is advisable that calves and heifers be separated from animals that are known to be infected.

Index

77431 O—51——35

430855°—42——33

○